Manual of
AVIAN PRACTICE

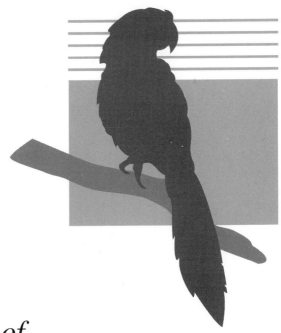

Manual of AVIAN PRACTICE

Agnes E. Rupley, DVM, ABVP Avian
Diplomate, American Board of Veterinary Practitioners
Certified in Avian Practice
College Station, Texas

W.B. SAUNDERS COMPANY
A Division of Harcourt Brace & Company
Philadelphia   London   Toronto   Montreal   Sydney   Tokyo

W.B. SAUNDERS COMPANY
A Division of Harcourt Brace & Company

The Curtis Center
Independence Square West
Philadelphia, Pennsylvania 19106

Library of Congress Cataloging-in-Publication Data

Rupley, Agnes E.
Manual of avian practice / Agnes E. Rupley.—1st ed.

p.   cm.

ISBN 0–7216–4083–4

1. Avian medicine—Handbooks, manuals, etc.   I. Title.
  [DNLM: 1. Bird Diseases—diagnosis.   2. Bird Diseases—therapy.
  3. Birds.   SF 994 R945m 1997]

SF994.R87   1997

636.5′089—dc20

DNLM/DLC   96-34618

MANUAL OF AVIAN PRACTICE   ISBN 0–7216–4083–4

Printed in the United States of America.

Last digit is the print number: 9   8   7   6   5   4   3   2   1

This book is dedicated with love to my husband, Bill,
who has encouraged me and has provided endless support;
to my children, Billy, Donald, Rose Marie, and Matt,
who bring me intense joy;
to my father, Don L. Emmott, who instilled in me the belief that
I can achieve my goals;
and to my mother, Marie Emmott, who has been a great source of
love and inspiration.

Preface

The goal of this book is to provide veterinarians the information they need to give quality avian medical care and to serve as a quick reference for use in practice. Because there is an increased need for veterinarians to provide quality avian medical care, now is an excellent time for veterinarians to make this service available. Quality avian medical care can be easily added to the existing practices of those doctors who have an interest in treating birds. This book presents material in a format that will enable a practitioner with little or no avian experience to begin seeing and treating birds with confidence while expanding an existing practice. A problem-oriented approach for veterinarians, veterinary students, and veterinary technicians is the overall focus of this book. Experienced avian veterinarians will find the complete list of differential diagnoses and information useful as an aid in making difficult diagnoses. This book is also useful in practices in which less experienced doctors occasionally treat birds for an experienced avian practitioner. Medical procedures, sample collection, clinical pathology, and nutrition, as well as general avian medicine, are of benefit to avian technicians.

In Chapter 1 the basic elements of the avian practice are discussed: history taking, performance of the avian physical examination, supportive care, nutrition, needed equipment, practice management, and continuing education. Chapters 2 through 8 provide problem-oriented diagnostic approaches to abnormal clinical signs, which are divided into general signs (Chapter 2), respiratory signs (Chapter 3), gastrointestinal signs (Chapter 4), ophthalmic signs (Chapter 5), neurologic signs (Chapter 6), musculoskeletal signs (Chapter 7), and dermatologic signs (Chapter 8). Each of these signs (Chapters) is divided into common clinical signs. Discussion of each clinical sign begins with an introduction and description of the clinical sign, followed by appropriate signalment information. Common causes of the clinical sign are presented for groups of pet birds. The history section is useful for exploration of important historical information. The physical examination section guides interpretation of the physical findings seen with the clinical sign of that section. An algorithm is included with each sign to provide quick reference for recommended tests. The diagnostic plan suggests useful tests. General treatments for each sign are discussed at the end of each chapter. References are listed to provide sources of further information.

Common diseases and treatments are discussed in Chapter 9. Chapter 10 provides a complete description of how to perform a necropsy on adult birds, chicks, and eggs. Grooming and complete descriptions of how to perform medical procedures are discussed in Chapter 11. Chapter 12 focuses on sample collection and clinical pathology and includes photographs of hematologic and cytologic specimens and of parasites, facilitating in-house performance of clinical pathology procedures. Selection of laboratory tests is discussed and information that may be gained with each test is furnished, along with the test's limitations and interpretations, rather than detailed descriptions of pathophysiology. Chapter 13 discusses the uses of radiology and other modes of imaging. Radiographs are provided of normal birds as well as of those with common abnormal findings. Chapter 14 is devoted to anesthesia, endoscopy, and surgery. Chapters 15 and 16 provide information concerning aviculture, obstetrics, and pediatrics. The formulary in Chapter 17 provides doses and treatment intervals for drugs commonly used in avian practice. Appendices include sources of equipment, typical weights of common pet birds, toxic plants, some plants suitable for use in aviaries, and schematics of skeletal and visceral anatomy.

New avian medical and surgical information is constantly evolving. As information and techniques are generated, these will be included in future editions. Comments, suggestions, and constructive criticisms for future editions are welcome and encouraged. The primary goal of this book is to provide a guide for the practice of quality avian medicine in a simple and useful format. This goal will be enhanced by the input and opinion of others.

AGNES E. RUPLEY, DVM, ABVP AVIAN

Acknowledgments

Many people helped me in the writing of this text. I want to thank the colleagues who reviewed manuscripts, including Drs. Stephen Fronefield, David Graham, Susan Orosz, Brian Speer, and especially Sue Sattler-Augustin. Their constructive criticism provided a more useful text. I want to thank Dr. Connie Orcutt for her contribution to the text. The support of Karl Storz Veterinary Endoscopy America, Ellman International, and AVID is appreciated. I would also like to thank the W. B. Saunders editors and staff who helped in the production of this book, especially Ray Kersey for his guidance, support, and belief in this project.

NOTICE

Avian practice is an ever-changing field. Standard safety precautions must be followed, but as new research and clinical experience grow, changes in treatment and drug therapy become necessary or appropriate. The authors and editors of this work have carefully checked the generic and trade drug names and verified drug dosages to assure that dosage information is precise and in accord with standards accepted at the time of publication. Readers are advised, however, to check the product information currently provided by the manufacturer of each drug to be administered to be certain that changes have not been made in the recommended dose or in the contraindications for administration. This is of particular importance in regard to new or infrequently used drugs. Recommended dosages for animals are sometimes based on adjustments in the dosage that would be suitable for humans. Some of the drugs mentioned here have been given experimentally by the authors. Others have been used in dosages greater than those recommended by the manufacturer. In these kinds of cases, the authors have reported on their own considerable experience. It is the responsibility of those administering a drug, relying on their professional skill and experience, to determine the dosages, the best treatment for the patient, and whether the benefits of giving a drug justify the attendant risk. The editors cannot be responsible for misuse or misapplication of the material in this work.

THE PUBLISHER

Contents

Chapter 1

History Taking, Physical Examination, Supportive Care, Nutrition, and Getting Started

The need for quality avian medical services is increasing rapidly. Now is an excellent time for veterinarians to make quality avian medical care available to their clients. With increased popularity of birds and increased public awareness of the availability of medical treatment, clients will seek out hospitals that offer both avian and small-animal medicine. This service can be incorporated into any small-animal veterinary hospital, with minimal expense.

Quality treatment of sick and apparently healthy birds requires a systematic, consistent, and thorough evaluation. This chapter provides a systematic approach to the evaluation of avian patients, beginning with important instructions the veterinarian or the receptionist should discuss with the bird owner when making an appointment. This is followed by a detailed discussion of history taking. Evaluation of the cage, cage contents, and droppings is discussed. The techniques of capture and restraint are detailed for species of birds commonly seen in pet-bird practice. Discussion of the physical examination provides detailed information on examining each part of the bird, how to examine the area, and what abnormalities to look for. When abnormalities are found, appropriate sections of this book should be consulted for differential diagnoses and assistance with making a diagnosis. The supportive care section discusses patient care before making a diagnosis and during treatment. The chapter concludes with discussions on nutrition, equipment, the hospital environment, practice management, and continuing education.

INSTRUCTIONS TO BIRD OWNERS WHEN MAKING APPOINTMENTS

The owner should bring the cage with the bird for examination, if possible. The cage should not be cleaned before the visit. If the appointment is scheduled for a later date, newspapers should be placed under the cage floor to collect the droppings for up to 24 to 48 hours before the appointment date. Ask the owner to place the newspapers in a Ziploc bag before transport and to bring them for examination with the bird.

If the owner cannot bring the cage, ask the owner to collect droppings on newspaper as above and to bring them to the appointment.

Before transport, water should be removed from the cage, and perches, swings, and toys should be removed if the bird is weak or severely ill. The owner should cover the cage for transport, which provides warmth and relieves stress. The bird needs to be kept warm during transport.

Ask the owner to bring in any medications being used.

HISTORY TAKING

The first step in evaluating a sick or healthy bird is taking a complete history, which includes topics such as exposure to infectious disease or toxins, environment, management practices, diet, reproductive status, and previous illnesses. Birds that are exposed to infectious disease are often ill as a result of infectious causes, including bacterial, chlamydial, viral, and parasitic infections. This may be the result of exposure to infectious agents as well as the stress of group contact. Familiarity with problems in local pet stores and local aviaries allows for specific testing to obtain a diagnosis. Isolated birds and those in aviaries where no new birds have been introduced are usually ill as a result of noninfectious causes. Gram-negative bacterial infections, diseases with carrier states (e.g., Pacheco's disease), and chronic diseases (e.g., chlamydiosis, mycobacteriosis (tuberculosis), aspergillosis, proventricular dilatation syndrome, and psittacine beak and feather disease) are also seen in aviaries where no new birds have been introduced.

Explore infectious and toxic causes of illness when more than one bird in the household is ill.

Important environmental history includes caging or lack of caging, cage contents, flight capabilities, exposure to natural sunlight, changes in the environment, and exposure or access to potential toxins. Trauma is common in birds allowed free flight. Lack of exposure to natural sunlight may result in general unthriftiness or dermatologic problems. Environmental low humidity may also result in dermatologic abnormalities. Changes in the environment may cause stress and result in feather picking, immunosuppression, or transient anorexia. Birds may compensate for mild disease states, thus hiding signs of disease. A change of environment may result in enough stress for a bird to begin showing signs of illness. Exposure to possible toxins should be explored historically. Lead, zinc, plants, insecticides, and vapors are common causes of toxicoses in pet birds.

Management practices that affect the health of the bird include hand-feeding practices, food preparation, sanitation, and exposure to disease vectors (wild birds, insects, rodents, etc.). Improper hand-feeding practices in chicks may adversely affect the health of the bird. Sanitation is important in prevention and control of disease. Food and water bowls need to be cleaned daily, and the bird must be given fresh food and water daily. These bowls should be placed appropriately to avoid contamination with droppings. Parasitic and other infectious diseases may be brought into or spread in an aviary by insects, arthropods, rodents, and wild birds. The introduction of apparently healthy pet birds can be a major source of infection.

The dietary history is extremely important in pet bird medicine. Many birds will choose to eat only seed when offered a variety of foods. Seed diets, as well as many homemade diets, lack important nutrients. The amount consumed, freshness of the diet, vitamin supplementation, and treats are all important aspects of the diet that must be explored.

A history of free-choice access to grit is important. Birds may ingest excessive grit, resulting in impaction. Grit should be offered in limited amounts. A few pieces each month are ample. Psittacines on a formulated diet do not require grit.

The reproductive status of the bird is historically important. Chronic egg laying, a recent history of egg laying, and dystocia may result in abnormalities and abnormal clinical signs.

Iatrogenic causes of illness must be explored during history taking.

Note previous illnesses, including signs, treatment, and response to treatment.

The duration of the present illness is important. Note the owner's description of the clinical signs and the course of the disease.

EVALUATION OF THE CAGE AND CAGE CONTENTS

The client should be instructed to bring the bird and the uncleaned cage to the hospital, when possible. Evaluate cage size, construction, and content. The cage should be of sufficient size for the bird to be comfortable, move around, and stretch without damaging feathers. Cages made from untreated hardware cloth can result in zinc toxicosis if the bird chews on the wire, which is typical of psittacines. Clamps to connect wire may also be a source of zinc. Treating hardware cloth with acetic acid (vinegar) and brushing or weathering decrease toxicity. Bowls and toys should be lead-free and appropriate for the size of the bird. Perches for pet birds should be of varying sizes and smooth. The shape and size of perches for raptors vary with the species.

Observe the cage for accumulation of discharges or vomitus on toys, mirrors, perches, etc.

EVALUATION OF THE DROPPINGS

Instruct the owner to remove the paper from the bottom of the cage and bring it to the hospital with the bird. This will allow evaluation of the droppings before transport, which often results in polyuria from the stress of transport. Evaluate the feces, urates, and urine portions of the droppings. The feces are the brown or green portion of the dropping. The urates are the white or light tan chalky substance in the dropping. And the urine is the liquid portion of the dropping. Evaluate the fecal portion of the dropping for amount, color, and consistency. Normal feces can be green to brown, depending on the diet. The consistency of normal feces can vary with the diet. Birds on seed diets typically have a formed green stool. Birds on formulated diets pass stools that are larger and contain more water, but are still somewhat formed. Fruits and vegetables in the diet can cause an increase in the size and water content of the feces. Pigments in the diet can result in the color of the feces being other than normal. Blood or undigested or partially digested food in the dropping or diarrhea is abnormal. The amount of feces is determined by intake of food. Lack of feces in the droppings or a decrease in feces production may occur when a bird is not eating. Consult Chapter 4 for the diagnostic plan for any abnormalities.

Normal urates are white to light tan. Any other color is abnormal. When abnormalities are found, consult Chapter 4 for assistance with making a diagnosis.

The urine in the droppings of normal birds is clear. An increase in urine or a change in the color is abnormal. Consult Chapter 4 if abnormalities are found.

OBSERVE THE BIRD IN THE CAGE

Before handling the bird, observe the bird in the cage. Observe the general attitude, respiratory effort, and stance. Normal birds are alert when out of their normal surroundings. Ill birds may sleep or close their eyes while in the examination room; healthy birds will not. Observe for the bird's sitting low on the perch, fluffing of feathers, and perching or grasping with only one foot. Observe the respiratory rate. Normal rates are listed in Table 1–1. Observe the wing positions and symmetry and the tail position. Sitting on the bottom of the cage, dyspnea, open-mouth breathing, and tail bobbing are signs of a critically ill bird. Tail bobbing is the rhythmic movement of the tail feathers with each inspiration or expiration. Any degree of tail bobbing is abnormal.

If abnormalities are noted, consult appropriate chapters for assistance with making a diagnosis.

CAPTURE AND RESTRAINT

The capture and restraint method used is determined by the type of bird. Never capture a bird while it is perching on the owner. Use either disposable

TABLE 1–1 Approximate Heart and Respiratory Rates of Normal Birds

	Resting Heart Rate* (Per Minute)	Resting Respiratory Rate† (Per Minute)
Finch	300–350	90–110
Canary	265–325	60–80
Budgie	260–270	60–75
Lovebird	240–250	50–60
Cockatiel	210–220	40–50
Small conure	205–220	40–50
Large conure	165–205	30–45
Toucan	130–165	15–45
Amazon parrot	125–160	15–45
Cockatoo	125–170	15–40
Macaw	115–135	20–25

*Restraint can increase heart rate 2 to 3 times resting rate.

(Data from Ritchie BW, Harrison GJ, Harrison LR (eds): *Avian Medicine: Principles and Application.* Lake Worth, FL, Wingers Publishing, 1994, p 148.)

†Restraint can increase respiratory rate 1.5 to 2 times resting rate.

Note: Estimation of resting heart rate may be calculated: heart rate (beats/minute) = $720 \times (4 \times \text{weight in grams})^{-0.209}$.

(Data from West NH, Langille BL, Jones DR: Cardiovascular system. In King AS, McLelland J (eds): *Form and Function in Birds,* vol 2. New York, Academic Press, 1981, p 319.)

materials to catch birds, or clean and disinfect towels and nets between each use. Do not use gloves except when capturing and handling raptors. Nets are useful for escaped birds and in aviary situations. Capture and restrain birds in a safe environment: covered windows, ceiling fans off, and door closed. Have all needed materials at hand before catching the bird. Restrain birds with a firm grip to prevent escape and decrease straining, but a bird must be able to move the sternum to breathe. Bruising may occur in birds with facial patches lacking feathers (e.g., macaws). If pressure is placed on the globe, the eye may appear shrunken when the bird is released. The eye will return to normal within minutes.

To catch a psittacine bird from a cage, remove perches and toys from the cage if needed. Use the towel to position the bird against the side of the cage. When the bird bites the side of the cage, catch the bird across the back of the head with the covered hand (Fig. 1–1). Small psittacines and passerines can be caught more easily with the lights dimmed or off. A pen light can be used to orient the person catching the bird. These small birds can be caught using paper towels. Use hand towels for catching medium-sized psittacines and bath towels for catching large psittacines. Once the head is restrained, the bird can be lifted from the cage with the towel wrapped around the wings and feet. Once the bird is caught, the bird is restrained by controlling the beak, wings, and feet. Birds may be restrained in the towel or taken out of the towel and held directly. Restraint in towels makes it easier to control the wings, but it may result in overheating and more difficult observation of some areas during the physical examination. Small birds may be restrained holding the head with the thumb and index finger and cupping the body with the palm and other fingers (Fig. 1–2). Medium-sized birds are restrained by holding the bird's mandible with the thumb and middle finger and placing the index finger on the top of the bird's head (Fig. 1–3). The wings and feet are controlled with the other hand. To help prevent the wings from flapping, the bird is wrapped in a towel or held close to the restrainer's body. Large psittacines are restrained by holding the head just

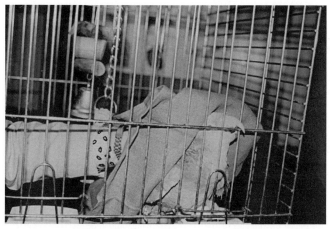

Figure 1–1. Catch the bird across the back of the head with a covered hand when the bird bites the side of the cage.

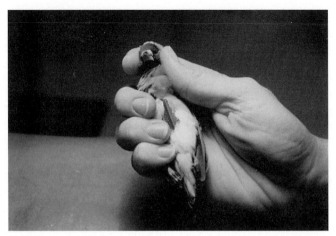

Figure 1-2. Small birds are restrained by holding the head with the thumb and index finger and cupping the body with the palm and other fingers. This method works well for small psittacines and passerines.

underneath the beak (Fig. 1-4). The body can be wrapped in a towel and cradled under the arm of the restrainer, if needed, to control the wings.

Toucans can be captured with a towel or net, similar to psittacines; however, the body, wings, and feet must be restrained as well. Hold the beak closed or tape it closed to prevent biting. The beak is held with one hand, and the body and wings are controlled with the other hand. Never handle toucans by the head and neck alone.

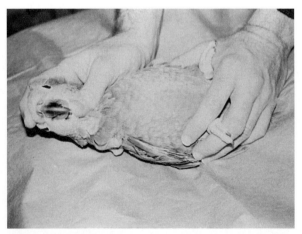

Figure 1-3. Medium-sized birds are restrained by holding the mandible with the thumb and middle finger and placing the index finger on the top of the head. The wings and feet are controlled with the other hand. Flapping of the wings can be controlled by holding the bird close to the restrainer's body.

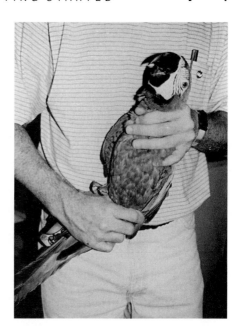

Figure 1-4. Large psittacines are restrained by holding the head just underneath the beak. The body can be wrapped in a towel and cradled under the arm of the restrainer, if needed, to control the wings.

When capturing raptors, the talons (nails) are the major source of injury. The view of the bird is obstructed with paper, board, or towel, and the feet are caught with a gloved hand; then the head and wings are restrained. A hood may be used to calm nervous raptors during restraint. Ball bandages may be applied to the feet after they are inspected for problems. This allows easier handling and capture during hospitalization. Some birds, such as eagles and owls, readily use their mouths for protection as well.

Waterfowl may be netted or driven into a corner to capture. Restrain these birds by grasping the base of the wings with one hand and supporting the body with the other hand. Some, especially geese, may bite.

Handle dyspneic birds minimally. Place dyspneic birds in an oxygen cage as needed. Budgies, especially obese ones on a poor diet that are never handled by their owner, will occasionally die when restrained. Warn the owner of this possibility before capturing such budgies.

To get a bird to release its grip when it bites, blow in its face. Gently tapping the base of beak may also cause the bird to open its beak. If this is unsuccessful in getting the bird to let go, release the bird completely. Prying the beak open may damage the beak.

PHYSICAL EXAMINATION

Equipment and supplies that may be needed during the examination are placed within the examiner's reach before the bird is captured.

A complete physical examination is important to identify the extent of the problem and to determine which systems are involved. Birds often can hide signs of illness and may be very ill by the time the owner observes that there is a problem. Tame birds may show signs at home, but they may hide these signs when out of their normal environment.

Consult appropriate chapters for assistance with making a diagnosis when abnormalities are noted.

Dyspneic or debilitated birds must be handled with care. The physical examination should be performed quickly and with the least possible amount of stress. Oxygen can be administered with a mask during examination, if necessary. The bird may need to be placed in an oxygen cage before handling and returned to the cage to recover during the examination if needed.

The first step of the physical examination is weighing the bird. Special scales allow accuracy and make it easier to weigh the bird (see Equipment). An accurate weight is necessary for drug dose calculations and to monitor patients. Evaluation of pectoral muscling is necessary to determine if this is the normal weight for the bird. Fluctuations of weight are significant even without loss of pectoral musculature. In normal chicks, pectoral muscles are less developed. Weight gain, general attitude, crop emptying, feeding response, and the presence of food in the duodenal loop are important in evaluating chick weight.

Develop a systematic approach and use it every time a physical examination is performed on a bird. Evaluate the entire bird. A stamp, such as the one in Figure 1–5, may be useful to reinforce and record a complete physical examination.

A systematic approach is presented and common abnormal findings are discussed below. Consult appropriate chapters when abnormalities are observed.

Eyes

The eyes of a normal bird are clear, symmetrical, and centered in the socket. The normal conjunctiva is pale pink and moist. Hydration is evaluated by tenting the skin over the eyelids. Note the color of the conjunctiva.

Assess the periorbital area for swelling, discoloration, pustules, scars, scabs, or abnormal growths. Conjunctivitis, sunken eyes, and ocular discharges are abnormal. Pale or white coloration of the conjunctiva can indicate anemia.

Note the iris color. The color is an indication of age or sex in many species of birds. Young Amazon parrots have brown irises that become red-orange as they age. Young African gray parrots have brown irises that change to gray, then white. Young macaws have brown irises that change to gray within the first year, and then between 1 and 3 years of age the color changes from gray to yellow. Young cockatoos have brown irises, adult female cockatoos have red-brown irises, and adult males have dark brown to black irises.

Infraorbital Sinus

The infraorbital sinus is the only paranasal sinus in most birds. It extends from the nasal cavity medially and from the oral cavity ventrally, and it communicates with the cervicocephalic air sac system caudally (Fig. 1–6). It extends medial, cranial, and ventral to the eye. The sinus lacks bony walls; therefore,

Cage _____

Droppings _____

Attitude _____

Posture _____

Weight _____

Eyes _____

Sinuses _____

Nostrils/cere _____

Beak _____

Oropharynx _____

Head (skin/feathers) _____

Ears _____

Neck

    Crop/esophagus _____

    Trachea _____

Thorax

    Muscling _____

    Skin/feathers _____

Abdomen _____

Vent/cloaca _____ _____

Wings _____

Feet/legs _____

Leg band _____

Back (skin/feathers) _____

Tail/uropygial gland _____

Auscultation _____

Skin/feathers _____

Hydration status _____

Figure 1–5. Stamp for physical examination checklist.

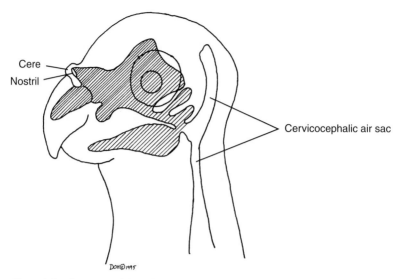

Cere
Nostril

Cervicocephalic air sac

DoH©1995

Figure 1–6. The extent of the infraorbital sinus varies between species of birds. It is an extensive sinus with diverticuli around the eyes and into bones of the head *(shaded area).*

swellings may be noted as fluctuant swellings around the eye or between the commissure of the beak and eye. Observe for swelling between the beak and eye and around the eyes. An asymmetry between the two sides of the face may be noted if one sinus is affected.

Nostrils and Cere

The cere is the raised sensitive area at the base of the upper beak surrounding the nares in psittacines, owls, and pigeons (see Fig. 1–6). The shape of the normal nostril varies with the species of bird and ranges from circular to slitlike. The cartilaginous structure forming the medial wall of the nostril is the operculum. The operculum prevents entry of foreign objects into the nasal cavity.

The nostrils of normal birds are symmetrical and patent. The opening is free of discharge. Patency of the nostril can be determined by placing a sterile drop of saline on the nostril. The fluid will be aspirated into the nasal cavity if the nostril is patent. Abnormalities of the cere and nostril include asymmetrical nostrils, deformed nostrils, nasal discharge, debris in the nostril and on the operculum, and, in budgies, thickening of the cere.

The color of the cere can indicate the sex of the bird in mature budgies. Immature budgies have a tan-colored cere. When mature, the cere is blue in male budgies and pink or tan colored in females. Cere color is undependable in color mutation budgies (e.g., yellow, white, blue).

Beak

The beak consists of the bones of the upper and lower jaws (the premaxilla, nasal, and maxilla above and the mandible below) and their keratinized sheaths (rhamphotheca). The rate of replacement of the rhamphotheca varies. In large parrots, the upper rhamphotheca (rhinotheca) is completely replaced in about 6 months. In toucans, the rhinotheca grows about 0.5 cm in 2 years. Caged birds may be classified as hardbills (e.g., psittacines) or softbills (e.g., mynahs).

The normal avian beak is smooth and symmetrical. In smaller species, transillumination of the beak with a bright light may be helpful.

Abnormalities of the beak include overgrown upper or lower beak, overgrown side of the beak, crossed upper and lower beaks (scissors beak), shortened upper beak (prognathism), and areas of swelling, grooves, or necrosis.

Mouth

The oral cavity and the pharynx are combined in birds to form the oropharynx. The oropharynx communicates with the sinuses through the median fissure in the palate, the choana. There are numerous caudally directed papillae associated with the choana in most species of birds. The glottis is located directly behind the tongue (birds do not have an epiglottis).

The psittacine tongue is muscular, blunt, and dexterous. Most passerines have a narrow, triangular tongue. The oropharynx is lined by stratified squamous epithelium that is keratinized in areas subject to abrasion (e.g., papillae). There are numerous mucus-secreting salivary glands in the lining of the oropharynx.

Evaluation of the mouth includes visualization of the choana and oropharynx and evaluation of jaw tone. Most birds will open their beaks when the beak is tapped with a pen light. This will allow a quick examination of the oral cavity. For an extensive examination, the beak is held open with an oral speculum or loops of gauze (Figs. 1–7 and 1–8). Gauze is preferable because most birds will

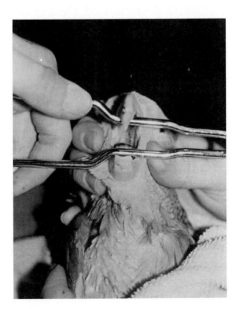

Figure 1–7. An oral examination using an oral speculum to hold the mouth open. Birds sometimes damage the edges of their beaks biting on the speculum.

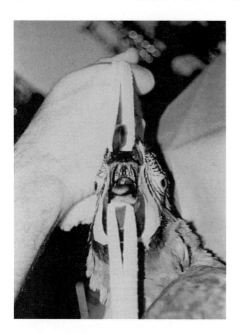

Figure 1–8. An oral examination using gauze loops to hold the mouth open. This method requires more assistance than the technique using an oral speculum but it does not damage the beak.

bite on the speculum, causing beak trauma; however, using gauze requires a technician to hold the loops of gauze. The oropharynx of normal birds is smooth, moist, and pink. The choana is sharp and clean and bordered by numerous sharp papillae. Dehydration can cause dry mucous membranes. Pale mucous membranes can indicate anemia. Abnormalities that may be observed in the oropharynx include inflammation, masses, swellings, abnormal coloration, accumulation of debris or food, blunting or missing papillae, and poor jaw tone.

Skin and Feathers of the Head

The feathers of the head of normal birds are smooth and symmetrical. Normal featherless areas in some species include the top of the head, cheeks, and around the eyes.

Abnormalities of the skin and feathers of the head include swellings, proliferations (common around the beak and cere), wet or sticky feathers, misshapen feathers, broken feathers, and feather loss (around the nostrils, increased area on top of the head, etc.). Examine the crest closely for abnormal feathers.

In budgies, immature birds will have horizontal bars across the top of the head. At about 6 months of age, these feathers are lost and replaced with solid-colored feathers.

Ears

The ear canals of birds can be examined with an otoscope and small cone or endoscope. Erythema, blood, and discharges are abnormal.

Neck: Crop, Esophagus, and Trachea

The esophagus courses down the right side of the neck in birds. It is thin walled and distensible. The crop (ingluvies) is a dilatation of the esophagus just cranial to the thoracic inlet that occurs in many species of birds. It is prominent in psittacines, pigeons, and doves and smaller in passerines and most raptors. Toucans and owls lack crops. The crops of chicks are much larger than those of adults.

Palpate the neck area from the intermandibular space to the thoracic inlet. The intermandibular space in normal birds is free of lumps and masses. The crop usually contains food, unless the bird is fasting or anorectic. In chicks, the crop can be distended with food and will require gentle palpation to prevent regurgitation and aspiration. Birds may swallow large food items whole, and these may be palpated in the crop. When empty, the normal crop feels thin and striated longitudinally. In pigeons, the crop mucosa becomes thickened when feeding their chicks. Observe the skin overlying the crop. Wet the feathers along the ventral neck and transilluminate the crop and esophagus with a small, bright light source if abnormalities are observed or suspected. If the crop is empty, it can be filled with air with a feeding tube. The air is held in the crop with digital pressure on the esophagus and the crop is transilluminated. This provides better visualization. The normal crop is of uniform thickness and vascularity. Observe peristalsis of the crop in neonates and birds with delayed crop emptying. Normal peristalsis is 1 to 3 contractions per minute when partially filled.

Transilluminate the trachea with a bright light source in passerines and, if respiratory signs are present, in budgies. Pinhead-sized black moving spots in the trachea of small passerines may indicate mites.

Abnormalities of the crop and esophagus include swellings, thickening, increased vascularity, foreign bodies, slow emptying of the crop, an enlarged crop that fails to empty, and lack of or a decrease in peristalsis. The consistency of the ingesta is usually thick and doughlike when crop stasis is present. The crop may be filled with fluid in some sick birds.

Abnormalities of the skin over the neck area include thickening, lumps, ulcerations, scabs, discoloration, masses, and emphysema. Subcutaneous emphysema may be noted as an accumulation of air under the skin. This can be the result of abnormal air sac function or fracture of pneumatic bones, such as the humerus. The air may be withdrawn with a needle and syringe or released through a small incision: make a 1-cm incision in an avascular area. Cauterize the incision and leave the incision open. The emphysema may return. Surgical procedures have been described for the placement of a stent if air continues to accumulate (see Harris 1991).

Pectoral Musculature, Skin, and Feathers

In normal birds, the sternum is straight and slightly elevated in comparison with the pectoral muscles. Passerines will normally have a more prominent sternum. The skin is smooth and free of masses or discoloration. Wetting of the skin and feathers over the pectoral area with alcohol will improve visualization, if needed. Normal feathers are smooth, symmetrical, and clean. Featherless areas between feather tracts are normal.

The normal muscling of the pectoral muscles is a better indicator of a normal weight of birds than is the actual weight.

Abnormalities include deviations of the sternum, muscle and fat mass even with or bulging above the sternum, prominence of the sternum (decreased muscle mass), scabs, ulcerations, swellings, subcutaneous hemorrhage, feather loss, and torn, frayed, or abnormally shaped feathers. Feather picking of the pectoral area is common in Amazon parrots. Excess fat is often deposited in the cranial pectoral area.

Abdomen

Observe and palpate the abdomen. Exercise caution when palpating a distended abdomen that may contain fluid. Rupture of the peritoneum can result in flooding of the air sacs and lungs with the fluid, resulting in death. The normal abdomen is slightly concave or flat. The normal liver cannot be palpated. Abdominal contents can be visualized through the skin in chicks and small passerines. In normal chicks, the ventriculus is proportionally large and protrudes slightly.

Abnormalities of the abdomen include bulging, palpable masses, the liver extending beyond the edge of the sternum, and fatty subcutaneous masses. In canaries and finches, hepatomegaly can often be visualized as a black mass just caudal to the sternum. Excess fat is common in the lateral flank areas. An increase in the distance from the sternum to the pubic bone in budgies can indicate organomegaly. The maximal normal distance is 4 to 5 mm. This distance can be quickly estimated with the fingertip.

Cloaca and Vent

The cloaca is a three-chambered terminal portion of the digestive, urinary, and reproductive tracts (Fig. 1–9). The vent is the opening of the cloaca to the outside. The rectum is continuous with the coprodeum. The coprodeum is separated from the urodeum with a fold of tissue and keeps feces separate from urinary and reproductive tract products. The presence of feces causes this membrane to bulge through the urodeum and proctodeum, allowing the feces to be deposited through the vent. The urodeum contains openings from the ureters and reproductive tract.

The normal pericloacal area is free of feces. The cloaca can be examined by gently everting it with a moistened cotton swab. The swab is gently inserted into the cloaca and slowly withdrawn while placing gentle pressure on one side of the cloaca with the tip of the swab by angling the swab to one side. The cloacal mucosa can also be exposed by bending the tail over the back and gently pinching the sides of the cloaca, causing the cloaca to evert. Normal cloacal mucosa is pink, moist, and relatively smooth.

Abnormalities of the vent include soiled feathers in the pericloacal area, proliferations, and protruding tissue. Abnormalities of the cloaca include prolifer-

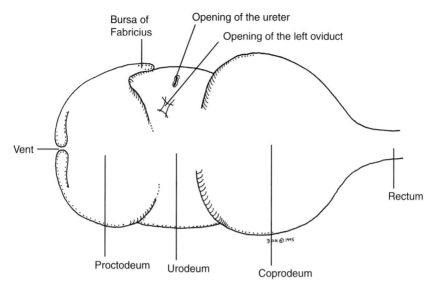

Figure 1–9. The cloaca consists of the coprodeum, urodeum, and proctodeum. The relative size of each chamber, folds, and exact location of orifices varies with age, sex, reproductive status, and species of bird.

ative lesions, erosions, hypertrophy, erythema, and uroliths. An acetic acid solution (apple-cider vinegar) can be applied to a suspected papilloma lesion and will cause papillomatous tissue to blanch to white from the pink or red original color. See Chapter 15 for diagnosis of abnormalities associated with tissue protruding through the vent (prolapse).

Wings

The wings are examined for symmetry, range of motion, and bony abnormalities. The skin and feathers are examined for color, shape, uniformity, and presence of parasites. Normal feathers are smooth and flat with unfrayed edges. Hydration status can be determined by observation of the basilic (wing) vein. Normal veins are turgid and refill immediately when depressed.

Abnormalities of the wings include asymmetry, a decrease in the range of motion, enlarged joints, ulcerations, swellings, bony abnormalities (crepitation, fractures, etc.), stress marks, parasites, retained feather sheaths, and bleeding, broken, missing, abnormally shaped, or chewed feathers. Stress marks are translucent lines across the feather. The wings are a common area of feather picking in cockatiels, cockatoos, African gray parrots, Quaker parrots, and gray-cheeked parakeets. When lice are present, they are often found on the long feathers of the wings.

Feet and Legs

The normal avian foot is uniform in color and texture. The dorsal and plantar surfaces have a prominent scale pattern. The grip is strong. The feathers are smooth and uniform.

Abnormalities of the feet and legs include abnormally shaped feathers, bald areas, swellings, constrictions, erythema, erosions, ulcers, proliferative lesions, broken nails, weak grip, swollen joints, and neurologic deficits.

Leg Bands

Leg bands are useful for identification of individual birds in aviaries. Banding of individual pet birds serves no useful purpose. Check the skin under leg bands for irritation or swelling. Necrosis, swelling, and trauma can be the result of leg bands that fit improperly or a trapped or caught band. In pet bird households, remove the band. Small bands may be cut. Large open bands are twisted in opposite directions with pliers or vise grips (Fig. 1–10). Careful, controlled removal is extremely important to avoid trauma to the leg or fractures. Large closed bands can sometimes be slipped over the foot when the toes facing cranially are placed along the tibiotarsus and the band is slipped over the foot. Tight-fitting closed bands must be cut with a dental blade attachment on a Dremel tool, jeweler's ring cutters, or other cutting devices. When using a Dremel tool to remove a band, protect the leg with a wooden tongue depressor and keep the band from becoming excessively hot with water from a syringe. Before removing the band, warn the owner that trauma may occur during band removal.

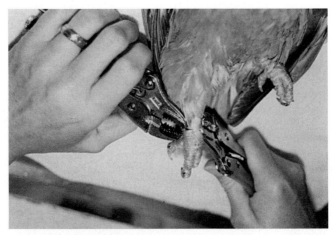

Figure 1–10. Leg band removal using vise grips, taking care to avoid traumatizing the leg. The band is carefully twisted with controlled force such that the leg can be slipped through the gap between the ends of the band.

Back: Skin, Feathers, and Musculature

The feathers and skin along the back of normal birds are smooth and uniformly shaped and colored.

Abnormalities include abnormally colored or shaped feathers, skin discoloration, swellings, and missing feathers.

Tail and Uropygial Gland

Normal tail feathers are clean, unbroken, and unfrayed. The uropygial (preen) gland is a secretory gland located dorsally at the base of the tail in some species of birds. Many pigeons and parrots lack this gland. Secretions from the uropygial gland are spread over the feathers during preening, keeping the feathers, beak, and scales waterproof and supple.

Abnormalities of the uropygial gland include swelling, erythema, ulceration, and rupture. Abnormalities of the tail include stress lines and broken, dirty, frayed, abnormally shaped, or discolored feathers.

Auscultation

In birds, the lungs adhere to the dorsal thorax extending from the first through the eighth rib. Left and right primary bronchi terminate in numerous secondary bronchi. Parabronchi (tertiary bronchi) anastomose with other parabronchi and extend from the secondary bronchi to air labyrinth (air capillaries), the site of gas exchange (Fig. 1–11). Parabronchi and air labyrinth branch and anastomose

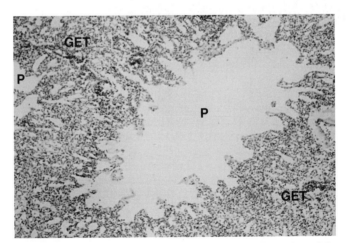

Figure 1–11. Gas exchange in the avian lung occurs at the interface of the air labyrinth (formerly incorrectly termed "air capillaries") and the pulmonary blood capillaries. Secondary bronchi connect with the parabronchi (*P*) (also called tertiary bronchi), which connect via atria in their walls with the air labyrinth of the gas exchange tissue *(GET)*. (Photo courtesy of David Graham, DVM, PhD, Department of Veterinary Pathobiology, Texas A&M University.)

extensively, forming an extensive network of tubules. Air sacs communicate with the lungs and aid in circulation of air. Air sac membranes are thin membranous structures located in various areas of the body. There are species variations in the number and size of air sacs. In general, there are three air sac systems: pharyngeal-tracheal, cervicocephalic, and pulmonary. The pharyngeal-tracheal air sac system is used for sexual display. The cervicocephalic air sac system extends from the infraorbital sinus, over the back of the head, and down the back of the neck and surrounds the crop. In most species of pet birds, the pulmonary air sac system consists of a singular clavicular air sac and paired cervical, cranial thoracic, caudal thoracic, and abdominal air sacs (Fig. 1–12). The clavicular air sac lies dorsal to the crop between the clavicles. Diverticula extend into the humerus, clavicles, coracoids, vertebrae, sternum, and ribs. The cervical air sacs are small and extend dorsally to the last few cervical vertebrae, with diverticula into pneumatized vertebrae, and cranially to the extrathoracic diverticula of the clavicular air sac.

Birds lack a diaphragm. Respiration is accomplished through movement of

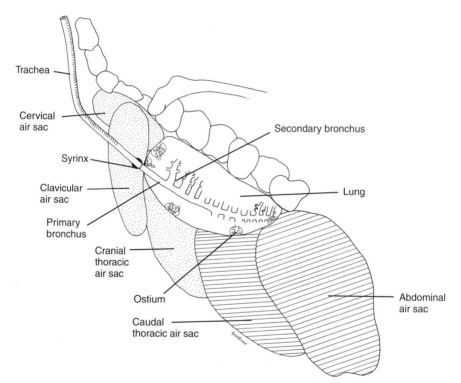

Figure 1–12. The pulmonary air sac system consists of the clavicular air sac and paired cervical, cranial thoracic, caudal thoracic, and abdominal air sacs in most species of pet birds. Circulation of inspired air requires two inspirations and two expirations. During inspiration, posterior air sacs receive fresh oxygen-rich air, and anterior air sacs receive oxygen poor air that has already passed through exchange tissue in the lungs. During expiration, lungs fill with oxygen-rich air from the posterior air sacs, and oxygen-poor air leaves the anterior air sacs into the bronchi and trachea, and is expired. *Hatchmarks* indicate posterior air sacs; *dots* indicate anterior air sacs.

the ribs and sternum. Circulation of inspired air requires two inspirations and two expirations. During inspiration, posterior air sacs (caudal thoracic and abdominal sacs) receive fresh, oxygen-rich air, and anterior air sacs (cranial thoracic, cervical, and clavicular air sacs) receive air that has already passed through exchange tissue in the lungs. During expiration, lungs fill with oxygen-rich air from posterior air sacs, and oxygen-poor air leaves anterior air sacs into bronchi and the trachea and is expired.

Auscultate the cranial thorax for cardiac and respiratory sounds. Normal heart and respiratory rates vary with the size of bird and level of excitement (see Table 1–1). The caudal thorax and back areas are ausculted for wheezes, crackles, pops, whistles, and gurgles.

Skin and Feathers

The feathers of birds provide insulation, waterproofing, and flight capabilities. They grow in tracts (pterylae) with featherless areas (apteria) between tracts. These featherless areas appear as bare skin and are normal. Feathers grow from follicles similar to hair follicles.

Birds may molt continuously or two to three times per year. Molting is influenced by light exposure and controlled by hormones. During molting, birds preen more to remove the feather shaft from newly erupted feathers. White flaking associated with this feather shaft material is normal. Growing feathers contain a vascular shaft that appears dark.

The general condition of the feathers and skin is evaluated. Normal feathers are smooth, uniform, and clean and lack stress bars. Some birds will develop a brood patch, a bare area on the ventral abdomen and lower legs.

Abnormalities of the feathers include stress marks and broken, malformed, dirty, missing, or abnormally colored feathers. Stress marks are translucent lines across the feather.

Abnormalities of the skin include swellings, discolorations, edema, thickening, bleeding, exudation, laceration, hyperkeratosis, bruising, proliferative lesions, and ulceration.

Hydration Status

Evaluation of the hydration status of the bird is based on turgidity and refill time of the basilic (wing) vein and artery. The vein will refill immediately in normal birds. A refill time of the basilic vein greater than 1 to 2 seconds indicates dehydration greater than 7%. Unfeathered areas of the skin (around the eyes, on legs, etc.) may also be tented and observed for return to a normal state. Mucous membranes will be moist when a bird is adequately hydrated. With dehydration, mucous membranes may be tacky. With severe dehydration, the eyes may be sunken, but the eyes may also be sunken as a result of other causes.

LABORATORY DIAGNOSTICS

Diagnostic testing is extremely important to diagnose or rule out disease in birds. Birds in the wild developed the ability to hide signs of illness to survive.

Pet birds have retained this ability and rarely show signs of illness until quite severely affected. Determination of a diagnosis through diagnostic testing allows for prompt correct treatment of the disease. Presumed diagnoses may lead to delayed treatment or even death. A diagnosis may be suspected, and treatment begun awaiting results of diagnostic tests, but diagnostic testing should always be used to determine a definitive diagnosis in all cases where an owner will allow. Always offer all diagnostic tests necessary to make a diagnosis. Let the owner make an informed decision and set financial limitations. Never assume an owner does not wish to pursue diagnostic testing based on the monetary value of the bird or for other reasons.

SUPPORTIVE CARE

Provide supportive care as needed until a diagnosis is made and during treatment.

Minimize stress and handling of sick birds. Separate ill birds from other birds to decrease stress, facilitate monitoring, and avoid the spread of disease. Provide a quiet environment. Weigh the bird daily before treatments and feeding. Lower perches or, if the bird is very weak or has neurologic signs, remove them.

If the bird is on a poor diet, a multivitamin injection should be administered.

Warmth

Provide ill birds with a warm, quiet, dimmed environment. Maintain an ambient temperature of 85° to 90°F. Birds with head trauma or hyperthermia need a cool environment, approximately 75°F.

Nutrition

Ill birds that are not eating are tube fed, which should be continued until the bird is eating on its own. Techniques of tube feeding are presented in Chapter 11. Table 1–2 suggests volumes and frequencies of tube feedings. When tube feeding is needed, perform other diagnostic maneuvers or sample collections before feeding to prevent regurgitation. Palpate the crop before each feeding. If food is present in the crop, do not tube feed (consult Chapter 4).

Commercial feeding formulas for birds are available (Table 1–3). Hand-feeding formulas, human enteral nutritional formulas, and homemade formulas may also be used. The commercial feeding formulas for birds and hand-feeding formulas are convenient and nutritionally balanced and will pass through a feeding needle. Caloric density and nutritional content vary with the human and homemade formulas, which are less desirable. The commercial feeding formulas for birds and hand-feeding formulas are mixed with warm water, heated under hot running water to a temperature between 101° and 104°F, and fed immediately. Tube feeding mixtures are always fed warmed to prevent delayed crop emptying. To prevent crop burns, do not warm food in a microwave, and always stir the formula before measuring the temperature.

TABLE 1–2 Guidelines for Volumes and Frequency for Tube Feeding of Warmed Formulas

Finch	.1–.5 ml 6×/day
Budgie	.5–3 ml QID
Lovebird	1–3 ml QID
Cockatiel	1–8 ml QID
Small conure	3–12 ml QID
Large conure	7–24 ml TID or QID
Amazon parrot	5–35 ml TID
Cockatoo	10–40 ml BID or TID
Macaw	20–60 ml BID or TID

Begin with frequent small amounts. As the crop accommodates larger volumes, adjust volume and frequency.

Anorectic raptors are fed pieces of prey. If the bird will not eat from the cage floor in a quiet room, the prey is offered dangling with forceps. Pieces of prey can be force fed with forceps, gently pushing the prey into the crop.

Fluid Therapy

Fluid therapy is used to replace losses or occasionally to maintain normal hydration. For rehydration, fluids are given intraosseously or intravenously. Subcutaneous fluid administration may be used when mild dehydration is present and the bird is not in critical condition. Lactated Ringer's solution or a similar balanced isotonic solution is used. Infuse fluids warmed to 100.4° to 102.2°F. A solution of 50% dextrose may be added to the lactated Ringer's solution to make a 5% dextrose solution for intravenous or intraosseous fluid administration. This may be important with chicks, raptors, septicemic birds, and cachectic birds.

Estimation of the fluid deficit is based on estimated dehydration and body weight:

$$\text{Estimated dehydration } (\%) \times \text{body weight } (g) = \text{fluid deficit } (ml)$$

Daily maintenance fluid requirements in most companion and aviary birds is 50 ml/kg/day. The daily maintenance fluid requirement and half of the fluid deficit is given during the first 12 to 24 hours, along with any estimated ongoing losses. The remaining half of the fluid deficit is given during the following 48 hours, along with the daily maintenance fluid requirement and estimated ongoing losses. Intravenous and intraosseous fluids can be administered as a bolus or constant

TABLE 1–3 Some Commercial Tube Feeding Formulas

Emeraid I.   LaFeber Co., Cornell, IL 61319; (815) 358-2301
Emeraid II.   LaFeber Co. (address above)
Formula AA. Roudybush Inc., Sacramento, CA 95821; (800) 326-1726
Hand-feeding formulas for chicks (Exact, Harrison's, LaFeber)

rate infusion. Because birds may chew at the catheter or extension tubing, cover the catheter with a bandage. The tubing may be placed inside corrugated tubing to prevent damage to the fluid line. Bolus administration of up to 10 ml/kg of warmed fluids given slowly over 5 to 7 minutes is usually well tolerated. For guidelines for volumes of bolus fluids for various species, see Table 1–4. Anesthesia is used during placement of catheters. Intravenous boluses may be administered without catheterization in calm patients; however, there are a limited number of veins for this use, and hematomas are common after fluid administration. Also, when catheters are used, other veins are left for obtaining blood samples for diagnostic testing.

Intraosseous catheter sites include the ulna and tibiotarsus. Catheters placed

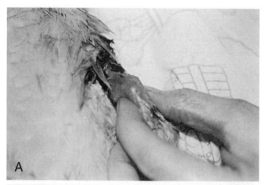

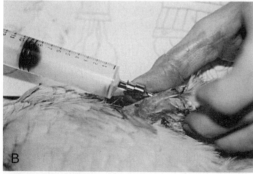

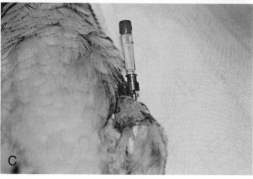

Figure 1–13. Placement of an intraosseous catheter in the tibiotarsus. The proximal cranial tibiotarsus is surgically prepped. The tibiotarsus is grasped in one hand, and the stifle is flexed (**A**). The needle is introduced into the cnemial crest (tibial crest) through the patellar tendon parallel to the tibiotarsus. Once the needle has been introduced into the medullary cavity to the level of the hub, a syringe is attached. If the needle is placed correctly, negative pressure will cause a small amount of blood to come into the hub of the needle and syringe (**B**). A prefilled adapter is placed if needed, and the needle and adapter are flushed (**C**).

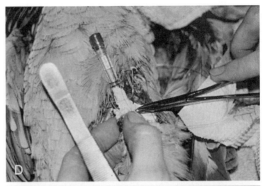

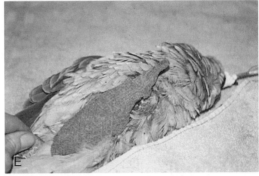

Figure 1–13 *Continued.* A butterfly tape is placed on the hub of the needle and sutured to the skin (**D**). A bandage is applied over the site (**E**).

in the ulna are usually better tolerated. Placement of an intraosseous catheter in the tibiotarsus is discussed in Figure 1–13 and placement in the ulna is shown in Figure 1–14.

When an intraosseous catheter is placed correctly, negative pressure will cause a small amount of blood to come into the hub of the needle and syringe. Resistance after entering the medullary cavity can indicate contact with cortical bone; if this happens, reposition the needle. Spinal needles and regular syringe needles may be used as intraosseous catheters.

Intravenous catheter sites include the right jugular and basilic veins. Placement of jugular catheters is discussed in Figure 1–15, and basilic catheterization is shown in Figure 1–16. Prefill the catheter and adapter.

The lateral and medial flank areas and the axilla are common sites for

TABLE 1–4 Volumes of Bolus Warmed Fluids for Various Species

Finch	.5–1 ml
Budgie	1–2 ml
Cockatiel	2–3 ml
Conure	3–4 ml
Amazon parrot	7–10 ml
Cockatoo	10–20 ml
Macaw	15–25 ml

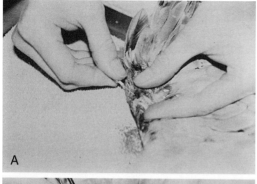

A

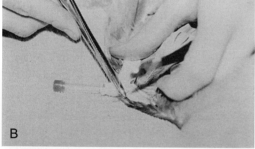

B

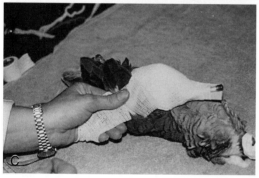

C

Figure 1–14. Placement of an intraosseous catheter in the ulna. The ulna is catheterized on the medial side of the wing. The distal carpus is surgically prepped. The ulna is supported with one hand, and the needle is introduced in the medial distal ulna parallel to the diaphysis **(A)**. A prefilled adapter is applied if needed, and the needle and adapter are flushed. A butterfly tape is sutured to the skin **(B)**, and the wing is immobilized with a figure-of-eight bandage. A wooden tongue depressor is incorporated into the bandage and extends beyond the tip of the catheter or adapter **(C)**.

subcutaneous fluid administration. Use a 25- to 27-gauge needle. Subcutaneous fluid administration is limited to 5 to 10 ml/kg per site.

Nebulization Therapy

Nebulization therapy is helpful in birds with upper and lower respiratory tract infections. Antibiotics may be nebulized for direct local action. A particle size less than 3 μm is required to have a local effect in the lungs and air sacs. Many inexpensive commercial nebulizers will not produce this small particle size. Some ultrasonic nebulizers produce particles of this size. Larger-sized particles are generally deposited in the nasal cavity or trachea.

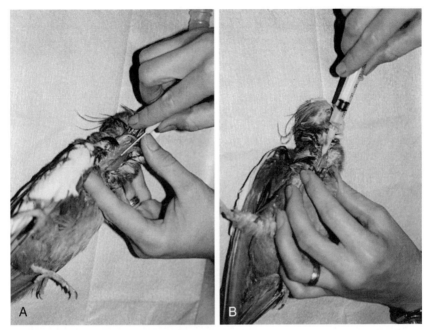

Figure 1–15. Placement of a jugular catheter. The catheter is prefilled. The right lateral neck area is surgically prepped, and the right jugular is catheterized (**A**). The catheter is flushed (**B**) and capped, and a light bandage is applied.

Most intravenous antibiotics can be mixed with saline for nebulization (see Table 11–1). Some antifungal medications have been nebulized and used in the treatment of mycotic airsacculitis (see Chapter 17).

Oxygen

Dyspneic birds are placed in a cage with oxygen supplementation (oxygen cage). Signs of dyspnea include open-mouth breathing, tail bobbing, cyanosis, and increased respiratory effort and rate. High levels of oxygen supplementation (up to 100%) for 12 hours can be provided without complications but should be limited to short-term exposures, because prolonged high oxygen concentrations can be harmful. Oxygen is delivered by face mask during physical examination, sample collection, and treatments as needed.

Oxygen may be supplemented in an aquarium, incubator, or a specialized hospitalization unit.

If an upper airway obstruction is suspected, based on clinical signs, an air sac breathing tube is placed (see Chapters 3 and 14).

Antibiotic and Antifungal Administration

Initial antibiotic or antifungal therapy may be indicated before obtaining culture and sensitivity results. Very ill birds and those with abnormal Gram's

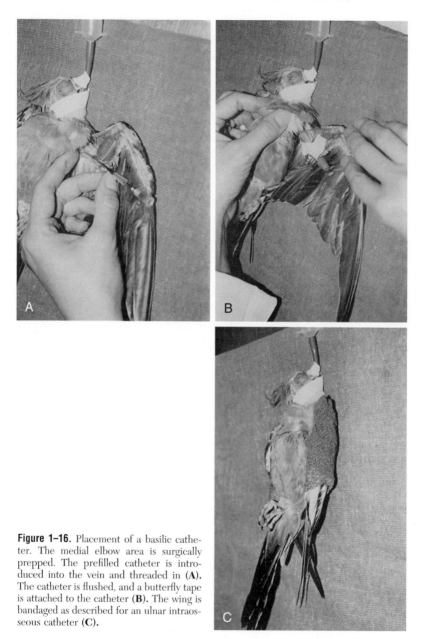

Figure 1–16. Placement of a basilic catheter. The medial elbow area is surgically prepped. The prefilled catheter is introduced into the vein and threaded in (**A**). The catheter is flushed, and a butterfly tape is attached to the catheter (**B**). The wing is bandaged as described for an ulnar intraosseous catheter (**C**).

stain results or other signs of bacterial infection often benefit from early administration of antibiotics.

In acutely ill birds, instigation of treatment may be important before completion of diagnostic testing. A broad-spectrum bactericidal antibiotic, an antifungal, and doxycycline may be initiated before obtaining a diagnosis. Cefotaxime, enrofloxacin, or amikacin can be used as an initial choice for injectable antibiotic therapy. Do not use amikacin in dehydrated birds. For very ill birds, parenteral administration of antibiotics is preferable. Orally administered antibiotics can be used once the bird is stabilized. Oral antibiotics may be used in conjunction with parenteral antibiotics with gastrointestinal infections. Birds with mild clinical signs often respond well to oral administration of antibiotics. Doxycycline is used to treat chlamydiosis, a common cause of acute illness in psittacines. Doxycycline administration may be beneficial in conjunction with other antibiotics before completion of diagnostics, before chlamydial status is known. Fluconazole, itraconazole, or flucytosine may be used orally to initiate antifungal therapy before completion of diagnostic tests when a fungal infection is suspected. Nystatin, ketoconazole, or fluconazole can be administered orally if large numbers of yeast are found in oral or fecal Gram's stains. *Collect laboratory samples before administration of antibiotics and antifungals whenever possible.*

Correct poor diet and husbandry problems in birds with bacterial infections.

Antibiotics are changed based on culture and sensitivity results, clinical response, or diagnostic testing results.

NUTRITION

Nutritional problems are common in pet birds. Some very common nutritional diseases include obesity, vitamin A deficiency, and poor feathering. Other conditions resulting from inadequate nutrition include brittle bones, splay leg, hepatic lipidosis, goiter, and many others. Consult appropriate chapters for further information about specific malnutrition conditions.

Commercial formulated diets are available for gallinaceous birds, finches, canaries, psittacines, toucans, mynahs, ratites, and waterfowl. Many formulated diets are available for different ages, activity levels, and reproductive periods.

At this time, exact nutritional requirements of psittacine birds are not known. However, field tests have been used to determine diets on which many birds perform well, determined by longevity and sustained reproductive success. Hand-feeding formulas are discussed in Chapter 16. Currently, adult commercial formulated diets appear to be superior to homemade diets and definitively superior to seed diets. Seed diets are deficient in many essential nutrients, and many seeds are excessively high in fat (e.g., sunflower, safflower, hemp, rape, and Niger). Birds will not choose a balanced diet if offered a variety of foods that include seeds or other unhealthy foodstuffs.

Current recommendations for psittacine diets are to feed a commercial formulated diet, fresh water, no seeds, no vitamins, no minerals, no grit, with or without supplementation with small amounts of vegetables and fruits (no more than 20% of the diet). Commercial formulated diets contain vitamins; therefore, supplementation with vitamins in birds eating formulated diets can result in vitamin toxicoses. Some commercial formulated diets are listed in Table 1–5. Some large psittacines such as macaws, palm cockatoos, and Queen of Bavaria conures appear to perform better on a high-fat and high-fiber formulated diet supplemented with nuts. Specially formulated commercial diets are available for macaws.

When commercial formulated diets are supplemented with vegetables and

TABLE 1–5 Some Commercial Formulated Diets

Exact Complete Daily Diets. Kaytee Products Inc., Chilton, WI 53014; (414) 849-2321; (800) 529-8331

Harrison's Bird Diets. HBD Inc., Omaha, NE 68106; (402) 397-9442; (800) 346-0269

LaFeber Bird Diets. LaFeber Co., Cornell, IL 61319; (815) 358-2301

Lakes Ultimate Avian Diets. Lakes Minnesota Macaws Inc., St. Paul, MN 55107; (800) 634-2473

Mazuri Cage Bird Diets. Purina Mills Inc., St. Louis, MO 63166; (800) 227-8941

Pretty Bird Daily Select Diets. Pretty Bird International Inc., Stacy, MN 55079; (800) 356-5020

Roudybush Maintenance Pellets. Roudybush Inc., Paso Robles, CA 93446; (800) 326-1726

Topper Bird Ranch Total Diets. Topper Bird Ranch, Modesto, CA 95351; (209) 524-2828

Tropican Lifetime Pellets and Granules. Rolf C. Hagen USA Inc., Mansfield, MA 02048; (800) 724-2436

Zeigler Parrot Diets. Zeigler Inc., Gardners, PA 17324; (800) 841-6800

fruits, offerings should be limited to fruits and dark green or dark yellow vegetables, such as greens, broccoli, carrots, sweet potatoes, spinach, beets, endive, escarole, cantaloupe, papayas, mango, apricot, pumpkin, Brussels sprouts, winter squash, dried peppers, and corn.

Converting birds to a commercial formulated diet can be challenging, but the benefits of adequate nutrition often result in a longer, healthier life. The total food consumption should be carefully monitored during diet changes. Many birds will not recognize new foodstuffs as food and may refuse to eat if only offered the new food. While trying to get the bird to eat a new food, always place the new food in the familiar feeding bowl. Many strategies have been suggested for conversion to a formulated diet; some are listed in Table 1–6. The technique that appears to be successful most often is placing the new food in the cage the entire day and limiting the normal diet to two 15-minute feedings, one late morning and the other in the evening. Birds offered mixtures of

TABLE 1–6 Some Strategies for Conversion to Commercial Formulated Diets

1. Place the new food in the regular feeding bowl for the entire day and offer the old diet for 15 minutes midmorning and evening (four meals per day for young birds). Access to the new diet in early morning is important because the natural habit of many birds is to eat a meal in the early morning and again in the early evening.

2. Place a healthy bird that is already eating the new diet near the bird that you want to eat the new diet. The bird eating the new diet will often prompt the new bird to try the new diet.

3. Mix the commercial formulated diet with the seed diet. Gradually increase the amount of formulated diet while decreasing the seed diet in the mix. When the bird begins eating the formulated diet, quit offering the seed diet.

4. Place the bird in unfamiliar surroundings, such as in an aquarium or new cage, and sprinkle the food on the bottom of the cage near a small container of water.

5. Hand feed the new diet as a treat until the bird readily accepts it as food.

6. Hospitalize the bird and offer only the commercial formulated diet. Monitor the bird for weight loss, activity levels, and any signs of illness. Do not allow a bird to lose more than 10% of its body weight. Most birds will not eat the new food for 1 to 3 days. Offer the bird's regular diet if the bird resists eating the new diet for 2 days or loses up to 10% of its body weight. Attempt this only with healthy birds. Second and third attempts are sometimes needed for successful diet conversion.

7. Offer commercial cakes of combined seeds and pellets while reducing the amount of seed offered. When the bird is eating the new diet, replace the seeds with pellets.

foodstuffs will often pick out favorite food items (e.g., seeds), resulting in inadequate nutrition. Do not offer seeds once a bird is eating a commercial formulated diet.

Birds may be fed a commercial formulated diet by free choice or limited to meals. In adult psittacines, morning and evening feedings mimic their natural foraging habits in the wild. Provide fresh food daily. If moist foods are fed, remove these from the cage and cage floor before their spoilage, which may occur in 4 hours in warm temperatures.

Birds not on a complete diet (i.e., not on a commercial formulated diet) should be given vitamins until the diet is corrected. Vitamins should not be placed in the bird's water because many vitamins quickly degrade in water, and vitamins promote bacterial growth in water.

Lories, lorikeets, and related birds require a diet that simulates nectar. A commercial formula can be offered dry or moist and supplemented with fresh fruits, vegetables, pollen, seeds, mealworms, and nontoxic branches with fresh leaves and blossoms.

Toucans and mynahs should be offered a commercial formulated low-iron diet, such as Harrison's Low Iron Formula, Kaytee Softbill Diet, or Bird of Paradise Diet (see Table 1–5). These birds should also be offered diced low-iron fruits and vegetables, such as boiled potatoes, corn, apples, bananas, pears, pineapples, plums, figs, berries, papayas, and melons. Avoid feeding foods high in iron, such as grapes, raisins, and dark green vegetables and greens.

Raptors may be fed a commercial formulated diet or whole prey items such as rodents, chicks, chickens, quail, or fish.

Fresh food and water should be provided in clean, nontoxic bowls. Glazed bowls can be tested for lead content with inexpensive screening kits available for testing children's toys. Bowls should be placed above perches to avoid contamination with feces. Food and water bowls should not be placed side by side, because some birds will dunk their food in the water, which promotes bacterial growth in the water and washes nutrients from the outer surface of some pellets. Bowls should be washed and disinfected daily.

Psittacine and passerine birds on commerical pelleted diets do not need any grit. Pigeons, doves, gallinaceous birds, cassowaries, and ratites need grit to aid in digestion of food in the ventriculus. Ingestion of excessive grit may result in hemorrhagic enteritis, gastrointestinal obstruction, and death and grit should not be offered to those species not requiring it for digestion.

EQUIPMENT

Much of the equipment needed for the practice of avian medicine is already present in the average veterinary practice, including radiographic equipment, isoflurane anesthesia, ophthalmic instruments, binocular microscope with oil immersion capability, centrifuge, hemocytometer, biochemistry testing system, and radiosurgery unit. Specialized items needed for avian practice include equipment to weigh, examine, collect samples, diagnose, and treat birds. Sources of equipment are listed in Appendix 1. A gram scale is important to obtain accurate weights in birds. Scales may be fitted with perches or lightweight containers or baskets to aid in weighing birds (Fig. 1–17). Paper bags may be used to hold

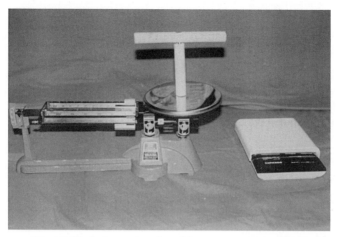

Figure 1–17. Scales can be adapted for easier weighing of birds.

small birds while weighing them. Pediatric stethoscopes are ideal for auscultation of respiratory and cardiac sounds in birds. Heavy ceramic bowls, gavage feeding tubes, and mouth speculums are needed. Perches must be made of nonporous materials such as PVC pipe or heavy plastic rods that can be disinfected. A hemocytometer, Gram's staining kit, small culturettes, and small blood-collecting tubes are needed for laboratory diagnostics. A dremel tool is necessary for beak and nail trimming. Specialized radiographic positioning boards aid in positioning and restraining birds during radiographic and surgical procedures. Isoflurane is necessary for the practice of avian medicine. A nonrebreathing apparatus and small endotracheal tubes are used for anesthesia in birds. Important surgical supplies include iris scissors, iris forceps, ophthalmic needle holders, and transparent avian drapes. Dental acrylics or methacrylate products are necessary for orthopedics and beak repair.

HOSPITALIZATION OR HOME CARE

Limit stress of ill birds as much as possible. For most birds, home care is much less stressful than hospitalization. Owners can be taught how to give oral medications or injections. Injectable medications can be premeasured in syringes for easier dosing. A warm environment is important. Heat supplementation may be provided in the home environment by placing a heating pad under one side of the cage floor and covering that half of the cage with a towel, or a light with a 75- to 100-watt bulb may be placed outside of the cage but close to one perch. Both of these methods allow the ill bird to regulate the amount of heat by moving to warmer or cooler areas of the cage.

Severely ill birds or those requiring more intense treatment are hospitalized. Birds that need tube feeding, fluid therapy, nebulization therapy, oxygen supplementation, or monitoring are hospitalized.

HOSPITAL ENVIRONMENT

Prevent the spread of disease by disinfecting equipment and surfaces that come in contact with each bird between each patient use. Remove feces, food, and other organic material from bowls and equipment before disinfecting. Cages, bowls, perches, other cage accessories, feeding equipment, capture nets, and grooming tools can be soaked in a phenol or quaternary ammonia solution for 30 minutes for disinfection. Thoroughly rinse equipment after the soak to remove all disinfectant. Disinfect tables and counters between patients. Wash hands between patients. Spray clothing and hair with disinfectant spray or change laboratory coats as needed between patients. Wear a mask and gown when handling highly infectious patients. With hospitalized patients, clean, feed, and treat the healthiest birds first and the contagious ones last.

Remove birds from cages only in safe environments, with windows covered, ceiling fans off, and door closed.

Hospitalization cages can include aquariums, small animal kennels, incubators, and specialized commercial avian cages. Cages require good ventilation and a heat source. An ambient temperature of 85° to 90°F is maintained for most ill birds. Removable perches that can be disinfected are used. Remove the perches if the bird is very ill, has difficulty perching, or has seizures. Line the cage with paper or nonwoven towels. Newspaper may stain feathers. Aquariums with screened covers are heated by placing a heating pad under one end of the cage. Use a thermometer in the cage to evaluate the temperature. Small animal kennels can be heated with heating pads or clamp-type lamps. Towels, acrylic, or Plexiglas can be placed across the front of the cage to retain heat.

Place food and water where they are easily accessible. Placing seeds, fruits, vegetables, and the regular diet of the bird around a nonperching bird may stimulate eating. Place the food and water containers next to the perches if the bird is still perching.

PRACTICE MANAGEMENT

Annual or semiannual examinations are recommended for birds. Detecting subclinical problems, monitoring the bird's weight, and evaluating the bird's nutritional status are the emphases of the routine visit. Nail, wing, and beak trims are performed as needed. A complete and thorough physical examination is used to detect physical abnormalities of which the owner is often unaware. Laboratory diagnostics are often performed to detect subclinical disease states. A complete blood count (CBC), plasma biochemistries, and Gram's stain and culture of the cloaca are indicated with routine examinations. Important plasma biochemistry tests to perform on apparently healthy birds include aspartate aminotransferase (AST or SGOT), uric acid, total protein, albumin, and creatinine kinase (CK). Radiography and other more extensive diagnostics are indicated when abnormalities are detected or suspected.

During the initial visit, nutrition and husbandry are discussed in detail. Instructions for emergency care and routine care are also provided. A complete physical examination is performed. Important laboratory diagnostics for the initial visit of an apparently healthy bird include cloacal and choanal Gram's stains; cloacal and choanal cultures; CBC; plasma biochemistries; and tests for specific infectious diseases as needed. Laboratory testing is important to find illness in birds that appear healthy, often allowing earlier treatment. Important plasma biochemistries for the initial examination of an avian patient include uric acid, AST, total protein, glucose, calcium, CK, and albumin. Measure bile acids if liver disease is suspected. Plasma protein electrophoresis (EPH) is valuable in identifying many disease states in apparently healthy birds (e.g., chlamydiosis, aspergillosis, mycobacteriosis, peritonitis, liver disease, kidney disease). After a client purchases a new bird, EPH is recommended for postpurchase testing. Important tests for infectious diseases include chlamydiosis testing and probe tests for psittacine beak and feather disease (PBFD) and polyomavirus. Radiography is used to detect organomegaly, airsacculitis, and other abnormalities, especially for a postpurchase examination. Other tests are performed as needed based on abnormal clinical signs or findings, as well as on exposure. Imported birds may benefit from routine deworming for tapeworms, particularly African gray parrots and cockatoos.

A bird cannot be determined to be healthy. A bird may be apparently healthy, with diagnostic tests to support that it is healthy.

Testing in some birds may be cost prohibitive, or sampling may be impossible. All reasonable options should be offered to every client. Allow owners to determine the amount of testing they wish to pursue.

Client education is a major part of the practice of avian medicine. Client educational materials aid in the education process. Important topics for printed educational material include nutrition, basic care, hand feeding, grooming, training, laboratory diagnostics, diseases, and special instruction sheets. Commercial client education brochures are available through the Association of Avian Veterinarians.°

Well-educated staff members can provide clients information on nutrition and husbandry, collect diagnostic samples, perform routine grooming procedures, and assist with radiology, anesthesia, and surgery. A well-trained avian technician can perform and assist with these procedures, providing the doctor more time to examine, diagnose, and treat patients.

Let clients know avian medicine is a part of the practice by displaying client educational brochures, avian pictures, and avian literature in the reception area and examination rooms of the clinic. Incorporate birds into the clinic logo. Let the public know you have an interest in the treatment of birds. Offer to give lectures at local bird clubs and speak to students at schools. Offer medical care and rehabilitation for injured avian wildlife. Working with local pet stores, aviaries, and breeders can provide abundant referrals. Avian veterinarians have much to offer pet stores. Many stores and aviaries would benefit greatly from information on sanitation, nutrition, and disease control. If a veterinarian is available to treat ill birds, pet stores are less likely to recommend treatments. Performing gross necropsies for a reduced fee for aviaries, breeders, or pet stores will supply abundant experience and education to the veterinarian.

Meticulous record keeping is imperative in avian practice. Avian cases are often involved and may require prolonged care.

°PO Box 618372, Orlando, FL 32861. Fax (407) 521-6401; phone (407) 521-6101.

CONTINUING EDUCATION

Continued education is extremely important in avian medicine. Join the Association of Avian Veterinarians (AAV). This organization offers an informative quarterly journal and an excellent yearly conference and proceedings. Both introductory and advanced lectures are provided in addition to hands-on laboratories. The published proceedings, available for purchase from the AAV, are a good source of information. Other national and regional veterinary conferences that offer avian programs include the North American Veterinary Conference, Western Veterinary Conference, American Animal Hospital Association, Mid-Atlantic Avian Veterinary Association, and American Association of Zoo Veterinarians. Many state associations and veterinary medical schools offer avian continuing education. Join aviary clubs, acquire pet birds, and breed and raise birds. Abundant books and journals are available to further explore avian medicine. *Parrots of the World* (Forshaw, Cooper, 1989) is an excellent source for species identification. Abstracts and indexes are available from *Quarterly Index, Veterinary Bulletin, Poultry Abstracts, Veterinary Update,* and *Small Animal Abstracts.* Telephone consultations, radiographic consultations, and computer on-line services are available for assistance with difficult cases. Use every case as a learning experience, and provide your technicians with continuing education. Referral of cases beyond the scope of the practice can also provide learning experiences and feedback. Always follow up on referrals. Another form of inexpensive continuing education is necropsies. Necropsy all birds that die in your clinic and client birds that die, and offer to necropsy birds that die in local pet stores and aviaries.

References and Additional Readings

Abou-Madi N, Kollias GV. Avian fluid therapy. In Kirk RW, Bonagura JD (eds): *Current Veterinary Therapy XI, Small Animal Practice.* Philadelphia, WB Saunders, 1992, pp 1154–1159.

Altman RB, Rowan E. Emergencies of avian species. In Morgan RV (ed): *Manual of Small Animal Emergencies.* Philadelphia, WB Saunders, 1985, pp 453–505.

Altman RB. Establishing an avian practice. *Proc Assoc Avian Vet* 1990;390–393.

Bauck L. Nutritional problems in pet birds. *J Avian Exot Pet Med* 1995;4(1):3–8.

Bond MW, Downs D, Wolfe S. Intravenous catheter therapy. *Proc Assoc Avian Vet* 1993;8–14.

Brown R. Client communications: Supportive care for the grieving client. *Proc Assoc Avian Vet* 1990;524–527.

Brue RN. Nutrition. In Ritchie BW, Harrison GJ, Harrison LR (eds): *Avian Medicine: Principles and Application.* Lake Worth, FL, Wingers Publishing, 1994, pp 63–95.

Castro L. Basic hospital equipment and supplies. *Proc Assoc Avian Vet* 1992;455–458.

Carpenter J, Hoefer H, Janeczek F, et al. Roundtable discussion on referral protocols and the basic exam. *J Assoc Avian Vet* 1994;4(1):35–40.

Clipsham R. Introduction to avicultural medicine. *Proc Assoc Avian Vet* 1989;223–238.

Clipsham R. Environmental preventive medicine: Food and water management for reinfection control. *Proc Assoc Avian Vet* 1990;87–105.

Clipsham R. Preventive medical management of aviary diseases. *Proc Parrot Mgmt Sem Avian Res Fund* 1991;23–56.

Clipsham RC. Restraint, sample collection and surgical preparation in the avian patient. *Proc Assoc Avian Vet* 1991;331–340.

Degernes LA, Davidson GF, Barnes HJ, et al. A preliminary report on intraosseous total parenteral nutrition in birds. *Proc Assoc Avian Vet* 1995;25–26.

Flammer K. Aviculture management. In Harrison GJ, Harrison LR (eds): *Clinical Avian Medicine and Surgery.* Philadelphia, WB Saunders, 1986, pp 601–612.

Forshaw JM, Cooper WT. *Parrots of the World.* Neptune, NJ, T.F.H. Publications, 1989.

Freedman AR. Marketing the veterinarian. *J Assoc Avian Vet* 1992;6(2):76.

Fudge AM. Avian practice tips. In Rosskopf WJ, Woerpel RW (eds): *The Veterinary Clinics of North America, Small Animal Practice* 1991;21(6):1121–1134.

Gallerstein GA, Acker H. Mixed avian/small animal practice management: Some of the critical components. *Proc Assoc Avian Vet* 1991;66–77.

Gould J. Fundamentals of avian practice. *Proc Am Animal Hosp Assoc* 1992;289–293.

Harris DJ. Avian restraint and physical exam. *Proceedings of the North American Veterinary Conference* 1995;561.

Harris DJ. Care of the critically ill patient. *Sem Avian Exot Pet Med* 1994;3(4):175–179.

Harris JM. Teflon dermal stent for the correction of subcutaneous emphysema. *Proc Assoc Avian Vet* 1991;20–21.

Harrison GJ, Harrison LR. Management procedures. In Harrison GJ, Harrison LR (eds): *Clinical Avian Medicine and Surgery.* Philadelphia, WB Saunders, 1986, pp 85–100.

Harrison GJ, Harrison LR, Fudge AM. Preliminary evaluation of a case. In Harrison GJ, Harrison LR (eds): *Clinical Avian Medicine and Surgery.* Philadelphia, WB Saunders, 1986, pp 101–114.

Harrison GJ, Ritchie BW. Making distinctions in the physical examination. In Ritchie BW, Harrison GJ, Harrison LR (eds): *Avian Medicine: Principles and Application.* Lake Worth, FL, Wingers Publishing, 1994, pp 144–175.

Hernandez M, Aguilar R. Steroids and fluid therapy for treatment of shock in the critical avian patient. *Sem Avian Exot Pet Med* 1994;3(4):190–199.

Huff DG. Avian fluid therapy and nutritional therapeutics. *Sem Avian Exot Pet Med* 1993;2(1):13–16.

Jenkins J. Promoting practice loyalty through an enhanced owner/bird bond. *J Assoc Avian Vet* 1992;6(2):79–80.

Johnson-Delaney C. Practice dynamics. In Ritchie BW, Harrison GJ, Harrison LR (eds): *Avian Medicine: Principles and Application.* Lake Worth, FL, Wingers Publishing, 1994, pp 132–143.

Johnson-Delaney CA. Adding birds to the small animal practice or emergency clinic. *Proc Assoc Avian Vet* 1995;319–326.

King AS, McLelland J. *Birds: Their Structure and Function,* ed 2. London, Baillier Tindall, 1984.

LaBonde J. Obesity in pet birds: The medical problems and management of the avian patient. *Proc Assoc Avian Vet* 1992;72–77.

Lightfoot TL. Avian practice tips. *Proc Assoc Avian Vet* 1992;94–97.

Loudis BG, Sutherland-Smith M. Methods used in the critical care of avian patients. *Sem Avian Exot Pet Med* 1994;3(4):180–189.

Lupu C. Clinical nutrition for psittacine birds. *Basic Avian Medicine Symposium. Proc Assoc Avian Vet* 1991;M1-1–M1-4.

Lyon K. Sources of information. In Rosskopf WJ, Woerpel RW (eds): *The Veterinary Clinics of North America, Small Animal Practice* 1991;21(6):1111–1120.

Macwhirter P. Malnutrition. In Ritchie BW, Harrison GJ, Harrison LR (eds): *Avian Medicine: Principles and Application.* Lake Worth, FL, Wingers Publishing, 1994, pp 842–861.

Marshall R. The management of diseases in the pet shop. *Proc Assoc Avian Vet* 1991;205–223.

McCluggage DM. Avian emergency medicine. *Proc Am Animal Hosp Assoc* 1995;319–324.

McDonald SE. Practice tips. *Proc Assoc Avian Vet* 1990;316–318.

McFadden CB. Anecdotal report: Caloric density requirements in neonatal blue and gold macaws. *Proc Assoc Avian Vet* 1993;240–243.

Murray MJ. Management of the avian trauma case. *Sem Avian Exot Pet Med* 1994;3(4):200–209.

Murray MJ. Physical examination and sample collection. *Proc N Am Vet Conf* 1994;794–795.

Nott HMR, Taylor EJ. The energy requirements of pet birds. *Proc Assoc Avian Vet* 1993;233–239.

Oglesbee BL. Avian techniques. In Birchard SJ, Sherding RG (eds): *Saunders Manual of Small Animal Practice*. Philadelphia, WB Saunders, 1994, pp 1249–1256.

Orosz SE. Applied avian anatomy and physiology. *Proc N Am Vet Conf* 1994;800–801.

Orosz SE. Supportive care of the hospitalized patient. *Proc Assoc Avian Vet* 1992;459–462.

Quesenberry K. Avian nutritional support. In Kirk RW, Bonagura JD (eds): *Current Veterinary Therapy XI, Small Animal Practice*. Philadelphia, WB Saunders, 1992, pp 1160–1163.

Quesenberry KE. Basic management and diagnostic techniques in caged bird medicine. *Waltham Focus* 1994;4(1):17–24.

Quesenberry KE, Hillyer E. Hospital management of the critical avian patient. *Proc Assoc Avian Vet* 1989;365–369.

Quesenberry KE, Mauldin G, Hillyer E. Nutritional support of the avian patient. *Proc Assoc Avian Vet* 1989;11–19.

Reavill DR. Psittacine pediatric emergency medicine. *Sem Avian Exot Pet Med* 1994;3(4):169–174.

Rich GA. Basic history taking and the avian physical examination. *Vet Clin North Am, Small Anim Pract* 1991;21(6):1135–1145.

Rich GA. Technicians' laboratory: The basics—restraint, sampling, tubing. *Proc Assoc Avian Vet* 1991;362–366.

Ritchie BW. Emergency care of avian patients. *Proc N Am Vet Conf* 1994;806–807.

Rosskopf WJ, Shindo MK. The laboratory workup: Tips on convincing the client of its necessity and value. *Proc Assoc Avian Vet* 1992;468–470.

Rosskopf WJ, Woerpel RW. Pet avian practice tips. *Proc Assoc Avian Vet* 1991;57–65.

Rosskopf WJ, Woerpel RW, Albright M, et al. Pet avian emergency care. *Proc Assoc Avian Vet* 1991;341–356.

Rosskopf WJ, Woerpel RW, Fudge AM, et al. Iron storage disease (hemochromatosis) in a citron-crested cockatoo and other psittacine species. *Proc Assoc Avian Vet* 1992;98–107.

Roudybush T. Psittacine nutrition. *Proc Parrot Mgmt Sem Avian Res Fund* 1991;95–103.

Smith J. Proper use of disinfectants. *J Assoc Avian Vet* 1990;4(4):212–213.

Spink RR. Aerosol therapy. In Harrison GJ, Harrison LR (eds): *Clinical Avian Medicine and Surgery*. Philadelphia, WB Saunders, 1986, pp 376–379.

Ullrey DE. Dietary husbandry of psittacines. *Proc Assoc Avian Vet* 1991;224–226.

Underwood MS, Polin D, O'Handley P, et al. Short term energy and protein utilization by budgerigars (*Melopsittacus undulatus*) fed isocaloric diets of varying protein concentrations. *Proc Assoc Avian Vet* 1991;227–237.

Williams DL. Start at square one: Avian history taking and clinical examination. *Proc N Am Vet Conf* 1993;717–718.

Wilson L. Care and handling of clients from phone calls to office calls. *Proc Assoc Avian Vet* 1989;449–453.

Chapter 2

General Signs

Birds are often first seen with general signs of illness. Usually, more specific signs accompany these general signs. Diagnostic plans are provided for three general signs in this chapter: anorexia, wasting, and swollen abdomen. When more specific signs are present, consult appropriate chapters to assist in making a diagnosis.

Each sign presented in this chapter begins with an introduction followed by a list of differential diagnoses. This list is followed by appropriate signalment information. Common causes of the clinical sign are presented for groups of pet birds. The history section is useful to explore important historical information. The physical examination section guides interpretation of the physical findings seen with the clinical sign of that section. An algorithm is included to provide quick reference for recommended tests. The diagnostic plan suggests useful tests. Consult Chapter 12 for techniques of sample collection and assistance with test interpretation. General treatments are discussed at the end of each sign. Once a diagnosis is made, refer to Chapter 9 for specific treatments. Consult the formulary in Chapter 17 for drug dosages.

ANOREXIA

Anorexia is a nonspecific clinical sign. It may be a normal behavior (e.g., immediately before egg laying) or the result of illness.

Anorexia in birds may be caused by psychologic or physiologic abnormalities. Stress or fear may cause a bird to quit eating for a day or two. No other signs will be present along with the anorexia if stress is the cause.

Physiologic abnormalities resulting in anorexia usually are seen with other concurrent abnormal clinical signs. Abnormalities affecting the gastrointestinal tract, liver, kidneys, reproductive tract, or systemic disease may cause anorexia. Multiple etiologies occur.

Differential Diagnoses for Anorexia

1. Infectious
   a. Bacterial: °gram-negative (*Borrelia, Campylobacter, Citrobacter, Esche-*

°Common causes.

richia coli, *Klebsiella, Salmonella, Yersinia*), gram-positive (*Enterococcus, Erysipelothrix,* megabacteria, *Mycobacterium, Staphylococcus aureus, Streptococcus*)
   b. Chlamydial: °*Chlamydia psittaci*
   c. Viral: adenovirus, avian influenza, duck viral enteritis, eastern and western equine encephalomyelitis, inclusion body hepatitis of pigeons, °Pacheco's disease, papillomavirus, paramyxovirus-1 (including Newcastle disease), polyomavirus, poxvirus, psittacine beak and feather disease, reovirus
   d. Fungal: *Aspergillus,* °*Candida*
   e. Parasitic: ascarids, *Atoxoplasma, Capillaria, Cryptosporidium, Eimeria,* flukes, *Giardia, Hemoproteus, Isospora, Leucocytozoon, Plasmodium, Sarcocystis,* tapeworms, *Trichomonas*
   f. Unclassified (probably viral): proventricular dilatation syndrome (PDS, neuropathic gastric dilatation, macaw wasting disease)
2. Metabolic: °hepatitis (bacterial, mycobacterial, Pacheco's disease, adenovirus, chlamydiosis, aspergillosis, flukes), °hepatic lipidosis, hepatic fibrosis, pancreatitis, renal disease
3. Nutritional: diet change
4. Toxic: aflatoxin, avocado, carbamate, cholecalciferol, ethylene glycol, °lead, mycotoxin, nitrate, organophosphate, °zinc
5. Physical: °oral abscess, fractured mandible, mouth trauma, paralysis of head muscles, food inaccessible, blindness, foreign body in mouth, °peritonitis, °egg binding
6. Trauma
7. Allergic: food
8. Behavioral: stress, environmental change, competition, brooding, imminent egg laying
9. Neoplastic: hepatic, renal, other

Signalment

Common causes of anorexia in large psittacines include chlamydiosis, gram-negative bacterial infections, lead or zinc toxicosis, and liver disease. Cockatiels and budgies are often anorectic as a result of gram-negative bacterial infections, egg binding, egg-related peritonitis, chlamydiosis, and candidiasis. Neoplasia is also common in older budgies. Common causes of anorexia in finches and canaries include bacterial infections, tapeworms, megabacteria, and egg binding or peritonitis. Mynahs are commonly anorectic as a result of liver disease (hemochromatosis, cirrhosis, neoplasia), heart failure, and gram-negative bacterial infections.

Common causes of anorexia in young birds include candidiasis, gram-negative bacterial infections, chlamydiosis, too low of an environmental temperature, polyomavirus, nutritional diseases, crop burns, and fractures; however, many young birds continue to maintain good appetites with crop burns, fractures, and nutritional diseases.

°Common causes.

History

Isolated birds and those in closed collections are commonly ill because of toxicoses, neoplasia, reproductive disorders, and management-related illnesses. Chronic bacterial and fungal diseases (chlamydiosis, mycobacteriosis, aspergillosis), gram-negative bacterial infections, and those diseases with carrier states (e.g., Pacheco's disease) are also seen.

Birds recently exposed to other birds are commonly ill as a result of infectious diseases, including bacterial, chlamydial, viral, and parasitic diseases. This is the result of stress and exposure to infectious disease. Chlamydiosis, mycobacteriosis, Pacheco's disease, paramyxovirus, polyomavirus, poxvirus, reovirus, and many parasitic diseases are commonly associated with group contact. Illnesses common in isolated birds may also be seen.

Significant dietary history for an anorectic bird includes type of diet, freshness of diet, and any change in type of food or treats. Candidiasis and crop burns are common in chicks being fed by hand. Mycotoxins may be present in moldy food and may be present even after signs of the mold have disappeared. Ingestion of a toxic dose of mycotoxin can result in death in a few days. Chronic exposure can cause liver disease and liver failure. High-fat diets (e.g., seed diets) and unbalanced diets (deficient in biotin, choline, or methionine) may lead to hepatic lipidosis.

Important environmental factors in an anorectic bird include changes in the environment, access to potential toxins, flight capabilities, sanitation, and exposure to wild birds or disease vectors. A new home or cagemate may cause anorexia in some birds, no other signs of illness will be present, and the bird should begin eating within 1 or 2 days. Birds allowed out of their cages are more susceptible to trauma. Free-flight episodes are conducive to collisions with windows, walls, and ceiling fans, resulting in trauma.

A history of exposure or access to a potential toxin is significant in an anorectic bird. Toxins that may cause anorexia are listed in the Differential Diagnoses for Anorexia (this chapter). Possible sources of lead are listed in Table 9–3. Some sources of zinc include pennies minted since 1982, staples, fertilizers, some paints, Monopoly game pieces, hardware cloth, and galvanized wire, mesh, containers, dishes, bolts, washers, and nails. Nitrates are found in fertilizers, and the pellets may be mistaken for food by birds.

Parasitic infections are most common in recently imported birds, birds that have access to the ground, and birds exposed to wild birds, wild bird droppings, rodents, and other parasite vectors.

Egg laying or nesting behavior before the episode of anorexia can be consistent with egg yolk peritonitis.

Infectious and toxic etiologies are suspected when multiple birds are affected.

The duration of the illness is important. Note the owner's description of the clinical signs and the course of the disease. Note previous illnesses, including signs, treatment, and response to treatment.

Physical Examination

A complete physical examination is important to identify abnormalities and to determine which systems are involved. Observation of oral lesions, crop abnormalities, trauma, abdominal swelling, respiratory signs, neurologic signs, or abnormal droppings will help to narrow differential diagnoses.

Algorithm for Anorexia or Decreased Appetite

See Figures 2–1 and 2–2.

Diagnostic Plan for Anorexia or Decreased Appetite

Stabilize severely ill birds before performing stressful diagnostic tests. Provide supportive care as needed (see Chapter 1).

If no other clinical signs are present and the diet and environment have not been altered, perform diagnostic tests to determine the etiology.

Selection of appropriate diagnostic tests is based on consideration of the signalment and history of the bird, findings of the physical examination, and evaluation of the droppings.

The most useful initial diagnostic tests are Gram's stains of the choana and cloaca. Collect and submit samples for culture and sensitivity testing also; many infections can be missed using Gram's stains alone. Abnormal Gram's stains will indicate a need for institution of therapy before culture results can be obtained. A crop wash and examination of the contents with a direct smear may reveal trichomoniasis or candidiasis. Fecal flotation, sedimentation, and direct smears are useful for identification of intestinal parasites. Hematology and biochemistry tests are important in the diagnosis of infectious, metabolic, inflammatory, and some toxic diseases. Useful biochemistry tests include aspartate transferase (AST or SGOT), creatinine kinase (CK), uric acid, total protein, and bile acids. Plasma protein electrophoresis (EPH) is useful in identifying many disease states (e.g., chlamydiosis, aspergillosis, mycobacteriosis, peritonitis, liver disease, and renal disease). Radiology is useful for the diagnosis of lead and zinc toxicoses and trauma, for providing information on liver size and proventriculus size, and for allowing evaluation of the respiratory tract and other abdominal structures. Lead or zinc toxicosis may be present without radiographic evidence of heavy metal densities in the gastrointestinal tract. Titers, cultures, special stains, virus tests, cholinesterase assays, and lead and zinc blood levels are used to rule in or out specific diseases.

Treatment of Anorexia or Decreased Appetite

Treat the underlying cause. Tube feeding and other supportive care are important while treating the underlying cause (see Chapter 1). Tube feeding is continued until the bird is eating on its own. If dehydration is present, administer intravenous, intraosseous, or subcutaneous fluids.

WASTING

Wasting is the state of emaciation that has occurred over a period of time. This is a chronic condition. Illnesses that cause an acute loss of weight are not

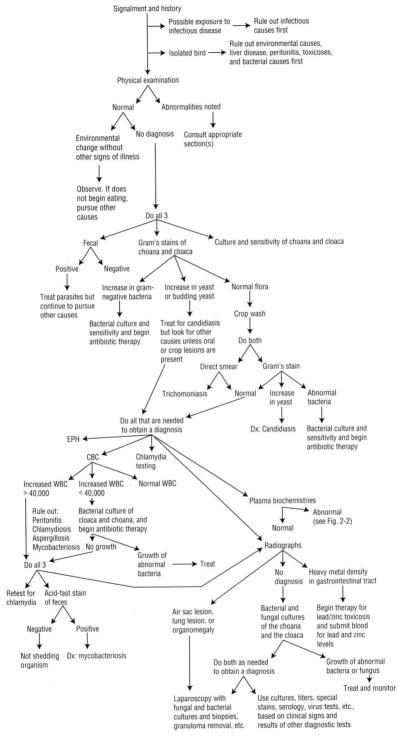

Figure 2–1. Algorithm for anorexia or decreased appetite.

considered in this section (see appropriate chapters). Wasting is indicated by a loss of breast muscle and protrusion of the keel (Fig. 2–3).

Differential Diagnoses for Wasting

1. Infectious
   a. Bacterial: gram-negative bacteria, gram-positive bacteria (megabacteria, *Mycobacterium*, others)
   b. Chlamydial: *Chlamydia psittaci*
   c. Fungal: *Aspergillus, Candida*
   d. Parasitic: *Amidostomum,* ascarids, *Capillaria,* cestodes, *Cryptosporidium, Cochlosoma,* *coccidia (*Eimeria, Isospora*),* Giardia, Hexamita, Histomo-nas,* spirurids, *Trichomonas*
   e. Unclassified: proventricular dilatation syndrome (PDS, neuropathic gastric dilatation, macaw wasting disease)
2. Metabolic: *chronic peritonitis, hemochromatosis
3. Nutritional: *starvation
4. Toxic: lead, zinc
5. Physical: *beak abnormality, *oral lesion
6. Neoplastic: papilloma, other

Signalment

Common causes of wasting in large psittacines include PDS, chlamydiosis, aspergillosis, and beak abnormalities. Common causes in small psittacines include candidiasis, chronic peritonitis, starvation, and giardiasis. Canaries and finches often show wasting as a result of megabacteria, endoventricular candidiasis, chronic peritonitis, starvation, mycobacteriosis, or *Cochlosoma* infection. Common causes of wasting in mynahs include mycobacteriosis, hemochromatosis, and aspergillosis. Common causes in toucans include hemochromatosis and diabetes mellitus. Wasting in raptors is commonly the result of aspergillosis, starvation, lead toxicosis, trichomoniasis, or other gastrointestinal parasites.

Wasting in young birds is commonly the result of candidiasis, PDS, chlamyd-iosis, or starvation.

History

Isolated birds and those in closed collections are commonly ill because of fungal infections, metabolic problems, nutritional problems, beak or oral lesions, or neoplasia. Bacterial infections are also common. Chronic illnesses occasionally occur in this group (e.g., chlamydiosis, mycobacteriosis, or PDS).

Birds recently exposed to other birds are commonly ill as a result of infectious diseases, including bacterial, chlamydial, and parasitic diseases. Proventricular

---

*Common causes.

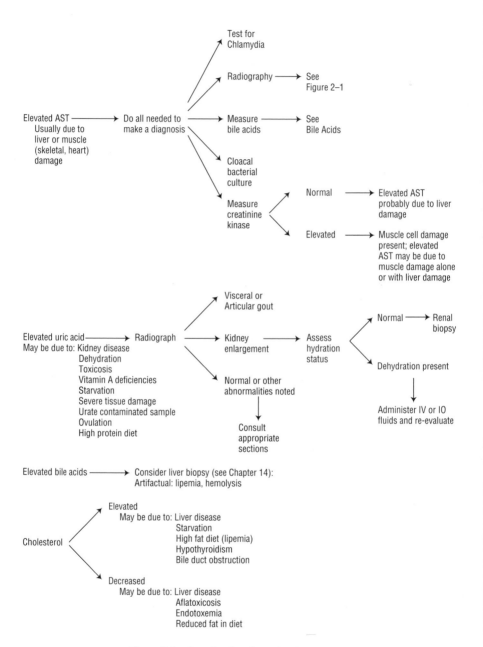

Figure 2–2. Algorithm for plasma biochemistries.

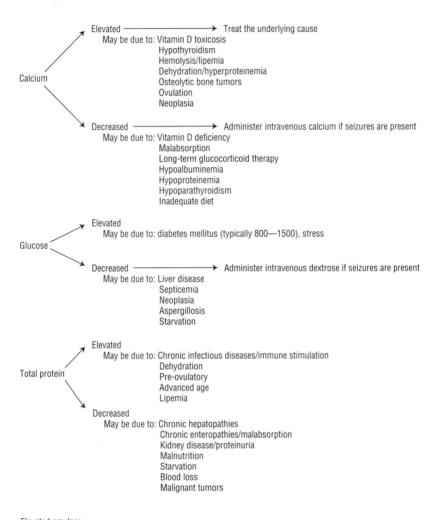

Calcium
  Elevated ─────────────────→ Treat the underlying cause
    May be due to: Vitamin D toxicosis
                   Hypothyroidism
                   Hemolysis/lipemia
                   Dehydration/hyperproteinemia
                   Osteolytic bone tumors
                   Ovulation
                   Neoplasia

  Decreased ─────────────────→ Administer intravenous calcium if seizures are present
    May be due to: Vitamin D deficiency
                   Malabsorption
                   Long-term glucocorticoid therapy
                   Hypoalbuminemia
                   Hypoproteinemia
                   Hypoparathyroidism
                   Inadequate diet

Glucose
  Elevated
    May be due to: diabetes mellitus (typically 800—1500), stress

  Decreased ─────────────────→ Administer intravenous dextrose if seizures are present
    May be due to: Liver disease
                   Septicemia
                   Neoplasia
                   Aspergillosis
                   Starvation

Total protein
  Elevated
    May be due to: Chronic infectious diseases/immune stimulation
                   Dehydration
                   Pre-ovulatory
                   Advanced age
                   Lipemia

  Decreased
    May be due to: Chronic hepatopathies
                   Chronic enteropathies/malabsorption
                   Kidney disease/proteinuria
                   Malnutrition
                   Starvation
                   Blood loss
                   Malignant tumors

Elevated amylase
  May indicate pancreatitis or enteritis

Elevated lipase
  May indicate pancreatitis

Figure 2–2 *Continued*

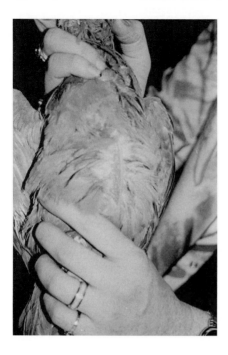

Figure 2–3. Wasting is indicated by loss of breast muscle and protrusion of the keel, as shown in this Amazon parrot.

dilatation syndrome is suspected to be infectious also and is a common cause of wasting. Illnesses occurring in isolated birds also occur in group situations.

Infectious and toxic etiologies are suspected when multiple birds are affected.

A history of previous egg laying activity and clinical signs associated with peritonitis is consistent with egg-related peritonitis. A history of prolonged antibiotic therapy can be consistent with a fungal infection.

Important environmental factors in birds with wasting include exposure to infectious diseases, a change of environment, exposure to lead or zinc, management practices, and sanitation. A change of environment can be stressful, leading to an increased susceptibility to bacterial and fungal diseases. Poor management practices and sanitation, in addition to exposure to infectious diseases, increases spread of disease (e.g., PDS, chlamydiosis, mycobacteriosis, megabacteria, and parasites). Sources of lead are listed in Table 9–3. Excessive or even normal iron content in mynah and toucan diets may be a factor in the development of hemochromatosis in mynahs and toucans.

The duration of the illness is important. Note the owner's description of the clinical signs and the course of the disease. Note previous illnesses, including signs, treatment, and response to treatment.

Physical Examination

Debilitated birds must be handled with care. The physical examination should be performed quickly and with the least amount of stress possible.

A complete physical examination is important to identify the extent of the problem and to determine which systems are involved. Observe for concurrent clinical signs, including gastrointestinal, respiratory, or neurologic signs. Common findings of birds with wasting are discussed below.

Check the cage for the presence of food. Some new owners may mistake seed hulls for intact seeds and not offer fresh food. Inspect the droppings for number of droppings, pigmented urates, abnormal size or consistency of feces, and unusual odor. Large, soft, foul-smelling droppings are often associated with maldigestion. Birds that are not eating produce few or no droppings. Consult Chapter 4 for further discussion of abnormal droppings.

Inspect the oral cavity and beak for lesions and palpate the crop. Misshapen beaks can cause difficulty in grasping food or cracking seed and lead to starvation. Fungal infections of the ventriculus often have associated oral and ingluvial (crop) lesions. Examine the skin over the abdomen. A bulging of the abdomen may be associated with ascites, peritonitis, or an abdominal mass (e.g., tumor, organomegaly). In canaries and finches, hepatomegaly can often be visualized as a black mass just caudal to the keel.

Palpate the abdomen; an enlarged liver and other organs may be palpable.

Neurologic signs may accompany wasting with PDS, chlamydiosis, lead or zinc toxicosis, and occasionally peritonitis. Feather picking may be noted in conjunction with giardiasis, especially in cockatiels.

Respiratory signs may accompany wasting with chlamydiosis, peritonitis, aspergillosis, hepatopathies, and some oral lesions.

Algorithm for Wasting

See Figure 2–4.

Diagnostic Plan for Wasting

Stabilize severely ill birds before performing stressful diagnostic tests. Provide supportive care as needed (see Chapter 1).

Consider the signalment and history. Dietary causes of wasting must be sought from the history. Exposure to infectious diseases and management-related problems may be exposed with a complete history. Candidiasis and liver disease are suspected based on physical examination findings and evaluation of the droppings.

Initial diagnostic tests include a Gram's stain of the cloaca, a fecal flotation, and wet mount. Bacterial gastroenteritis, megabacteria, or candidiasis may be diagnosed with the Gram's stain. Megabacteria and *Candida* organisms may be absent in the feces and still be causing proventriculitis or ventriculitis. A proventricular washing may better demonstrate megabacteria. A wet mount preparation may reveal the motile *Giardia* trophozoite in fresh feces or *Trichomonas* in a crop wash sample. If the trophozoite cannot be demonstrated in suspected giardiasis cases, a trichrome stain of pooled feces may reveal cysts. This organism may be shed in low numbers and is difficult to demonstrate.

If peritonitis is suspected based on physical examination findings, an abdominal tap is performed and the sample evaluated.

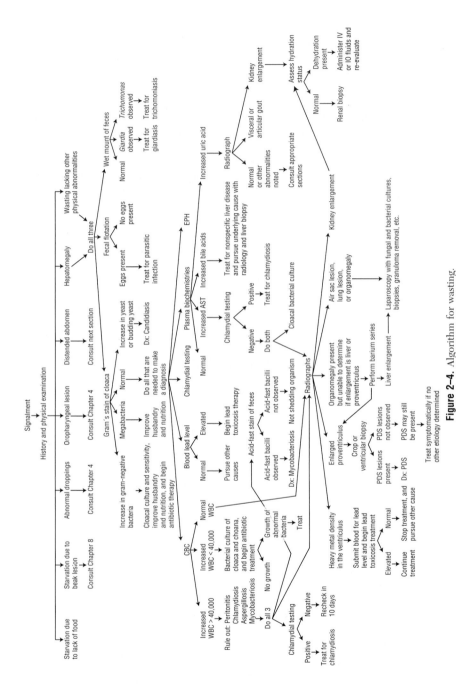

Figure 2–4. Algorithm for wasting.

If the problem is not obvious, radiology is the next step. Radiology is useful to observe heavy metal densities in the ventriculus; to evaluate proventricular, hepatic, and renal size; and to evaluate the gastrointestinal tract. A barium series may be needed to determine the location and size of some organs.

A complete blood count (CBC), biochemistry tests, and cloacal culture and sensitivity are the next step. A CBC is useful in supporting a diagnosis of infectious or inflammatory disease. Biochemistry tests are important to assess liver and kidney function. Important biochemistry tests include AST, CK, uric acid, albumin, bile acids, and total protein. Chlamydial testing is appropriate if exposure is possible or other clinical signs of infection are present. If the white blood cell (WBC) count is in excess of 40,000 WBC/μl, chlamydiosis, aspergillosis, mycobacteriosis, or peritonitis is suspected and tested for. Submit chlamydial and aspergillosis titers and a fecal acid-fast stain for mycobacteriosis, and perform an abdominal tap to check for peritonitis (if indicated).

An EPH is useful to detect and identify some disease states (e.g., chlamydiosis, aspergillosis, mycobacteriosis, peritonitis, liver disease, or renal disease).

If PDS is suspected based on radiology (i.e., distended proventriculus), a crop or ventricular biopsy may be performed for a definitive diagnosis. A negative biopsy result does not rule out PDS.

Submit a blood sample for lead and zinc levels.

If the diagnosis is still uncertain, perform endoscopy (proventricular, abdominal). During abdominal endoscopy, visualize the lungs, liver, air sacs, kidney, adrenal glands, gonads, and intestines. Biopsy abnormal tissues and submit samples for histopathology.

Group or flock situations benefit from complete necropsy examinations.

Treatment of Wasting

Treat the underlying cause. Tube feed the bird if the bird is not eating on its own. Provide other supportive care as needed. If dehydration is present, administer intravenous, intraosseous, or subcutaneous fluids.

DISTENDED ABDOMEN

The normal abdomen of birds is flat or slightly concave. Convex bulging of the abdominal wall is abnormal and indicates a space-occupying lesion (mass, fluid, or a combination).

Ascites and organomegaly are common causes of a distended abdomen in birds. Common causes of ascites in birds include liver disease, heart disease, and egg-related peritonitis. Organomegaly may involve any of the organs of the body cavity. The liver is often involved. The liver may be enlarged as a result of hepatitis, lipidosis, hemochromatosis, toxicosis, trauma, subcapsular hemorrhage, tumor, or portal hypertension caused by heart failure. Causes of hepatitis include bacterial, viral, chlamydial, fungal, and parasitic infections. Causes of viral hepatitis include adenovirus, avian viral serositis, coronavirus, duck viral hepatitis, Pacheco's disease, polyomavirus, and reovirus. Infectious hepatitis commonly results in other clinical signs in addition to abdominal swelling; therefore, specific bacterial and viral causes of hepatitis will not be discussed in this section.

Differential Diagnoses for Distended Abdomen

1. Infectious
   a. Bacterial: gram-negative, gram-positive (including *Mycobacterium,* others)
   b. Chlamydial: *Chlamydia psittaci*
   c. Viral: avian leukosis, avian viral serositis form of eastern equine encephalitis virus, Marek's disease, polyomavirus
   d. Fungal: *Aspergillus, Candida*
   e. Parasitic: *Atoxoplasma, Leucocytozoon, Microsporidium, Cryptosporidium*
   f. Other (probably viral): PDS (proventricular dilatation syndrome, macaw wasting disease, neuropathic gastric dilatation)
2. Metabolic: °hepatitis (bacterial, mycobacterial, chlamydial, viral, fungal, parasitic), °hepatic lipidosis, °hepatic fibrosis, pancreatitis, renal disease, °heart failure, amyloidosis, hypoproteinemia, hypoalbuminemia, gastrointestinal obstruction, ovarian cyst, °obesity, hemochromatosis
3. Toxic: mycotoxins
4. Physical: °impending normal egg laying, peritonitis (°egg related, bacterial), °egg binding, abdominal hernia, fecalith
5. Trauma: hemoperitoneum, hepatic hematoma
6. Neoplastic: hepatic, °renal, other

Signalment

Common causes of abdominal swelling in large psittacines include egg laying, hepatic lipidosis, and hepatitis. Macaws are often affected by egg-related peritonitis but produce little fluid. Cockatiels and budgies often have abdominal swelling as a result of egg binding, egg laying, egg-related peritonitis, hepatic lipidosis, or abdominal hernias. Renal and gonadal neoplasia are also common in older budgies. Common causes of abdominal swelling in finches and canaries include egg binding, egg-related peritonitis, *Atoxoplasma,* and leukosis. Common causes of distended abdomen in mynahs and toucans include liver disease (hemochromatosis, cirrhosis, neoplasia), heart failure, and mycobacteriosis.

Common causes of distended abdomen in young birds include hepatic lipidosis, gastrointestinal obstruction, and in budgies, polyomavirus.

History

Isolated birds and those in closed collections are commonly ill because of reproductive, metabolic, toxic, physical, and neoplastic disorders and trauma. Chronic bacterial and fungal diseases (chlamydiosis, mycobacteriosis, aspergillo-

---

°Common causes.

sis), gram-negative bacterial infections, and those diseases with carrier states (e.g., Pacheco's disease) are also seen.

Birds recently exposed to other birds are commonly ill as a result of infectious diseases, including bacterial, viral, and parasitic diseases. This is the result of stress and exposure to infectious disease. Chlamydiosis, mycobacteriosis, Pacheco's disease, polyomavirus, reovirus, and many parasitic diseases are commonly associated with group contact. Illnesses common in isolated birds may also be seen.

Significant dietary history for birds with a swollen abdomen includes type of diet and freshness. Mycotoxins may be present in moldy food and may be present even after signs of the mold have disappeared. Ingestion of a toxic dose of mycotoxin can result in death in a few days. Chronic exposure can cause liver disease and failure. High-fat diets (e.g., seed diets) and unbalanced diets (deficient in biotin, choline, or methionine) may lead to hepatic lipidosis. Excessive or even normal iron content in the diet may be a factor in the development of hemochromatosis in mynahs and toucans.

Important environmental factors in birds with abdominal swelling include flight capabilities, sanitation, and exposure to wild birds or disease vectors. Hand-raised chicks may ingest substrate. Inappropriate substrate materials may cause a gastrointestinal obstruction, especially corncob and wood shavings. Birds allowed out of their cages are more susceptible to trauma. Free-flight episodes are conducive to collisions with windows, walls, and ceiling fans, resulting in trauma. Parasitic infections are most common in recently imported birds, birds that have access to the ground, and birds exposed to wild birds or their droppings. Also, rodents and other vectors may spread parasitic infections.

Egg laying or nesting behavior before abdominal distention can be consistent with impending egg laying, egg binding, or egg-related peritonitis.

The duration of the illness is important. Note the owner's description of the clinical signs and the course of the disease. Note previous illnesses, including signs, treatment, and response to treatment.

Physical Examination

A complete physical examination is important to identify the extent of the problem and to determine which organs are involved. Observation of dyspnea, organomegaly, trauma, or abnormal droppings may help to narrow differential diagnoses. If abnormalities are present, consult the appropriate section to assist in making a diagnosis. Common findings in birds with swollen abdomens are discussed below.

Examine the cage and droppings. Abnormal colored urates can occur in conjunction with a distended abdomen with hepatitis (bacterial, chlamydial, viral, parasitic, fungal, and toxic) and hepatic lipidosis. Diarrhea may occur with abdominal distention with chlamydiosis, hepatitis, hepatic lipidosis, renal disease, pancreatitis, gastrointestinal obstruction, abdominal hernia, impending egg laying, egg binding, and egg-related peritonitis. Consult Chapter 4 for further discussion of abnormal droppings.

Observe the bird in the cage. Note the attitude, respiratory rate, respiratory effort, and stance. Observe for sitting low on the perch, dyspnea, open-mouth breathing, tail bobbing, and perching or grasping with only one foot.

Examine the bird. Debilitated birds must be handled with care. The physical examination should be performed quickly and with the least amount of stress possible. Assess hydration status. Auscultate the heart and lungs. Murmurs may be noted. A decrease of air sounds on auscultation may indicate ascites. Evaluate musculature over the keel, and observe for fatty deposits. Palpate the crop for abnormalities. Gently palpate the abdomen for abdominal masses, organomegaly, or ascites. Exercise caution when palpating an abdomen that may contain fluid. Rupture of the peritoneum can result in flooding of the air sacs and lungs with fluid, leading to death. In small birds, the abdominal contents may be viewed through the skin. In canaries and finches, an enlarged liver may be seen as a dark area just caudal to the keel. Wetting the skin with alcohol and parting the feathers will help visualization. In normal chicks, the ventriculus is large and protrudes slightly. Abdominal effusions can often be observed through the abdominal wall when present in chicks. Examine the vent for pasting of feces causing an obstruction, and examine the cloaca for papillomas, fecalith, etc.

Algorithm for Distended Abdomen

See Figure 2–5.

Diagnostic Plan for Distended Abdomen

Stabilize severely ill birds before performing stressful diagnostic tests. Provide supportive care as needed (see Chapter 1).

Selection of appropriate diagnostic tests is based on consideration of the signalment and history of the bird, findings of the physical examination, and evaluation of the droppings.

Differentiation between abdominal distention caused by ascites from organomegaly or an abdominal mass can often be made by physical examination. Radiology or ultrasonography is useful when the distinction is not obvious. A minimum database is important with either cause. A minimum database consists of a CBC, plasma biochemistries, and radiography. A CBC is useful in the diagnosis of inflammatory or infectious causes. If the WBC is in excess of 40,000/μl, rule out peritonitis, chlamydiosis, aspergillosis, and mycobacteriosis. Useful plasma biochemistries in birds with abdominal distention include total protein, albumin, uric acid, AST, CK, lactate dehydrogenase (LDH), and, if liver disease is suspected, bile acids. Radiology will allow determination of organ sizes and location. A barium series may be helpful to determine the location and size of some organs. Ascites may result in a loss of serosal detail and a hazy appearance in the abdomen. Removal of some of the fluid by abdominocentesis will improve radiographic visualization. If the bird is not in critical condition, administration of furosemide for several days will often improve visualization of organ detail.

An EPH is useful to identify many disease states (e.g., chlamydiosis, aspergillosis, mycobacteriosis, peritonitis, liver disease, or renal disease).

Fecal flotation and evaluation of the sediment are useful to evaluate for the

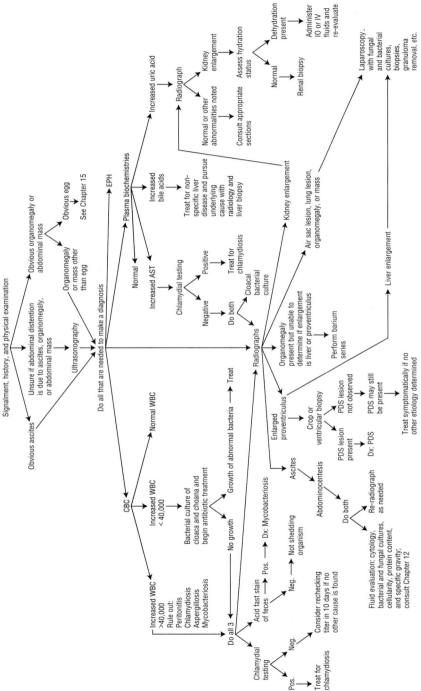

Figure 2–5. Algorithm for distended abdomen.

presence of intestinal parasites. Chlamydial testing is appropriate if exposure is possible or other clinical signs of the disease are present.

If ascites is present, abdominocentesis is performed. Remove only the amount of fluid necessary for evaluation and to relieve life-threatening dyspnea, if present. The fluid is evaluated with cytology, and protein content and cellularity are determined. Submit a sample for culture.

Ascites and peritonitis are common in pet birds. Hemoperitoneum is uncommon. Hemoperitoneum appears as free blood. Ascitic fluid is typically yellow to clear. Abdominal fluid as a result of peritonitis may be opaque, yellow, white, or reddish brown. Ascites can be the result of liver disease, heart failure, or neoplasia. Peritonitis may be the result of bacterial or *Aspergillus* infection or urate contamination or may be egg related. Abdominal infections may be the result of gastrointestinal perforation or secondary from lung, air sac, pericardium, female reproductive tract, or gastrointestinal tract. Hemoperitoneum is usually the result of trauma. Cytologic evaluation is required to determine the cause. Consult Chapter 12 for evaluation of abdominal fluids.

Organ biopsies may be necessary to determine the underlying cause of organomegaly or ascites. Hepatic and renal biopsies may be performed endoscopically. Make the incision into the body cavity for hepatic biopsies close to the caudal border of the sternum to avoid entering the abdominal air sacs in birds with ascites. Flow of ascitic fluid into the air sacs can result in death. Abdominocentesis before surgery will decrease the likelihood of this complication. Ventricular or crop biopsy may provide a diagnosis of PDS and may be indicated when proventricular dilatation is noted radiographically or with ultrasonography.

Treatment of Distended Abdomen

Treat the underlying cause. Tube feeding and other supportive care are important while treating the underlying cause. Tube feeding is continued until the bird is eating on its own. If dehydration is present, administer intravenous, intraosseous, or subcutaneous fluids.

References and Additional Readings

Bond MW, Downs D, Wolf S. Screening for psittacine proventricular dilatation syndrome. *Proc Assoc Avian Vet* 1993;92–97.

Campbell TW. Cytology in avian diagnostics. In Kirk RW (ed): *Current Veterinary Therapy IX, Small Animal Practice*. Philadelphia, WB Saunders, 1986, pp 725–731.

Campbell TW. Cytology of abdominal effusions. *Avian Hematology and Cytology*, ed 2. Ames, Iowa, Iowa State University Press, 1995, pp 43–46.

Cray C, Bossart G, Harris D. Plasma protein electrophoresis: Principles and diagnosis of infectious disease. *Proc Assoc Avian Vet* 1995;55–59.

Degernes LA. A clinical approach to ascites in pet birds. *Proc Assoc Avian Vet* 1991;131–136.

Degernes LA, Flammer K, Fisher P. Proventricular dilatation syndrome in a green-winged macaw. *Proc Assoc Avian Vet* 1991;45–49.

Filippich LJ, Parker MG. Megabacteria and proventricular/ventricular disease in psittacines and passerines. *Proc Assoc Avian Vet* 1994;287–293.

Gaskin JM, Homer BL, Eskelund KH. Preliminary findings in avian viral serositis: A newly recognized syndrome of psittacine birds. *J Assoc Avian Vet* 1991;5(1):27–34.

Graham DL. Endoventricular mycosis: An avian pathologist's perspective. *Proc Assoc Avian Vet* 1994;279–282.

Graham DL. Wasting/proventricular dilation disease: A pathologist's view. *Proc Assoc Avian Vet* 1991;43–44.

Gregory CR, Latimer KS, Niagro FD, et al. A review of proventricular dilatation syndrome. *J Assoc Avian Vet* 1994;8(2):69–75.

King AS, McLelland J. Digestive system. In *Birds: Their Structure and Function*, ed 2. London, Bailliere-Tindall, 1984, pp 84–109.

LaBlonde J. Pet avian toxicology. *Proc Assoc Avian Vet* 1988;159–174.

MacWhirter P. A review of 60 cases of abdominal hernias in birds. *Proc Assoc Avian Vet* 1994;27–37.

Morris PJ, Avgeris SE, Baumgartner RE. Hemochromatosis in a greater Indian hill mynah (*Gracula religiosa*): Case report and review of the literature. *J Assoc Avian Vet* 1989;3(2):87–92.

Murphy J. Psittacine fatty liver syndrome. *Proc Assoc Avian Vet* 1992;78–82.

Oglesbee BL, McDonald S, Warthen K. Avian digestive system disorders. In Birchard SJ, Sherding RG (eds): *Saunders Manual of Small Animal Practice*. Philadelphia, WB Saunders, 1994, pp 1290–1301.

Orosz SE. Fungal and mycobacterial diseases. *Proc N Am Vet Conf* 1995;569–570.

Ritchie BW, Harrison GJ, Harrison LR (eds): *Avian Medicine: Principles and Application*. Lake Worth, FL, Wingers Publishing, 1994.

Rosenthal K, Stefanacci J, Quesenberry K, et al. Ultrasonic findings in 30 cases of avian coelomic disease. *Proc Assoc Avian Vet* 1995;303.

Rosskopf WJ, Woerpel RW, Fudge AM, et al. Iron storage disease (hemochromatosis) in a citron-crested cockatoo and other psittacine species. *Proc Assoc Avian Vet* 1992;98–107.

Suedmeyer WK. Diagnosis and clinical progression of three cases of proventricular dilatation syndrome. *J Assoc Avian Vet* 1992;6(3):159–163.

Van Sant F. Zinc toxicosis in a hyacinth macaw. *Proc Assoc Avian Vet* 1991;255–259.

Worell AB. Further investigations in rhamphastids concerning hemochromatosis. *Proc Assoc Avian Vet* 1993;98–107.

Chapter 3

Respiratory Signs

Respiratory disease is a common cause of illness in pet birds. This chapter presents a diagnostic approach for respiratory signs commonly seen in pet birds. It is divided into five sections, by signs that are grouped according to the diagnostic approach required to diagnose the cause of the illness. Each section begins with general information and definitions of terms, followed by a list of differential diagnoses. This is followed by appropriate signalment information. Common causes of the group of clinical signs are presented for each group of pet birds. Pertinent information as to which species and ages of birds may be affected by the diseases in the differential diagnosis is also given. The history section is useful to explore important historical information that may narrow the differential diagnosis. The physical examination section guides interpretation of the physical findings seen with the clinical signs of that section. An algorithm is included in each section to provide a quick reference for recommended tests. The diagnostic plan suggests useful tests. Consult Chapter 12 as needed for techniques of sample collection and assistance with test interpretation. Treatments are found in Chapter 9. Additional general treatments are discussed at the end of each section. Consult the formulary in Chapter 17 for drug dosages. This chapter concludes with additional readings and references for further information.

Clinical signs of respiratory disease vary with the cause of illness and its location within the respiratory tract. Because signs may be overt or hidden, close observation is needed. Upper and lower respiratory signs are listed in Tables 3–1 and 3–2. Ill birds may exhibit one or more signs. Normal respiratory and heart rates of birds are listed in Table 1–1.

TABLE 3–1 Upper Respiratory Tract Signs

Sneezing	Coughing
Nasal discharge	Abnormal breathing sounds
Head shaking	Abnormally shaped nostril
Scratching beak	Longitudinal groove in beak
Swollen infraorbital sinus	Loss of vocalization
Sunken eye	Voice change

TABLE 3–2 Lower Respiratory Tract Signs

Sneezing	Increased respiratory rate
Nasal discharge	Labored breathing
Coughing	Dyspnea
Abnormal breathing sounds	Tail bobbing
Open-mouth breathing	Cyanosis

SNEEZING, NASAL DISCHARGE, HEAD SHAKING, OR SINUSITIS

All birds sneeze occasionally. However, an increase in the frequency or repeated sneezing warrants investigation. Sneezing is caused by irritation or infection. Sneezing and nasal discharge are signs of nasal or sinus disease or may be caused by lower respiratory or systemic disease. Sinusitis may be localized or accompanied by lower respiratory tract or systemic disease. Head shaking may be associated with sinusitis or nasal, sinus, or choanal foreign bodies or tumors.

Differential Diagnoses for Sneezing, Nasal Discharge, Head Shaking, or Sinusitis

1. Infectious
   a. Bacterial: °gram-negative (*Escherichia coli*, *Haemophilus*, *Klebsiella*, *Pasteurella*, *Pseudomonas*, *Salmonella*, *Yersinia*, other), gram-positive (*Mycobacterium*, *Streptococcus*, *Staphylococcus*, other)
   b. Chlamydial: °*Chlamydia psittaci*
   c. Mycoplasma: °*Mycoplasma*
   d. Fungal: °*Aspergillus*, *Candida*, *Cryptococcus*
   e. Viral: Amazon tracheitis, Pacheco's disease, poxvirus, reovirus, infectious laryngotracheitis, avian influenza
2. Allergic: tobacco, other
3. Neoplastic: papilloma, other
4. Nutritional: †vitamin A deficiency
5. Physical: foreign body, trauma
6. Metabolic: coagulopathy
7. Iatrogenic: prolonged antibiotic treatment
8. Other: conure bleeding syndrome

Signalment

Common causes of sneezing, nasal discharge, head shaking, or sinusitis in larger psittacines include chlamydiosis, gram-negative bacteria, and aspergillosis.

°Common causes.
†Vitamin A deficiency is often a primary or concurrent problem.

Cockatiels and budgies are commonly affected by gram-negative bacteria, chlamydiosis, and *Mycoplasma*. Vitamin A deficiency is often a primary cause or concurrent problem in all psittacines. Common infections in passerines include gram-negative bacteria, *Mycoplasma*, and aspergillosis.

Pacheco's disease affects only psittacines. Conure bleeding syndrome affects only conures. The cutaneous form of poxvirus is rare except in blue-fronted Amazons, lovebirds, passerines, raptors, and pigeons. Reovirus is commonly reported in imported birds and primarily affects African gray parrots, cockatoos, and other Old World psittacines. Avian mycobacteriosis is most commonly associated with the intestinal tract in psittacines but affects the respiratory tract in pigeons, some finches, and some other species. Infectious laryngotracheitis affects gallinaceous species and canaries. Avian influenza may cause respiratory signs in gallinaceous birds and waterfowl.

History

A complete history may reveal trauma; allergic, iatrogenic, or nutritional problems; or exposure to infectious diseases. Birds recently exposed to other birds are commonly ill as a result of infectious diseases, including bacterial, chlamydial, *Mycoplasma*, and viral infections. Some diseases have carrier states. Previously infected birds, especially conures, can be carriers of Pacheco's disease, which can cause illness and death in exposed susceptible birds.

Birds recently acquired from a pet store or aviary may be at a higher risk of having been exposed to contagious pathogens. Many birds in this category are also stressed by prior group contact and a change of environment, predisposing them to disease. Knowledge of common diseases in the breeder facility or pet store may provide insight to the possible cause of disease.

Infectious and toxic etiologies are suspected when multiple birds are affected.

Isolated birds and those in closed collections are commonly ill as a result of vitamin A deficiency, trauma, neoplasia, allergic disease, or chronic infections such as chlamydiosis and aspergillosis. Some bacterial diseases are also common, especially gram-negative infections.

Stress may play a role in precipitating clinical signs. Chronic diseases such as chlamydiosis may go undetected until the bird is stressed. Stressful situations for birds include going to a new home, the addition of a new bird, changing to a new cage, a change in diet, or temperature extremes.

The diet can affect the health of the bird. Diets deficient in vitamin A, such as an all-seed diet, can lead to vitamin A deficiency. Vitamin A deficiency causes squamous metaplasia of mucous membranes, causing sinusitis, obstructing airways, or increasing susceptibility to respiratory tract infections.

Consider the bird's environment. Birds allowed out of their cages are more susceptible to trauma. Contact with tobacco smoke or other allergens can cause an allergic reaction and rhinorrhea.

The duration of the illness is important. Note the owner's description of the clinical signs and the course of the disease. Note previous illnesses, including signs, treatment, and response to treatment. A history of worsening of signs during treatment with antibiotics is common with aspergillosis.

Physical Examination

The physical examination may reveal obvious trauma or vitamin A deficiency. Common findings in birds with sneezing, nasal discharge, head shaking, or sinusitis are discussed below.

Observe the bird in the cage before handling. The normal bird shows little movement while breathing. Open-mouth breathing or rhythmic movement of the tail is abnormal. Note the posture. Rapid breathing after the examination is normal. A healthy bird should completely recover from the stress of examination within 5 minutes of release.

Nasal discharges are characterized as serous, mucopurulent, or hemorrhagic. Serous discharges occur with viral and bacterial infections, allergies, and nutritional deficiencies. Mucopurulent discharges occur with viral, bacterial, and fungal infections; neoplasia; sinus foreign bodies; and lower respiratory tract infections. Hemorrhagic or serosanguinous discharges occur with sinus foreign bodies, neoplasia, trauma, reovirus, conure bleeding syndrome, and coagulopathies.

Nasal discharges may be unilateral or bilateral. Diseases that can result in a unilateral discharge include fungal infections, bacterial infections, and neoplasia. Trauma and sinus foreign bodies also may cause unilateral discharges.

Differential diagnoses for a nonpatent nostril include sinusitis, granuloma, foreign body, or neoplasia.

Swellings around the eye or between the eye and beak may be caused by sinusitis, trauma, or neoplasia. The infraorbital sinus is lateral to the nasal cavity and lacks outer bony walls. Externally, it occupies the area between the commissure of the beak and the eye. The sinus has diverticula into the upper beak, mandible, around the eye, and pneumatized bones of the skull.

The choana can become inflamed or contain a discharge caused by viral, yeast, or primary bacterial infections or be secondarily infected because of vitamin A deficiency, neoplasia, or allergies. Granulomas in the mouth are common with vitamin A deficiency. A thick, white oral exudate can be caused by yeast or bacterial infections. See Chapter 4 for diagnostic tests for oral lesions.

Vitamin A deficiency causes squamous metaplasia of mucous membranes. On physical examination, this is evidenced by swollen margins of the choana in the roof of the mouth. Associated papillae may be blunted or absent, and sterile granulomas of the oral and lingual mucosa and sinuses may be present.

Viral infections often are seen with signs of involvement of multiple body systems. Cutaneous or diphtheritic poxvirus lesions may be seen on physical examination. Signs of poxvirus vary with the type of poxvirus and species of bird. There are cutaneous and diphtheroid forms. The diphtheroid form is characterized by gray or brown fibrinous lesions in the oropharynx and larynx. Clinical signs include nasal discharge, coughing, and dyspnea. The cutaneous form is characterized by cutaneous proliferative growths or scabs on featherless areas of skin and around eyes, nares, beak, and feet (see Figure 9–1).

Signs of Pacheco's disease include acute onset of anorexia, biliverdinuria, polyuria, diarrhea, sinusitis, and sometimes central nervous system (CNS) signs. Sudden death without premonitory signs is common. The course of the disease is frequently swift, such as a bird appearing normal in the morning and being found dead by evening.

Reovirus presents with a bloody brown nasal discharge, diarrhea, labored breathing, and ataxia.

Signs of Amazon tracheitis include nasal and ocular discharges, dyspnea, and coughing. The disease may be peracute, acute, subacute, or chronic.

Signs of infectious laryngotracheitis in canaries include severe dyspnea, inspiratory wheeze, expectoration of bloody mucus, ocular and nasal discharge, and sinusitis.

Signs of avian influenza in gallinaceous birds and waterfowl include depression, dyspnea, sinusitis, diarrhea, and anorexia. Lethargy, CNS signs, and diarrhea may occur in psittacines infected by avian influenza.

Signs of conure bleeding syndrome include periodic recurrences of bleeding, epistaxis, dyspnea, polyuria, diarrhea, and occasionally ataxia.

Gastrointestinal signs in conjunction with sneezing, nasal discharge, head shaking, or sinusitis may occur with bacterial infections, chlamydiosis, candidiasis, aspergillosis, coagulopathies, *Cryptococcus*, *Mycoplasma*, conure bleeding syndrome, Pacheco's disease, reovirus, and papillomas.

Neurologic signs may accompany sneezing, nasal discharge, head shaking, or sinusitis with chlamydiosis, Pacheco's disease, reovirus, or *Cryptococcus* infection.

Algorithm for Sneezing, Nasal Discharge, Head Shaking, or Sinusitis

See Figure 3–1.

Diagnostic Approach for Sneezing, Nasal Discharge, Head Shaking, or Sinusitis

Provide supportive care as needed during diagnostic testing (see Chapter 1).

Obtaining a complete history and performing a complete physical examination are the first steps in evaluating the bird with sneezing, nasal discharge, head shaking, or sinusitis. Dietary and iatrogenic causes must be sought from the history. Trauma, papillomas, poxvirus lesions, and typical vitamin A or candidiasis lesions may be suspected based on physical examination findings. Vitamin A deficiency is diagnosed through diet history and physical examination. Cytology of aspirates of keratin cysts reveal cornified epithelial cells and debris. Biopsy of keratin cysts may reveal hyperkeratosis or squamous metaplasia.

Allergic disease is suspected based on clinical signs and history, e.g., exposure to tobacco smoke or cockatoo feather dust. If allergic disease is suspected and cytology of sinus aspirate is not diagnostic, confine the bird to an allergen-free environment for a trial period. A reduction in clinical signs can take weeks to months.

After signalment and history are considered and the physical abnormalities are noted, cytology of the sinus is usually the most useful diagnostic test. Infectious, allergic, and neoplastic diseases may be identified with cytology. Sinus aspirates are superior to nasal exudates for sample evaluation because nasal exudates may be contaminated by insignificant bacteria in or around the nostril.

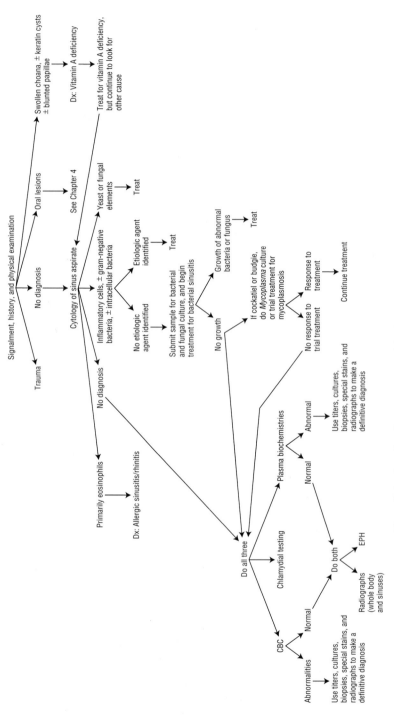

Figure 3–1. Algorithm for sneezing, nasal discharge, head shaking, or sinusitis.

Sampling of one sinus is usually adequate in psittacine birds; both sinuses may need to be sampled in some passerines when signs are bilateral.

If an adequate sample cannot be obtained with a sinus aspiration, flush the nostril with sterile saline (0.5–1 ml) and collect a sample with a sterile swab from the rostral choana. The mouth is held open with a speculum or gauze to collect the sample. This sample is usually adequate for Gram's staining, cytology, and culturing. Contamination by oral and nasal bacteria and yeast must be considered. Normal flora of the choana are gram-positive bacteria, including *Bacillus* spp., *Corynebacterium* spp., *Lactobacillus* spp., *Staphylococcus epidermidis*, and *Streptococcus* spp.

Cytology of sinus aspirates is discussed in Chapter 12. Aspirates may contain inflammatory cells without an etiologic agent being apparent. Cultures or other diagnostic tests are used to make a diagnosis.

Aspirates and swabs can also be evaluated with Gram's stain. Normal flora of sinuses and the choana are gram-positive rods and cocci; an occasional gram-negative bacterial rod or *Candida* organism can be seen in normal birds. Yeast stain deeply basophilic. An increase in gram-negative bacteria or yeast is abnormal. An increase in gram-negative bacteria can be the result of either primary bacterial infection or secondary to vitamin A deficiency, nasal or sinus foreign body, or neoplasia. Cultures must be performed to identify the bacteria and susceptibility. A Gram's stain is useful if bacterial or yeast sinusitis is suspected. Initial antibiotic therapy can be chosen based on Gram's staining characteristics. The staining procedure is quick, and results are easy to interpret (see Chapter 12). However, because limited information is obtainable with a Gram's stain, cytology is often much more informative.

If conjunctivitis is present and chlamydiosis is suspected, a conjunctival smear will sometimes reveal intracytoplasmic inclusion bodies in macrophage-like cells.

A complete blood count (CBC) and plasma biochemistries rarely provide a diagnosis, but they are useful in supporting the diagnosis of infectious and systemic diseases and aid in evaluating the general health of the bird. Perform a CBC when systemic disease is suspected, when a bird is unresponsive to treatment, or to help determine the general health of the bird. Changes in the hemogram commonly seen in birds with sneezing, nasal discharge, head shaking, or sinusitis are detailed below.

Leukocytosis may be caused by stress, inflammatory diseases, or neoplasia. Many normal young psittacines have a mild heterophilia. Regenerative left shifts may be seen with chronic or severe bacterial sinusitis, aspergillosis, chlamydiosis, and neoplasia. Differentials to consider with a white blood cell (WBC) count between 25,000 and 40,000 WBC/μl include *Pseudomonas*, salmonellosis, chlamydiosis, aspergillosis, and mycobacteriosis. *Chlamydia*, *Aspergillus*, and *Mycobacterium* infections often cause a WBC count in excess of 40,000/μl in larger psittacines. Toxic heterophils and monocytosis may occur with severe bacterial, chlamydial, viral, and *Aspergillus* infections. Toxic changes include degranulation, vacuolation, increased cytoplasmic basophilia, and nuclear degeneration. Lymphocytosis can be associated with infectious agents. Monocytosis is common with chronic fungal and bacterial infections (e.g., chlamydiosis, mycobacteriosis) and tissue necrosis. Basophilia may be seen with chlamydiosis.

Leukopenia may be associated with overwhelming bacterial or viral infection, chlamydiosis, or aspergillosis.

Nonregenerative anemias may be seen with chronic inflammatory diseases such as chlamydiosis, aspergillosis, mycobacteriosis, and neoplasia. Regenerative anemias may be seen with coagulopathies, trauma, and neoplasia.

Perform plasma biochemistries when systemic disease is suspected, when a bird is unresponsive to treatment, or to help determine the general health of the bird. Hyperproteinemia may be seen with dehydration or chronic diseases such as chlamydiosis, aspergillosis, and mycobacteriosis. A decrease in total proteins may be seen with trauma, stress, coagulopathies, neoplasia, or poor nutrition. Normal young psittacines often have total protein levels lower than adults.

An elevation in aspartate transferase (AST or SGOT) is usually the result of liver or muscle damage. Heart, brain, and kidney damage may also result in an elevation of AST. Because of liver damage, AST may be elevated in chlamydiosis and Pacheco's disease. Muscle damage caused by trauma and irritating intramuscular injections also cause an elevation in AST. Creatinine kinase activity increases with muscle damage and may be used to differentiate an increase in AST caused by liver disease from an increase caused by muscle damage.

Hypoglycemia may be seen with Pacheco's disease, neoplasia, septicemia, aspergillosis, or anorexia.

Plasma protein electrophoresis (EPH) is useful in identifying many disease states (e.g., chlamydiosis, aspergillosis, mycobacteriosis).

Radiography is useful in diagnosing sinus and choana foreign bodies and granulomas. Lesions associated with systemic diseases may be noted radiographically. Radiograph birds with suspected systemic disease and birds with infections unresponsive to appropriate antibiotic therapy, based on culture and sensitivity results. Generalized soft tissue opacity within the infraorbital sinus may be seen with vitamin A deficiency or sinusitis. Circumscribed tissue densities within the sinus may be caused by neoplasia, aspergillosis, or granulomas. These conditions cannot be differentiated radiographically. Sinus aspirates, cytology, or biopsy of the lesion is used to obtain a diagnosis.

Thickening of the caudal thoracic and abdominal air sacs on lateral radiographs and diffuse increased opacity of these air sacs on ventrodorsal views indicate airsacculitis. Splenomegaly, hepatomegaly, and airsacculitis support a diagnosis of chlamydiosis (see Chapter 13). *Aspergillus* infection may be visualized radiographically as focal densities in the sinus, trachea, air sac (most common), or lung. Lesions may be present in more than one site. Tumors and some sinus, nasal, and choana foreign bodies may be visualized with radiography.

Cultures and titers are useful to rule in or out specific diseases. Aspergillosis can sometimes be demonstrated with a fungal culture. Useful samples to culture include sinus aspirates, tracheal washes, and swabs of the choana. Samples should be sent to a laboratory familiar with avian aspergillosis. False-negative results occur. False-positive results occur if the sample is contaminated with *Aspergillus* from the environment. Serologic testing is available for raptors and psittacines.

Diagnosis of chlamydiosis can be difficult. No single test or combination of tests can detect *Chlamydia* infection in all infected or carrier birds and not result in false-positive results in uninfected birds (see Chapter 9). Antigen tests are useful in-house tests in birds showing clinical signs of infection, although false-negative results occur. Serology is useful in birds large enough to provide a blood sample adequate for evaluation (cockatiel or larger birds). False-negative results can occur early in the disease before antibody production and in some species of birds (e.g., cockatiels). Low serology may be difficult to interpret. The laboratory performing the serology will aid in interpretation of results. Chlamydial cultures of nasal or ocular discharges or feces may provide a diagnosis if shedding of the organism is occurring at the time of sampling. Obtain culture samples before beginning antibiotic therapy. False-negative cultures occur. Plasma protein electrophoresis is useful for chlamydial diagnosis.

Acid-fast staining can be used to identify acid-fast *Mycobacterium*. *Mycobacterium* affects the digestive tract in most birds. Feces or liver biopsy samples may reveal acid-fast organisms. Samples from the trachea are useful if the organism is causing a respiratory infection.

Various tests are available to aid in diagnosis of viral infections (see Chapter 12). A suspicion of infection is based on signalment, history, and clinical signs.

Antemortem diagnosis of Pacheco's disease is difficult. Intermittent shedding by carrier birds may be detected by virus isolation. Histology (hepatic necrosis, eosinophilic intranuclear inclusion bodies), virus neutralization, enzyme-linked immunosorbent assay (ELISA), and immunofluorescence may be useful postmortem.

Cloacal swabs and samples from affected organs may be used for reovirus isolation and culture. Viral antigen may be detected by immunofluorescence in affected tissue.

Pharyngeal swabs are useful for culture of Amazon tracheitis.

Intranuclear inclusion bodies may be found postmortem in respiratory epithelial cells of canaries with infectious laryngotracheitis. Virus isolation is required for definitive diagnosis.

Diagnosis of poxvirus is based on clinical signs, cytology and histopathology of cutaneous lesions, or culture. Cytology and histopathology may reveal pathognomonic Bollinger bodies, eosinophilic intracytoplasmic inclusion bodies (see Fig. 12–24). Virus culture is required for diagnosis in acute cases lacking lesions.

Swabs from the cloaca and upper respiratory tract may be used for direct virus demonstration from live birds infected with avian influenza. Liver, lung, spleen, and brain are the best postmortem samples for virus isolation.

Anemia, heterophilia, hypoproteinemia, and large numbers of immature erythrocytes are common laboratory findings with conure bleeding syndrome. Bone marrow aspirates show erythemic myelosis. Diagnosis is based on history, clinical signs, laboratory findings, and necropsy.

Trial treatment with tetracyclines, macrolides, or enrofloxacin for *Mycoplasma* infection may allow a presumed diagnosis; however, response to treatment is not definitive.

Aviaries or flock situations benefit from complete necropsy examinations. Submit adequate samples for histopathology, microbiology, and virus isolation, especially when infectious disease is suspected.

Treatment

Once a diagnosis is made, treat the underlying cause. Provide supportive care as needed (see Chapter 1). Severely ill birds may die as a result of the treatment if not stabilized with supportive care before beginning curative therapy.

Treatment of bacterial rhinitis and sinusitis includes oral or parenteral antibiotics (based on culture and sensitivity results) and local treatment (nasal flushes or nebulization therapy). Systemic therapy can be initiated with later-generation beta-lactams (e.g., piperacillin, cefotaxime), fluroquinolones (e.g., enrofloxacin), or trimethoprim-sulfa combinations (e.g., trimethoprim/sulfadiazine, trimethoprim/sulfamethoxazole) until sensitivity can be determined. Nasal or sinus flushes or nebulization with saline and antibiotics will increase efficacy of treatment. Birds with minor, non–life-threatening illness usually respond well to appropriate oral antibiotics and twice daily nasal flushes containing diluted antibiotics (see Chapter 11). Hospitalize very ill birds, begin parenteral antibiotics and nebulization therapy, and provide supportive care as needed. Heat, oxygen, intravenous or intraosseous fluids, and tube feeding should be provided as needed. Nasal flushes are started when the bird is strong enough to survive the stress of the procedure.

Sinus, nasal, and choanal foreign bodies may dislodge with nasal or sinus flushes. Some foreign bodies require either flushing through a catheter placed surgically in the infraorbital sinus or surgical removal. Surgery in this area is complicated by the vascularity of the tissue.

Allergic disease responds to removal of the offending substance, which in some instances may require a new home. The owner should limit smoking to outdoors and wash hands and arms before contact with the bird. Symptomatic therapy using an antihistamine or bronchodilator is sometimes useful.

Vitamin A deficiency requires parenteral vitamin A initially, then oral supplementation and correction of the diet. Keratin cysts and sterile abscesses are debrided. Treat any secondary infections.

Management of viral infections includes symptomatic therapy and prevention of secondary bacterial infection and contagion. Isolate ill birds. Chlorhexidine in the drinking water is used to decrease spread in flock situations. Antibiotics may be used to prevent and treat secondary bacterial infections.

ABNORMALLY SHAPED NOSTRIL OR GROOVE IN BEAK

An abnormally shaped nostril or a groove in the beak originating at the base of the beak near the nostril may be the result of chronic sinusitis or damage to the germinal tissue of the beak by a previous infection or trauma (Fig. 3–2).

Differential Diagnoses

1. Sinusitis
2. Trauma

Signalment

The signalment will not provide a diagnosis, but may help identify common problems. Refer to the previous section for a discussion of signalment for sinusitis.

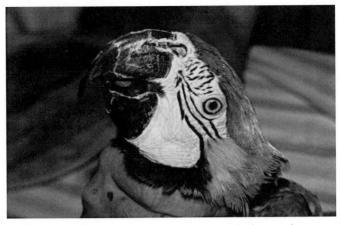

Figure 3–2. An abnormal longitudinal groove in the beak, as in this macaw, may be caused by chronic sinusitis or damage to the germinal tissue of the beak by a previous infection or trauma. (Photo courtesy of Brian L. Speer, DVM, ABVP-avian.)

History

History of a previous trauma may be determined by questioning the owner. The trauma will have occurred some time before the examination because it takes time for the beak to grow. Damage to the germinal cells of the growing portion of the beak causes a longitudinal groove to form in the beak. If trauma is the cause, no sign of sinusitis or rhinitis will be present.

Physical Examination

The physical examination may reveal signs of sinusitis or previous trauma, e.g., old fractures. If the nostril is larger than the one on the unaffected side, pursue diagnostic tests for sinusitis. Consult the previous section for additional physical examination findings.

Diagnostic Approach for Abnormally Shaped Nostril or Groove in Beak

If there is no history of trauma, the diagnostic approach for sinusitis is performed (see the previous section).

COUGHING OR VOICE CHANGE

Coughing is a relatively rare clinical sign in pet birds. Coughing indicates irritation or infection of the respiratory tract, or it may be a learned vocalization imitating a human cough. A change in voice is common in pet birds and is associated with pathology of the syrinx, the organ of vocalization at the distal trachea.

Differential Diagnoses for Coughing or Voice Change

1. Infectious
   a. Bacterial: °gram-negative bacteria (*Escherichia coli, Klebsiella pneumoniae, Pasteurella multocida, Pseudomonas aeruginosa, Salmonella* spp., *Yersinia pseudotuberculosis*, other), gram-positive bacteria (*Mycobacterium*, other)
   b. Chlamydial: °*Chlamydia psittaci*
   c. Fungal: °*Aspergillus, Candida*
   d. Viral: Amazon tracheitis, infectious laryngotracheitis, poxvirus
   e. Parasitic: *Cytodites nudus* (air sac mites), °*Sternostoma tracheocolum* (tracheal mites), *Syngamus trachea* (gapeworms)
2. Nutritional: vitamin A deficiency
3. Physical: °foreign body, ascites, peritonitis
4. Trauma
5. Allergic
6. Neoplastic: metastatic, papilloma, other
7. Other: °mimicking human cough, conure bleeding syndrome

Signalment

Common causes of coughing in larger psittacines include a tracheal foreign body, mimicking, chlamydiosis, aspergillosis, and gram-negative bacterial infection. Cockatiels and budgies commonly cough because of chlamydiosis, a tracheal foreign body, or gram-negative bacterial infections. Tracheal mites and bacterial upper respiratory tract infections are common causes of coughing in canaries and finches. Ascites, aspergillosis, and bacterial infections are common causes of coughing in mynahs. Aspergillosis and bacterial infections are common causes of coughing in raptors. A common cause of change in voice in pet birds is aspergillosis.

Aspergillosis is common in African gray parrots and raptors, but it may cause illness in any species of bird. Conure bleeding syndrome affects only conures. The cutaneous form of poxvirus is rare except in blue-fronted Amazons, lovebirds, passerines, raptors, and pigeons. Infectious laryngotracheitis affects canaries and gallinaceous species. Gapeworm infections are common in gallinaceous birds and rare in pet birds. Tracheal mites and air sac mites may affect budgies and cockatiels, but they are a common cause of coughing in canaries and Gouldian finches. Avian mycobacteriosis is most commonly associated with the intestinal tract in psittacines, but it commonly affects the respiratory tract in pigeons, some finches, and some other species.

°Common causes.

History

A complete history may reveal allergic or nutritional problems, possible exposure to infectious diseases, or recent trauma. A history of acute dyspnea and coughing that started while the bird was eating is consistent with inhalation of a seed. Inhalation of other foreign bodies (e.g., granulomas from vitamin A deficiency or infection) also occurs. Tracheal blockage is an emergency (see below).

Birds recently exposed to other birds are commonly ill as a result of infectious diseases, including bacterial, chlamydial, viral, and parasitic infections.

Birds recently acquired from a pet store or aviary may be at a higher risk of having been exposed to contagious pathogens. Many birds in this category are also stressed by prior group contact and a change of environment, predisposing them to disease. Knowledge of common diseases in the breeder facility or pet store may provide insight to the possible cause of disease.

Infectious and toxic etiologies are suspected when multiple birds are affected.

Stress may play a role precipitating clinical signs. Chronic diseases such as chlamydiosis may go undetected until the bird is stressed. Stressful situations for birds include going to a new home, the addition of a new bird, changing to a new cage, a change in diet, or temperature extremes.

Isolated birds and those in closed collections are commonly ill because of foreign body inhalation, nutritional deficiencies, trauma, reproductive problems, neoplasia, allergic disease, or chronic infections such as chlamydiosis and aspergillosis. Some bacterial diseases are also common, especially gram-negative infections.

The diet affects the health of the bird. Diets deficient in vitamin A, such as an all-seed diet, can lead to vitamin A deficiency. Vitamin A deficiency causes squamous metaplasia of mucosal surfaces, increasing susceptibility to respiratory tract infections. Keratin cysts at the glottal opening can cause coughing.

Consider the bird's environment. Birds allowed out of their cages are susceptible to trauma. Contact with tobacco smoke or other allergen can cause an allergic reaction and coughing. Gapeworms are most common in outdoor aviaries because of the life cycle of the parasite.

The duration of the illness is important. Note the owner's description of the clinical signs and the course of the disease. Note previous illnesses, including signs, treatment, and response to treatment. A history of worsening of signs while on antibiotics is common with aspergillosis.

Physical Examination

The physical examination may reveal obvious trauma or vitamin A deficiency. Observations may help to narrow the differential diagnoses. Descriptions follow of common findings in birds with coughing or a change in voice.

Acute dyspnea is an emergency situation. Birds with tracheal blockage from a foreign body, fungal granuloma, or other inhaled material will benefit greatly from placement of an air sac breathing tube. A chronic respiratory condition will not respond to air sac breathing tube placement. A decision to place an air sac breathing tube is based on history and clinical signs, and in emergency situations in which tracheal blockage is suspected the tube is placed before other diagnostic tests are done. The technique is detailed in Chapter 14.

Nasal discharge is a sign of nasal or sinus disease or tracheal, lower respiratory, or systemic disease. When a nasal discharge is present in a coughing bird, the nasal discharge is often caused by tracheal or lower respiratory disease.

The choana can become inflamed or contain a discharge resulting from viral, yeast, or primary bacterial infections, or it may be secondarily infected because of vitamin A deficiency, neoplasia, or allergies. Granulomas in the mouth are common with vitamin A deficiency. A thick, white oral exudate can result from yeast or bacterial infections. See Chapter 4 for a discussion of oral lesions.

Oral mucous membranes may be cyanotic, indicating a lack of oxygenation of the blood. This may be seen with tracheal foreign bodies or diseases affecting the trachea or lower respiratory tract.

Vitamin A deficiency causes squamous metaplasia of mucous membranes. On physical examination, this is evidenced by swollen margins of the choana in the roof of the mouth. Associated papillae may be blunted or absent, and sterile keratin cysts may be present in the oral and lingual mucosa and sinus.

Cutaneous or diphtheritic poxvirus lesions may seen on physical examination. The diphtheroid form is characterized by gray or brown fibrinous lesions in the oral cavity, pharynx, and larynx. The cutaneous form is characterized by cutaneous proliferative growths on featherless areas of skin (around eyes, nares, beak, and feet).

Gapeworms may be visualized in the glottal opening. They are large, red helminths. Transillumination of the trachea with a bright light in passerines may reveal tracheal or air sac mites. The mites appear as dark, moving, pinhead-sized spots. To improve visualization, wet the feathers over the trachea.

Auscultation of the lungs, air sacs, and heart may reveal abnormal respiratory sounds, cardiac murmur, or arrhythmia.

A distended abdomen may be seen with ascites, egg binding, hepatomegaly, distended proventriculus, or large abdominal tumors.

Signs of Amazon tracheitis include nasal and ocular discharges, dyspnea, and coughing. The disease may be peracute, acute, subacute, or chronic.

Signs of poxvirus vary with the type of poxvirus and species of bird. There are cutaneous and diphtheroid forms. The diphtheroid form is characterized by gray or brown fibrinous lesions in the oropharynx and larynx. Clinical signs include nasal discharge, coughing, and dyspnea. The cutaneous form is characterized by cutaneous proliferative growths or scabs on featherless areas of skin (around eyes, nares, beak, and feet).

Signs of conure bleeding syndrome include periodic recurrence of bleeding, epistaxis, dyspnea, polyuria, diarrhea, and occasionally ataxia.

Signs of infectious laryngotracheitis in canaries include severe dyspnea, inspiratory wheeze, expectoration of bloody mucus, ocular and nasal discharge, and sinusitis.

Illnesses that can cause gastrointestinal signs with coughing or a change in voice include chlamydiosis, bacterial infections, aspergillosis, candidiasis, conure hemorrhagic syndrome, peritonitis, and papillomas.

Neurologic signs may accompany coughing or a change in voice with chlamydiosis or bacterial infections.

Ophthalmic signs may accompany coughing or a change in voice with chlamydiosis, bacterial infections, candidiasis, aspergillosis, poxvirus, Amazon tracheitis, trauma, and vitamin A deficiency.

Algorithm for Coughing or Voice Change

See Figure 3–3.

Diagnostic Approach for Coughing or Voice Change

Stabilize severely ill birds before performing stressful diagnostic tests. Provide supportive care as needed (see Chapter 1).

If severe inspiratory dyspnea is present and an upper airway obstruction is suspected, placement of an air sac canula will allow easier breathing and oxygen administration (see Chapter 14). This is discussed further below.

If a coughing bird has a distended abdomen, follow the diagnostic approach for the distended abdomen in Chapter 2. Birds do not have a diaphragm; therefore, illnesses causing abdominal distension (e.g., organomegaly, ascites, peritonitis) can affect the respiratory tract.

A complete history and physical examination are the initial diagnostic steps for a coughing bird or a bird with a change in voice. Vitamin A deficiency may be diagnosed through diet history and physical examination. Poxvirus lesions, mites, trauma, ascites, or papillomas may be suspected based on physical examination findings.

Fecal flotation or direct smears of pharyngeal mucus in gallinaceous birds and passerines may reveal gapeworm eggs. Tracheal and air sac mite eggs may be found in the feces of infected birds.

After signalment and history are considered, the physical abnormalities noted, and the fecal test performed, cytology of a tracheal washing is usually the most useful diagnostic test. A minimum database is also obtained. Infectious, allergic, and neoplastic diseases may be identified with cytology of a sample from the trachea. With the bird's mouth held open with a speculum or gauze, a sample is collected at the laryngeal opening. If the bird can withstand anesthesia, sampling from the trachea and tracheal washes may be performed (see Chapter 12). Many unanesthetized birds will tolerate tracheal aspiration with adequate restraint. This sample is useful for cytology, culture, and sensitivity testing.

Radiography is useful for visualization of tracheal foreign bodies, tumors, and granulomas and to check for lower respiratory involvement. Lesions associated with systemic diseases may be noted radiographically. Tracheal foreign bodies can often be visualized radiographically. Tissue densities in the tracheal lumen, such as tumors, aspergillosis granulomas, bacterial granulomas, and abscesses, may be visualized, but they must be differentiated with endoscopy and biopsy. Thickening of the caudal thoracic and abdominal air sac on lateral radiographs and diffuse increased opacity of the caudal thoracic and abdominal air sac region on ventrodorsal views indicate airsacculitis. The airsacculitis differential diagnoses include bacterial infection, chlamydiosis, and aspergillosis. Nodular densities on the air sacs can be bacterial or *Aspergillus* granulomas. Splenomegaly, hepatomegaly, and airsacculitis are consistent with chlamydiosis (see Chapter

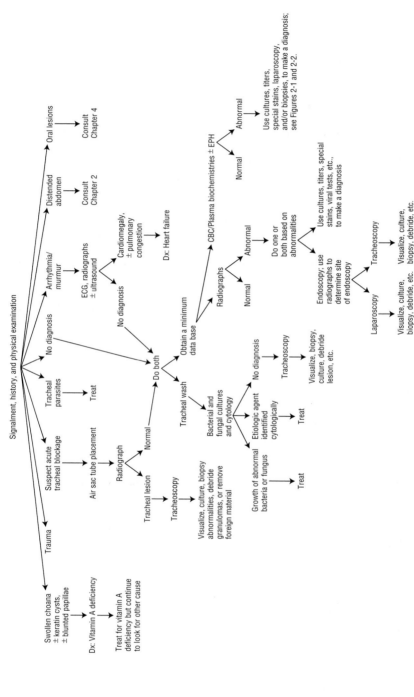

Figure 3-3. Algorithm for coughing or voice change.

13). Metastatic neoplasia can be visualized as multiple, variably sized nodules. Differentiation among types of neoplasms requires biopsy. Ascites and peritonitis cause an overall loss of organ detail. On the ventrodorsal view, this loss of detail may be difficult to distinguish from hepatomegaly. On the lateral view, ascites and peritonitis will cause loss of detail in the celomic cavity, with the lung, intestinal gas, and grit in the ventriculus often being the only identifiable features.

A CBC and plasma biochemistries rarely provide a diagnosis but are useful in supporting infectious and systemic diseases. These tests may reveal unsuspected organ involvement or allow monitoring of the success of treatment in some disease states. Perform a CBC when systemic disease is suspected, when a bird is unresponsive to treatment, or to help determine the general health of the bird. CBCs are also useful to monitor treatment success in disease states that cause elevated WBC counts (e.g., aspergillosis, chlamydiosis) or plasma protein abnormalities. Changes in the leukogram commonly seen with diseases that cause coughing or a change in voice are detailed below.

Leukocytosis may be due to stress, inflammatory diseases, or neoplasia. Differentials for a WBC count between 25,000 to 40,000 WBC/μl include *Pseudomonas*, salmonellosis, chlamydiosis, aspergillosis, mycobacteriosis, and peritonitis. White blood cell counts in excess of 40,000/μl can occur with chlamydiosis, aspergillosis, mycobacteriosis, or peritonitis. Heterophilia can be seen with bacterial, fungal, and parasitic infections and with trauma or stress. Many normal young psittacines have a mild heterophilia. Regenerative left shifts are common with chronic or severe bacterial infections (mycobacteriosis, *Pseudomonas*, *Salmonella*), chlamydiosis, aspergillosis, and neoplasia. Toxic heterophils and monocytosis occur with severe bacterial, chlamydial, viral, and *Aspergillus* infections. Toxic changes include degranulation, vacuolation, increased cytoplasmic basophilia, and nuclear degeneration. Lymphocytosis can be associated with infectious agents. Monocytosis is common with chronic fungal and bacterial infections (chlamydiosis, mycobacteriosis) and tissue necrosis. Basophilia may be seen with chlamydiosis. Eosinophilia may be seen with parasitic infections and allergic reactions. Lymphocytosis may be present in canaries and finches with air sac mites.

Leukopenia occurs with overwhelming bacterial and viral infections.

Nonregenerative anemias may be seen with chronic inflammatory diseases such as chlamydiosis, aspergillosis, mycobacteriosis, and neoplasia. Regenerative anemias may be seen with blood loss, trauma, and neoplasia.

Plasma biochemistries are useful but rarely diagnostic. Perform plasma biochemistries when systemic disease is suspected, when a bird is unresponsive to treatment, or to help determine the general health of the bird. Unsuspected organ involvement may be found. Changes in biochemistry test results commonly seen in birds with diseases that cause coughing or a change in voice are detailed below.

Hyperproteinemia may be seen with dehydration and chronic diseases such as chlamydiosis, aspergillosis, and mycobacteriosis. A decrease in total proteins may be seen with trauma, stress, coagulopathy, neoplasia, chronic disease, and poor nutrition. Young psittacines often have total protein levels lower than those of adults.

An elevation in AST is usually the result of liver or muscle damage. Heart, brain, and kidney damage may also result in an elevation of AST, and AST may be elevated with chlamydiosis. Muscle damage caused by trauma and irritating intramuscular injections also causes an elevation in AST. Creatinine kinase activity increases with muscle damage and may be used to differentiate an increase in AST caused by liver disease from an increase caused by muscle damage.

Hypoglycemia may be seen with neoplasia, anorexia, septicemia, or aspergillosis.

Plasma protein electrophoresis is useful in identifying many disease states (e.g., chlamydiosis, aspergillosis, or mycobacteriosis).

Tracheal endoscopy is used to visualize and to obtain biopsy samples and to culture intratracheal lesions and to visualize and remove tracheal foreign bodies. Tracheoscopy is practical in Amazon parrots or larger birds. Look for inflammation, exudates, foreign bodies, granulomas, and tumors. Collect bacterial and viral culture samples from the tip of the endoscope after the examination. If a foreign body is suspected based on acute severe inspiratory dyspnea, endoscopy is performed early in the diagnostic scheme to look for and remove a foreign body after an air sac breathing tube has been placed.

Laparoscopy (abdominal endoscopy) is used to visualize air sacs, lungs, and other organs and to collect biopsy samples and cultures of air sacs, liver, and lungs. Excellent equipment designed for use in birds is available (Karl Storz Veterinary Endoscopy). An otoscope with a sterile speculum can be used if an endoscope is unavailable. For details on the procedure, see Chapter 14. The normal air sac is transparent with little vascularity. The normal lung is pink. Thickened, opaque air sacs with increased vascularity indicate airsacculitis. Granulomas may be visualized.

Cultures and titers are useful to rule in or out specific diseases. Fungal cultures, in addition to cytology, radiographs, hematology, endoscopy, and biopsy, are useful to help diagnose aspergillosis. Useful samples for fungal culture include tracheal wash samples and air sac wash samples. Positive culture of *Aspergillus* without typical lesions is not diagnostic because contamination with this ubiquitous organism occurs. Samples should be sent to a laboratory familiar with avian aspergillosis. False-negative results occur. Serologic testing is available for raptors and pet birds.

Diagnosis of chlamydiosis can be difficult. No single test or combination of tests can detect *Chlamydia* infection in all infected or carrier birds and not result in false-positive results in uninfected birds (see Chapter 9). Antigen tests are useful in-house tests in birds showing clinical signs of infection. False-negative results occur. Serology is useful in birds large enough to provide a blood sample adequate for evaluation (cockatiel or larger birds). False-negative results can occur early in the disease before antibody production and in some species of birds (e.g., cockatiels). Low titers may be difficult to interpret. The laboratory performing the test will aid in interpretation of results. Chlamydial cultures of nasal or ocular discharges or feces may provide a diagnosis if shedding of the organism is occurring at the time of sampling. Obtain culture samples before beginning antibiotic therapy. False-negative culture results occur. Plasma protein electrophoresis is useful for chlamydial diagnosis.

Use acid-fast staining to identify acid-fast *Mycobacterium*. *Mycobacterium* affects the digestive tract in most birds. Feces or biopsy samples (liver, lung) may reveal acid-fast organisms. Samples from the trachea are useful if the organism is causing a respiratory infection. A negative result does not rule out mycobacteriosis because the bird must be shedding the organism in numbers high enough to produce a positive result.

Various tests are available for aid in diagnosis of viral infections (see Chapter 12). A suspicion of infection is based on signalment, history, and clinical signs. Concurrent signs are usually present with viral infections.

Pharyngeal swabs are useful for culture of Amazon tracheitis.

Definitive diagnosis of poxvirus is based on clinical signs, cytology, and histopathology of cutaneous lesions, or culture. Cytology and histopathology may reveal eosinophilic intracytoplasmic inclusion bodies, Bollinger bodies. Virus culture is required for diagnosis in acute cases lacking lesions.

Anemia, heterophilia, hypoproteinemia, and large numbers of immature erythrocytes are common laboratory findings in birds affected with conure bleeding syndrome. Bone marrow aspirates show erythemic myelosis. Diagnosis is based on history, clinical signs, laboratory findings, and necropsy.

Intranuclear inclusion bodies may be found in respiratory epithelial cells in canaries infected with infectious laryngotracheitis. Virus isolation is required for definitive diagnosis.

Allergic disease is suspected from clinical signs and history, e.g., exposure to cigarette smoke or cockatoo feather dust. If allergic disease is suspected and cytology of the tracheal wash is not diagnostic, confine the bird to an allergen-free environment for a trial period. Weeks to months may be required to see an improvement in clinical signs.

Aviaries or flock situations benefit from complete necropsy examinations. Submit adequate samples for histopathology, microbiology, and virus isolation, especially when infectious disease is suspected.

Treatment for Coughing or Voice Change

Once a diagnosis is made, treat the underlying cause.

Provide supportive care as needed (see Chapter 1). Severely ill birds may die as a result of the treatment if they are not stabilized with supportive care before beginning curative therapy. Selection of antibiotics for treatment of bacterial tracheitis and tracheobronchitis is based on culture and sensitivity results. Therapy can be initiated with fluroquinolones (e.g., enrofloxacin), later-generation beta-lactams (e.g., piperacillin, cefotaxime), or trimethoprim-sulfa combinations (e.g., trimethoprim/sulfadiazine, trimethoprim/sulfamethoxazole) until sensitivity can be determined.

A combination of systemic antibiotics and nebulization of antibiotics is most effective. The route of administration of systemic antibiotics is based on the severity of clinical signs. Use parenteral antibiotics until the bird is stabilized. Oral or parenteral antibiotics are used to continue treatment. Nebulization is beneficial in treating bacterial tracheitis and tracheobronchitis because it delivers the antibiotic to the site of infection and increases the humidity of inspired air (see Chapter 11).

Tracheal foreign bodies are removed using endoscopy, transtracheal flush, or surgical tracheotomy. Place an air sac breathing tube to provide ventilation and anesthesia. Use an endoscope to view the foreign body while it is grasped with forceps, or remove the foreign body with suction in birds weighing more than 300 g. A small-gauge needle placed through the trachea distal to the foreign body will prevent further movement. In smaller birds, suction applied to a tube passed blindly to the approximate level of the foreign body is sometimes successful. A transtracheal flush will sometimes dislodge a tracheal foreign body. A needle is passed distal to the foreign body, and sterile saline is infused while holding the bird upside down. Perform a tracheotomy if these methods are unsuccessful.

Allergic disease responds to removal of the offending substance, and in some instances the bird may require a new home. The owner should limit smoking to outdoors and wash hands and arms before contact with the bird. Symptomatic therapy with an antihistamine or bronchodilator is sometimes useful.

Vitamin A deficiency requires parenteral vitamin A initially, then oral supplementation and correction of the diet. Keratin cysts and abscesses are cultured and debrided; antibiotic selection is based on sensitivity results.

Management of viral infections includes symptomatic therapy and prevention of secondary bacterial infection and contagion. Isolate ill birds. Chlorhexidine in the drinking water is used to decrease spread in flock situations. Antibiotics may be used to treat or prevent secondary bacterial infections.

ABNORMAL BREATHING SOUNDS

The normal bird does not produce any noise when breathing. Abnormal respiratory sounds include cheeps, clicks, gurgles, and wheezes.

Differential Diagnoses for Abnormal Breathing Sounds

1. Infectious
   a. Bacterial: *gram-negative, gram-positive
   b. Viral: infectious laryngotracheitis, poxvirus
   c. Parasitic: *Syngamus trachea* (gapeworms), *Sternostoma tracheocolum* (tracheal mites), *Cytodites nudus* (air sac mites).
2. *Metabolic: goiter

Signalment

A common cause of clicks and cheeps in budgies is goiter. Air sac mites are a common cause of abnormal breathing sounds in canaries and Gouldian finches.

Air sac mites can cause disease in canaries, finches, and budgerigars. Gapeworm infections occur primarily in gallinaceous birds and rarely in pet birds. Thyroid hyperplasia causing goiter is most common in budgerigars but may occur in pigeons, cockatiels, canaries, and lovebirds. Infectious laryngotracheitis

---

*Common causes.

affects gallinaceous birds and canaries. The cutaneous form of poxvirus is rare except in blue-fronted Amazons, lovebirds, passerines, raptors, and pigeons.

History

A complete history may reveal nutritional problems or possible exposure to infectious diseases. Birds recently exposed to other birds commonly have abnormal breathing sounds as a result of infectious diseases, including viral, bacterial, and parasitic infections.

Isolated birds and those in closed collections are commonly ill because of nutritional deficiencies (e.g., goiter) and chronic diseases. Parasitic infections can be chronic.

Birds recently acquired from a pet store or private breeder may be at a higher risk of having been exposed to contagious pathogens. Many birds in this category are also stressed by prior group contact and a change of environment, predisposing them to disease. Knowledge of the breeder facility or pet store may provide insight to the possible cause of disease.

Infectious and toxic etiologies are suspected when multiple birds are affected.

Stress may play a role in precipitating clinical signs. Chronic infections, such as air sac mites, may go undetected until the bird is stressed. Stressful situations for birds include going to a new home, the addition of a new bird, changing to a new cage, a change in diet, or temperature extremes.

The diet affects the health of the bird. Goiter is associated with a seed diet deficient in iodine.

The duration of the illness is important. Note the owner's description of the clinical signs and the course of the disease. Note previous illnesses, including signs, treatment, and response to treatment.

Physical Examination

The physical examination may reveal obvious poxvirus lesions or tracheal parasites. If other clinical signs are also present, consult appropriate chapters for assistance in making a diagnosis.

Cutaneous or diphtheritic poxvirus lesions may be seen on physical examination. The diphtheroid form is characterized by gray or brown fibrinous lesions in the oropharynx and larynx. A nasal discharge, coughing, and dyspnea often accompany these lesions. The cutaneous form is characterized by cutaneous proliferative growths on featherless areas of skin (around eyes, nares, beak, and feet).

Gapeworms may be visualized in the glottal opening. They are large, red helminths. Gapeworms embed in the tracheal wall, causing irritation, mucus production, coughing, and granulomatous inflammation. Pneumonia may develop after migration of the larvae. Transillumination of the trachea with a bright light may allow visualization of the helminth in the larynx.

Transillumination of the trachea in passerines may reveal tracheal or air sac mites. The mites appear as dark, pinhead-sized spots. To improve visualization, wet the feathers over the trachea. Clinical signs include loss of condition, loss of vocalization, respiratory distress, coughing, or sudden death. A nasal discharge can be present with tracheal mites.

A respiratory chirp on expiration, especially in budgies, is suggestive of goiter. Regurgitation or a pendulous crop often accompany respiratory sounds. Enlarged thyroid glands are intrathoracic and cannot be palpated.

A wheezing sound during inspiration in canaries or gallinaceous birds is suspicious of infectious laryngotracheitis. Additional clinical signs include dyspnea, coughing, expectoration of bloody mucus, ocular and nasal discharge, and sinusitis.

Illnesses that can cause gastrointestinal signs and abnormal breathing sounds include bacterial infections and goiter.

Algorithm for Abnormal Breathing Sounds

See Figure 3–4.

Diagnostic Approach for Abnormal Breathing Sounds

Stabilize severely ill birds before performing stressful diagnostic tests. Provide supportive care as needed (see Chapter 1).

The signalment, history, and physical examination often provide a diagnosis. Fecal flotation or direct smears of pharyngeal mucus may reveal parasite eggs. Use fecal flotation to visualize gapeworm, tracheal mite, and air sac mite eggs in the feces of infected birds. Flotation of pharyngeal mucus may demonstrate eggs.

Cytology is useful to identify suspicious poxvirus lesions. Aspirate or scrape cutaneous proliferative growths that may be caused by poxvirus. Cytology may reveal pathognomonic Bollinger bodies (eosinophilic intracytoplasmic inclusion bodies) in lesions caused by poxvirus. Histopathology may also reveal Bollinger bodies. Virus culture is required for diagnosis of poxvirus in acute cases lacking lesions.

Tracheal washes may be used to obtain a tracheal sample for cytology and culture (see previous section on coughing).

Trial treatment may be necessary to support a diagnosis of goiter. Response to iodine supplementation supports a diagnosis of goiter. If improvement is not seen within 3 days of initiating treatment, re-evaluate the diagnosis.

Virus isolation is required for a definitive diagnosis of infectious laryngotracheitis.

Treatment for Abnormal Breathing Sounds

Once a diagnosis is made, treat the underlying cause. Provide supportive care as needed. Severely ill birds may die of the treatment if not stabilized with supportive care before beginning curative therapy (see Chapter 1).

Management of viral infections includes symptomatic therapy and prevention of secondary bacterial infection and contagion. Isolate ill birds. Chlorhexidine in

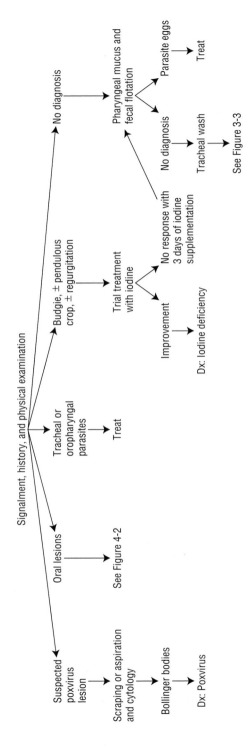

Figure 3–4. Algorithm for abnormal breathing sounds.

the drinking water is used to decrease spread in flock situations. Antibiotics may be used to treat or prevent secondary bacterial infections.

DYSPNEA, TAIL BOBBING, OR CYANOSIS

Tail bobbing is the rhythmic movement of the tail feathers with each inspiration or expiration. Any degree of tail bobbing is abnormal.

Birds showing signs of dyspnea, tail bobbing, or cyanosis are critically ill. Open-mouth breathing is a clinical sign associated with dyspnea or excessive heat. Upper respiratory signs often accompany dyspnea.

Differential Diagnoses for Dyspnea, Tail Bobbing, or Cyanosis

1. Infectious
   a. Bacterial: °gram-negative bacteria (*Escherichia coli, Klebsiella pneumoniae, Pasteurella multocida, Pseudomonas aeruginosa, Salmonella* spp., *Yersinia pseudotuberculosis*, other), gram-positive bacteria (*Streptococcus* spp., *Staphylococcus aureus, Mycobacterium, Enterococcus,* other)
   b. Chlamydial: °*Chlamydia psittaci*
   c. Mycoplasma: *Mycoplasma* spp.
   d. Fungal: °*Aspergillus, Cryptococcus*
   e. Viral: °Pacheco's disease, Amazon tracheitis, °reovirus, Newcastle disease, °poxvirus, avian viral serositis form of eastern equine encephalitis, infectious laryngotracheitis, avian influenza
   f. Parasitic: *Cytodites nudus* (air sac mites), °*Sternostoma tracheocolum* (tracheal mites), *Syngamus trachea* (gapeworms), *Knemidokoptes pilae* (scaly face mites), *Sarcocystis falcatula, Cryptosporidium, Toxoplasma, Atoxoplasma*
2. Metabolic: liver disease, kidney disease, heart failure, coagulopathies, anemia, gout, °hemochromatosis
3. Nutritional: malnutrition, °thyroid hyperplasia (goiter), °obesity
4. Toxins: polytetrafluoroethylene (Teflon), zinc, smoke inhalation
5. Physical: °aspiration pneumonia, trauma (ruptured air sac, humoral fracture with ascending infection), °tracheal foreign body, °ascites, °peritonitis
6. Neoplastic
7. Other: conure bleeding syndrome

Signalment

Common causes of dyspnea, tail bobbing, or cyanosis in large psittacines include chlamydiosis, aspergillosis, gram-negative bacterial infections, Pacheco's disease, Amazon tracheitis, obesity, peritonitis, allergy, and poxvirus. Conures,

---

°Common causes.

lovebirds, and gray-cheek parakeets with these signs are commonly ill because of chlamydiosis or gram-negative bacterial infections. Cockatiels and budgies often have chlamydiosis, gram-negative bacterial infections, *Mycoplasma* infection, obesity, tracheal foreign bodies, and egg-related peritonitis. Canaries and finches are often affected by air sac mites, gram-negative and gram-positive bacterial infections, poxvirus, and peritonitis. Mynahs often suffer from hemochromatosis, heart failure, aspergillosis, and bacterial infections. Raptors are often dyspneic as a result of aspergillosis, bacterial infections, or trauma.

Gram-negative bacterial infections, aspiration pneumonia caused by feeding formula, and poxvirus are common causes of dyspnea in young birds. Gapeworms and *Atoxoplasma* primarily affect young birds.

Aspergillosis is common in African gray parrots, but it may cause illness in any type of bird. The cutaneous form of poxvirus is rare except in blue-fronted Amazons, lovebirds, passerines, raptors, and pigeons. Reovirus is commonly reported in imported birds and primarily affects African gray parrots, cockatoos, and other Old World psittacines. Conure bleeding syndrome is a disease of conures. *Enterococcus faecalis* has been associated with chronic tracheal, lung, and air sac infections in canaries. Gapeworm infections are common in gallinaceous birds but can also occur in pet birds. Tracheal mites and air sac mites may affect budgies and cockatiels, but they are a common cause of dyspnea in canaries and Gouldian finches. Mycobacteriosis is most commonly associated with the intestinal tract in psittacines, but it commonly affects the respiratory tract in pigeons, some finches, and some other species. *Atoxoplasma* affects canaries and other passerines, but toxoplasmosis can affect all birds. *Cryptosporidium*-associated respiratory disease occurs in gallinaceous birds and budgies. It affects the gastrointestinal tract and urinary tract in other psittacines and passerines. *Cryptococcus* is a rare fungal infection that can affect many species of birds. Infectious laryngotracheitis affects gallinaceous species and canaries. Avian influenza may cause respiratory signs in gallinaceous birds and waterfowl.

History

A complete history may reveal allergic or nutritional problems, possible exposure to infectious diseases, toxins, or recent trauma. A history of acute dyspnea that started while the bird was eating is consistent with inhalation of a seed. Inhalation of other foreign bodies (e.g., granulomas from vitamin A deficiency or infection) also occurs. Acute dyspnea after overheating of a nonstick surface such as Teflon cookware is consistent with polytetrafluoroethylene gas toxicosis. Tracheal blockage is an emergency (see Physical Examination section below).

Birds recently exposed to other birds are commonly ill as a result of infectious diseases, including bacterial, chlamydial, *Mycoplasma*, viral, and parasitic infections.

Birds recently acquired from a pet store or aviary may be at a higher risk of having been exposed to contagious pathogens. Many birds in this category are also stressed by prior group contact and a change of environment, predisposing them to disease. Knowledge of common diseases in the breeder facility or pet store may provide insight to the possible cause of disease.

Infectious and toxic etiologies are suspected when multiple birds are affected.

Stress may play a role in precipitating clinical signs. Chronic diseases such as chlamydiosis may go undetected until the bird is stressed. Stressful situations for birds include being taken to a new home, the addition of a new bird, being changed to a new cage, a change in diet, or temperature extremes.

Isolated birds and those in closed collections are commonly ill because of nutritional deficiencies, trauma, toxicoses, reproductive problems, neoplasia, allergic disease, or chronic infections such as chlamydiosis and aspergillosis. Some bacterial diseases are also common, especially gram-negative infections.

The diet affects the health of the bird. Diets deficient in vitamin A, such as an all-seed diet, can lead to vitamin A deficiency. Vitamin A deficiency causes squamous metaplasia of mucosal surfaces, increasing susceptibility to respiratory tract infections. Keratin cysts at the glottal opening can cause dyspnea.

Consider the bird's environment. Birds allowed out of their cages are susceptible to trauma and heavy metal toxicosis. Sources of zinc are listed in Chapter 9. *Sarcocystis* occurs most often in outdoor aviaries where birds can come in contact with opossum feces. Cockroaches can serve as transport hosts. Contact with cigarette smoke or other allergen can cause an allergic reaction and dyspnea.

The duration of the illness is important. Note the owner's description of the clinical signs and the course of the disease. Note previous illnesses, including signs, treatment, and response to treatment. A history of worsening of signs while on antibiotics is common with aspergillosis.

Physical Examination

The physical examination may reveal obvious trauma, obesity, vitamin A deficiency, or *Knemidokoptes* lesions. Common findings in birds with dyspnea, tail bobbing, or cyanosis are discussed below.

Severely dyspneic birds must be handled with care. The physical exam and obtaining of diagnostic samples must be done as the condition of the bird allows. Place the bird in a warmed oxygen cage before handling. Oxygen delivered by face mask during the physical examination and during sample collection will increase survival. Severely dyspneic birds that are unaccustomed to being handled should be anesthetized with isoflurane before diagnostic procedures are performed.

Acute dyspnea is an emergency situation. Dyspnea from tracheal blockage by a foreign body, fungal granuloma, or other inhaled material will benefit greatly from placement of an air sac breathing tube. A chronic respiratory condition will not respond to air sac breathing tube placement. A decision to place an air sac breathing tube is made based on history and clinical signs, and the tube is placed before other diagnostics are performed in emergency situations in which tracheal blockage is suspected. The technique is detailed in Chapter 14.

Proliferative growths on the beak, feet, and legs are seen with scaly face mites. Lesions can also occur around the eyes and vent. The proliferative tissue has a characteristic honeycombed appearance. Dyspnea occurs when the proliferative tissue impedes air movement through the nares.

Upper respiratory signs are common in conjunction with lower respiratory disease. Conjunctivitis and nasal discharge are often present with bacterial, chlamydial, *Mycoplasma*, and viral infections.

Nasal discharge is a sign of nasal or sinus disease or may be caused by tracheal, lower respiratory, or systemic disease. When a nasal discharge is present in a dyspneic bird, the nasal discharge is often the result of tracheal or lower respiratory disease.

The choana can become inflamed or contain a discharge caused by viral, yeast, or primary bacterial infections, or it can be secondarily infected because of vitamin A deficiency, neoplasia, or allergies. Granulomas in the mouth are common with vitamin A deficiency. A thick, white oral exudate can be the result of yeast or bacterial infections.

Oral mucous membranes may be cyanotic, indicating lack of oxygenation of the blood. This may be seen with tracheal foreign bodies or diseases affecting the trachea or lower respiratory tract.

Gapeworms may be visualized in the glottal opening. They are large, red helminths. Transillumination of the trachea with a bright light may reveal helminths in the larynx. In passerines, transillumination of the trachea may reveal tracheal or air sac mites. The mites appear as dark, moving, pinhead-sized spots. To improve visualization, wet the feathers over the trachea.

Goiter often causes enough pressure on the esophagus to cause a pendulous crop in affected budgies. Enlarged thyroid glands are intrathoracic and cannot be palpated.

Auscultation of the lungs, air sacs, and heart may reveal abnormal respiratory sounds, cardiac murmur, or arrhythmia.

A distended abdomen may be seen with ascites, egg binding, hepatomegaly, peritonitis, serositis, or large abdominal tumors. Hepatomegaly, common with *Atoxoplasma* infection, may be visualized as a dark mass in the cranial abdomen viewed through the skin in canaries and finches.

Signs of Pacheco's disease include acute onset of anorexia, biliverdinuria, polyuria, diarrhea, and sometimes CNS signs. Sudden death without premonitory signs is common.

Birds with reovirus have a bloody brown nasal discharge, diarrhea, labored breathing, and ataxia.

Signs of Amazon tracheitis include nasal and ocular discharges, dyspnea, and coughing. The disease may be peracute, acute, subacute, or chronic.

Signs of infectious laryngotracheitis in canaries include severe dyspnea, inspiratory wheeze, expectoration of bloody mucus, ocular and nasal discharge, and sinusitis.

Signs of poxvirus vary with the type of poxvirus and species of bird. There are cutaneous and diphtheroid forms. The diphtheroid form is characterized by gray or brown fibrinous lesions in the oropharynx and larynx. Clinical signs include nasal discharge, coughing, and dyspnea. The cutaneous form is characterized by cutaneous proliferative growths or scabs on featherless areas of skin (around eyes, nares, beak, and feet).

Signs of avian influenza in gallinaceous birds and waterfowl include depression, dyspnea, sinusitis, diarrhea, and anorexia. Lethargy, CNS signs, and diarrhea may occur in psittacines infected by avian influenza.

Signs of conure bleeding syndrome include periodic recurrence of bleeding, epistaxis, dyspnea, polyuria, diarrhea, and occasionally ataxia.

Respiratory signs in birds infected with Newcastle disease virus include nasal exudate, cyanosis, and dyspnea.

Clinical signs associated with avian viral serositis include acute death or weight loss, abdominal distention caused by ascitic fluid, and respiratory distress.

Illnesses that may cause gastrointestinal signs in conjunction with dyspnea, tail bobbing, or cyanosis include bacterial infections, chlamydiosis, *Mycoplasma*, aspergillosis, Pacheco's disease, reovirus, Newcastle disease, avian influenza, conure bleeding syndrome, *Cryptosporidium*, *Sarcocystis*, *Atoxoplasma*, goiter, ascites, peritonitis, liver disease, renal disease, hemochromatosis, and zinc toxicosis.

Neurologic signs may accompany dyspnea, tail bobbing, or cyanosis with bacterial infections, chlamydiosis, *Mycoplasma*, Pacheco's disease, aspergillosis, *Cryptococcus*, reovirus, Newcastle disease, *Sarcocystis*, liver disease, and zinc toxicosis.

Algorithm for Dyspnea, Tail Bobbing, or Cyanosis

See Figure 3–5.

Diagnostic Approach for Dyspnea, Tail Bobbing, or Cyanosis

Stabilize severely ill birds before performing stressful diagnostic tests (see Chapter 1). Sample collection and diagnostic tests must be done as the condition of the bird will allow. Place the bird in a warmed oxygen cage before handling. Provide supportive care as needed during the diagnostic evaluation. Oxygen delivered by face mask during diagnostic tests will increase survival. Severely dyspneic birds that are not used to being handled are anesthetized with isoflurane before these procedures. Do not use injectable sedatives.

If severe inspiratory dyspnea is present and an upper airway obstruction is suspected, placement of an air sac canula will allow easier breathing and oxygen administration (see Chapter 14). This is further discussed in the preceding Physical Examination section.

If a dyspneic bird has a distended abdomen, follow the diagnostic approach for the distended abdomen in Chapter 2. Birds do not have a diaphragm; therefore, illnesses causing abdominal distention (e.g., organomegaly, ascites, peritonitis) can affect the respiratory tract.

Consider the signalment, obtain a complete history, and perform a complete physical examination. A sample or skin scraping may reveal parasites or eggs. Fecal flotation or direct smears of pharyngeal mucus in gallinaceous birds and passerines may reveal gapeworm eggs or tracheal or air sac mite eggs. Use fecal flotation to visualize gapeworm eggs or tracheal and air sac mite eggs, and *Atoxoplasma* eggs in the feces of infected birds. Birds infected with *Atoxoplasma* may show clinical signs without shedding oocysts in the feces.

If typical mite lesions are present, a skin scraping sample is placed in oil and examined microscopically for scaly face mites and eggs. Useful samples include scrapings of affected beak, feet, legs, and cloaca.

Allergic disease is suspected by clinical signs and history, e.g., exposure to tobacco smoke or cockatoo feather dust. If allergic disease is suspected and

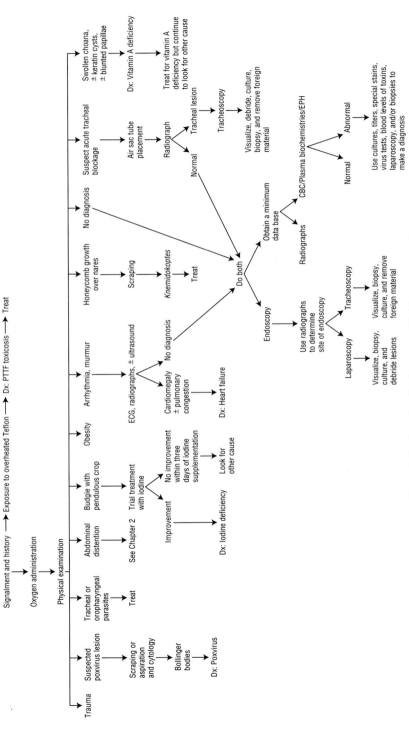

Figure 3–5. Algorithm for dyspnea, tail bobbing, or cyanosis.

cytology of the tracheal wash is not diagnostic, confine the bird to an allergen-free environment for a trial period.

After signalment and history are considered and the physical abnormalities are noted, collection of a minimum database is the next step. The minimum database in a bird with dyspnea includes CBC, plasma biochemistries, and radiographs of the upper and lower respiratory tract. Although these tests may not be diagnostic, they provide important information on the general health of the bird; they may localize lesions, allowing determination of those that need to be visualized endoscopically; and they allow for monitoring of some disease states.

A CBC provides information on the general health of the bird, may support a diagnosis of infectious or systemic disease, and allows monitoring of treatment of some diseases. Changes in the leukogram commonly seen with diseases with dyspnea, tail bobbing, or cyanosis are detailed below.

Leukocytosis may be caused by stress, inflammatory diseases, or neoplasia. Heterophilia can be seen with bacterial, chlamydial, mycoplasma, fungal, and parasitic infections, and with trauma or stress. Differentials to be considered when the WBC count is between 25,000 and 40,000 WBC/μl include *Pseudomonas*, salmonellosis, chlamydiosis, aspergillosis, mycobacteriosis, and peritonitis. Consider chlamydiosis, aspergillosis, mycobacteriosis, and peritonitis as possible causes with WBC counts in excess of 40,000/μl. Many normal young psittacines have a mild heterophilia. Regenerative left shifts are common with chronic or severe bacterial infections (chlamydiosis, mycobacteriosis, *Pseudomonas, Salmonella*), aspergillosis, and neoplasia. Toxic heterophils and monocytosis occur with severe bacterial, chlamydial, viral, and *Aspergillus* infections. Toxic changes include degranulation, vacuolation, increased cytoplasmic basophilia, and nuclear degeneration. Lymphocytosis can be associated with infectious agents. Monocytosis is common with chronic fungal, chlamydial, and bacterial infections (e.g., chlamydiosis, mycobacteriosis) and tissue necrosis. Basophilia may be seen with chlamydiosis. Eosinophilia may be seen with parasitic infections and allergic reactions. Lymphocytosis may be present in canaries and finches with air sac mites.

Leukopenia occurs with overwhelming bacterial and viral infections.

Nonregenerative anemias may be seen with chronic inflammatory diseases such as chlamydiosis, aspergillosis, mycobacteriosis, and neoplasia. Regenerative anemias may be seen with blood loss, coagulopathies, trauma, and neoplasia.

Atoxoplasma intracytoplasmic inclusion bodies may be found in mononuclear cells on blood smears or buffy coat smears. They stain reddish with Giemsa stain.

Plasma biochemistries are rarely diagnostic but are an important part of a minimum database. Useful plasma biochemistries for birds with dyspnea, tail bobbing, or cyanosis include AST, total protein, uric acid, creatinine kinase, glucose, and, if liver disease is suspected, bile acids. Important information obtained will be organ involvement and function, and the tests may support a diagnosis of infectious or systemic disease. Changes in plasma biochemistry test results commonly seen in birds with diseases causing dyspnea, tail bobbing, or cyanosis are detailed below.

Hyperproteinemia may be seen with dehydration and chronic diseases such as chlamydiosis, aspergillosis, and mycobacteriosis. A decrease in total proteins may be seen with trauma, stress, coagulopathies, neoplasia, some chronic diseases, and poor nutrition. Young psittacines often have normal total protein levels lower than those of adults.

An elevation in AST is usually the result of liver or muscle damage. Heart, brain, or kidney damage can also result in an increase in AST, and the AST may be elevated with chlamydiosis, Pacheco's disease, or septicemia. Muscle damage caused by trauma and irritating intramuscular injections also causes an elevation in AST. Creatinine kinase activity increases with muscle damage and may be used to differentiate an increase in AST caused by liver disease resulting from muscle damage.

Hypoglycemia may be seen with liver disease, septicemia, neoplasia, anorexia, aspergillosis, chlamydiosis, or Pacheco's disease.

Radiography is used to visualize tracheal lesions, pulmonary lesions, or systemic disorders in dyspneic birds. Tissue densities in the tracheal lumen such as tumors, parasites, foreign bodies, aspergillosis granulomas, bacterial granulomas, and abscesses may be visualized, but they must be differentiated with endoscopy and biopsy. An enhancement of the normal reticular pattern of the lungs indicates an infiltration, as in pneumonia. Pneumonia is most readily seen in the posterior and mid to lateral aspects of the lungs. A blotchy mottled appearance occurs when the lumen fills with exudate. Obliteration of the normal reticular pattern occurs with pulmonary consolidation (exudate, blood, abscesses, granulomas). Differential diagnoses for pneumonia are numerous, including bacterial, chlamydial, *Mycoplasma*, viral, fungal, and parasitic infections; inhalation of foreign material; heart failure; and toxicoses.

Thickening of the caudal thoracic and abdominal air sac membranes on lateral radiographs and diffuse increased density of these air sac regions on ventrodorsal views indicate airsacculitis. Splenomegaly, hepatomegaly, and airsacculitis are consistent with chlamydiosis (see Chapter 13). Hepatomegaly, splenomegaly, and pulmonary congestion are consistent with *Sarcocystis* infection. Hepatomegaly with pulmonary congestion and consolidation may be seen with toxoplasmosis. Differentials for soft tissue masses in air sac or lung regions include granuloma and neoplasia. Granulomas can result from bacteria, aspergillosis, or foreign bodies. Metastatic neoplasia can be visualized as multiple, variably sized nodules. Differentiation between types of neoplasms and granulomas requires biopsy. Ascites and peritonitis cause an overall loss of organ detail. On the ventrodorsal view, this loss of detail may be difficult to distinguish from hepatomegaly. On the lateral view, ascites and peritonitis will cause loss of detail in the celomic cavity, with the lung, intestinal gas, and grit in the ventriculus often being the only identifiable features.

Plasma protein electrophoresis is useful in detecting and identifying many disease states (e.g., chlamydiosis, aspergillosis, peritonitis, mycobacteriosis, liver disease, kidney disease).

Endoscopy of the celomic cavity (laparoscopy) is the next step unless tracheal pathology is present, based on radiography. Tracheal endoscopy may also be performed and is indicated when there is radiographic evidence of a tracheal lesion. Air sac washes are indicated when there is air sac pathology, and tracheal washes are indicated in birds that are too small to allow tracheoscopy.

Laparoscopy is used to visualize air sacs, lungs, other organs, and abnormalities seen on radiographs. Laparoscopy allows collection of biopsy samples and cultures of air sacs and lungs. Excellent equipment designed for use in birds is available. For the procedure, see Chapter 14. The normal air sac is transparent with little vascularity. The normal lung is pink. Thickened, opaque air sacs with increased vascularity indicates airsacculitis. Granulomas may be visualized, biopsied, debrided, and cultured.

Tracheoscopy (tracheal endoscopy) is used to visualize, biopsy, and culture intratracheal lesions and to visualize and remove tracheal foreign bodies. Tracheal endoscopy is practical in Amazon parrots or larger birds. Bacterial and viral culture samples are collected from the tip of the endoscope after the examination. If a foreign body is suspected based on acute severe inspiratory dyspnea, endoscopy may be performed early in the diagnostic scheme to find and remove a foreign body.

Samples for air sac cytology can be obtained with an air sac wash or swabs. An air sac wash is performed by passing a tube through an endoscopic canula. The air sac is lavaged with sterile saline and is immediately aspirated. A sterile swab can be passed through an endoscope canula or otoscope speculum to obtain a sample. Abnormal cytologic samples may result from bacterial, viral, or fungal infections or inhalation of foreign bodies.

Abnormal tracheal washes may be caused by bacterial, chlamydial, *Mycoplasma*, viral, or fungal infections. Parasite eggs (tracheal and air sac mites and gapeworms) and neoplastic cells also may be found in washes from affected birds. To obtain a tracheal sample, the bird's mouth is held open with a speculum or gauze and a sample is collected at the laryngeal opening. If the bird can withstand anesthesia, tracheal washes can be performed (see Chapter 12). Some unanesthetized birds will tolerate tracheal aspiration with adequate restraint. This sample will be useful for cytology, culture, and sensitivity testing.

More specialized testing is necessary if the diagnosis is still uncertain. Cultures, titers, virus tests, blood zinc levels, and special stains are useful to rule in or out specific diseases. Fungal cultures are useful to help diagnose aspergillosis and can be used in addition to cytology, radiographs, hematology, endoscopy, and biopsy. Useful samples for fungal culture include tracheal wash samples and air sac wash samples. Positive culture of *Aspergillus* without typical lesions is not diagnostic because contamination with this ubiquitous organism often occurs. Samples should be sent to a laboratory familiar with avian aspergillosis. False-negatives occur. Serologic testing is available for raptors and psittacines.

Diagnosis of chlamydiosis can be difficult. No single test or combination of tests can detect *Chlamydia* infection in all infected or carrier birds without false-positive results occurring in some uninfected birds (see Chapter 9). Antigen tests are useful in-house tests in birds showing clinical signs of infection. False-negative results occur. Serology is useful in birds large enough to provide a blood sample adequate for evaluation (cockatiels or larger birds). False-negative results can occur early in the disease before antibody production and in some species of birds (e.g., cockatiels). Low titers may be difficult to interpret. The laboratory performing the test will aid in interpretation of results. Chlamydial cultures of nasal or ocular discharges or feces may provide a diagnosis if shedding of the organism is occurring at the time of sampling. Obtain culture samples before beginning antibiotic therapy. False-negative cultures occur. Plasma protein electrophoresis is useful for chlamydial diagnosis.

Mycobacteriosis may be identified with acid-fast staining. *Mycobacterium* affects the digestive tract in most birds. Feces or liver or intestine biopsy samples may reveal acid-fast organism. Samples from the trachea are useful if the organism is causing a respiratory infection. A negative fecal result does not rule out mycobacteriosis, because the bird must be shedding the organism in high enough numbers to produce a positive result.

Definitive diagnosis of viral infections requires specific viral isolation or cultures. A suspicion of infection is based on signalment, history, and clinical signs. Viral infections usually have multiple signs.

A suspicion of Pacheco's disease is based on history and clinical signs. Antemortem diagnosis is difficult. Intermittent shedding by carrier birds may be detected by virus isolation. Histology (hepatic necrosis, eosinophilic intranuclear inclusion bodies), virus neutralization, ELISA, and immunofluorescence may be useful postmortem.

Cloacal swabs and samples from affected organs may be used for reovirus isolation and culture. Viral antigen may be detected by immunofluorescence in affected tissue.

Pharyngeal swabs are useful for culture of Amazon tracheitis virus.

Intranuclear inclusion bodies may be found in respiratory epithelial cells in birds infected with infectious laryngotracheitis. Virus isolation is required for definitive diagnosis.

A diagnosis of poxvirus is based on clinical signs, cytology, and histopathology of cutaneous lesions, or on culture results. Cytology and histopathology may reveal pathognomonic Bollinger bodies (eosinophilic intracytoplasmic inclusion bodies). Virus culture is required for diagnosis in acute cases lacking lesions.

Feces, tracheal swabs, and nasal discharges are useful for culturing Newcastle disease virus. Serology is useful in some birds; contact a laboratory familiar with Newcastle disease for recommendations.

Swabs from the cloaca and upper respiratory tract may be used for direct virus demonstration from live birds infected with avian influenza. Liver, lung, spleen, and brain are the best postmortem samples for virus isolation.

Anemia, heterophilia, hypoproteinemia, and large numbers of immature erythrocytes are common laboratory findings in birds affected with conure bleeding syndrome. Bone marrow aspirates show erythemic myelosis. Diagnosis is based on history, clinical signs, laboratory findings, and necropsy.

In flock situations, a complete necropsy is important in the control of disease.

Treatment for Dyspnea, Tail Bobbing, or Cyanosis

Place the bird in a warmed oxygen cage. Provide supportive care as needed (see Chapter 1). If severe inspiratory dyspnea is present and an upper airway obstruction is suspected, placement of an air sac canula may relieve dyspnea and allow oxygen administration (see Chapter 14). This is also discussed in the above Physical Examination section.

Once a diagnosis is made, treat the underlying cause.

Selection of antibiotics for treatment of bacterial airsacculitis and pneumonia is based on culture and sensitivity results. Therapy can be initiated with fluoroquinolones (e.g., enrofloxacin), later-generation beta-lactams (e.g., piperacillin, cefotaxime), or trimethoprim-sulfa combinations (e.g., trimethoprim/sulfadiazine, trimethoprim/sulfamethoxazole) until sensitivity can be determined. The route of administration is based on the severity of clinical signs. Use parenteral antibiotics until the bird is stabilized. Nebulization therapy used in conjunction with systemic therapy is often beneficial. Oral or parenteral antibiotics are used to continue treatment. Granulomas must be surgically debrided, in conjunction with administration of systemic antibiotics.

Tracheal foreign bodies are removed using endoscopy, transtracheal flush, or surgical tracheotomy. An air sac breathing tube is placed to provide ventilation and anesthesia. An endoscope can be used to view the foreign body while it is grasped with forceps or removed with suction in birds weighing more than 300 g. A small-gauge needle placed through the trachea distal to the foreign body will prevent further movement. In smaller birds, suction applied to a tube passed blindly to the approximate level of the foreign body is sometimes successful. A transtracheal flush will sometimes dislodge a tracheal foreign body. A needle is passed distal to the foreign body, and sterile saline is infused while holding the bird upside down. Tracheotomy is used if these methods are unsuccessful.

Allergic disease responds to removal of the offending substance, which in some instances may require placing the bird in a new home. The owner should limit smoking to outdoors and wash hands and arms before contact with the bird. Symptomatic therapy using an antihistamine or bronchodilator may be effective.

Management of viral infections includes symptomatic therapy and prevention of secondary bacterial infection and contagion. Isolate ill birds. Antibiotics may be useful for prevention and treatment of secondary bacterial infections. Chlorhexidine in the drinking water may decrease spread to other birds. Acyclovir may be useful in herpesvirus (Pacheco's disease) infections. Conure hemorrhagic syndrome sometimes responds to calcium supplementation. Newcastle disease is a reportable disease. There are no effective treatments.

References and Additional Readings

Bauck L. Rhinitis: Case reports. *Proc Assoc Avian Vet* 1992;134–139.

Baumgartner R, Hoop RK, Widmer R. Atypical nocardiosis in a red-lored Amazon parrot. *J Assoc Avian Vet* 1994;8(3):125–127.

Bennett RA. Thoracic surgery and biopsy. *Proc Assoc Avian Vet* 1995;297–299.

Brown PA, Newman JA. Diagnosis of avian chlamydiosis: Questions, answers, questions. *Proc Assoc Avian Vet* 1992;42–47.

Brown PA, Redig PT. Aspergillus ELISA: A tool for detection and management. *Proc Assoc Avian Vet* 1994;295–300.

Campbell TW. *Avian Hematology and Cytology*, ed 2. Ames, Iowa, Iowa State University Press, 1995.

Campbell TW. Cytology in avian diagnostics. In Kirk RW (ed): *Current Veterinary Therapy IX, Small Animal Practice*. Philadelphia, WB Saunders, 1986, pp 725–731.

Clubb SL. Viscerotropic velogenic newcastle disease in pet birds. In Kirk RW (ed): *Current Veterinary Therapy VIII, Small Animal Practice*. Philadelphia, WB Saunders, 1983, pp 628–630.

Cray C, Bossart G, Harris D. Plasma protein electrophoresis: Principles and diagnosis of infectious disease. *Proc Assoc Avian Vet* 1995;55–59.

Cross GM. Newcastle disease. *Vet Clin North Am Small Anim Pract* 1991;21(6):1231–1239.

Dustin LR. Surgery of the avian respiratory system. *Sem Avian Exot Pet Med* 1993;2(2):83–90.

Flammer K. An overview of antifungal therapy in birds. *Proc Assoc Avian Vet* 1993;1–4.

Flammer K. An update on the diagnosis and treatment of avian chlamydiosis. In Kirk RW, Bonagura JD (eds): *Current Veterinary Therapy XI, Small Animal Practice*. Philadelphia, WB Saunders, 1992, pp 1150–1153.

Flammer K. Avian chlamydiosis. *Proc N Am Vet Conf* 1994;787–788.

Flammer K. Oropharyngeal diseases in caged birds. In Kirk RW (ed): *Current Veterinary Therapy IX, Small Animal Practice*. Philadelphia, WB Saunders, 1986, pp 699–702.

Flammer K. The biology of avian chlamydiosis: Know the enemy! *Proc Assoc Avian Vet* 1992;412–419.

Fudge AM. Clinical observations with avian chlamydial infections. *Proc Assoc Avian Vet* 1992;48–58.

Fudge AM, Reavill DR, Rosskopf WJ. Diagnosis and management of avian dyspnea: A review. *Proc Assoc Avian Vet* 1993;187–195.

Galvin C. Acute hemorrhagic syndrome of birds. In Kirk RW (ed): *Current Veterinary Therapy VIII, Small Animal Practice*. Philadelphia, WB Saunders, 1983, pp 617–619.

Greenacre CB, Watson E, Ritchie BW. Choanal atresia in an African grey parrot (*Psittacus erithacus*) and an umbrella cockatoo (*Cacatua alba*). *J Assoc Avian Vet* 1993;7(1):19–22.

Grimes JE. Elementary body agglutination: A rapid clinical diagnostic aid for avian chlamydiosis. *Proc Assoc Avian Vet* 1993;30–40.

Grimes JE. Evaluation and interpretation of serologic responses in psittacine bird chlamydiosis and suggested complementary diagnostic procedures. *J Avian Med Surg* 1996;10(2):75–83.

Kennedy-Stoskopf S. Avian pox in caged birds. In Kirk RW (ed): *Current Veterinary Therapy VIII, Small Animal Practice*. Philadelphia, WB Saunders, 1983, pp 628–630.

King AS, McLelland J. *Birds: Their Structure and Function*, ed 2. Philadelphia, WB Saunders, 1983.

LaBonde J. Obesity in pet birds: The medical problems and management of the avian patient. *Proc Assoc Avian Vet* 1992;72–77.

Ley DH, Flammer K, Cowen P, et al. Performance characteristics of diagnostic tests for avian chlamydiosis. *J Assoc Avian Vet* 1993;7(4):203–207.

McMillan MC. Aspergillosis in pet birds: A review of 45 cases. *Proc Assoc Avian Vet* 1988;35.

McMillan JC, Petrak ML. Retrospective study of aspergillosis in pet birds. *J Assoc Avian Vet* 1989;3(4):211–215.

Miller MS. Avian cardiology. *Proc N Am Vet Conf* 1993;706–708.

Morris PJ, Avgeris SE, Baumgartner RE. Hemochromatosis in a greater Indian hill mynah (*Gracula religiosa*): Case report and review of the literature. *J Assoc Avian Vet* 1989;3(2):87–92.

Murphy J. Psittacine fatty liver syndrome. *Proc Assoc Avian Vet* 1992;78–82.

Nye RR. Avian respiratory system. In Birchard SJ, Sherdig RG (eds): *Saunders Manual of Small Animal Practice*. Philadelphia, WB Saunders, 1994, pp 1282–1289.

Olsen GH. Avian respiratory system disorders. *Proc Assoc Avian Vet* 1989;433–435.

Orosz SE. Fungal and mycobacterial diseases. *Proc N Am Vet Conf* 1994;569–570.

Orosz SE. Respiratory system: Anatomy, physiology and disease response. *Proc N Am Vet Conf* 1994;804.

Paul-Murphy J. Avian respiratory system (with emphasis on cage bird species). *Proc Assoc Avian Vet* 1992;398–411.

Pitts C. Hypovitaminosis A in psittacines. In Kirk RW (ed): *Current Veterinary Therapy VIII, Small Animal Practice*. Philadelphia, WB Saunders, 1983, pp 622–625.

Quesenberry K. Avian respiratory disease. *Proc N Am Vet Conf* 1992;653–654.

Rae MA, Rosskopf WJ. Mycobacteriosis in passerines. *Proc Assoc Avian Vet* 1992;234–243.

Redig PL. Aspergillosis. In Kirk RW (ed): *Current Veterinary Therapy VIII, Small Animal Practice*. Philadelphia, WB Saunders, 1983, pp 611–613.

Redig PT. Avian aspergillosis. In Fowler ME (ed): *Zoo and Wild Animal Medicine, Current Therapy 3.* Philadelphia, WB Saunders, 1993, pp 178–181.

Ritchie BW, Harrison GJ, Harrison LR (eds): *Avian Medicine: Principles and Application.* Lake Worth, FL, Wingers Publishing, 1994.

Rosenthal K, Stamoulis M. Diagnosis of congestive heart failure in an Indian hill mynah bird (*Gracula religiosa*). *J Assoc Avian Vet* 1993;7(1):27–30.

Rosskopf WJ. Abdominal air sac breathing tube placement in psittacines and raptors: Its use as an emergency airway in cases of tracheal obstruction. *Proc Assoc Avian Vet* 1990;215–217.

Rosskopf WJ, Woerpel RW: Successful treatment of avian tuberculosis in pet psittacines. *Proc Assoc Avian Vet* 1991;238–251.

Rosskopf WJ, Woerpel RW, Fudge AM, et al. Iron storage disease (hemochromatosis) in a citron-crested cockatoo and other psittacine species. *Proc Assoc Avian Vet* 1992;98–107.

Spink RR. Aerosol therapy. In Harrison GJ, Harrison Lr (eds): *Clinical Avian Medicine and Surgery.* Philadelphia, WB Saunders, 1986, pp 376–379.

Tully TN. Avian respiratory diseases: Clinical overview. *J Avian Med Surg* 1995;9(3):162–174.

Tully TN, Harrison GJ. Pneumonology. In Ritchie BW, Harrison GJ, Harrison LR (eds): *Avian Medicine: Principles and Application.* Lake Worth, FL, Wingers Publishing, 1994, pp 556–581.

Tully TN, Carter JD. Bilateral supraorbital abscesses associated with sinusitis in an orange-winged Amazon parrot (*Amazona amazonica*). *J Assoc Avian Vet* 1993;7(3):157–158.

VanDerHeyden N. Aspergillosis in psittacine chicks. *Proc Assoc Avian Vet* 1993;207–212.

VanDerHeyden N. Evaluation and interpretation of the avian hemogram. *Sem Avian Exot Pet Med* 1994;3(1):5–24.

Westerhof I. Treatment of tracheal obstruction in psittacine birds using a suction technique: A retrospective study of 19 birds. *J Avian Med Surg* 1995;9(1):45–49.

Worell AB. Further investigations in rhamphastids concerning hemochromatosis. *Proc Assoc Avian Vet* 1993;98–107.

Chapter 4

Gastrointestinal Signs

Gastrointestinal signs are a common presenting complaint in pet bird practice. One or more signs may be present. Emaciation is often present with chronic diseases. Common gastrointestinal signs are listed in Table 4–1. Anorexia is discussed in Chapter 2. Infectious and toxic causes are most common, but metabolic, physical, and other problems also cause gastrointestinal signs.

This chapter presents a diagnostic approach for gastrointestinal signs commonly seen in pet birds. The chapter is divided by common gastrointestinal signs. Each section begins with general information and definitions of terms, followed by a list of differential diagnoses. This is followed by appropriate signalment information. Common causes of the clinical sign are presented for each group of pet birds. Use the history section to explore important historical information that may narrow differential diagnoses. The physical examination section guides interpretation of the physical findings occurring with the clinical signs of that section. If other abnormalities are noted, consult appropriate chapters to assist in making a diagnosis. An algorithm is included in each section to provide a quick reference for recommended tests and interpretation of tests. The diagnostic plan suggests useful tests. Consult Chapter 12 for techniques of sample collection and for assistance with test interpretation. General treatments conclude each section of signs. Specific treatments are found in Chapter 9. Consult the formulary in Chapter 17 for drug dosages. This chapter concludes with additional readings and references, which can be consulted for further information.

VOMITING OR REGURGITATION

Regurgitation is the expulsion of ingesta from the crop. It may be a normal physiologic process (e.g., courtship behavior, weaning) or it may be pathologic.

TABLE 4–1 Gastrointestinal Signs

Anorexia	Abnormal droppings
Regurgitation	Polyuria
Vomiting	Abnormal color of urates
Oral lesions	Diarrhea
Crop abnormalities	Blood in droppings
Emaciation	Undigested food in droppings
Wasting	

Vomiting is the expulsion of ingesta from the proventriculus and is associated with illness. Depression and dehydration commonly accompany vomiting. Vomiting or regurgitation may occur alone or in conjunction with other gastrointestinal signs (e.g., diarrhea) or systemic illness.

Signs associated with regurgitation or vomiting include food on the feathers of the face, or partially digested food may be found on the floor, perches, or walls of the cage.

Differential Diagnoses for Vomiting or Regurgitation

1. Infectious
   a. Bacterial: °gram-negative bacteria, gram-positive bacteria (°megabacteria, other)
   b. Fungal: °*Candida, Aspergillus*
   c. Viral: avian viral serositis form of eastern equine encephalitis, inclusion body hepatitis in pigeons (pigeon herpesvirus), Pacheco's disease, polyomavirus, poxvirus
   d. Parasitic: *Capillaria, Plasmodium,* °tapeworms, °*Trichomonas*
   e. Other (probably viral): °proventricular dilatation syndrome (PDS, psittacine dilatation syndrome, macaw wasting disease, neurotropic gastric dilatation, NGD)
2. Metabolic: °goiter, heart failure, °liver disease, kidney disease, pancreatitis, egg binding, °peritonitis, ileus, electrolyte imbalance
3. Nutritional: high protein diet
4. Toxic: arsenic, carbamate, chocolate, cholecalciferol, copper, organochlorine (lindane), organophosphate, °lead, nicotine, nitrate, phosphorus, rotenone, rubbing alcohol, salt, thallium, °zinc, plants (philodendron, rhododendron, Solanaceae, yew)
5. Physical: crop/ventricular/intestinal impaction, °foreign body, ascites, overheated or underheated formula, improper formula consistency, °overfeeding, aerophagia, °cast formation, °goiter, intussusception, volvulus, stricture of gastrointestinal tract, stenosis, hernia
6. Trauma: crop burn
7. Allergic: food
8. Behavioral: excitement, stress, °courtship behavior, °normal weaning behavior, crop milk feeding in pigeons
9. Neoplastic: papilloma, other
10. Iatrogenic: °doxycycline, fenbendazole, fluconazole, itraconazole, ketoconazole, levamisole, polymyxin B, praziquantel, °trimethoprim/sulfadiazine
11. Other: motion sickness

Signalment

Common causes of vomiting or regurgitation in Amazon parrots include gram-negative bacterial infection, liver disease (lipidosis, mycotoxicosis, hepatitis), lead

---

°Common causes.

and zinc toxicoses, and doxycycline and other medications. Common causes in African gray parrots include gram-negative bacterial infection, tapeworms, and lead and zinc toxicoses. Vomiting or regurgitation is often the result of gram-negative bacterial infection, PDS, lead or zinc toxicosis, doxycycline, trimethoprim/sulfadiazine, or a behavioral response in macaws. Cockatoos often regurgitate or begin vomiting as a result of gram-negative bacterial infection, tapeworms, or lead or zinc toxicosis. Common causes of vomiting or regurgitation in smaller psittacines include gram-negative bacterial infections, giardiasis, megabacterial infection, trichomoniasis, and candidiasis. Also consider neoplasia, hepatic disease, and goiter in budgies. Canaries and finches often regurgitate or vomit as a result of bacterial infections, megabacterial infections, egg binding, and trichomoniasis. Bacterial infections, liver disease (hemochromatosis, cirrhosis, hepatitis), and heart failure are common causes of vomiting in mynahs and toucans. Pigeons vomit or regurgitate most commonly as a result of trichomoniasis or crop milk feeding. Common causes of vomiting or regurgitation in raptors include normal cast formation, trichomoniasis, and bacterial infections.

Common causes of vomiting and regurgitation in young birds being hand fed, fledglings, and recently weaned birds include candidiasis, gram-negative bacterial infections, crop burns, crop foreign bodies, overheated or underheated formula, excessively thin formula, overfeeding, and weaning. Crop and gastrointestinal *Candida* and gram-negative bacterial infections are very common in birds being hand fed.

Polyomavirus and Pacheco's disease affect psittacines. Birds that recover from Pacheco's disease may become carriers. Patagonian and Nanday conures are common asymptomatic carriers of the virus causing Pacheco's disease.

Trichomoniasis occurs in passerines, psittacines, pigeons, and raptors. Tapeworm infections are most common in imported African gray parrots, cockatoos, finches, and eclectus parrots. *Capillaria* infections are most common in budgies, macaws, canaries, pigeons, and gallinaceous birds.

History

Isolated birds and those in closed collections are commonly ill because of toxicoses, reproductive disorders, nutritional imbalances, neoplasia, or management-related disorders. Gram-negative bacterial infections, candidiasis, chronic diseases (e.g., PDS), and those diseases with carrier states (e.g., Pacheco's disease) are also seen.

Birds recently exposed to other birds are commonly ill as a result of infectious diseases, including bacterial, viral, and parasitic diseases. This is the result of stress and exposure to infectious disease. Illnesses occurring in isolated birds also occur in group situations.

Infectious and toxic etiologies are suspected when multiple birds are affected.

Significant dietary history for a vomiting or regurgitating bird includes the type of diet, freshness, and any change in type of food or treats. In chicks being hand fed, crop burns, candidiasis, and gram-negative bacterial infections are common. Overheated, underheated, or excessively thin formula may cause vomiting in hand-fed birds. Excessive or even normal iron content in the diet may be a factor in the development of hemochromatosis in mynahs or toucans. High-protein diets can cause vomiting in cockatiels. High-fat diets (e.g., seed diets) and unbalanced diets (biotin, choline, methionine deficient) may cause hepatic lipidosis.

Mycotoxins may be present in moldy food and may be present even after signs of the mold have disappeared. Ingestion of a toxic dose of mycotoxin can result in death in a few days. Chronic exposure can cause liver disease and death.

Grit impaction may occur when grit is offered free choice.

Important environmental factors in a vomiting or regurgitating bird include access to potential toxins, sanitation, and exposure to wild birds or disease vectors. In chicks, ingestion of the nest substrate may lead to impaction, especially corncob. Toxins that may cause vomiting are listed in the differential diagnoses. Some sources of lead are listed in Table 9–3. Sources of zinc include pennies minted since 1982, Monopoly game pieces, and galvanized materials. Nitrates are found in fertilizers, and the pellets may be mistaken for food by birds. Ornamental dough and sea sand used for grit or nesting substrate are common sources of salt ingested by birds, leading to salt toxicosis. A history of doxycycline, ketoconazole, itraconazole, fluconazole, levamisole, amphotericin B, polymyxin B, or trimethoprim/sulfadiazine is consistent with an iatrogenic cause of vomiting.

Poxvirus is transmitted by mosquitoes and other biting arthropods; therefore, poxvirus infection is more common in outside aviaries. Parasitic infections are most common in recently imported birds, birds that have access to the ground, and birds exposed to wild birds, wild bird feces, rodents, and other parasite vectors. Tapeworms are most common in imported birds. Trichomoniasis is commonly transmitted through ingestion of contaminated food or water or parental feeding of young chicks.

Egg laying or nesting behavior before the onset of vomiting can be consistent with egg binding or peritonitis.

The duration of the illness is important. Note the owner's description of the clinical signs and the course of the disease. Note previous illnesses, including signs, treatment, and response to treatment.

Physical Examination

A complete physical examination may reveal oral lesions (plaques, ulcers, granulomas, papilloma), poxvirus lesions, crop burn or trauma, crop impaction, or crop foreign body as the cause of vomiting or regurgitation. Clinical signs that may occur concurrently with vomiting or regurgitation include weight loss, distended abdomen, other gastrointestinal signs (abnormal droppings, tenesmus, crop abnormalities), respiratory signs, neurologic signs, or abdominal swellings. If abnormalities are present, see the appropriate chapter for additional assistance with making a diagnosis.

Vomiting and neurologic signs may occur with Pacheco's disease, polyomavirus, PDS, liver disease, kidney disease, and peritonitis and with mycotoxin, insecticide, salt, lead, and zinc toxicoses.

Respiratory signs and vomiting may occur with bacterial infections, aspergillosis, avian viral serositis, Pacheco's disease, poxvirus, ascites, goiter, egg binding, peritonitis, zinc toxicosis, and heart, liver, and kidney disease.

Algorithm for Vomiting or Regurgitation

See Figure 4–1.

Diagnostic Plan for Vomiting or Regurgitation

Stabilize severely ill birds before performing stressful diagnostic tests, and provide supportive care as needed (see Chapter 1).

Selection of appropriate diagnostic tests is based on consideration of the signalment and history of the bird and the findings of the physical examination and evaluation of the droppings.

The most useful initial diagnostic tests are a wet-mount and Gram's stain of a crop aspirate or wash. Submit a sample of the aspirate or wash for bacterial culture and sensitivity testing and fungal culture. A wet-mount of crop contents may reveal trichomoniasis or candidiasis. Gram-negative bacterial, megabacterial, and *Candida* infections may be identified with Gram's staining. Flotation of feces and crop aspirate samples are useful for identification of intestinal parasites. Hematology and biochemistry tests are important in the diagnosis of infectious, metabolic, inflammatory, and some toxic diseases. Perform a complete blood count (CBC) and biochemistry tests when systemic disease is suspected, when a bird is unresponsive to treatment, or to help determine the general health of the bird. Useful biochemistry tests for vomiting birds include aspartate aminotransferase (AST or SGOT), uric acid, creatinine kinase (CK), total protein, calcium, amylase, and lipase. Measure bile acids if liver disease is suspected. Plasma protein electrophoresis (EPH) is useful in identifying many diseases (e.g., chlamydiosis, aspergillosis, mycobacteriosis, peritonitis, liver disease, and renal disease). Radiology is useful for diagnosis of lead and zinc toxicoses, grit impaction, enteritis, crop calculi and foreign bodies, and trauma. Radiographs can provide information on liver and proventriculus size and allow evaluation of the respiratory tract and abdominal organs. Lead and zinc toxicoses can occur without radiographic signs. Titers, cultures, special stains, virus tests, cholinesterase assays, and lead and zinc blood levels are used to rule in or out specific diseases.

Treatment for Vomiting or Regurgitation

Treat the underlying cause. Provide supportive care while treating the cause of vomiting. Withhold food until clinical signs of vomiting have been controlled. Dehydration is common with vomiting, and fluids are replaced intravenously or intraosseously. Alert and active birds may be rehydrated with subcutaneous fluids.

To remove a crop foreign body, the bird is anesthetized and an endotracheal tube is placed. Alligator forceps are carefully passed into the crop. The foreign body is held in one hand through the skin and grasped with the forceps. Take care to avoid damaging the crop. The foreign body is then withdrawn through the mouth. Large foreign bodies and calculi may require an ingluvotomy (see Chapter 14).

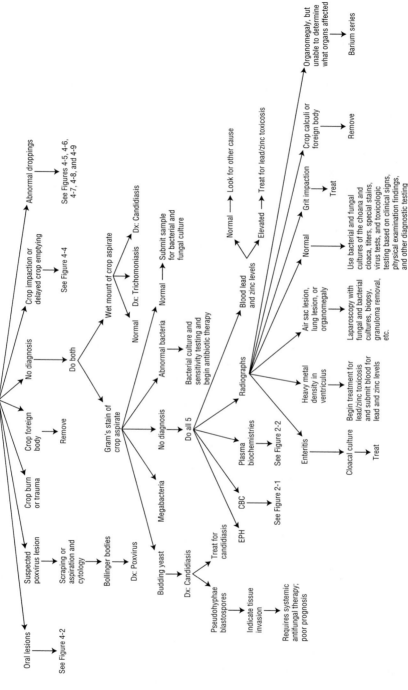

Figure 4–1. Algorithm for vomiting or regurgitation.

OROPHARYNGEAL LESIONS

The oral cavity and the pharynx are combined in birds to form the oropharynx. The oropharynx communicates with the sinuses through the median fissure in the palate called the choana. There are numerous caudally directed papillae associated with the choana. The glottis is located directly behind the tongue, and birds do not have an epiglottis.

The psittacine tongue is muscular, blunt, and dexterous. Most passerines have a narrow and triangular tongue. The oropharynx is lined with stratified squamous epithelium that is keratinized in areas subject to abrasion (e.g., papillae). There are numerous mucus-secreting salivary glands in the lining of the oropharynx. These glands may undergo squamous metaplasia with vitamin A deficiency, leading to keratin- and debris-filled cysts that may become infected.

Oropharyngeal lesions are common in pet birds. Clinical signs associated with abnormalities of the oropharynx include swellings, growths, abscesses, granulomas, ulcers, diphtheritic membranes, and discharges. Neurologic abnormalities such as the inability to swallow or move the tongue or jaw are discussed in Chapter 6.

Differential Diagnoses for Oropharyngeal Lesions

1. Infectious
   a. Bacterial: gram-negative bacteria, gram-positive bacteria (*Mycobacterium*, other)
   b. Viral: *poxvirus, duck viral enteritis (duck plague), owl herpesvirus, pigeon herpesvirus
   c. Fungal: *Candida*
   d. Parasitic: *Trichomonas, Capillaria*
2. Nutritional: *vitamin A deficiency
3. Toxic: trichothecenes (T_2 toxin)
4. Physical: trauma, foreign bodies, irritating substances (hot foods, silver nitrate sticks)
5. Neoplastic: *papilloma, other
6. Other: pigeon sialolith

Signalment

Common causes of lesions of the oropharynx in large psittacines include vitamin A deficiency, papillomas, and abscesses. Cockatiels and budgies are commonly affected by candidiasis, trichomoniasis, and vitamin A deficiency. Common causes of oropharyngeal lesions in small passerines include hyperkeratosis of the tongue and poxvirus. Trichomoniasis, candidiasis, and poxvirus are common causes of oropharyngeal lesions in raptors. Pigeons commonly have oropharyngeal lesions as a result of trichomoniasis and poxvirus.

---

*Common causes.

Young hand-fed birds, fledglings, and recently weaned birds commonly have oropharyngeal lesions as a result of candidiasis, poxvirus, or trauma. Gram-negative bacterial infections are also common.

Trichomoniasis is most common in pigeons (canker) and raptors (frounce), but it also occurs in passerines (especially canaries and zebra finches) and psittacines (especially budgies and cockatiels). *Capillaria* infections are most common in budgies, macaws, canaries, pigeons, and gallinaceous birds.

History

Isolated birds and those in closed collections are commonly ill because of nutritional deficiencies, candidiasis, trauma, oropharyngeal foreign bodies, neoplasia, and management-related and chronic debilitating diseases. Chronic diseases (e.g., mycobacteriosis, aspergillosis, psittacine beak and feather disease [PBFD]) and gram-negative bacterial infections are also seen.

Birds recently exposed to other birds are commonly ill as a result of infectious diseases, including bacterial, viral, and parasitic diseases. This is the result of stress and exposure to infectious disease. Illnesses occurring in isolated birds also occur in group situations.

Infectious and toxic etiologies are suspected when multiple birds are affected.

Significant dietary history for a bird with oropharyngeal lesions includes type of diet, freshness, vitamin supplementation, and hand-feeding techniques. Diets deficient in vitamin A, such as an all-seed diet, can lead to vitamin A deficiency. Vitamin A deficiency causes squamous metaplasia of mucosal surfaces and metaplasia of the salivary glands.

T_2 toxin can cause ulcerative lesions in the mouth. Grains heavily damaged by insects may have a higher incidence of the presence of this toxin.

Hand-fed birds are often affected by trauma associated with feeding practices, excessively hot formula, candidiasis, and bacterial infections associated with poor hygiene.

Consider the bird's environment. Poxvirus is transmitted by mosquitoes and other biting arthropods; therefore, poxvirus infection is more common in outside aviaries. *Capillaria* eggs require approximately 2 weeks to embryonate and become infectious. Because they can remain infectious in the environment for several months, poor sanitation increases spread and exposure. Overcrowding and poor hygiene may increase the incidence of trichomoniasis in flocks.

The duration of the illness is important. Note the owner's description of the clinical signs and the course of the disease. Note previous illnesses, including signs, treatment, and response to treatment.

Physical Examination

A complete physical examination may reveal trauma, poxvirus lesions, vitamin A deficiency lesions, oropharyngeal foreign bodies, or papillomas. Common findings in birds with oropharyngeal lesions are discussed below.

Stomatitis may be the result of ingestion of hot food, silver nitrate, or T_2 toxin. The choana can become inflamed or contain a discharge caused by viral, yeast, or primary bacterial infections, or it may be secondarily infected because of vitamin A deficiency, neoplasia, or allergies. A thick, white oral exudate can be the result of yeast or bacterial infections.

Oropharyngeal ulcers may be associated with candidiasis, PBFD, *Capillaria*, T_2 toxin, or duck viral enteritis. Diphtheritic membranes may be the result of infection with poxvirus, pigeon herpesvirus, duck viral enteritis, trichomoniasis, candidiasis, or *Capillaria*.

Clinical signs associated with candidiasis include focal areas of thickened oral mucosa with a mucoid exudate. Diphtheritic membranes or white caseated plugs may form with severe infections. Anorexia, weight loss, and vomiting may occur. Hand-fed baby birds may show a poor feeding response.

T_2 toxin can cause ulceration of the oropharyngeal mucosa with yellow erosive and exudative plaques. Crusts of exudate can accumulate along the anterior margin of the beak.

Diphtheritic lesions may occur in the oropharynx as a result of *Capillaria* infection. This parasite may also cause hemorrhagic inflammation in the commissure of the beak. This tiny, threadlike nematode may be found embedded in the associated exudate.

Clinical signs of duck viral enteritis include oropharyngeal ulcers, depression, hematochezia, photophobia, and epiphora.

Cutaneous or diphtheritic pox lesions may be seen on physical examination. The diphtheroid form is characterized by gray or brown fibrinonecrotic lesions in the oropharynx. The cutaneous form is characterized by cutaneous proliferative growths on featherless areas of skin (around eyes, nares, beak, feet, and vent).

Diphtheritic membranes may also be associated with pigeon herpesvirus infection (Smadel's disease). Other clinical signs include dyspnea, conjunctivitis, and rhinitis, with a mucopurulent discharge from the eyes and nostrils.

Clinical signs of trichomoniasis include white caseous plaques, proliferative necrotic lesions, or ulcerative lesions in the mouth, esophagus, and crop; depression, vomiting, and diarrhea also may occur.

Granulomas in the mouth are common with vitamin A deficiency, but they may also result from foreign bodies, mycobacteriosis, or bacterial infections.

Vitamin A deficiency causes squamous metaplasia of mucous membranes. On physical examination, this is evidenced by swollen margins of the choana in the roof of the mouth. Associated papillae may be blunted or absent, and sterile granulomas of the oral or lingual mucosa may be present. These granulomas may become secondarily infected.

Clinical signs associated with owl herpesvirus infection include yellowish, 1- to 2-mm nodules on the pharyngeal mucosa, depression, anorexia, and weakness.

Sialoliths in pigeons are white lesions occurring on the palate. They contain a proteinaceous substrate and cellular debris.

Papillomas are proliferative growths that may occur in the oral cavity, cloaca, gastrointestinal tract, or on unfeathered skin. Lesions are wartlike proliferations. They occur as single or multiple slow-growing masses.

Psittacine beak and feather disease can cause oral ulceration and necrosis of the mucosa in the dorsum of the mouth. The beak may become elongated and may contain fractures. Abnormal feathers may be present, including short, clubbed, deformed, or curled feathers, retained feather sheaths, circumferential constrictions, or hemorrhage within the pulp cavity. Nails may become fractured, necrotic, or deformed, or slough.

Oropharyngeal lesions may occur in conjunction with respiratory signs with bacterial infections, poxvirus, candidiasis, trichomoniasis, duck viral enteritis, pigeon herpesvirus, and PBFD.

Neurologic signs and oral lesions may occur with duck viral enteritis and pigeon herpesvirus.

Dermatologic abnormalities may occur with oropharyngeal lesions with PBFD and trichothecene toxin.

Algorithm for Oropharyngeal Lesions

See Figure 4–2.

Diagnostic Plan for Oropharyngeal Lesions

Stabilize severely ill birds before performing stressful diagnostic tests, and provide supportive care as needed (see Chapter 1).

Selection of appropriate diagnostic tests is based on consideration of the signalment and history of the bird and the findings of the physical examination and evaluation of the droppings.

The most useful initial diagnostic test is cytologic evaluation of a scraping or aspirate of the lesion. Cytologic evaluation of scrapings of ulcerative, proliferative, or diphtheritic lesions may reveal candidiasis, trichomoniasis, or bacterial infection. Hyperkeratosis and hyperplasia indicate vitamin A deficiency. Bollinger bodies are associated with poxvirus infection. Bacterial cultures and sensitivity are used to detect primary or secondary bacterial infections. A Gram's stain of a smear from a scraping or aspiration from the lesion may reveal budding yeast, pseudohyphae, blastophores, or gram-negative bacteria. A saline wet mount of crop wash or esophageal smear is best for detection of trichomoniasis and may be used to detect *Capillaria* eggs. Application of an acetic acid solution (apple cider vinegar) to a suspected papilloma will cause papillomatous tissue to blanch to white from the pink or red original color. Biopsy of proliferative lesions may reveal papillomas, other neoplasms, vitamin A deficiency, abscesses, poxvirus lesions, and sialoliths. Acid-fast stains are used to detect *Mycobacterium* in exudate from mycobacterial granulomas. Virus tests are used to identify suspected viral infections. Radiology may be useful for diagnosis of a foreign body lodged in the oral mucosa.

Treatment for Oropharyngeal Lesions

Treat the underlying cause. Tube feed the bird if the bird is not eating on its own. Provide other supportive care as needed. If dehydration is present, administer intravenous, intraosseous, or subcutaneous fluids.

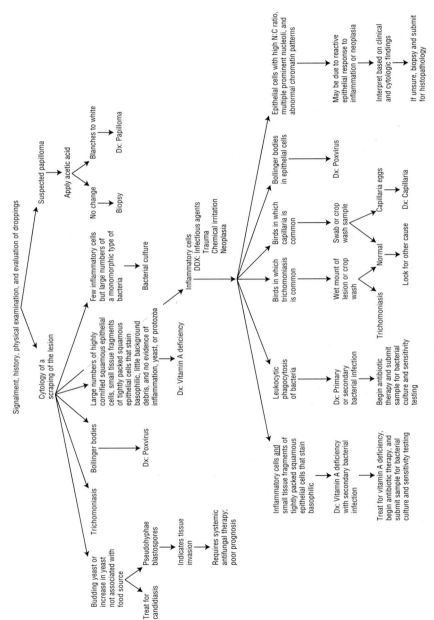

Figure 4–2. Algorithm for oral lesions.

ESOPHAGEAL OR CROP DISORDERS

Disorders of the crop are common in pet birds. Clinical signs that may occur with esophageal or crop disorders include delayed crop emptying, crop stasis, vomiting, regurgitation, dysphagia, and anorexia. Delayed crop emptying occurs when an enlarged crop empties more slowly than normal. Crop stasis occurs when an enlarged crop fails to empty. Crop stasis in chicks is often referred to as sour crop. Any disease or illness that causes a severely debilitated state has the potential to cause crop stasis.

The esophagus courses down the right side of the neck in birds. It is thin walled and distensible. The crop (ingluvies) is a dilatation of the esophagus just cranial to the thoracic inlet that occurs in many species of birds. It is prominent in psittacines, pigeons, and doves and smaller in passerines and most raptors. Toucans and owls lack crops. The crops of young birds are much larger than those in adult birds.

Differential Diagnosis for Esophageal or Crop Disorders

1. Infectious
   a. Bacterial: °gram-negative bacteria, gram-positive bacteria (megabacteria, others)
   b. Viral: avian viral serositis form of eastern equine encephalitis, °polyomavirus, PBFD
   c. Fungal: °*Candida*
   d. Parasitic: °*Trichomonas, Capillaria, Cryptosporidium*
   e. Unclassified: °proventricular dilatation syndrome (PDS)
2. Nutritional: high-fiber diet, excessive fat in diet, excessive protein in diet, °foreign material ingestion, excessive grit consumption, °infrequent feeding of large amounts, vitamin E/selenium deficiency, hypervitaminosis D
3. Toxic: °lead, zinc, organophosphate, carbamate
4. Physical: ingluvioliths (crop calculi), °overheated or underheated formula, °improper consistency of formula, °overfeeding, aerophagia, °foreign body, goiter, °cold environment, callus formation after a coracoid fracture
5. Trauma: °crop burn, °crop laceration
6. Behavioral: fear, excitement
7. Neoplastic: papilloma, other
8. Iatrogenic: °feeding tube trauma/laceration
9. Other: dehydration, paralytic ileus

Signalment

Common causes of disorders of the crop or esophagus in adult large psittacines include polyomavirus, PDS, lead toxicosis, and bacterial infections. Cockatiels are commonly affected by candidiasis, gram-negative bacterial infections, and

---

°Common causes.

lead toxicosis. Esophagus and crop disorders are commonly associated with candidiasis, trichomoniasis, goiter, and gram-negative bacterial infections in budgies. Common causes of esophageal or crop lesions in raptors include trichomoniasis, trauma, candidiasis, and bacterial infections. Pigeons and doves commonly have crop or esophagus disorders as a result of trichomoniasis or trauma. Crop and esophageal disorders are uncommon in finches, canaries, mynahs, and toucans.

Young birds being hand fed, fledglings, and recently weaned birds commonly have esophageal or crop disorders as a result of overheated or underheated formula, improper consistency of formula, overfeeding, cold environment, crop burns, candidiasis, ingestion of substrate, polyomavirus, or gram-negative bacterial infections. Nutritional deficiencies are common in young birds. Young and growing birds have smaller body stores of vitamin E.

Trichomoniasis is most common in doves and pigeons (canker), and raptors (frounce), but it also occurs in passerines (especially canaries and zebra finches) and psittacines (especially budgies and cockatiels). Capillaria is most common in budgies, macaws, canaries, pigeons, and gallinaceous birds. Thyroid hyperplasia that causes goiter is most common in budgies, but it may occur in pigeons, cockatiels, canaries, or lovebirds.

Psittacine dilatation syndrome affects psittacines. Psittacine beak and feather disease can affect psittacine species, and the acute disease causing crop stasis is most common in young sulfur-crested cockatoos and lovebirds. Larger psittacines may have delayed crop emptying as a result of polyomavirus.

History

Isolated birds and those in closed collections are commonly ill as a result of management-related problems, nutritional deficiencies, candidiasis, trauma, foreign bodies, neoplasia, and chronic debilitating diseases (e.g., PDS). Gram-negative bacterial infections are also seen.

Birds recently exposed to other birds are commonly ill as a result of infectious diseases, including bacterial, viral, and parasitic diseases. This is the result of stress and exposure to infectious disease. Illnesses occurring in isolated birds also occur in group situations.

Infectious and toxic etiologies are suspected when multiple birds are affected.

Significant dietary history for a bird with esophageal or crop disorders includes type of diet, intake, vitamin supplementation, and hand-feeding diet consistency, temperature, amounts fed, feeding techniques, and formula heating techniques. Diets deficient in vitamin A, such as an all-seed diet, can lead to vitamin A deficiency. Vitamin A deficiency causes hyperkeratosis of mucosal surfaces and metaplasia of the salivary glands.

Seed diets are high in fat and may be deficient in vitamin E and selenium. Birds on high-fat diets are more likely to show signs of vitamin E deficiency than are birds on diets low in fat. Goiter is associated with a seed diet deficient in iodine.

Hand-fed birds are often affected by trauma associated with feeding practices, crop burns, candidiasis, and bacterial infections associated with poor hygiene. Cold formula and cold environmental temperature can also slow crop emptying.

Infrequent feeding of large amounts of feeding formula may increase incidence of crop impaction, especially in macaws, Queen of Bavaria conures, and pionus parrots. Aerophagia may occur when improper techniques are used to hand feed young psittacines. Excessively high-fiber diets may also lead to crop impaction. Formula heated in a microwave often develops areas of excessively high temperatures, while other portions may be much lower in temperature. Crop burns are common in chicks fed formula warmed in microwave ovens.

Important environmental factors include management practices, access to potential toxins, nest substrate material, and exposure to other animals. Evaluate management practices, including environmental temperature, feeding formula, sanitation, and bedding substrates. Some birds will become impacted with grit when allowed unrestricted access to grit. Chicks will ingest bedding material, which can lead to crop impaction. Bedding materials that commonly cause problems and should not be used include crushed walnut shell, ground corncob, shredded paper pulp, and styrofoam packing material. Crop emptying may slow in chicks at low environmental temperatures. Proper temperatures for chicks are as follow: up to 7 days old, 94° to 97°F; 7 to 14 days old, 90° to 94°F; more than 14 days old, 85° to 90°F.

Capillaria eggs require approximately 2 weeks to embryonate and become infectious. Because they can remain infectious in the environment for several months, poor sanitation increases spread and exposure. Overcrowding and poor hygiene may increase the incidence of trichomoniasis in flocks.

Access or exposure to potential toxins is significant in a bird with delayed crop emptying or crop stasis. Toxins that may cause crop emptying abnormalities include lead, zinc, and organophosphate and carbamate insecticides. Some sources of lead are listed in Table 9–3. Sources of zinc include pennies minted since 1982, Monopoly game pieces, and galvanized materials.

Crop injuries are common with dog and cat bites.

The duration of the illness is important. Note the owner's description of the clinical signs and the course of the disease. Note previous illnesses, including signs, treatment, and response to treatment.

Physical Examination

A complete physical examination is important to determine the extent of the problem and to determine if there is involvement of other body systems. Common findings in birds with esophageal or crop disorders are discussed below.

Examine the mouth for oropharyngeal lesions. Esophageal or crop disorders may have concurrent oral lesions with diseases that can affect both areas, such as candidiasis, trichomoniasis, bacterial infections, and papillomas.

Palpate the crop to determine the amount and consistency of the ingesta and whether foreign material is present. The normal crop wall is thin and difficult to palpate. Thickened or fibrous areas of the crop wall are abnormal. Examine the skin and feathers over the crop. Part the feathers and moisten the skin with alcohol to allow better visualization of the skin for evidence of lacerations, erythema, or discolorations. Look for evidence of crop burns, trauma, or subcutaneous food that has been deposited after penetrating the crop mucosa with tube feeding. Crop burns may be noted as skin lesions just cranial to the thoracic inlet. Evidence of a crop burn may not be apparent for 3 to 5 days after the bird has been fed hot food. Erythema or edema of the area over the affected portion of the crop is usually the first sign. The skin then blanches, and the texture of the skin changes. Feathers over the burned area often fall out. With severe burns, the skin becomes leathery and black (Fig. 4–3). In 7 to 14 days after the injury, the devitalized tissue becomes well demarcated. The necrotic tissue will slough, and food and fluid may leak onto the chest.

Transillumination of the esophagus and crop may allow visualization of some lesions. Observe for peristaltic contractions. A partially filled psittacine crop should average one or two contractions per minute. An enlarged crop that fails to empty indicates crop impaction. The consistency of the ingesta is usually thick and doughlike when crop stasis is present.

Other gastrointestinal signs may occur concurrently and may help to narrow differential diagnoses; consult appropriate sections.

Clinical signs associated with viral infections often involve multiple systems. Clinical signs associated with PBFD include dyspnea, diarrhea, depression, crop stasis, and feather abnormalities (see Chapter 9).

Large psittacines infected with polyomavirus may die peracutely or develop depression, anorexia, delayed crop emptying, regurgitation, diarrhea, dyspnea, weight loss, and subcutaneous hemorrhages. Ataxia, tremors, and paralysis may also occur.

Clinical signs associated with avian viral serositis include weight loss, dyspnea, and abdominal distention.

Birds with proventricular dilatation syndrome may show depression, weight

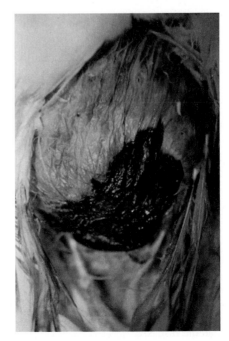

Figure 4–3. An advanced crop burn in an umbrella cockatoo. (Photo courtesy of Brian L. Speer, DVM, ABVP–avian.)

loss, vomiting, or passing undigested food in the droppings. Polyuria and neurologic signs (paresis, ataxia) may also occur.

A respiratory chirp on expiration, especially in budgies, is suggestive of goiter. Regurgitation and a pendulous crop often accompany respiratory sounds. Enlarged thyroid glands are intrathoracic and cannot be palpated.

Concurrent neurologic signs may be seen with polyomavirus, avian viral serositis, PDS, vitamin E/selenium deficiency, and toxins (lead, zinc, organophosphate, carbamate).

Respiratory signs may accompany esophageal or crop lesions with goiter, bacterial infections, avian viral serositis, polyomavirus, PBFD, candidiasis, trichomoniasis, and *Capillaria* infection.

Dermatologic signs may occur with esophageal or crop disorders with PBFD and polyomavirus in large psittacines.

Algorithm for Esophageal or Crop Disorders

See Figure 4–4.

Diagnostic Plan for Esophageal or Crop Disorders

Stabilize severely ill birds before performing stressful diagnostic tests. Provide supportive care as needed (see Chapter 1).

Dietary and management problems must be sought from the history. A thorough history may reveal feeding of formula at an improper temperature or consistency, exposure to infectious disease, or other management or dietary problems. Crop burns and crop foreign bodies may be noted on the physical examination.

Selection of appropriate diagnostic tests is based on consideration of the signalment and history of the bird and the findings of the physical examination.

The most useful initial diagnostic tests are a wet mount and Gram's stain of a crop aspirate. Gram-negative bacteria, megabacteria, and *Candida* infections may be identified with the Gram's stain. Submit a sample of the aspirate for bacterial culture and sensitivity testing. A wet mount of crop contents may reveal trichomoniasis or candidiasis. Flotation of feces and crop contents is useful for identification of parasites. Hematology and biochemistry tests are important in the diagnosis of infectious, metabolic, inflammatory, and some toxic diseases. Perform a CBC and biochemistry tests when systemic disease is suspected, when a bird is unresponsive to treatment, or to help determine the general health of the bird. Useful biochemistry tests for birds with esophageal or crop disorders include AST, uric acid, CK, total protein, and calcium. EPH is useful in identifying many diseases. Radiology is useful for diagnosis of lead and zinc toxicoses, grit impaction, enteritis, crop calculi and foreign bodies, and trauma. Radiographs provide information on liver and proventriculus size and allow evaluation of the respiratory tract and other celomic structures. Lead and zinc toxicoses can occur without radiographic signs. Titers, cultures, special stains, virus tests, cholinesterase assays, and lead and zinc blood levels are used to rule in or out specific diseases.

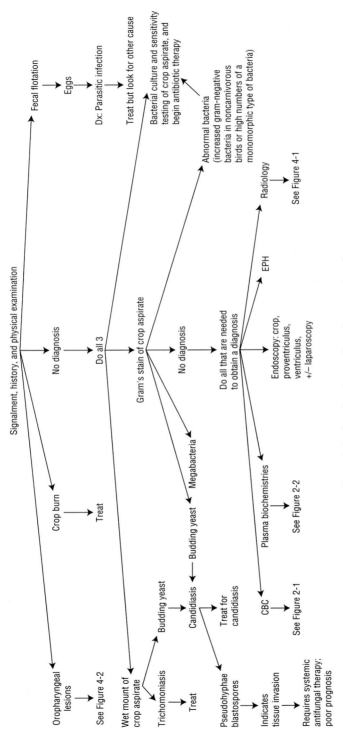

Figure 4-4. Algorithm for esophageal or crop disorder.

Endoscopy can be useful for examining the crop, proventriculus, ventriculus, and other intracelomic structures.

Treatment for Esophageal or Crop Disorders

Treat the underlying cause.

If crop stasis is present, it must be treated intensively. Impacted material may be softened with warm water or lactated Ringer's solution, massaged, and withdrawn from the crop with a large catheter. Because this requires multiple administrations and withdrawals to remove all the contents, it may be extremely stressful for debilitated birds. An ingluviotomy (crop incision) is usually the treatment of choice to quickly remove crop contents in debilitated birds. Begin therapy with a systemic broad-spectrum antibiotic (e.g., enrofloxacin, cefotaxime) until culture and sensitivity results are obtained. Lactated Ringer's solution or Pedialyte is tube fed until crop motility returns. Antibiotics and an antifungal (e.g., trimethoprim/sulfadiazine and nystatin) are added to the fluids for a local effect if abnormal bacteria are noted with Gram's stain of crop contents. When motility returns, dilute hand-feeding formula or garden vegetable or oatmeal baby food is fed. If crop emptying remains normal, feed half-strength hand-feeding formula mixed with fluids, gradually increasing the consistency until a normal consistency is tolerated. Metoclopramide may act as a crop stimulant. Adult birds and severely debilitated chicks may require tube feeding of formula.

Dehydration is common with crop stasis. Fluids are replaced intravenously or intraosseously. Alert and active birds may be rehydrated with subcutaneous fluids.

Repeated overstretching of the crop from overfeeding or pronged crop stasis may cause a pendulous crop. Support can be provided with elastic bandage material or infant tube socks. Apply the support while the crop is full to avoid too tight a fit. A proventricular feeding tube may be placed and used for nutritional support instead of a crop bandage (see Chapter 14).

Treatment of crop burns includes feeding reduced volumes of food more frequently, placing the bird on antibiotics and antifungals (e.g., enrofloxacin and ketoconazole), and monitoring the bird until the wound contracts and a fistula appears (7–14 days after injury). Food and water may leak from the fistula. When the wound contracts and a fistula forms, the scab is removed and the necrotic portions of the skin and crop are surgically excised (see Chapter 14). Surgery before wound contraction is often unsuccessful because devitalized and healthy tissue cannot be differentiated. Surgical adhesives can be used to close the wound if food begins to leak before wound contracture. Severe burns may require feeding via a proventricular feeding tube before surgery (see Chapter 14).

Treatment of crop foreign bodies and calculi is discussed in the section on treatment of regurgitation or vomiting.

A proventricular feeding tube may be placed to provide nutritional support while crop abnormalities are treated (see Chapter 14). Feed the amount the proventriculus will accommodate every 2 hours (approximately 20 ml in macaws).

ABNORMAL DROPPINGS

The normal avian dropping consists of three components: feces, urates, and urine. Normal feces vary in color from green to brown, and they are slightly loose to firm in consistency, depending on the diet. Normal urates are white to light beige, and normal urine is clear.

Abnormal droppings include polyuria, a color of urates other than white or light beige, diarrhea, and droppings containing blood or undigested food. Polyuria is an increase in the amount of urine present in the droppings. Diarrhea is an increase in fluid in the fecal component of the dropping. Bubbles are common in feces of birds with diarrhea.

The bird's diet affects the droppings. Consumption of large amounts of fruits and vegetables or formulated diets will produce large, loose feces and more urine than does consumption of seed diets. Consumption of some formulated diets and monkey biscuits results in brown feces. Consumption of a seed diet results in green feces. Liquid or nectar diets result in loose, watery feces, which are normal in lorikeets. Soft, large feces are normal in hand-fed chicks, hens immediately before and after egg laying, and the first morning droppings in some birds.

POLYURIA

Polyuria is common in birds. Most owners mistake polyuria for diarrhea, unaware that the increase in the dropping or stain on the cage floor is the result of an increase in urine rather than watery feces. Polyuria may be physiologic or result from illness. Normal physiologic polyuria occurs with stress, egg laying, feeding chicks, hot environments, hand-fed chicks, and birds on diets with a high water content (e.g., fruits and vegetables). Most birds seen in the exam room will have polyuria caused by the stress associated with travel and different surroundings. Have the owner remove and bring in the paper from the bottom of the cage, if present, before travel. This will provide a sample of droppings prior to the stress of transport for evaluation.

Illness may cause an increase in urine production as a result of a direct effect on the kidney or be the result of stress-induced polyuria. Examples of illnesses that cause an increase in urine production include diabetes, kidney disease, and liver disease. Any illness that causes stress may cause polyuria. Illnesses associated primarily with polyuria are discussed in this section. If other signs are present, consult those areas of the text for diagnosis and treatment.

Differential Diagnoses for Polyuria

1. Metabolic: °kidney disease (neoplasia, nephritis—bacterial, viral, fungal, parasitic, toxic), °liver disease, °peritonitis, diabetes mellitus, diabetes insipidus, renal glucosuria, gout

---

°Common causes.

2. Nutritional: excessive dietary protein, °vitamin A deficiency, °hypervitaminosis D₃, excessive dietary calcium, excessive dietary salt, formulated diets in chicks, high-fiber diets, °high fruit/vegetable content in diet
3. Toxic: salt, cholecalciferol, °lead, °zinc, arsenic, mycotoxins, ethylene glycol, other
4. Behavioral: psychogenic polydipsia, °fear, °excitement, °nervousness
5. Neoplastic: °renal neoplasia
6. Iatrogenic: °aminoglycoside antibiotics, corticosteroids, progesterone, amphotericin B, diuretics, allopurinol, sulfonamide antibiotics
7. Other: °stress (illness, psychologic), pigeons feeding squabs, normal chick droppings

Signalment

Common causes of polyuria in adult large psittacines include bacterial and viral induced kidney disease, liver disease, hypervitaminosis D₃, vitamin A deficiency, high fruit and vegetable content of diet, lead and zinc toxicoses, and stress. Cockatiels are commonly affected by lead and zinc toxicoses, egg-laying–related polyuria, peritonitis, liver and kidney disease, vitamin A deficiency, and stress-associated polyuria. Polyuria is often the result of kidney neoplasia, nephritis, liver disease, peritonitis, vitamin A deficiency, or stress in budgies. Polyomavirus infection is a common cause of polyuria in young budgies. Common causes of polyuria in raptors include kidney and liver disease, aminoglycoside antibiotic administration, and stress. Pigeons and doves commonly are polyuric as a result of feeding their young, kidney disease, or liver disease. Paramyxovirus is a common cause of polyuria in racing pigeons. Common causes of polyuria in finches and canaries include bacterial nephritis, liver disease, stress, and egg-related peritonitis. Mynahs and toucans are often polyuric as a result of liver disease (especially hemochromatosis), nephritis, high fruit or vegetable content of their diet, or stress. Diabetes mellitus is also fairly common in mynahs and toucans.

Young birds being hand fed, fledglings, and recently weaned birds commonly have polyuria as a result of formulated diets, hypervitaminosis D₃, bacterial or viral nephritis, or stress.

History

Isolated birds and those in closed collections are commonly ill because of nutritional problems, toxicoses, neoplasia, reproductive disorders, and management-related and chronic debilitating diseases. Chronic bacterial diseases (e.g., chlamydiosis, mycobacteriosis), gram-negative bacterial infections, and those diseases with carrier states (e.g., Pacheco's disease) are also seen.

Birds recently exposed to other birds are commonly ill as a result of infectious diseases, including bacterial, viral, and parasitic diseases. This is the result of

---

°Common causes.

stress and exposure to infectious disease. Illnesses occurring in isolated birds also occur in group situations.

Infectious and toxic etiologies are suspected when multiple birds are affected.

Significant dietary history for a polyuric bird includes type of diet, intake, changes in diet, freshness of diet, treats, vitamin supplementation, whether the bird is being hand fed, and the formula being hand fed. Droppings of birds on formulated diets, diets with large amounts of fruits and vegetables, and diets with excessive fiber, calcium, salt, or protein have an increased water content. Excessive vitamin supplementation may lead to hypervitaminosis D. Vitamin supplementation in birds on formulated diets can result in toxicosis. Nephrocalcinosis, visceral calcinosis, urate nephrosis, and visceral gout are frequent complications of excessive supplementation with vitamin D. Moldy or previously moldy foods may contain mycotoxins that may cause kidney failure. Feeding salty treats can cause an excessive salt intake.

Diets deficient in vitamin A, such as an all-seed diet, can lead to vitamin A deficiency. Vitamin A deficiency can cause metaplasia of the epithelium of the ureters and collecting ducts.

Important environmental factors in birds with polyuria include management practices and access to potential toxins. Polyuria is common with a change in surroundings, as a result of stress. Toxins that may cause polyuria include lead, zinc, salt, cholecalciferol, mycotoxins, and ethylene glycol. Some sources of lead are listed in Table 9–3. Sources of zinc include pennies minted since 1982, Monopoly game pieces, and galvanized materials. Ornamental dough is a common source of salt, and sea sand used as a source of grit or in nest boxes is another source.

A history of administration of aminoglycoside antibiotics, corticosteroids, progesterone, amphotericin B, or diuretics is consistent with iatrogenic causes.

Egg laying or nesting behavior before the onset of polyuria can be consistent with egg-related peritonitis.

The duration of the illness is important. Note the owner's description of the clinical signs and the course of the disease. Note previous illnesses, including signs, treatment, and response to treatment.

Physical Examination

A complete physical examination is important to identify the extent of the problem and to determine which systems are involved. If other clinical signs are present, consult appropriate chapters to assist in making a diagnosis. Common findings in birds with polyuria are discussed below.

Nonspecific signs such as lethargy and a decreased appetite are common. Birds may be too weak to fly. Dehydration may be present with serious illnesses. Evidence of dehydration includes slow refill of the basilic (wing) artery and vein, reduced skin elasticity, and dry mucous membranes. Subcutaneous tophi may be observed in joints if articular gout is present.

Changes in the oral cavity that may occur as a result of vitamin A deficiency include swollen margins of the choana, blunted or absent choanal papillae, or granulomas of the oral and lingual mucosa, periorbital area, or sinuses.

A bulging of the abdomen may be associated with ascites or an abdominal mass (e.g., egg, tumor, organomegaly). Abdominal palpation may reveal ascites, retained egg, or other abdominal mass. The maximal distance from the keel to the pubic bone in budgies is 4 to 5 mm. An increase in this distance is common with abdominal masses.

In large birds, palpation of the caudal division of the kidney can be performed. A lubricated, gloved finger is inserted gently into the cloaca. The kidney is palpated dorsally. Any swelling, asymmetry, or tenderness may indicate renal disease.

Neurologic signs may accompany polyuria. Renal neoplasia, internal trauma associated with egg laying, gout, liver disease, mycotoxicosis, salt toxicosis, and amphotericin B administration can cause polyuria and neurologic signs. Liver diseases that commonly cause both include lipidosis, mycotoxicosis, and hemochromatosis. Renal neoplasia may cause unilateral or bilateral paresis of the legs, especially common in budgies. Leg paresis can also be the result of internal trauma associated with egg laying. Gout can cause gait abnormalities that may appear neurologic in origin.

Algorithm for Polyuria

See Figure 4–5.

Diagnostic Plan for Polyuria

Provide supportive care as needed during the diagnostic evaluation (see Chapter 1).

History taking, physical examination, and evaluation of the droppings are the first steps in evaluating the polyuric bird. Dietary and iatrogenic causes must be sought from the history. Exposure to infectious diseases or toxins or management-related problems may be exposed with a complete history. Egg-related peritonitis is suggested by history (recent egg laying) and physical examination findings (swollen abdomen, palpable egg). If in doubt, CBC, radiographs, and abdominocentesis are usually definitive. The physical examination may reveal vitamin A deficiency, ascites, an abdominal mass, or articular gout.

If the cause is not obvious, perform urinalysis, plasma biochemistry tests, CBC, and EPH. Glucosuria suggests diabetes mellitus. Hyperglycemia must be present in conjunction with glucosuria for a diagnosis of diabetes mellitus. Glucosuria frequently accompanies egg-related peritonitis and may also be associated with a rare syndrome similar to Fanconi's syndrome (renal glycosuria). Important biochemistry tests in polyuric birds include uric acid, glucose, AST, calcium, albumin, and total protein. If liver disease is suspected, bile acids should be measured. Uric acid is usually elevated with gout. Other causes of elevated uric acid include renal disease, ovulation, starvation, liver disease, tissue damage, or decreased glomerular filtration. An elevation of glucose may be associated with diabetes mellitus. An elevation of AST can be associated with muscle or liver damage. Hypercalcemia occurs with dehydration, vitamin D toxicosis, ovulation, and bone osteolytic activity. Total protein increases occur with immune stimulation, dehydration, and chronic infections. Hypoalbumi-

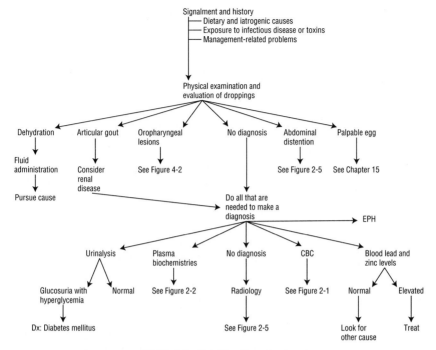

Figure 4–5. Algorithm for polyuria.

nemia may be the result of decreased production from liver disease or increased losses through the intestinal tract or kidneys. Bile acid increases are the result of reduced liver function; however, liver disease may be present with normal bile acid concentrations. Plasma protein electrophoresis is useful in identifying many diseases (e.g., liver disease, kidney disease, peritonitis).

Radiology aids in the diagnosis of lead and zinc toxicoses, gout, and hypervitaminosis D. Lead and zinc toxicoses can occur without radiographic evidence; however, metallic densities are often observed. Liver and kidney size and shape, peritonitis, and retained eggs may also be observed.

More specialized testing is necessary if the diagnosis is still uncertain. Titers, cultures, special stains, virus tests, and lead and zinc blood levels are used to rule in or out specific diseases. Endoscopy and renal or hepatic biopsy may also be used to determine the etiology of the polyuria.

Treatment for Polyuria

Treat the underlying cause. Provide other supportive care as needed. If dehydration is present, administer intravenous, intraosseous, or subcutaneous fluids.

ABNORMAL COLOR OF URATES

The normal color of avian urates is white, off-white, or light beige. Abnormal colors occurring in birds include red, yellow, brown, and green. Pigmented foods, medications, blood, hemolysis, and liver disease can alter the color of the urates. Yellow urates indicate hemolysis or liver disease or may occur as a result of vitamin B supplementation or ingestion of yellow vegetables. Green urates may occur with liver disease (biliverdinuria) or hemolysis. Brown urates may occur in some hand-fed chicks on an animal protein–based diet, with lead toxicosis, and with vitamin B supplementation. Red pigments can be the result of intake of colorful foods such as berries and dyed treats or the presence of hemoglobin, myoglobin, or blood. Hematuria is abnormal. Sources of blood in urates include the gastrointestinal tract, reproductive tract, urinary tract, and cloaca.

Differential Diagnoses for Abnormal Color of Urates

1. Infectious
   a. Bacterial: gram-negative bacteria, gram-positive bacteria
   b. Chlamydial: °*Chlamydia*
   c. Viral: adenovirus, °Pacheco's disease virus, acute PBFD
2. Metabolic: °hepatic lipidosis, hemochromatosis, hemolysis, hepatitis (°bacterial, °mycobacterial, °Pacheco's disease, adenovirus, °chlamydial, aspergillosis, flukes)
3. Nutritional: hand feeding of some chicks, vitamin B supplementation, °food dyes, °berries, °other brightly colored fruits, °vegetables, °or treats
4. Toxic: °lead, mercury
5. Physical: cloacal papilloma
6. Unclassified: conure bleeding syndrome

Signalment

Common causes of abnormally colored urates in psittacines include chlamydiosis, Pacheco's disease, lead toxicosis, pigmented foods, and liver disease. Liver disease and bacterial infections are common causes of abnormally colored urates in passerines (finches, canaries, and mynahs).

History

Isolated birds and those in closed collections commonly have abnormally colored urates caused by toxicoses, diet-related pigments, and liver disease.

°Common causes.

Chronic bacterial diseases (e.g., chlamydiosis), gram-negative bacterial infections, and diseases with carrier states (e.g., Pacheco's disease) are also seen.

Birds recently exposed to other birds are commonly ill as a result of infectious diseases, including bacterial and viral diseases. This is the result of stress and exposure to infectious disease. Illnesses occurring in isolated birds also occur in group situations.

Infectious and toxic etiologies are suspected when multiple birds are affected.

Significant dietary history for a bird with abnormally colored urates includes type of diet, treats, vitamin supplementation, and hand-feeding formula. Dyes contained in treats may pass through the digestive tract and stain the urates when feces and urates come in contact in the cloaca. Some fruits and vegetables contain pigments that may stain urates. Vitamin B supplementation can result in urates that are yellow or brown.

Hand-fed chicks being fed an animal protein–based diet may have reddish-brown urates. In some cases, urates will return to a normal color when the bird is switched to a plant protein–based formula.

High-fat diets (e.g., seed diets) and unbalanced diets (biotin, choline, methionine deficient) may lead to hepatic lipidosis. Excessive or even normal iron content in the diet may be a factor in the development of hemochromatosis in mynahs and toucans.

Important environmental factors in birds with abnormally colored urates include management practices and access to potential toxins. Failure to isolate new birds before their entry into an aviary allows introduction of infectious diseases. Overcrowding and poor sanitation increase exposure to and spread of infectious diseases. Toxins that may cause red pigmented urates are lead and mercury. Some sources of lead are listed in Table 9–3.

The duration of the illness is important. Note the owner's description of the clinical signs and the course of the disease. Note previous illnesses, including signs, treatment, and response to treatment.

Physical Examination

A complete physical examination is important to identify the extent of the problem and to determine which systems are involved.

Examine the cloacal mucosa for tumors and papillomas. The cloacal mucosa is exposed by bending the tail over the back and gently pinching the sides of the cloaca. Normal cloacal mucosa is pink, moist, and smooth. Papilloma lesions are wartlike proliferations. They occur as single or multiple slow-growing masses. Application of an acetic acid solution (apple cider vinegar) to a suspected papilloma will cause papillomatous tissue to blanch to white from the original pink or red color.

Abnormally colored urates in conjunction with respiratory signs may occur with chlamydiosis, bacterial infections, conure hemorrhagic syndrome, Pacheco's disease, adenovirus, and liver disease.

Neurologic signs may accompany abnormally colored urates with lead toxicosis, liver disease, chlamydiosis, and Pacheco's disease.

Algorithm for Abnormal Color of Urates

See Figure 4–6.

Diagnostic Plan for Abnormal Color of Urates

Stabilize severely ill birds before performing stressful diagnostic tests. Provide supportive care as needed (see Chapter 1).

History taking, evaluation of the droppings, and physical examination are the first steps in evaluating the bird with abnormally colored urates. Dietary causes must be sought from the history. Exposure to infectious diseases or toxins or management-related problems may be revealed with a complete history. Papillomas or cloacal tumors are diagnosed by physical examination.

If the cause is not obvious, next perform a CBC, biochemistry tests, and EPH. A CBC is useful in supporting infectious, inflammatory, and some toxic diagnoses. Biochemistry tests are important in the diagnosis of metabolic diseases. Important biochemistry tests for birds with abnormally colored urates include AST, uric acid, albumin, total protein, and bile acids. Because of the incidence of chlamydiosis, chlamydial testing is warranted. If lead or zinc toxicosis is suspected, blood is submitted for lead and zinc level determinations. Fecal flotation may reveal fluke eggs in cockatoos. Electrophoresis can be used to identify many diseases (e.g., chlamydiosis, mycobacteriosis, liver and kidney disease).

Radiology is useful to evaluate liver size, look for metal densities in the ventriculus indicative of lead or zinc toxicosis, and evaluate the gastrointestinal tract. Bacterial culture and sensitivity of the cloaca may reveal bacterial pathogens susceptible to antibiotic therapy.

More specialized testing is necessary if the diagnosis is still uncertain. Virus tests and acid-fast stains of feces are used to rule in or out specific diseases. Acid-fast stains are used to detect mycobacteria. Endoscopy and hepatic biopsy may also be used to determine the etiology. Biopsy of proliferative lesions may reveal papillomas, neoplasms, or granulomas.

Treatment for Abnormal Color of Urates

Treat the underlying cause.

DIARRHEA

Diarrhea is an increase in water content of the fecal portion of the dropping. The pericloacal area, the area surrounding the vent, is often soiled with feces accumulated on the feathers and skin. The feces may contain bubbles, blood, or mucus and may be malodorous. In many cases, the bird owner believes the bird has diarrhea when the bird actually has polyuria, an increase in urine in the dropping.

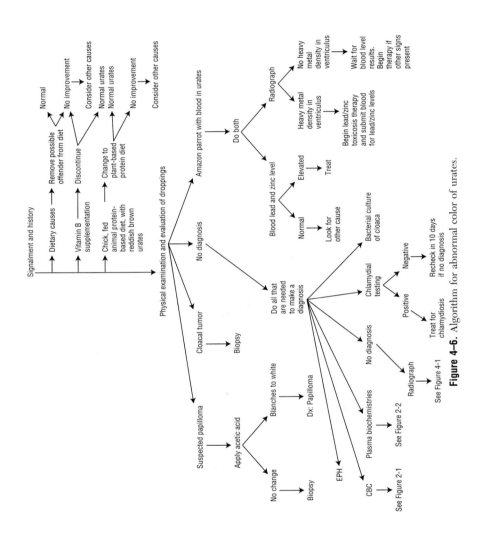

Figure 4-6. Algorithm for abnormal color of urates.

117

Differential Diagnoses for Diarrhea

1. Infectious
    a. Bacterial: °gram-negative bacteria (*Borrelia, Campylobacter, Citrobacter, Escherichia coli, Pasteurella, Salmonella, Yersinia*, other), gram-positive bacteria (*Clostridium*, megabacteria, *Mycobacterium, Streptococcus*, other)
    b. Chlamydial: °*Chlamydia psittaci*
    c. Mycoplasma: *Mycoplasma*
    d. Viral: adenovirus, astrovirus, calicivirus, coronavirus, duck viral enteritis, enterovirus, inclusion body hepatitis of pigeons (herpesvirus), influenza, Marek's disease, orthovirus, °Pacheco's disease, parvovirus, °polyomavirus, paramyxoviruses 1, 3, and 5 (including Newcastle disease), PBFD, °reovirus, rotavirus, togavirus-like agent, retrovirus (leukosis/sarcoma group)
    e. Fungal: °*Candida*
    f. Parasitic: °ascarids, °*Atoxoplasma, Capillaria,* °coccidia, *Cochlosoma, Cryptosporidium,* °flukes, *Giardia, Hexamita, Histomonas, Microsporum, Sarcocystis,* tapeworms, *Toxoplasma, Trichomonas*
2. Metabolic: °liver disease (lipidosis, hepatitis), kidney disease, pancreatitis, pancreatic insufficiency
3. Nutritional: diet change, chronic malnutrition, low-fiber or high-fat foods, °high water content diet (fruits, vegetables)
4. Toxic: carbamate, chocolate, cholecalciferol, °lead, nicotine, nitrates, organophosphate, salt, shampoo, °zinc
5. Physical: gastrointestinal obstruction, °foreign body, abdominal hernia, fecalith, grit impaction, °impending egg laying, egg binding/peritonitis
6. Behavioral: stress
7. Neoplastic: cloacal papilloma
8. Iatrogenic: antibiotics
9. Unclassified: conure bleeding syndrome

Signalment

Common causes of diarrhea in psittacines include chlamydiosis, bacterial enteritis, lead or zinc toxicosis, ascarids, and hepatic disease, and, in imported cockatoos and African gray parrots, flukes. Pacheco's disease, polyomavirus, reovirus, and candidiasis are also fairly common causes in psittacines. Canaries and finches commonly have diarrhea as a result of bacterial enteritis or coccidiosis. Diarrhea in mynahs and toucans is commonly the result of hemochromatosis, bacterial enteritis, or coccidiosis. Coccidia is a major cause of diarrhea in pigeons and backyard poultry.

Common causes of diarrhea in young birds include bacterial enteritis, candidiasis, polyomavirus, and gastrointestinal foreign bodies. In general, young birds show more severe signs of infection with parasitic and viral diseases.

°Common causes.

History

Isolated birds and those in closed collections are commonly ill because of bacterial enteritis, toxicoses, liver disease, nutritional diseases, neoplasia, candidiasis, and foreign bodies. Chronic bacterial and viral diseases (e.g., chlamydiosis, mycobacteriosis, PDS) and diseases with carrier states (e.g., Pacheco's disease) are also seen.

Birds recently exposed to other birds are commonly ill as a result of infectious diseases, including bacterial, viral, and parasitic diseases. This is the result of stress and exposure to infectious disease. Illnesses occurring in isolated birds also occur in group situations.

Poor management techniques, such as lack of quarantine procedures, buying birds from unfamiliar sources, and poor sanitation, increase the spread of infectious diseases. Poor diets may increase susceptibility to disease.

Infectious and toxic etiologies are suspected when multiple birds are affected.

Significant dietary history for a bird with diarrhea includes type of diet, freshness, and treats. Low-fiber diets, high-fat foods, and diets with a high water content (e.g., abundant fruits and vegetables) will result in loose stools. Unrestricted access to grit can result in grit impaction. Moldy or previously affected foods may contain mycotoxins that may cause liver disease. High-fat diets (e.g., seed diets) and unbalanced diets (biotin, choline, methionine deficient) may lead to hepatic lipidosis.

Important environmental factors include access to potential toxins, sanitation, and exposure to wild birds or disease vectors. Some toxins that may cause diarrhea are listed in the differential diagnoses. Some sources of lead are listed in Table 9–3. Sources of zinc include pennies minted since 1982, Monopoly game pieces, and galvanized materials. Nitrates are found in fertilizers, and the pellets are often mistaken for food by birds. Ornamental dough and sea sand are common sources of salt ingested by birds. Sources of cholecalciferol include vitamin D supplements and some rodenticides.

Onset of diarrhea after initiating antibiotic therapy is consistent with an iatrogenic cause. Trimethoprim-sulfa often causes diarrhea, especially in macaws and pigeons.

Loose stools associated with egg laying or nesting behavior can be normal or the result of egg-related peritonitis.

The duration of the illness is important. Note the owner's description of the clinical signs and the course of the disease. Note previous illnesses, including signs, treatment, and response to treatment.

Physical Examination

A complete physical examination is important to identify the extent of the problem and to determine which systems are involved. Debilitated birds must be handled with care. The physical examination and obtaining of diagnostic samples must be done as the condition of the bird allows. Place the bird in a warmed humidified cage.

Birds with diarrhea are often dehydrated. Hydration is determined based on skin elasticity in an unfeathered area, filling time of the basilic (wing) vein and artery, and the presence of sunken eyes and dry mucous membranes.

A distended abdomen may be associated with ascites or an abdominal mass (e.g., egg, tumor, organomegaly). Palpate the crop and abdomen. Abdominal palpation may reveal ascites, retained egg, or other abdominal mass. Palpate the keel. Loss of breast muscle and protrusion of the keel indicate emaciation and chronicity.

Examine the cloacal mucosa for tumors and papillomas. The cloacal mucosa is exposed by bending the tail over the back and gently pinching the sides of the cloaca. Normal cloacal mucosa is pink, moist, and smooth. Papilloma lesions are wartlike proliferations. They occur as single or multiple slow-growing masses. Application of an acetic acid solution (apple cider vinegar) to a suspected papilloma will cause papillomatous tissue to blanch to white from the original pink or red color.

Diarrhea in conjunction with respiratory signs may occur with chlamydiosis, bacterial infections, liver disease, kidney disease, heart failure, coagulopathies, peritonitis, malnutrition, mycoplasmosis, conure hemorrhagic syndrome, Pacheco's disease, reovirus, paramyxovirus 1 (including Newcastle disease), and some parasitic infections (e.g., *Toxoplasma, Atoxoplasma, Cryptosporidium,* and *Sarcocystis*).

Neurologic signs may accompany diarrhea with some bacterial infections, chlamydiosis, liver disease, Pacheco's disease, paramyxovirus, reovirus, duck viral enteritis, Marek's disease, polyomavirus, toxicoses (e.g., lead, zinc, mycotoxins, insecticides, salt), and parasitic infections *(Toxoplasma, Sarcocystis)*.

Illnesses that may result in both diarrhea and ophthalmic signs include chlamydiosis, reovirus, Pacheco's disease, paramyxovirus, lead toxicosis, botulism, and some parasitic infections *(Cryptosporidium, Giardia, Toxoplasma)*.

Algorithm for Diarrhea

See Figure 4–7.

Diagnostic Plan for Diarrhea

Stabilize severely ill birds before performing stressful diagnostic tests. Provide supportive care as needed (see Chapter 1).

History taking and physical examination are the first steps in evaluating the bird with diarrhea. Dietary and iatrogenic causes must be sought from the history. Exposure to infectious diseases or toxins or management-related problems may be exposed with a complete history. Impending egg laying or egg-related peritonitis is suspected based on behavior and recent egg laying. Papillomas, other cloacal tumors, fecaliths, and abdominal hernias are suspected based on physical examination findings. A Gram's stain of the cloaca and analysis of feces for parasites (direct smear, sedimentation, and flotation) are performed.

If the cause is not obvious, culture and sensitivity of the cloaca, CBC, biochemistry tests, and EPH are the next step. A CBC is useful in supporting infectious, inflammatory, and some toxic diagnoses. Biochemistry tests are im-

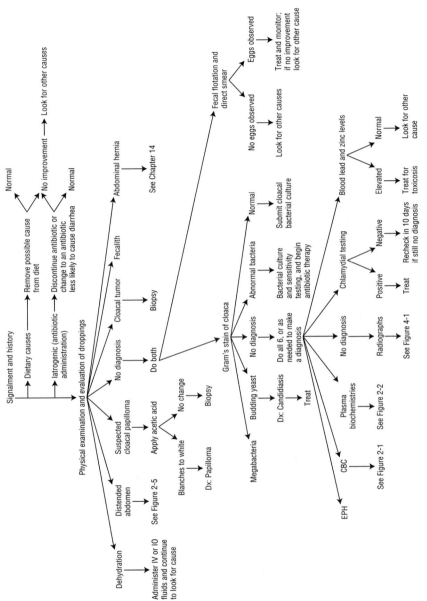

Figure 4-7. Algorithm for diarrhea.

121

portant in the diagnosis of metabolic diseases. Important biochemistry tests for birds with diarrhea include AST, uric acid, albumin, total protein, calcium, and, if liver disease is suspected, bile acids. Electrophoresis can be used to identify many diseases (e.g., chlamydiosis, mycobacteriosis, peritonitis, and liver and kidney disease). Because of the incidence of chlamydiosis, chlamydial testing is warranted. If lead or zinc toxicosis is suspected, blood is submitted for lead and zinc level determinations.

Radiology is useful to evaluate liver size, look for gastrointestinal foreign bodies or metal densities in the ventriculus (indicative of lead or zinc toxicosis), and evaluate the gastrointestinal tract. Lead or zinc toxicosis can occur without radiographic evidence; however, metallic densities are often present. Abnormalities to look for include changes in the position of organs, abnormal distention of the proventriculus, intestines, or cloaca, or the presence of gas. A barium series aids in determination of the location and size of organs of the gastrointestinal tract.

More specialized testing is necessary if the diagnosis is still uncertain. Virus tests, acid-fast stains of feces, fecal trichrome stains of pooled feces, and cholinesterase assay are used to rule in or out specific diseases. Endoscopy and liver biopsy may also be used to determine the etiology. Biopsy of proliferative lesions may reveal papillomas, neoplasia, or granulomas. Acid-fast stains are used to detect mycobacteria. Virus tests are used to identify suspected viral infections.

Group or flock situations benefit from complete necropsy examinations. Submit adequate samples for histopathology, microbiology, and virus isolation, especially when infectious diseases are suspected.

Treatment for Diarrhea

Treat the underlying cause. Provide supportive care as needed. If dehydration is present, administer intravenous or intraosseous fluids.

If the bird is eating well, eating an adequate diet, and maintaining its weight, continue the same diet. If not, feed a low-fiber, easily digested carbohydrate and highly digestible protein diet.

If severe diarrhea is present, administer intravenous or intraosseous fluids, one dose of rapidly acting corticosteroids, and parenteral bactericidal antibiotics with a broad gram-negative spectrum (e.g., enrofloxacin, cefotaxime) pending culture results.

BLOOD IN DROPPINGS

Blood in the droppings is abnormal and may originate from the gastrointestinal tract, reproductive tract, urinary tract (kidneys), or cloaca. Bleeding from the distal gastrointestinal tract, urinary tract, reproductive tract, or cloaca will be bright red and appear as fresh blood. Bleeding higher in the gastrointestinal tract can appear dark and tarry. Red, blue, or purple pigments from treats or berries may result in red droppings that do not contain blood.

Differential Diagnoses for Blood in Droppings

1. Infectious
   a. Bacterial: °gram-negative bacteria, gram-positive bacteria (*Clostridium*, other)
   b. Chlamydial: *Chlamydia psittaci*
   c. Viral: duck virus enteritis (duck plague), °Pacheco's disease, paramyxovirus 1 (Newcastle disease), PBFD, reovirus
   d. Parasitic: ascarids, *Capillaria*, cestodes (tapeworms), °coccidia, *Cryptosporidium*
2. Metabolic: liver disease (hepatitis), coagulopathies, vitamin K deficiency, nephritis
3. Toxic: aflatoxins, °lead, zinc, warfarin
4. Physical: °before or after egg laying, ulcer, °gastrointestinal foreign body, cloacal cyst
5. Trauma
6. Neoplastic: °papilloma, cloacal, other
7. Iatrogenic: trauma during examination
8. Unclassified: conure bleeding syndrome

Signalment

Common causes of blood in the droppings in adult psittacines include bacterial enteritis, Pacheco's disease, cloacal papillomas, and lead toxicosis (Amazon parrots). Passerines commonly have blood in their droppings as a result of bacterial enteritis, coccidiosis, or liver disease. Bacterial and parasitic infections are common causes of bloody droppings in pigeons, ducks, geese, and gallinaceous birds.

Young birds being hand fed, fledglings, and recently weaned birds commonly have bloody droppings as a result of bacterial enteritis, ingestion of substrate, or viral infections. Poor hygienic practices associated with hand feeding are a common cause of bacterial enteritis.

History

Isolated birds and those in closed collections are commonly ill because of bacterial infections, toxicoses, liver disease, kidney disease, neoplasia, foreign bodies, or reproductive-related illnesses. Chronic bacterial and viral diseases (e.g., chlamydiosis, mycobacteriosis, PBFD) and diseases with carrier states (e.g., Pacheco's disease) are also seen.

Birds recently exposed to other birds are commonly ill as a result of infectious diseases, including bacterial, viral, and parasitic diseases. This is the result of stress and exposure to infectious disease. Illnesses occurring in isolated birds also occur in group situations.

Poor management techniques, such as lack of quarantine procedures, buying

---

°Common causes.

birds from unfamiliar sources, and poor sanitation, increase the spread of infectious diseases.

Infectious and toxic etiologies are suspected when multiple birds are affected.

Imported birds are commonly exposed to infectious diseases. Chlamydiosis is common in imported birds. Tapeworms are common in imported cockatoos and African gray parrots.

Significant dietary history for a bird with blood in the droppings includes type of diet, freshness, and treats. Pigmented fruits, vegetables, and treats can result in droppings that appear to contain blood but actually contain a pigment from the food. Unrestricted access to grit can result in grit impaction. Moldy or previously moldy foods may contain mycotoxins that may cause liver disease. Excessive or even normal iron content in the diet may be a factor in the development of hemochromatosis in mynahs and toucans. High-fat diets, such as all-seed diets, and those deficient in biotin, choline, or methionine may lead to hepatic lipidosis.

Important environmental factors include access to potential toxins, sanitation, and exposure to wild birds or disease vectors. Some sources of lead are listed in Table 9–3. Sources of zinc include pennies minted since 1982, Monopoly game pieces, and galvanized materials. Warfarin is found in some rodenticides. Overcrowding and poor hygienic practices may increase the incidence and spread of infectious diseases.

Hemorrhage with egg laying occurs with trauma from oviposition or infection.

Blood in the droppings that occurs after abdominal or cloacal endoscopy is consistent with iatrogenic kidney or cloacal hemorrhage. Cloacal hemorrhage may also occur with trauma to the cloaca during examination or sample collection.

Vitamin K deficiency may occur with prolonged antibiotic therapy; intestinal bacterial flora are the source of vitamin K. This has not been proved to occur in pet birds.

The duration of the illness is important. Note the owner's description of the clinical signs and the course of the disease. Note previous illnesses, including signs, treatment, and response to treatment.

Physical Examination

A complete physical examination is important to identify the extent of the problem and to determine which systems are involved. Debilitated birds must be handled with care. The physical examination and obtaining of diagnostic samples must be done as the condition of the bird allows. Provide supportive care as needed.

Examine the cage. Pigmented treats and foods may be present in the cage. Observe the droppings. In addition to the blood, evaluate the color, consistency, and fluid content of the droppings. Observe the bird in the cage for abnormal clinical signs.

Palpate the keel. Loss of breast muscle and protrusion of the keel indicate emaciation and chronicity. Palpate the crop and observe the skin overlying the abdomen. A bulging of the abdomen may be associated with ascites, peritonitis, or an abdominal mass (e.g., egg, tumor, organomegaly). An enlarged liver can often be observed as a dark area distal to the keel in finches and canaries. Palpate the abdomen. Abdominal palpation may reveal ascites, retained egg, or other abdominal mass. Eggs lower in the reproductive tract are easily palpable.

Examine the cloacal mucosa for tumors, papillomas, cysts, and trauma. Normal cloacal mucosa is pink, moist, and smooth. Papilloma lesions are wartlike proliferations. They occur as single or multiple slow-growing masses. Application of an acetic acid solution (apple cider vinegar) to a suspected papilloma will cause papillomatous tissue to blanch to white from the original pink or red color.

Blood in the droppings in conjunction with respiratory signs may occur with chlamydiosis, bacterial infections, liver disease, kidney disease, coagulopathies, peritonitis, malnutrition, conure bleeding syndrome, Pacheco's disease, paramyxovirus 1 (including Newcastle disease), reovirus, and some parasitic infections (e.g., coccidia).

Neurologic signs may accompany blood in the droppings with some bacterial infections, chlamydiosis, liver disease, Pacheco's disease, paramyxovirus, reovirus, duck viral enteritis, toxicoses (e.g., lead, zinc, mycotoxins, rodenticide), coagulopathies, and some parasitic infections (coccidia).

Illnesses that may result in blood in the droppings and ophthalmic signs include chlamydiosis, reovirus, Pacheco's disease, paramyxovirus, lead toxicosis, and some parasitic infections (e.g., coccidia).

Concurrent feather abnormalities may occur with PBFD.

Algorithm for Blood in Droppings

See Figure 4–8.

Diagnostic Plan for Blood in Droppings

Provide supportive care as needed (see Chapter 1). The first steps in evaluating the bird with blood in the droppings are consideration of the signalment, taking a complete history, performing a complete physical examination, and evaluating the droppings. A history of exposure to infectious diseases or toxins and the reproductive history may narrow differential diagnoses. Pigments from foods or treats may be found in the cage. Cloacal papillomas, tumors, cysts, or lacerations are diagnosed by physical examination. An abdominal mass or enlarged liver may be suspected based on physical examination findings. If there is a question whether the pigment in the dropping is blood or pigment, a direct smear will reveal red blood cells, if present. A fecal occult blood test may also be used.

If the cause is not obvious, a fecal flotation, wet mount, and Gram's stain are performed. If the bird is an Amazon parrot, perform radiography, looking for metal densities in the ventriculus; lead toxicosis sometimes results in hematuria in these birds.

A CBC and cloacal bacterial culture are the next step. A CBC is useful in supporting infectious, inflammatory, and some toxic diagnoses. Bacterial culture and sensitivity are used to detect primary or secondary bacterial infections. The culture will detect bacteria that may have been missed on the Gram's stain.

If a diagnosis is still unclear, biochemistry tests, radiographs, chlamydial testing,

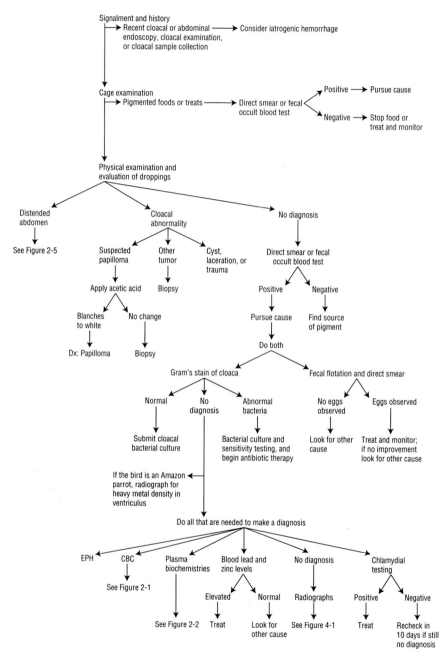

Figure 4–8. Algorithm for blood in droppings.

EPH, and lead and zinc blood levels are performed. Useful biochemistry tests for birds with blood in the droppings include AST, uric acid, total protein, and albumin; if liver disease is suspected, measure bile acids. Electrophoresis is useful to aid in identifying many diseases (e.g., chlamydiosis, liver disease). Radiology is useful to evaluate liver and kidney size, look for gastrointestinal foreign bodies or metal densities in the ventriculus indicative of lead or zinc toxicosis, and evaluate the gastrointestinal tract. Some abnormalities to look for include changes in the position of organs; abnormal distention of the proventriculus, intestines, and cloaca; metal densities in the gastrointestinal tract; and the presence of gas. A barium series may be required to aid in the determination of location and size of some organs.

Virus tests are required to definitively diagnose viral infections.

Group or flock situations benefit from complete necropsy examinations. Submit adequate samples for histopathology, microbiology, and virus isolation.

Treatment for Blood in Droppings

Provide other supportive care as needed. Treat the underlying cause. Document the presence of blood with cytology or a fecal occult blood test before aggressive therapy.

UNDIGESTED FOOD IN DROPPINGS

The presence of undigested seed or other food in the droppings is abnormal. Feces that contain undigested or partially digested food indicate a digestive or hypermotility problem.

Differential Diagnoses for Undigested Food in Droppings

1. Infectious
   a. Bacterial: °gram-negative bacteria, gram-positive bacteria (°megabacteria, other)
   b. Fungal: °*Candida*
   c. Parasitic: ascarids, °*Cochlosoma*, °*Giardia*
   d. Unclassified: °PDS
2. Metabolic: °pancreatitis, liver disease, dehydration, °proventriculitis, °ventriculitis, °intestinal disease, lack of grit (passerines)
3. Nutritional: vitamin E/selenium deficiency
4. Physical: foreign body, ingestion of oil, dehydration
5. Allergic: food
6. Neoplastic: upper gastrointestinal papilloma, other
7. Iatrogenic: °antibiotics

°Common causes.

Signalment

Common causes of undigested or partially digested food in the droppings in large psittacines include PDS, dehydration, and bacterial gastroenteritis. Common causes in small psittacines include fungal ventriculitis (candidiasis), megabacteria, giardiasis, bacterial gastroenteritis, PDS, and dehydration. Passerines are commonly affected by *Cochlosoma* infection, megabacteria, fungal ventriculitis, bacterial gastroenteritis, dehydration, or lack of grit.

Young birds being hand fed, fledglings, and recently weaned birds commonly have partially digested food in the droppings as a result of ingestion of foreign bodies, dehydration, or swallowing of unhulled seeds. Bacterial gastroenteritis and candidiasis are also common.

History

Isolated birds and those in closed collections are commonly ill because of fungal infections, metabolic problems, ingestion of oil or foreign bodies, food allergies, neoplasia, or iatrogenic causes. Bacterial infections are also common. Chronic illnesses also occur in this group (e.g., PDS).

Birds recently exposed to other birds are commonly ill as a result of infectious diseases, including bacterial and parasitic diseases. Proventricular dilatation syndrome is also suspected to be infectious, and it is a common cause of undigested food in the droppings in multiple bird environments. Illnesses occurring in isolated birds also occur in group situations.

Infectious and toxic etiologies are suspected when multiple birds are affected.

Significant dietary history for a bird with undigested or partially digested food in the droppings includes type of diet, freshness, and techniques associated with the preparation of hand-feeding diets. Hand-fed birds are often affected by candidiasis and bacterial infections, which are often associated with improper handling of hand-feeding formula. See Chapter 16 for proper handling of hand-feeding formula.

Seed diets are high in fat and may be deficient in vitamin E and selenium. Birds on high-fat diets are more likely to show signs of vitamin E deficiency than are birds on diets low in fat. High-fat diets (e.g., seed diets) and unbalanced diets (biotin, choline, methionine deficient) may lead to hepatic lipidosis. High-fat foods may also result in pancreatitis.

Important environmental factors in birds with undigested food in the droppings include exposure to infectious diseases, a change of environment, management practices, and sanitation. Also, the substrate in the nest box or cage is important in young birds, because young birds will often ingest this material. A change of environment can be stressful, leading to an increased susceptibility to bacterial and fungal diseases. Poor management practices and sanitation and exposure to infectious diseases increase illnesses (e.g., PDS, megabacteria, giardiasis, and ascarid infection). Ingestion of oil may cause passing of whole seed.

Iatrogenic causes include prolonged antibiotic therapy and administration of oil orally.

The duration of the illness is important. Note the owner's description of the clinical signs and the course of the disease. Note previous illnesses, including signs, treatment, and response to treatment.

Physical Examination

Debilitated birds must be handled with care. The physical examination is performed quickly and with the least amount of stress possible.

A complete physical examination is important to identify the extent of the problem and to determine which systems are involved. Common findings of birds with undigested or partially digested food in droppings are discussed below.

Inspect the droppings for pigmented urates, abnormal size or consistency of feces, and unusual odor. Large, soft, foul smelling droppings are often associated with maldigestion. Abnormally colored urates are discussed in a previous section.

Inspect the cage and observe the bird in the cage. Examine the bird for dehydration. Hydration is determined based on skin elasticity in an unfeathered area, filling time of the basilic (wing) vein and artery, and the presence of sunken eyes and dry mucous membranes.

Inspect the oral cavity and palpate the crop. Fungal infection of the ventriculus often has associated oral and ingluvial (crop) lesions. Palpate the keel. Loss of pectoral muscle and protrusion of the keel indicate emaciation and chronicity. Palpate the abdomen; an enlarged liver and other organs may be palpable. Examine the skin over the abdomen. Hepatomegaly can often be visualized in canaries and finches as a dark mass just distal to the keel.

Neurologic signs may accompany undigested food in the droppings with NGD, liver disease, kidney disease, and vitamin E/selenium deficiency.

Feather picking may be noted in conjunction with giardiasis, especially in cockatiels.

Algorithm for Undigested Food in Droppings

See Figure 4–9.

Diagnostic Plan for Undigested Food in Droppings

Stabilize severely ill birds before performing stressful diagnostic tests. Provide supportive care as needed (see Chapter 1).

Consider the signalment and history. Dietary or iatrogenic causes of undigested food in the droppings must be obtained from the history. Exposure to infectious diseases and management-related problems may be revealed with a complete history. Dehydration, candidiasis, and liver disease are suspected based on physical examination and evaluation of the droppings.

Initial diagnostics include a Gram's stain of the cloaca and a fecal flotation and wet mount. Megabacteria or candidiasis may be diagnosed with a Gram's stain; however, these organisms may be absent in the feces and still be causing

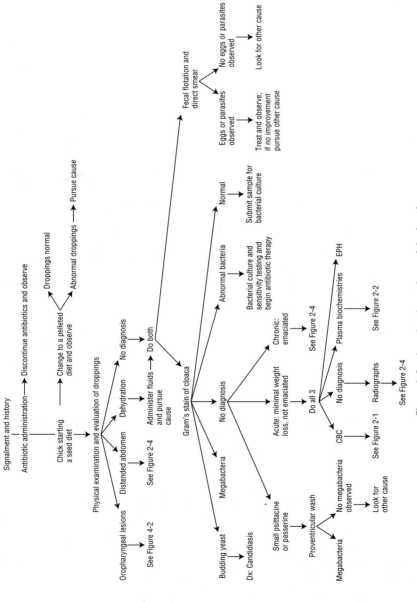

Figure 4-9. Algorithm for undigested food in droppings.

proventriculitis or ventriculitis. A proventricular washing may better demonstrate megabacteria. A wet mount preparation to reveal the motile *Giardia* trophozoite requires just-passed, fresh droppings. The cyst may be better visualized with a trichrome stain. This organism may be shed in low numbers and difficult to demonstrate.

If the problem is not obvious and if the problem appears acute (minimal weight loss, not emaciated), then a CBC, biochemistry tests, EPH, and cloacal culture and sensitivity are the next tests performed. A CBC is useful in diagnosing dehydration and supporting a diagnosis of infectious or inflammatory disease. Biochemistry tests are important in the diagnosis of metabolic diseases. Important biochemistry tests include AST, CK, uric acid, amylase, lipase, albumin, total protein, and, if liver disease is suspected, bile acids. Electrophoresis is useful in identifying many diseases (e.g., liver and kidney disease, peritonitis, mycobacteriosis).

If the problem appears chronic (the bird is emaciated), radiology is the next step. Radiology is useful to evaluate proventricular, liver, and kidney size and to evaluate the gastrointestinal tract. A barium series may be needed to determine the location and size of different organs. Radiology is helpful in determining possible etiologies, but supportive diagnostic tests are required for a definitive diagnosis.

If PDS is suspected based on radiology, a ventricular biopsy may be performed for a definitive diagnosis. If crop signs are also present, a crop biopsy is a less invasive and technically simpler procedure that may provide a diagnosis of PDS. A negative biopsy of any organ does not rule out PDS.

Other diagnostic tests that may be required if the diagnosis is uncertain include endoscopy (proventricular, abdominal) and liver or kidney biopsy.

Group or flock situations benefit from complete necropsy examinations.

Treatment for Undigested Food in Droppings

Treat the underlying cause. If the diet is poor, place the bird on an appropriate diet. Tube feed the bird if the bird is not eating on its own. Provide other supportive care as needed. If dehydration is present, administer intravenous or intraosseous fluids.

References and Additional Readings

Altman RB. Avian neonatal and pediatric surgery. *Semin Avian Exot Pet Med* 1992;34–39.

Anderson NL. Candida/megabacteria proventriculitis in a lesser sulphur-crested cockatoo (*Cacatua sulphurea sulphurea*). *J Assoc Avian Vet* 1993;7(4):197–201.

Bauck L. Vomiting in the young macaw. *Proc Assoc Avian Vet* 1992;126–133.

Bond MW, Downs D, Wolf S. Screening for psittacine proventricular dilatation syndrome. *Proc Assoc Avian Vet* 1993;92–97.

Campbell TW. Cytology in avian diagnostics. In Kirk RW (ed): *Current Veterinary Therapy IX, Small Animal Practice*. Philadelphia, WB Saunders, 1986, pp 725–731.

Campbell TW. *Avian Hematology and Cytology*, ed 2. Ames, Iowa State University Press, 1995.

Clipsham R. Noninfectious diseases of pediatric psittacines. *Semin Avian Exot Pet Med* 1992;22–33.

Clubb SL, Cray C, Greiner E, et al. Cryptosporidiosis in a psittacine nursery. *Proc Assoc Avian Vet* 1996;177–185.

Clyde VL, Patton S. Diagnosis, treatment, and control of common parasites in companion and aviary birds. *Semin Avian Exot Pet Med* 1996;5(2):75–84.

Cray C, Bossart G, Harris D. Plasma protein electrophoresis: Principles and diagnosis of infectious disease. *Proc Assoc Avian Vet* 1995;55–59.

Degernes LA, Davidson GF, Barnes HJ, et al. A preliminary report on intraosseous total parenteral nutrition in birds. *Proc Assoc Avian Vet* 1995;25–26.

Degernes LA, Flammer K. Proventricular dilatation syndrome in a green-winged macaw. *Proc Assoc Avian Vet* 1991;45–49.

Doolen M. Crop biopsy: A low risk diagnosis for neuropathic gastric dilatation. *Proc Assoc Avian Vet* 1994;193–196.

Ekstrom DD, Degernes L. Avian gout. *Proc Assoc Avian Vet* 1989;130–138.

Filippich LJ, Parker MG. Megabacteria and proventricular/ventricular disease in psittacines and passerines. *Proc Assoc Avian Vet* 1994;287–293.

Flammer K. Oropharyngeal diseases in caged birds. In Kirk RW (ed): *Current Veterinary Therapy IX, Small Animal Practice*. Philadelphia, WB Saunders, 1986, pp 699–702.

Goodwin M, McGee ED. Herpes-like virus associated with a cloacal papilloma in an orange-fronted conure (*Aratinga canicularis*). *J Assoc Avian Vet* 1993;7(1):23–25.

Gould J. Liver disease in psittacines. *Proc Assoc Avian Vet* 1989;125–129.

Gould J. Liver disease in psittacines. *Proc Am Animal Hosp Assoc* 1992;314–318.

Gould WJ. Liver disease in psittacines. In Kirk RW, Bonagura JD (eds): *Current Veterinary Therapy XI, Small Animal Practice*. Philadelphia, WB Saunders, 1992, pp 1145–1150.

Graham DL. Internal papillomatous disease: A pathologist's view. *Proc Assoc Avian Vet* 1991;141–143.

Graham DL. "Wasting/proventricular dilation disease": A pathologist's view. *Proc Assoc Avian Vet* 1991;43–44.

Graham DL. Endoventricular mycosis: An avian pathologist's perspective. *Proc Assoc Avian Vet* 1994;279–282.

Gregory CR, Latimer KS, Niagro FD, et al. A review of proventricular dilatation syndrome. *J Assoc Avian Vet* 1994;8(2):69–75.

Hoefer HL, Orosz S, Dorrestein GM. The gastrointestinal tract. In Altman RB, Clubb SL, Dorrestein GM, Quesenberry K (eds): *Avian Medicine and Surgery*. Philadelphia, WB Saunders, 1997, pp 412–453.

Ingram IA. Proventricular foreign body mimicking proventricular dilatation in an umbrella cockatoo. *Proc Assoc Avian Vet* 1990;314–315.

Kennedy FA, Sattler-Augustin S, Mahler JR, et al. Oropharyngeal and cloacal papillomas in two macaws (*Ara* spp.) with neoplasia with hepatic metastasis. *J Avian Med Surg* 1996;10(2):89–95.

King AS, McLelland J. Digestive system. In *Birds: Their Structure and Function*, ed 2. London, Baillier Tindall, 1984, pp 84–109.

LaBlonde J. Pet avian toxicology. *Proc Assoc Avian Vet* 1988;159–174.

Latimer KS, Niagro FD, Campagnoli RP, et al. Diagnosis of concurrent avian polyomavirus and psittacine beak and feather disease virus infections using DNA probes. *J Assoc Avian Vet* 1993;7(3):141–146.

Lloyd M. Heavy metal ingestion: Medical management and gastroscopic foreign body removal. *J Assoc Avian Vet* 1992;6(1):25–29.

Lumeij JT. Gastroenterology. In Ritchie BW, Harrison GJ, Harrison LR (eds): *Avian Medicine: Principles and Application*. Lake Worth, FL, Wingers Publishing, 1994, pp 482–521.

Mautino M. Avian lead intoxication. *Proc Assoc Avian Vet* 1990;245–247.

McCluggage D. Proventriculotomy: A study of select cases. *Proc Assoc Avian Vet* 1992;195–200.

McDonald SE. Lead poisoning in psittacine birds. In Kirk RW, Bonagura JD (eds): *Current Veterinary Therapy IX, Small Animal Practice.* Philadelphia, WB Saunders, 1986, pp 713–718.

Meier JE. Salmonellosis and other bacterial enteritides in birds. In Kirk RW (ed): *Current Veterinary Therapy VIII, Small Animal Practice.* Philadelphia, WB Saunders, 1983, pp 637–646.

Mohan R. Dursban toxicosis in a pet bird breeding operation. *Proc Assoc Avian Vet* 1990;112–114.

Mohan R. Evaluation of immunofluorescent and ELISA tests to detect *Giardia* and *Cryptosporidium* in birds. *Proc Assoc Avian Vet* 1993;62–64.

Murphy J. Diabetes in toucans. *Proc Assoc Avian Vet* 1992;165–179.

Murphy J. Psittacine fatty liver syndrome. *Proc Assoc Avian Vet* 1992;78–82.

Murphy J. Psittacine trichomoniasis. *Proc Assoc Avian Vet* 1992;21–24.

Murray MJ, Taylor M. Retrieval of proventricular and ventricular foreign bodies with rigid endoscopic equipment. *Proc Assoc Avian Vet* 1995;281–284.

Oglesbee BL, McDonald S, Warthen K. Avian digestive system disorders. In Birchard SJ, Sherding RG (eds): *Saunders Manual of Small Animal Practice.* Philadelphia, WB Saunders, 1994, pp 1290–1301.

Pare JA, Hunter DB. Ingluviolith in a cockatiel *(Nymphicus hollandicus). J Assoc Avian Vet* 1993;7(3):139–140.

Paster MB. A brief overview: The avian crop. *J Assoc Avian Vet* 1992;6(4):229–230.

Patton S. An overview of avian coccidia. *Proc Assoc Avian Vet* 1993;47–51.

Phalen DN, Wilson VG, Graham DL. A practitioner's guide to avian polyomavirus testing and disease. *Proc Assoc Avian Vet* 1994;251–257.

Ramsay EC, Drew ML, Johnson B. Trichomoniasis in a flock of budgerigars. *Proc Assoc Avian Vet* 1990;309–311.

Rich GA. Classic and atypical cases of proventricular dilatation disease. *Proc Assoc Avian Vet* 1992;119–125.

Ritchie BW, Harrison GJ, Harrison LR (eds): *Avian Medicine: Principles and Application.* Lake Worth, FL, Wingers Publishing, 1994.

Romagnano A, Grindem GB, Degernes L, et al. Treatment of a hyacinth macaw with zinc toxicity. *J Avian Med Surg,* 1995;9(3):185–189.

Rosskopf WJ, Shindo MK. Crop disorders in pet avian species. *Proc Assoc Avian Vet* 1993;263–267.

Rosskopf WJ, Woerpel RW. Cloacal conditions in pet birds with a cloaca-pexy update. *Proc Assoc Avian Vet* 1989;156–163.

Rupiper DJ. Hemorrhagic enteritis in a group of great billed parrots *(Tanygnathus megalorynchos). J Assoc Avian Vet* 1993;7(4):290.

Shivaprasad HL, Barr BC, Woods LW, et al. Spectrum of lesions (pathology) of proventricular dilatation syndrome. *Proc Assoc Avian Vet* 1995;505–506.

Steinohrt LA. Microsporidiosis in budgerigars. *Proc Assoc Avian Vet* 1995;341–343.

Suedmeyer WK. Diagnosis and clinical progression of three cases of proventricular dilatation syndrome. *J Assoc Avian Vet* 1992;6(3):159–163.

Taylor M. Biopsy techniques in avian medicine. *Proc Assoc Avian Vet* 1995;275–280.

Tully TM. Acute salmonellosis in a breeding facility of eclectus parrots. *Proc Assoc Avian Vet* 1990;119–121.

VanDerHeyden N. Update on avian mycobacteriosis. *Proc Assoc Avian Vet* 1994;53–61.

Van Sant F. Zinc toxicosis in a hyacinth macaw. *Proc Assoc Avian Vet* 1991;255–259.

Chapter 5

Ophthalmic Signs

Abnormal ocular clinical signs are common in pet birds. Clinical signs of ophthalmic disease include conjunctivitis, blepharitis, keratitis, ocular discharge, exophthalmos, periorbital swelling, buphthalmos, and impaired vision. Multiple or single signs may occur. Clinical signs of involvement of other body systems are common. The infraorbital sinus is closely associated with the eye and is a common source of infection.

This chapter presents a diagnostic approach for ophthalmic signs commonly seen in pet birds. The chapter is divided into four sections. Signs are grouped according to etiology and the diagnostic approach required to diagnose the cause of the illness. Each section begins with general information and definitions of terms, followed by a list of differential diagnoses and appropriate signalment information. Common causes of the clinical sign are presented for each group of pet birds. Pertinent information regarding which species and ages of birds may be affected by the diseases in the differential diagnoses section is also given. The history section can be used to explore important historical information. The physical examination section guides interpretation of the physical findings. If other abnormalities are noted, consult appropriate sections of the text to assist in making a diagnosis. An algorithm is included in each section to provide a quick reference to which tests are recommended. The diagnostic plan suggests useful tests. Consult Chapter 12 for techniques of sample collection and assistance with test interpretation. Once a diagnosis is made, general treatments are provided at the end of each section. Treatments for specific diseases are found in Chapter 9. Consult Chapter 17 for drug dosages. This chapter concludes with additional readings and references, which can be consulted for further information.

OPHTHALMIC EXAMINATION

A complete ophthalmic examination is required to determine the extent of the lesion. Intraocular abnormalities can accompany periorbital and corneal lesions. A physical examination is important because many ocular abnormalities are caused by systemic disease. Neurologic examination is important when vision is impaired or other signs of neurologic disease are present.

Assess the periorbital area for swelling, discoloration, or abnormal growths.

Samples of ocular discharges are obtained for cytology and culture. Abnormal masses are aspirated and evaluated cytologically.

Schirmer's test may be performed in cases of suspected keratoconjunctivitis sicca (e.g., vitamin A deficiency). A cutdown strip is used. Normal results vary between species. A normal bird of the same species or the normal eye in a bird with unilateral signs may be used for comparison. Zero or reduced readings are common with vitamin A deficiency–associated xerophthalmia.

The anterior chamber is examined with a bright pen light, binocular loupe, operating microscope, slit lamp, or ophthalmoscope. Evaluate the clarity of the cornea, aqueous, and lens and the color and vascularization of the iris. If blepharospasm is present, instill a topical anesthetic and examine the conjunctival fornix and behind the nictitating membrane for foreign bodies. Aqueous flare is seen as a cloudy appearance of the aqueous or as a scattering of the light beam with a slit lamp. Aqueous flare is associated with anterior uveitis.

Note the iris color. The color is an indication of age or sex in many species of birds. Young Amazon parrots have brown irises that become red-orange as they age. Young African gray parrots have brown irises that change to gray, then white. Young macaws have brown irises that change to gray within the first year; then, between 1 and 3 years of age, the color changes from gray to yellow. Young cockatoos have brown irises. Adult female cockatoos have red irises, and adult males have dark brown to black irises.

Evaluate pupillary light reflexes. Birds have some voluntary control of pupillary constriction due to skeletal muscles in the iris. Birds will constrict and dilate their pupils when excited. A consensual response is absent in birds but pupillary constriction may occur in the opposite eye from light that traverses the thin septum between the eyes.

Corneal swabs or scrapings are then obtained, if needed.

Fluorescein stain is used to visualize corneal ulceration and to determine the extent of an injury. Ultraviolet light aids in detecting small lesions with dye retention.

Intraocular pressure can be measured in larger birds with a tonometer. Uveitis causes reduced intraocular pressure. Glaucoma is rare in birds.

Visualization of the posterior segment is hindered by the small size of the avian eye and the presence of skeletal muscle in the iris, making mydriasis difficult to achieve consistently. Several topical applications of d-tubocurarine (3 mg/ml) is often successful in dilating the pupil. General anesthesia will also cause mydriasis.

Retinal lesions and the pectin may be examined with an indirect ophthalmoscope or a 28- or 40-diopter lens. The pectin is a black structure projecting from the retina into the vitreous. Look for pigmentation of the normally unpigmented peripheral retina, scarring, preretinal membranes, opacities in the vitreous, and inflammation.

Vision is assessed by observation. In unfamiliar surroundings, birds with visual deficits will be more timid and may walk or fly into objects. A bird without vision deficits will alternate eyes to observe while being caught. Test vision by slowly moving a hand or object toward the bird from behind on each side. The menace response requires vision, but absence of the menace response does not indicate an abnormality.

CONJUNCTIVITIS, BLEPHARITIS, KERATITIS, OR OCULAR DISCHARGE

Conjunctivitis is inflammation of the conjunctiva. Conjunctivitis is character-ized by a red or swollen conjunctiva. It is usually accompanied by an ocular discharge. The character of the discharge varies with the etiology. Conjunctivitis is a common disorder in birds and often has multiple etiologies. It often accompanies respiratory infections. Many organisms causing systemic disease can cause conjunctivitis. Intraocular disease may also be present.

Blepharitis is inflammation of the eyelids. Clinical signs of blepharitis include crusting of the eyelids and lashes with mucopurulent exudate and erythema and swelling of the eyelids. Conjunctivitis is usually associated with blepharitis, and keratitis may be present. Blepharitis may also be caused by an inflammatory skin disease (pyoderma, scaly face mites, or allergy).

Keratitis is inflammation of the cornea. Blepharospasm, photophobia, and epiphora are signs of keratitis.

Differential Diagnoses for Conjunctivitis, Blepharitis, Keratitis, or Ocular Discharge

1. Infectious
   a. Bacterial: °gram-negative bacteria (*Escherichia coli, Haemophilus* spp., *Klebsiella pneumoniae, Pasteurella multocida, Pseudomonas aeruginosa, Salmonella* spp., other), gram-positive bacteria (*Streptococcus* spp., *Staphylococcus aureus, Mycobacterium*, other)
   b. Chlamydial: °*Chlamydia psittaci*
   c. Mycoplasma: °*Mycoplasma* spp.
   d. Viral: °poxvirus, Pacheco's disease, Gouldian finch herpesvirus, paramyxovirus (PMV), quail bronchitis, Amazon tracheitis, infectious laryngotracheitis (ILT)
   e. Fungal: *Candida*
   f. Parasitic: *Cryptosporidium, Giardia, Oxyspirura mansoni, Thelazia, Philophthalmos*
2. Nutritional: °vitamin A deficiency
3. Toxic: botulism
4. Physical: foreign body, °handling, °trauma, °corneal ulcer, °disinfectants, ectropion, lid abnormalities, °chronic exposure to cigarette smoke
5. °Allergic
6. Unclassified: lovebird eye disease

Signalment

Common causes of conjunctivitis, blepharitis, keratitis, and ocular discharge in large psittacines include bacterial infections, trauma, allergic reactions, and

---

°Common causes.

vitamin A deficiency. Common causes in cockatiels include *Chlamydia*, *Mycoplasma*, and bacterial sinusitis. Budgies are commonly affected by bacterial infections, *Mycoplasma*, and trauma. Keratitis is common in recently captured and transported mynahs. The keratitis is usually related to corneal scratches associated with handling. Some Amazon parrots (Central American and South American) are prone to keratitis of unknown origin. Common causes of conjunctivitis, blepharospasm, keratitis, or ocular discharge in passerines include poxvirus, *Mycoplasma*, and bacterial infections. *Mycoplasma* is a common cause in pigeons, and less common are *Salmonella* and *Chlamydia*. Trauma is a common cause of these signs in raptors.

Diseases common in young birds include bacterial infections, trauma, poxvirus infection, and candidiasis. Lid abnormalities may be noted.

Conjunctivitis is common in cockatiels. Often, no infectious agent can be isolated. *Chlamydia* and *Mycoplasma* are suggested agents. Ectropion resulting in secondary keratitis occurs in cockatiels.

Keratoconjunctivitis in Australian parakeets is frequently caused by *Chlamydia*. *Chlamydia* causes a localized infection and conjunctivitis in finches and pigeons without other signs.

Conjunctivitis and nasal discharge are characteristic of chlamydiosis in domestic pigeons, and conjunctivitis may be the predominant clinical sign of chlamydiosis in infected ducks and geese.

Poxvirus lesions involving the eyes are most common in blue-fronted Amazon parrots and passerines (canaries, mynahs). Amazon tracheitis affects Amazon parrots and gallinaceous birds. A similar herpesvirus affects Bourke's parrots.

Lovebird eye disease is most common and most severe in peach-faced lovebirds. Amazon tracheitis causes severe disease in Amazon parrots. Paramyxovirus 3 causes conjunctivitis in finches. Botulism is uncommon in companion birds, but it is common in waterfowl. *Oxyspirura* infection is most common in cockatoos and mynahs.

Pacheco's disease affects only psittacines. Birds that recover from Pacheco's disease may become carriers. Patagonian and Nanday conures are common asymptomatic carriers.

Infectious laryngotracheitis affects canaries and gallinaceous birds and primarily adult or growing birds older than 8 weeks. Quail bronchitis is a highly infectious disease of young bobwhite quail. The severity of the disease depends on the age of the bird. Birds older than 3 weeks demonstrate milder signs.

Cryptosporidium causes conjunctivitis in budgies and gallinaceous birds, ducks, and geese and can be a cause of diarrhea in psittacines and gallinaceous birds.

Gouldian finch herpesvirus can cause disease in Gouldian, crimson, and zebra finches and red-faced waxbills.

History

Birds recently exposed to other birds are commonly ill as a result of infectious diseases, including bacterial, viral, and parasitic diseases. This is the result of stress and group contact.

Isolated birds and those in closed collections are commonly ill because of allergic disease, vitamin A deficiency, trauma, foreign bodies, neoplasia, or poor management practices. Chronic bacterial infections (e.g., chlamydiosis), gram-negative bacterial infections, and diseases with carrier states (e.g., Pacheco's disease) are also seen.

Infectious and toxic etiologies are suspected when multiple birds are affected.

Consider the bird's diet. Diets deficient in vitamin A, such as an all-seed diet, can lead to vitamin A deficiency. Intoxication with botulism toxins occurs after ingestion of contaminated food such as decaying organic matter or maggots that contain the toxin.

Consider the bird's environment. Birds allowed out of their cages are more susceptible to trauma. Contact with cigarette smoke or other allergens can cause conjunctivitis. Recent transport of mynahs commonly results in keratitis. Consider exposure to wild birds or disease vectors. Poxvirus can be transmitted by mosquitoes.

The duration of the illness is important. Note the owner's description of the clinical signs and the course of the disease. Note previous illnesses, including signs, treatment, and response to treatment.

Physical Examination

Complete physical and ophthalmic examinations are important to identify other ophthalmic and physical abnormalities. Intraocular abnormalities are common with keratitis (e.g., uveitis). The ophthalmic examination is discussed in a previous section.

A complete examination may reveal trauma, conjunctival worms, corneal ulcers, or characteristic poxvirus lesions or vitamin A deficiency. Clinical signs that may be noted on physical examination include ocular discharge, blepharospasms, conjunctival hyperemia, swelling of the eyelids, and corneal ulcers, masses, opacity, or vascularization. Chronic ocular discharges may result in loss of feathers around the eyes (Fig. 5–1).

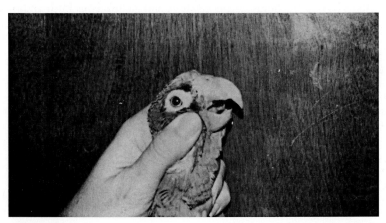

Figure 5–1. Feather loss around the eyes in an Amazon parrot caused by chronic conjunctivitis and ocular discharge.

The cutaneous form of poxvirus is characterized by cutaneous proliferative growths on featherless areas of skin (around eyes, nares, beak, vent, and feet). Early signs of the disease include unilateral or bilateral blepharitis, lid edema, and a serous ocular discharge. With progression, ulcers appear at the lid margins or medial or lateral canthus. Scabs form and may seal the eye or eyes shut. Scabs fall off within 2 weeks. Secondary bacterial infections are common, often causing severe sequelae.

Clinical signs of Amazon tracheitis include ocular, nasal, and oral discharges, open-mouth breathing, and coughing. The disease may be peracute, acute, subacute, or chronic (up to 9 months' duration). The disease in Bourke's parrots in general is less severe.

Birds with Pacheco's disease have lethargy, anorexia, fluffing, and intermittent diarrhea, polyuria, and polydipsia and a high mortality rate. Biliverdinuria, sinusitis, conjunctivitis, and convulsions may occur.

Clinical signs of Gouldian finch herpesvirus include dyspnea and slight nasal discharge, edematous eyelids, and conjunctivitis. The eyes may be crusted closed.

Clinical signs associated with quail bronchitis include coughing, sneezing, increased lacrimation, conjunctivitis, or sudden death.

Birds with PMV-1 infections may have ataxia, torticollis, tremors, leg paralysis, conjunctivitis, and occasionally dyspnea and diarrhea. Paramyxovirus 3 causes conjunctivitis, diarrhea, dyspnea, and dysphagia in finches.

Clinical signs associated with *Cryptosporidium* infection include depression, anorexia, rhinitis, conjunctivitis, sinusitis, tracheitis, airsacculitis, coughing, sneezing, diarrhea, and dyspnea.

Signs of ILT include dyspnea, nasal and ocular discharge (mucoid, purulent, or hemorrhagic), sinusitis, coughing, hemoptysis, and wheezing.

Lovebird eye disease is an infectious disease that initially is seen with depression, blepharitis, and serous ocular discharge. The disease progresses to hyperemia and edema of the periorbital area, with a mucopurulent ocular discharge.

Mild periorbital and conjunctival swelling, xerophthalmia, and ocular discharge may be seen with vitamin A deficiency. Xerophthalmia is abnormal dryness and thickening of the conjunctiva and cornea. Vitamin A deficiency causes squamous metaplasia of mucous membranes. Other signs that may be seen on physical examination include swollen margins of the choana in the roof of the mouth. Associated papillae may be blunted or absent, and granulomas of the oral and lingual mucosa, periorbital area, and sinuses may be present.

Oxyspirura, *Thelazia*, and *Philophthalmus* parasites may be present under the nictitating membrane, in the conjunctival fornix, or in the lacrimal duct. Birds scratch at affected eyes.

Botulism toxin causes a peripheral neuropathy. Leg paresis is usually the earliest clinical sign, characterized by the bird sitting on its sternum with legs extended caudally. Leg paresis is followed by wing paresis. Loss of control of the neck and head occurs in the terminal stages, resulting in the term *limber neck disease*. Diarrhea, chemosis, swelling of the eyelids and nictitating membrane, ocular discharge, and salivation may also occur.

Blepharospasm and conjunctival hyperemia are common with keratitis. Mynah keratitis syndrome is often related to corneal scratches from handling and shipping. The keratitis and ulcers usually regress spontaneously in a few weeks, and severe ulcers may scar. Chronic keratoconjunctivitis develops in some cases, leading to conjunctival masses and corneal vascularization.

Early Amazon keratitis syndrome is characterized by blepharospasm and serous ocular discharge. The lesions are bilateral and normally start in the medial cornea, and they usually progress to cover the cornea. Lesions usually resolve within 2 weeks. Occasionally, deep corneal ulcers and anterior uveitis occur, and sinusitis may develop.

Algorithm for Conjunctivitis, Blepharitis, Keratitis, or Ocular Discharge

See Figure 5–2.

Diagnostic Plan for Conjunctivitis, Blepharitis, Keratitis, or Ocular Discharge

Stabilize severely ill birds before performing diagnostic tests, and provide supportive care as needed during the diagnostic evaluation (see Chapter 1).

Selection of diagnostic tests is based on consideration of the signalment and history of the bird and the findings of the physical and ophthalmic examinations. Conjunctival or nictitating membrane foreign bodies and parasites, trauma, vitamin A deficiency, corneal ulcers, and involvement of other body systems may be identified during a complete physical examination. Poxvirus may be suspected based on characteristic lesions. Fluorescein stain is used to identify corneal ulcers.

Cytology is usually the most useful initial diagnostic test. Infectious and allergic conditions may be identified with cytology. To obtain a sample, a sterile moistened swab or a metal or plastic spatula is used to gently scrape the conjunctiva or the margins of the cornea. A topical ophthalmic anesthetic may be necessary before the scraping.

Samples from normal avian conjunctiva contain a few epithelial cells and clear background. Epithelial cells may occur singly or in small sheets. They have an eccentric, round to oval nucleus with coarse nuclear chromatin and abundant weakly basophilic cytoplasm with distinct margins. These cells may contain intracytoplasmic orange to brown pigmented granules.

Samples from normal avian cornea contain a few noncornified squamous epithelial cells with a central vesicular nucleus.

Increased cellularity and the presence of inflammatory cells indicates conjunctivitis or keratoconjunctivitis. Phagocytosis of bacteria may be seen with bacterial infections. Epithelial cells may show degenerative changes (cytoplasmic vacuolation, karyolysis, or karyorrhexis). Inflammatory cells and degenerative changes may be caused by primary or secondary bacterial, chlamydial, mycoplasmal, or viral infections; conjunctival or nictitating membrane foreign bodies; trauma; or neoplasia.

Intracytoplasmic inclusions in macrophages or epithelial cells may be seen with *Chlamydia* or *Mycoplasma* infections. Inclusions appear as small blue or

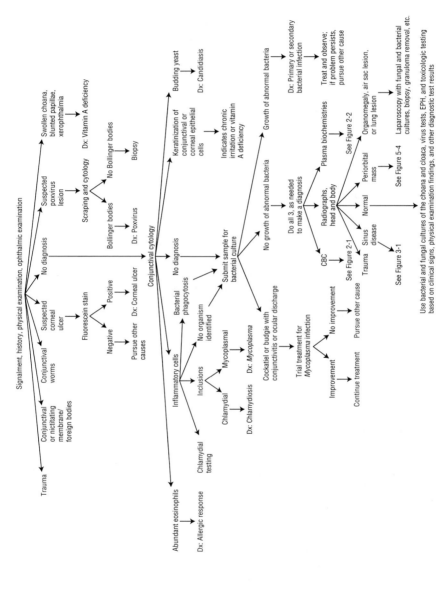

Figure 5–2. Algorithm for conjunctivitis, blepharitis, keratitis, or ocular discharge.

purple spherules when stained with Wright's or Diff-Quick stain (see Figure 12–19). *Mycoplasma* infection may be identified by basophilic coccoid intracytoplasmic inclusions when stained with Wright's or Diff-Quick stain similar to chlamydial inclusions. Gimenez or Macchiavello's stain aids in cytologic identification of *Chlamydia* inclusions.

An increase in mononuclear leukocytes, especially lymphocytes and plasma cells, indicates chronic inflammation. Mucous and conjunctival goblet cells may also be present. Goblet cells have abundant foamy cytoplasm with large secretory vacuoles and eccentric nuclei.

Keratinization of conjunctival or corneal epithelial cells indicates chronic irritation or vitamin A deficiency. Keratinization is indicated by cornified squamous epithelial cells. Keratinized cells may result from pathology or contamination. Interpret keratinization along with clinical signs. Corneal keratinization is usually associated with increased corneal opacity.

The presence of numerous eosinophils is suggestive of an allergic response.

Rare *Candida* conjunctivitis or keratitis may be identified by the presence of many oval budding yeasts (see Figure 12–20). Yeast cells stain basophilic with Wright's or Diff-Quick stain.

A bacterial culture and sensitivity will determine if bacteria are present as a primary or secondary infection. To obtain a sample, a sterile swab moistened with transport medium is inserted into the upper conjunctival fornix and moved from side to side two or three times.

Normal ocular bacteria include *Staphylococcus* and *Corynebacterium*. Other bacteria may be responsible for primary or secondary infections. Secondary bacterial infections are common. *Chlamydia*, *Mycoplasma*, and *Haemophilus* require special culture media and will not grow on routine culture media.

If there is involvement of other body systems or no growth of abnormal bacteria, then viral, chlamydial, *Mycoplasma*, *Haemophilus*, or parasitic diseases are suspected. A complete blood count (CBC) and plasma biochemistry tests rarely provide a diagnosis, but they are useful in supporting infectious and systemic diseases. Perform a CBC if septic or systemic disease is suspected, when a bird is unresponsive to treatment, or to help determine the general health of the bird. Changes in the hemogram commonly seen in birds with these ophthalmic signs are detailed below.

Nonregenerative anemias are usually normocytic and normochromatic, but hypochromasia, anisocytosis, and poikilocytosis frequently occur in birds. Nonregenerative anemias may occur with chronic inflammatory diseases, including chlamydiosis and mycobacteriosis.

Leukocytosis and heterophilia may be caused by stress or inflammatory diseases (e.g., bacteria, chlamydiosis, fungi). Differential diagnoses to consider in a bird with conjunctivitis or ocular discharge and a white blood cell (WBC) count in excess of 40,000/µl include chlamydiosis and mycobacteriosis. Monocytosis may occur with chlamydiosis, mycobacteriosis, and chronic bacterial infections.

Leukopenia may be associated with an overwhelming bacterial, fungal, chlamydial, or viral septicemia and endotoxemia. Leukopenia is common with Pacheco's disease.

Plasma biochemistry tests are important in the diagnosis of metabolic disease. The most useful biochemistries for birds with conjunctivitis or ocular discharge include aspartate transferase (AST or SGOT), total protein, and uric acid.

An elevation in AST is usually the result of liver or muscle damage. The AST may be elevated in birds with conjunctivitis, blepharitis, keratitis, or ocular discharge due to liver damage caused by Pacheco's disease, chlamydiosis, or hepatitis caused by a bacterial infection.

Radiology is useful for diagnosing periorbital, sinus, and systemic disease and trauma, and it is often the next step in the evaluation of birds with sinusitis, blepharitis, keratitis, or ocular discharge. Radiographic abnormalities in birds with ophthalmic abnormalities include trauma lesions, periocular masses, and organomegaly. Fractures of the skull or scleral ossicles indicate head trauma. Fractures elsewhere in the body may indicate trauma.

Evaluation of the hepatic silhouette may reveal hepatomegaly. Radiographic evidence of hepatomegaly in the ventrodorsal view includes loss of the hourglass silhouette between the heart and liver, compression of the abdominal air sacs, and extension of the liver lateral to a line drawn from the coracoid to the acetabulum. On the lateral view, hepatomegaly is indicated by the cranial displacement of the heart, dorsal elevation of the proventriculus, and caudodorsal displacement of the ventriculus. Hepatomegaly may be the result of chlamydiosis, mycobacteriosis, or bacterial infections.

If a diagnosis cannot be made based on previous tests, fecal tests, titers, cultures, special stains, plasma protein electrophoresis (EPH), and virus identification tests may be useful to determine the cause of the illness. Choose tests based on signalment and signs of other systems involved. Chlamydial titer, antigen testing, culture, and EPH are useful when chlamydiosis is suspected based on clinical signs or cytology. *Mycoplasma* is difficult to culture. Response to trial treatment may provide a presumed diagnosis. Acid-fast staining of feces or ocular discharges may reveal positive staining *Mycobacterium.*

Direct fecal smears may be used to demonstrate *Giardia* trophozoites or cysts. The preparation must be examined within 10 minutes of collection, and false-negative results are common. Flotation of feces with zinc sulfate will better concentrate cysts.

Cryptosporidium is small (4 to 6 μm) and is shed at a low rate. Diagnose by centrifuging diluted feces with a highly concentrated salt solution or Sheather's flotation. Oocysts may be demonstrated on fecal smears stained with Giemsa, carbolfuchsin, or periodic acid–Schiff stain.

Various methods are available to detect viral infections (see Chapter 12). A suspicion of infection is based on signalment, history, and clinical signs. Concurrent signs are usually present with viral infections.

Poxvirus may be diagnosed with cytology, histopathology, virus culture, or virus detection in feces by culture or electron microscopy. Asymptomatic carriers intermittently shed the virus in the feces and may be identified with repeated culturing of the feces.

Diagnosis of PMV is based on isolation of the virus from cloacal swabs in live birds. Hemagglutination inhibition serologic testing can be used to detect antibodies to PMV. Antibodies appear approximately 8 days after infection. Postmortem cases may be diagnosed through isolation of the virus from the brain or organs.

Antemortem definitive diagnosis of Pacheco's disease is difficult. Intermittent shedding by carrier birds may be detected by virus isolation. Histology (hepatic necrosis, eosinophilic intranuclear inclusion bodies), virus neutralization, enzyme-linked immunosorbent assay (ELISA), and immunofluorescence may be useful postmortem.

Pharyngeal swabs are useful for culture of Amazon tracheitis.

Intranuclear inclusion bodies may be seen in tracheal and bronchial epithelium 2 to 5 days after infection with quail bronchitis. Proliferation of lymph follicles and lymphocytic infiltrations also occur.

Histopathology is used to diagnose Gouldian finch herpesvirus. The disease is characterized by ballooning degeneration of conjunctival and respiratory epithelial cells. These epithelia may be thickened by increased numbers of ballooning cells and may detach from the basal membrane. Intranuclear inclusion bodies are characteristic.

Treatment for Conjunctivitis, Blepharitis, Keratitis, or Ocular Discharge

Provide supportive care as needed (see Chapter 1).

Corneal lacerations are sutured and treated with topical antibiotics, often successfully. Lens luxations are a surgical emergency requiring immediate referral.

Bacterial conjunctivitis or blepharitis is treated with antibiotic ophthalmic drops or ointment, used three times daily. Choice of antibiotic is based on culture and sensitivity results. Treatment may be initiated with gentamicin, chloramphenicol, or tetracycline, pending sensitivity results.

Keratitis is treated with antibiotic ophthalmic drops or ointment. Some keratitis syndromes (e.g., Amazon keratitis) are not altered by the use of antibiotics or antiviral drugs. If there is concurrent intraocular inflammation without corneal ulceration, topical corticosteroids are used. Systemic corticosteroids are used if corneal ulcers are present.

Corneal ulcers are treated with topical antibiotics. Acetylcysteine is sprayed into the eye every few hours if ulcers are severe. If intraocular inflammation is present, systemic corticosteroids are also used. Deep or severe ulcers may benefit from a temporary tarsorrhaphy. One or two horizontal mattress sutures with 4-0 or 6-0 nylon will provide a corneal bandage.

Mycoplasma infections are treated with tetracycline, a macrolide, or enrofloxacin. Tylosin is commonly used.

Allergic disease responds to removal of the offending substance, which in some instances may require moving the bird to a new home. Symptomatic therapy using antihistamines is sometimes successful.

Vitamin A deficiency requires parenteral vitamin A initially, then oral supplementation and correction of the diet. Keratin cysts and abscesses are debrided and cultured.

Ocular candidiasis is treated with 1% nystatin ointment topically or amphotericin B injected subconjunctivally.

Symptomatic therapy for lovebird eye disease consists of a stress-free environment. Although antibiotics have been suggested, they are usually not effective.

Small numbers of conjunctival, nictitating membrane, and lacrimal duct parasites are manually removed or flushed out. Heavy infestations are treated with a single topical dose of ivermectin. Repeated applications of topical carbamate powder may eliminate *Philophthalmus* flukes.

Some cockatiels and budgies with conjunctivitis, partial lid paralysis, and reduced jaw tone respond to treatment with metronidazole and vitamin E. *Giardia* is a possible cause.

Management of viral infections includes symptomatic therapy and prevention of secondary bacterial infection and contagion. Chlorhexidine in the drinking water is used to decrease spread in flock situations. Specific treatments are discussed in Chapter 9.

Treat other disorders according to their primary causes (see Chapter 9).

EXOPHTHALMOS OR PERIORBITAL SWELLING

Exophthalmos is abnormal protrusion of a normal-sized eye. Periorbital structures include the upper and lower eyelids, nictitating membrane, lacrimal gland, and structures surrounding the deep surface of the globe.

Differential Diagnoses for Exophthalmos or Periorbital Swelling

1. Infectious
   a. Bacterial: °gram-negative bacteria, gram-positive bacteria (*Mycobacterium avium*, other)
   b. Viral: °poxvirus, papilloma, avian sarcoma/leukosis
   c. Fungal: *Aspergillus*, *Cryptococcus*
   d. Parasitic: °*Knemidokoptes pilae* (scaly face mites), *Oxyspirura*, *Thelazia*, *Philophthalmus*
2. Nutritional: vitamin A deficiency
3. Physical: trauma, retrobulbar hematoma, lid abnormalities, periorbital infraorbital sinus inflation
4. Neoplastic: papilloma, other

Signalment

Common causes of exophthalmos or swellings around the eye are periorbital abscesses, infraorbital sinusitis, and abscesses of the lacrimal gland. Trauma is a common cause of exophthalmos in raptors.

Knemidokoptes mites are often the cause of proliferative lesions around the eyes, beak, cere, and vent and on the feet in budgies. These mites affect primarily budgies, but they also occur in other psittacines and passerines. Papillomas are common in finches. The cutaneous form of poxvirus is rare except in blue-fronted Amazon parrots, lovebirds, passerines, raptors, and pigeons. Avian

---

°Common causes.

sarcoma/leukosis virus generally affects birds at sexual maturity or later. Females are more susceptible than males.

History

Birds recently exposed to other birds are commonly ill as a result of infectious diseases, including bacterial, viral, and parasitic diseases, and from stress and group contact.

Isolated birds and those in closed collections are commonly ill because of trauma, vitamin A deficiency, or neoplasia. Chronic bacterial infections are also common.

Infectious and toxic etiologies are suspected when multiple birds are affected. Avian sarcoma/leukosis virus is transmitted vertically as well as horizontally. Feces and saliva are sources of horizontal transmission.

The diet may be of historical significance. Diets deficient in vitamin A, such as an all-seed diet, can lead to vitamin A deficiency.

Consider the bird's environment. Birds allowed out of their cages are more susceptible to trauma. Poxvirus is transmitted by mosquitoes; therefore, poxvirus infection is more common in outside aviaries.

The duration of the illness is important. Note the owner's description of the clinical signs and the course of the disease. Note previous illnesses, including signs, treatment, and response to treatment.

Physical Examination

The physical examination may reveal obvious trauma, abscesses, poxvirus lesions, *Knemidokoptes* lesions, or vitamin A deficiency. Common findings in birds with exophthalmos or periorbital masses are discussed below.

Swellings around the eye covered by skin may be abscesses, granulomas, tumors, or the result of trauma. Poxvirus often appears as a scab. Papillomas and *Knemidokoptes* lesions are proliferative.

Periorbital abscesses may be within the infraorbital sinus or involve orbital tissues. The infraorbital sinus is lateral to the nasal cavity and lacks outer bony walls. Externally, it occupies the area between the commissure of the beak and the eye. This sinus has extensive diverticula into the upper beak, mandible, around the eye, and pneumatized bones of the skull (see Fig. 1–6). Periorbital abscesses are often the result of chronic sinusitis (Fig. 5–3). Cellulitis or abscesses of orbital tissue can be the result of a primary bacterial or fungal infection or extension from the infraorbital sinus. Trauma may also cause orbital cellulitis, hematomas, or abscesses.

Lacrimal sac abscesses appear as mobile swellings at the medial canthus. Purulent material can sometimes be expressed through the lacrimal punctum.

Mild periorbital and conjunctival swelling, xerophthalmia, and ocular discharge may be seen with vitamin A deficiency. Xerophthalmia is abnormal dryness and thickening of the conjunctiva and cornea. Vitamin A deficiency causes squamous metaplasia of mucous membranes and salivary gland ducts and hyperkeratosis. Another sign of vitamin A deficiency that may be seen on physical examination

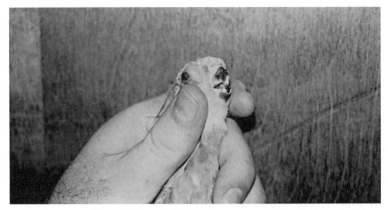

Figure 5–3. A periorbital abscess in a cockatiel.

is swollen margins of the choana in the roof of the mouth. Associated papillae may be blunted or absent, and sterile granulomas of the oral and lingual mucosa, periorbital area, and sinuses may be present.

The cutaneous form of poxvirus is characterized by cutaneous proliferative growths on featherless areas of skin (around eyes, nares, beak, vent, and feet). Early signs of the disease include unilateral or bilateral blepharitis, lid edema, and a serous ocular discharge. With progression, ulcers appear at the lid margins or medial or lateral canthus. Scabs form and may seal the eye or eyes shut. Scabs fall off within 2 weeks. Secondary bacterial infections are common, often causing severe sequelae.

Proliferative growths on the beak, feet, legs, and around the eyes and vent are seen with scaly face mites. The proliferative tissue has a characteristic honeycombed appearance.

Papillomas are also proliferative growths that may occur on eyelids and other unfeathered skin, oral cavity, cloaca, and gastrointestinal tract. Lesions are wartlike epithelial proliferations. They occur as single or multiple slow-growing masses.

Avian sarcoma/leukosis virus induces various types of neoplasia (e.g., fibrosarcoma, mesothelioma, endothelioma, chondroma). Periorbital tumors may be caused by this virus. Abdominal distention and dyspnea may be present because of abdominal tumors. The liver may be enlarged. Multiple tumors, often involving multiple organs, usually occur with this infection.

Oxyspirura, Thelazia, and *Philophthalmus* parasites may be present under the nictitating membrane, in the conjunctival sac, or in the lacrimal duct. Birds scratch at affected eyes.

Strabismus may occur with space-occupying lesions within the orbit (e.g., neoplasia, hematoma, or abscess).

Periorbital dermatitis may cause thickened skin around the eye. Bacterial or fungal infections or allergic reactions are possible etiologies. These lesions are often pruritic.

Check for signs of involvement of other body systems. Sinusitis often accompanies exophthalmos and may require additional treatment (see Chapter 3).

Algorithm for Exophthalmos or Periorbital Swelling

See Figure 5–4.

Diagnostic Plan for Exophthalmos or Periorbital Swelling

Stabilize severely ill birds before performing diagnostic tests, and provide supportive care as needed during the diagnostic evaluation (see Chapter 1).

Selection of diagnostic tests is based on consideration of the signalment and history of the bird and the findings of the physical and ophthalmic examinations. Trauma, vitamin A deficiency, poxvirus lesions, papillomas, *Knemidokoptes* lesions, hematomas, lid abnormalities, infraorbital sinus inflation, and involvement of other body systems may be identified during a complete physical examination. A scraping is used to visualize *Knemidokoptes* mites. Useful samples include scrapings of affected hyperkeratotic lesions around the cere, eyes, and vent and on the feet.

Cytology and culture of periorbital aspirates are often the most useful initial diagnostic tests. Periorbital cutaneous and subcutaneous lesion cytology is useful in the diagnosis of bacterial infections, foreign body granulomas, and poxvirus lesions. Squamous epithelial cells, debris, and extracellular bacteria may be seen in samples from normal birds. Phagocytosed bacteria indicate a primary or secondary bacterial infection. Macrophages and multinucleated giant cells indicate a foreign body reaction or mycobacteriosis. A mixed cell inflammatory response may be seen if a secondary bacterial infection has developed because of a foreign body. Poxvirus lesions contain squamous epithelial cells that contain large cytoplasmic vacuoles (Bollinger bodies) that push the cell nucleus to the cell margin (see Fig. 12–24). The vacuoles may contain small, pale eosinophilic inclusions. An inflammatory response is often present as a result of the secondary bacterial infections common with poxvirus lesions.

Sample collection for cytology, culture, and acid-fast staining of a retrobulbar mass is done by aspiration. The direction of the deviation of the eye suggests the location of the mass and the site for needle entry (e.g., lateral deviation indicates a medial mass). The globe is large and snugly fills the orbit, making retrobulbar sample collection difficult. Large masses may cause enough deviation to be reached with a needle. To sample a medial mass, insert the needle medial to the nictitating membrane, penetrate the conjunctiva, and aspirate along the medial orbital wall. Other areas are sampled similarly. Anesthesia is required. Ultrasound-guided orbital aspiration, if available, minimizes complications and ensures accurate needle placement.

Retrobulbar masses that may be differentiated cytologically include bacterial abscesses, fungal granulomas, hematomas, and neoplasia. Heterophils, lymphocytes, plasma cells, macrophages, and bacterial phagocytosis indicate septic inflammation. Macrophages, lymphocytes, plasma cells, and fungal elements indicate a fungal infection. *Aspergillus* is characterized by branching septate hyphae (see Fig. 12–29). Hyphae may stain poorly or basophilic with Wright's or Diff-Quick stain. Methylene blue stain may be used to better visualize hyphae. *Cryptococcus* is an oval to round yeast with a mucopolysaccharide capsule. Yeast cells stain basophilic with Wright's or Diff-Quick stain. The *Cryptococcus* capsule

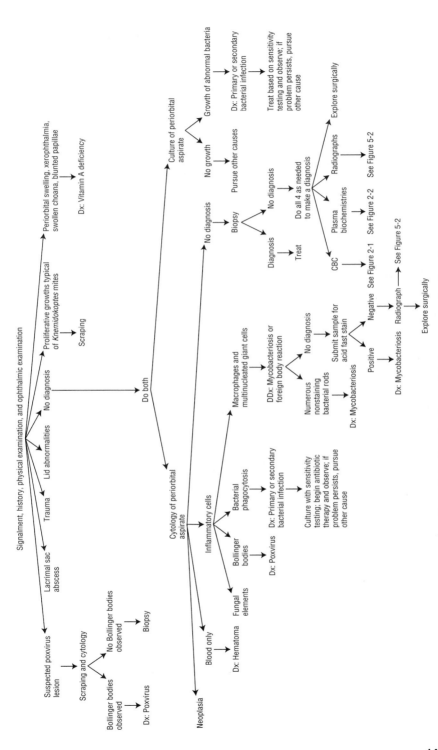

Figure 5–4. Algorithm for exophthalmos or periorbital swelling.

149

portion of the yeast does not stain with these stains, but forms a clear halo around the yeast.

Macrophages, multinucleated giant cells, and neutrophils may occur with *Mycobacterium* granulomas or foreign material. Macrophages and multinucleated giant cells may contain phagocytosed debris. With mycobacteriosis, the background may contain numerous bacterial rods that do not stain with Wright's or Diff-Quick stains (see Fig. 12–28). Acid-fast staining is used to identify the acid-fast bacteria.

Acute hematomas contain erythrocytes and may resemble peripheral blood. Thrombocytes are usually absent. Erythrophagocytosis, red cell fragments, and iron pigment with predominantly macrophages are characteristic of older hematomas.

Characteristics of neoplasia include cytoplasmic basophilia, increased N:C ratio, nuclear anisocytosis, nuclear pleomorphism, abnormal nucleoli, multinucleation, and abnormal mitotic figures. A combination of abnormalities is required for a diagnosis of neoplasia. Characteristics vary with the type and location of the neoplasm. Avoid false-positive diagnoses. Consult with an avian pathologist when the diagnosis is unclear.

When a diagnosis cannot be obtained with cytology, submit material from lesions for biopsy. Histopathology is useful for definitive diagnosis involving poxvirus lesions, papillomas, and avian sarcoma/leukosis virus–induced tumors. Differentiation among bacterial, vitamin A deficiency, and foreign body abscesses and granulomas may be accomplished.

Hematology may be helpful in inflammatory or infectious diseases. Perform a CBC if septic or systemic disease is suspected, when a bird is unresponsive to treatment, or to help determine the general health of the bird. Changes in the hemogram commonly seen in birds with exophthalmos or periorbital swelling are detailed below.

Nonregenerative anemias are usually normocytic and normochromatic, but hypochromasia, anisocytosis, and poikilocytosis frequently occur in birds. Nonregenerative anemias may occur with chronic inflammatory diseases, including aspergillosis, mycobacteriosis, and neoplasia.

Leukocytosis and heterophilia may be the results of stress, neoplasia, avian sarcoma/leukosis virus, or inflammatory diseases (e.g., bacteria or fungi). Differential diagnoses to consider in a bird with exophthalmos or periorbital swelling with a WBC count in excess of 40,000/µl include mycobacteriosis and aspergillosis. Monocytosis may occur with mycobacteriosis, aspergillosis, and chronic bacterial infections.

Leukopenia may be associated with an overwhelming bacterial, fungal, or viral septicemia and endotoxemia.

Plasma biochemistry tests are important in birds with exophthalmos or periorbital swelling to determine the general health of the bird and to test for elevation of liver enzymes. General tests are useful, such as AST, uric acid, total protein, and creatine kinase (CK). Bile acid concentrations may be useful to evaluate liver function, if needed. With impaired function, bile acids may increase.

An elevation in AST is usually the result of liver or muscle damage. The AST may be elevated in birds with exophthalmos or a periorbital swelling from hepatitis-induced liver damage caused by bacterial infections (e.g., *Mycobacterium*).

Radiology may reveal periorbital masses, trauma, or systemic involvement. Radiographic abnormalities in birds with exophthalmos or periorbital swelling include trauma lesions, periocular masses, and organomegaly. Fractures of the skull or scleral ossicles indicate head trauma. Fractures elsewhere in the body may indicate trauma.

Retrobulbar masses may be evaluated for location and size, and periorbital and sinus lesions may be detected. Pulmonary tissue is evaluated for the presence of metastatic disease when neoplasia is present.

Evaluation of the hepatic silhouette may reveal hepatomegaly. Hepatomegaly may be the result of bacterial infections.

If a diagnosis is still uncertain based on these tests, more specific testing is performed. Special stains, titers, cultures, and virus testing are used to rule in or out specific diseases. Acid-fast stains may be required to identify mycobacteriosis granulomas. Acid-fast staining can be used to identify acid-fast *Mycobacterium*, which affects the digestive tract in most birds. Feces or biopsy samples may reveal acid-fast organisms.

Ultrasonography is useful in larger birds to view orbital or ocular lesions. Magnetic resonance imaging and computed tomography are useful for imaging lesions that may not be visible with plain radiographs.

Serologic testing for aspergillosis is available for pet birds. A periorbital fungal granuloma may produce adequate antibodies for a positive diagnosis. False-negative results occur. Aspergillosis can sometimes be demonstrated with a fungal culture. Useful samples to culture include swabs of suspect lesions, sinus aspirates, tracheal washes, and swabs of the choana, if respiratory signs are also present. Samples should be sent to a laboratory familiar with avian aspergillosis. False-negative results occur. False-positive results occur if the sample is contaminated with *Aspergillus* from the environment.

Various methods are available to detect viral infections (see Chapter 12). A suspicion of infection is based on signalment, history, and clinical signs. Concurrent signs are usually present with viral infections.

Poxvirus may be diagnosed by histopathology, virus culture, virus detection in feces by culture, or electron microscopy. Asymptomatic carriers intermittently shed the virus in the feces and may be identified with repeated culturing of the feces.

Plasma, serum, or neoplastic tissue is best for demonstrating the presence of avian sarcoma/leukosis virus.

Treatment for Exophthalmos or Periorbital Swelling

Provide supportive care as needed (see Chapter 1).

Hematomas resolve without treatment.

Periorbital abscesses are debrided, and systemic antibiotics are used based on culture and sensitivity results. Therapy may be initiated with enrofloxacin or cefotaxime before sensitivity results. If sinusitis is present, treat with nasal flushes (see Chapters 3 and 11).

Lacrimal sac abscess contents are expressed through the lacrimal punctum or may require cannulation and flushing to remove. Flush with an antibiotic solution twice daily. Selection of an antibiotic is based on culture and sensitivity. Surgical removal of the nictitating membrane is not recommended.

Inflation of the portion of the infraorbital sinus surrounding the eye is not pathologic and requires no treatment.

Treatment of malignant tumors is usually unrewarding. Various combinations of surgery, chemotherapy, and radiation therapy have been used. If the tumor can be surgically removed, surgery is usually the treatment of choice. Papillomas will recur if excision is incomplete.

Vitamin A deficiency requires parenteral vitamin A initially, then oral supplementation and correction of the diet. Keratin cysts and abscesses are debrided and cultured.

Growths are surgically removed. Surgical reconstruction of congenital abnormalities is usually unsuccessful. Ectropion is surgically corrected with lateral canthoplasty.

Small numbers of conjunctival, nictitating membrane, or lacrimal duct parasites are manually removed or flushed out. Heavy infestations are treated with a single topical dose of ivermectin. Repeated applications of topical carbamate powder may eliminate *Philophthalmus* flukes.

Management of viral infections includes symptomatic therapy and prevention of secondary bacterial infection and contagion. Chlorhexidine in the drinking water is used to decrease spread in flock situations. Specific treatments are discussed in Chapter 9.

Treat other disorders according to their primary causes.

INTRAOCULAR ABNORMALITIES, SHRUNKEN GLOBE, OR BUPHTHALMOS

Intraocular abnormalities are common in birds. Uveitis, cataracts, and lens luxation are frequently encountered in pet bird practice. Retinal diseases, glaucoma, and intraocular tumors also occur.

Anterior uveitis is inflammation of the anterior uvea, which consists of the iris, ciliary body, and the choroid.

Buphthalmos, an abnormal enlargement of the globe, occurs when there is increased pressure in the globe or inflammation.

The anterior chamber on the down side of recumbent birds during anesthesia may collapse, causing a shrunken globe. Digital pressure during restraint may also result in this temporary condition. Posttraumatic lesions may result in a smaller-than-normal eye. Sunken eyes with normal globe size are common in macaws with chronic sinusitis because of loss of the periorbital fat pad (see Chapter 3).

Differential Diagnoses for Intraocular Abnormalities, Shrunken Globe, or Buphthalmos

1. Infectious
   a. Bacterial: gram-negative, gram-positive

b. Viral: avian picornavirus encephalomyelitis, reovirus, °poxvirus, PMV 3
c. Parasitic: *Toxoplasma*, ocular nematodiasis
2. Physical: °trauma, °corneal ulcer
3. Neoplastic
4. Anomalous: °cataracts, microphthalmos
5. Iatrogenic: °anesthesia, °handling, glaucoma after cataract surgery

Signalment

Common causes of anterior uveitis in pet birds include corneal ulcers and trauma. Less common causes include systemic disease (e.g., septicemia, PMV 3, reovirus, poxvirus), ocular nematodiasis, lens rupture, and intraocular bacterial infections.

Cataracts are commonly the result of trauma, old age, or intraocular inflammation. They may also be congenital. Congenital cataracts occur in canaries and macaws. Trauma is a common cause of cataracts in raptors.

Lens luxation is usually the result of trauma.

Retinal diseases are commonly the result of trauma, toxoplasmosis, reovirus, inflammation, and idiopathic causes.

Glaucoma is rare in birds. It is usually the result of trauma or lens luxation or may be associated with cataract surgery.

Intraocular tumors are rare in birds.

Buphthalmos is uncommon in birds. Inflammation and glaucoma are possible causes. Buphthalmos associated with avian picornavirus encephalomyelitis occurs primarily in pigeons and gallinaceous birds.

Shrunken globes are most commonly associated with anesthesia or restraint in pet birds. Traumatic rupture of the globe is a common cause of shrunken globes in raptors.

Toxoplasmosis primarily affects gallinaceous and passerine birds. The cutaneous form of poxvirus is rare except in blue-fronted Amazons, lovebirds, raptors, pigeons, and passerines (including mynahs). Reovirus is commonly seen in imported birds and primarily affects African gray parrots, cockatoos, and other Old World psittacines. African gray parrots may develop uveitis, retinal hemorrhages, and fibrinous exudate in the anterior chamber when infected with PMV 3.

History

A complete history may reveal trauma, exposure to infectious diseases, or previous cataract surgery. Infectious diseases are seen most frequently in birds recently exposed to other birds. Isolated birds and those in closed collections are commonly ill because of trauma, aging, transport, or iatrogenic causes. Bacterial infections are also seen in this group.

Exposure to cat feces is of historical importance. Toxoplasmosis is acquired

---

°Common causes.

through the ingestion of oocysts in the feces of infected cats, exposure to coprophagic arthropods, or food or water supplies contaminated with feces from infected cats.

The duration of the illness is important. Note the owner's description of the clinical signs and the course of the disease. Note previous illnesses, including signs, treatment, and response to treatment.

Physical Examination

A complete physical examination and ophthalmic examination may reveal obvious trauma, poxvirus lesions, cataracts, and ocular nematodes. Observations may help to narrow differentials. Common findings in birds with intraocular abnormalities, shrunken globes, or buphthalmos are discussed below.

A bright light source (e.g., pen light) is used to evaluate the pupil size, symmetry, and response to light. Aqueous flare and presence of hypopyon or hyphema are noted. Aqueous flare is seen clinically as a decrease in clarity of iris detail and pupil margin. The clarity of the cornea, aqueous humor, lens, and vitreous is also assessed. Cataracts and intraocular nematodes may be identified.

Poxvirus lesions are characterized by cutaneous proliferative growths on featherless areas of skin (around eyes, nares, beak, vent, and feet). Early signs of the disease include unilateral or bilateral blepharitis, lid edema, and a serous ocular discharge. With progression, ulcers appear at the lid margins or medial or lateral canthus. Scabs then form and may seal the eye or eyes shut. Scabs fall off within 2 weeks. Secondary bacterial infections are common, often causing severe sequelae.

Clinical signs associated with reovirus include ataxia, diarrhea, dyspnea, uveitis, retinal hemorrhage, hypopyon, intraocular fibrinous exudates, and fixed, dilated pupils.

African gray parrots may develop uveitis, retinal hemorrhages, and fibrinous exudate in the anterior chamber when infected with PMV 3. Paralysis and a hemorrhagic nasal discharge may also occur.

Avian picornavirus encephalomyelitis can cause enlargement of the globe, cataracts, fixed pupils, and blindness. Tremors and ataxia may also occur.

Clinical signs associated with toxoplasmosis include anorexia, diarrhea, conjunctivitis, blindness, head tilt, circling, and ataxia.

Algorithm for Intraocular Abnormalities, Shrunken Globe, or Buphthalmos

See Figure 5–5.

Diagnostic Plan for Intraocular Abnormalities, Shrunken Globe, or Buphthalmos

Stabilize severely ill birds before performing diagnostic tests, and provide supportive care as needed during the diagnostic evaluation (see Chapter 1).

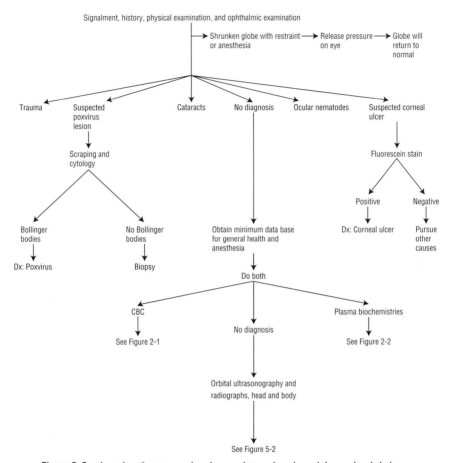

Figure 5–5. Algorithm for intraocular abnormalities, shrunken globe, or buphthalmos.

Selection of appropriate diagnostic tests is based on consideration of the signalment and history of the bird and the findings of the physical and ophthalmic examinations. Use the history to rule out trauma, exposure to infectious diseases, and previous cataract surgery. Trauma, poxvirus lesions, cataracts, ocular nematodes, and involvement of other body systems may be identified during a complete physical examination. Fluorescein stain is used to identify corneal ulcers. Systemic disease is suspected when there are clinical signs of involvement of other body systems.

Hematology and biochemistry tests rarely provide a diagnosis but are useful in supporting infectious, inflammatory, and some toxic diagnoses. Perform a CBC if septic or systemic disease is suspected, when a bird is unresponsive to treatment, or to help determine the general health of the bird. Changes in the hemogram commonly seen in birds with intraocular abnormalities are detailed below.

Nonregenerative anemias may occur with chronic inflammatory diseases. Leukocytosis and heterophilia may be caused by stress, neoplasia, or inflammatory diseases (e.g., bacteria). Leukopenia may be associated with an overwhelming bacterial or viral septicemia or endotoxemia.

Plasma biochemistry tests are important in the diagnosis of metabolic disease and to evaluate the general health of the bird. Useful biochemistries include AST, uric acid, total protein, glucose, and CK. Toxoplasmosis, bacterial hepatitis, and reovirus can cause an elevation of AST in a bird with intraocular abnormalities.

Orbital ultrasonography is useful in larger birds to view orbital or ocular lesions. Radiology is useful for diagnosing periorbital and systemic disease and trauma. Radiographic abnormalities in birds with intraocular abnormalities include trauma lesions and organomegaly. Fractures of the skull or scleral ossicles indicate head trauma. Fractures elsewhere in the body may indicate trauma.

Evaluation of the hepatic silhouette may reveal hepatomegaly. Hepatomegaly may occur with toxoplasmosis, reovirus infection, or bacterial infections.

Various tests are available for diagnosis of viral infections (see Chapter 12). A suspicion of infection is based on signalment, history, and clinical signs. Concurrent signs are usually present with viral infections. Choose tests based on signalment and clinical signs.

Poxvirus may be diagnosed by histopathology, virus culture, virus detection in feces by culture, or electron microscopy. Asymptomatic carriers intermittently shed the virus in the feces and may be identified with repeated culturing of the feces.

Diagnosis of PMV is based on isolation of the virus from cloacal swabs in live birds. Hemagglutination inhibition serologic testing can be used to detect antibodies to PMV. Antibodies appear approximately 8 days after infection. Postmortem cases may be diagnosed through isolation of the virus from the brain or organs.

Diagnosis of avian picornavirus encephalomyelitis is based on postmortem histology. Histologic changes include neuronal degeneration with lymphocytic perivascular cuffing and gliosis in the brain and spinal cord.

Cloacal swabs and samples from affected organs may be used for virus isolation and culture for identification of reovirus infection. Viral antigen may be detected by immunofluorescence in affected tissues.

A small sample of aqueous humor can be collected using a 27-gauge needle. This sample is examined cytologically and cultured. Complications are common with intraocular sample collection; however, this test may be warranted if a diagnosis cannot be made using less invasive techniques.

Treatment for Intraocular Abnormalities, Shrunken Globe, or Buphthalmos

Provide supportive care as needed (see Chapter 1).

Corneal lacerations are sutured and treated with topical antibiotics, often successfully. Lens luxations are surgical emergencies requiring immediate referral.

Corneal ulcers are treated with topical antibiotics. Acetylcysteine is sprayed into the eye every few hours if ulcers are severe. If intraocular inflammation is present, systemic corticosteroids are also used. Deep or severe ulcers may benefit from a temporary tarsorrhaphy. One or two horizontal mattress sutures with 4-0 or 6-0 nylon will provide a corneal bandage.

If uveitis is present, treat the primary cause. Corticosteroids are used topically if corneal ulceration is not present.

Treatment of malignant tumors is usually unrewarding. Various combinations of surgery, chemotherapy, and radiation therapy have been used. If the tumor can be surgically removed, surgery is usually the treatment of choice. Enucleation is complicated by a very short optic nerve.

Cataracts may impair vision. Most pet birds do well with limited or no vision, except passerines. Some raptors will survive in the wild with vision in only one eye (e.g., owls); others cannot catch prey.

Intraocular parasites require surgical removal if they are problematic.

Management of viral infections includes symptomatic therapy and prevention of secondary bacterial infection and contagion. Chlorhexidine in the drinking water is used to decrease spread in flock situations. Specific treatments are found in Chapter 9.

Treat other disorders according to their primary causes.

BLINDNESS

Blindness is uncommon in birds. It may be caused by central or peripheral lesions. Peripheral lesions include opacity of the visual media (e.g., cornea, lens) or retinal lesions.

Blindness as a result of encephalitis may result in other neurologic signs. Consult Chapter 6 for assistance with neurologic signs.

Differential Diagnoses for Blindness

1. Infectious: any organism causing encephalitis
   a. Bacterial: organisms causing encephalitis
   b. Chlamydial: *Chlamydia psittaci*
   c. Viral: avian picornavirus encephalomyelitis, others causing encephalitis
   d. Fungal: organisms causing encephalitis
   e. Parasitic: *Toxoplasma*, others causing encephalitis
2. Metabolic: °hepatic encephalopathy (hepatic lipidosis, mycotoxicosis, hemochromatosis, and vaccine-induced hepatopathy)
3. Toxic: °lead, organochlorine, cephaloridine
4. Physical: °cerebral vascular accident, ischemic infarction, cataracts, °trauma, atherosclerosis
5. Neoplasia: pituitary, ocular
6. Developmental: cryptophthalmos; microphthalmos; maldevelopment of ciliary body, retina, and pectin; retinal dysplasia; congenital cataracts

---

°Common causes.

Signalment

Common causes of blindness in psittacines include trauma, lead toxicosis, and hepatic encephalopathy. Cerebrovascular accidents are also a common cause of blindness in budgies. Passerines are commonly affected by cataracts, hepatic lipidosis, or hemochromatosis. Raptors are commonly blind as a result of trauma.

Cataracts are commonly the result of trauma, old age, or intraocular inflammation or are congenital. Trauma is a common cause of cataracts in raptors. Congenital cataracts are common in canaries and macaws.

Toxoplasmosis primarily affects gallinaceous and passerine birds. Avian picornavirus encephalomyelitis may cause blindness in pigeons and gallinaceous birds. Pituitary adenomas are common in budgies. Affected birds are usually about 4 years old and most often male.

History

A complete history may reveal trauma or access to potential toxins or infectious diseases. Isolated birds and those in closed collections are commonly ill because of toxicoses, trauma, metabolic problems, neoplasia, or cerebrovascular accidents. Birds recently exposed to other birds may become ill as a result of infectious diseases, including viral, chlamydial, parasitic, and bacterial infections, or those problems occurring in isolated birds. Toxic and infectious causes are suspected when multiple birds are affected.

A history of exposure or access to a potential toxin is significant in a blind bird. Toxins that may cause blindness include lead, organochlorines, cephaloridine, and mycotoxins. Some sources of lead are listed in Table 9–3.

Diets contaminated with mycotoxin can result in abnormalities that cause blindness. Ingestion of a toxic dose of mycotoxin can result in death in a few days. Chronic exposure can cause liver disease, leading to hepatic encephalopathy and associated blindness.

Onset of signs after food intake may indicate hepatic encephalopathy.

Exposure to cat feces is of historical importance. Toxoplasmosis is acquired through the ingestion of oocysts in the feces of infected cats, exposure to coprophagic arthropods, or food or water supplies contaminated with feces from infected cats.

The duration of the illness is important. Note the owner's description of the clinical signs and the course of the disease. Note previous illnesses, including signs, treatment, and response to treatment.

Physical Examination

Complete physical, ophthalmic, and neurologic examinations are important in blind birds. The physical examination may reveal obvious eyelid lesions (e.g., fused eyelid margins), periorbital or orbital masses, and corneal or lens opacities. Retinal lesions are more difficult to observe because of the size of the avian eye and presence of skeletal muscle in the iris. A complete ophthalmic examination requires anesthesia and examination of the retina. Other systems are often affected when central blindness occurs, resulting in associated clinical signs.

Blood in the mouth, ears, or eyes indicates head trauma. Look at the skin at the top of the head; meningeal hematomas may be visualized through the calvarium in some cases. Fractures or bruises anywhere in the body can indicate that trauma has occurred.

Evaluation of the droppings may help narrow differential diagnoses. Polyuria or hematuria may indicate lead toxicosis. Biliverdinuria (green-colored urates) may indicate liver disease, which may occur from lead toxicosis, hepatic lipidosis, or hemochromatosis.

Neurologic signs other than blindness occur with lead and organochlorine toxicoses, encephalitis, hepatopathies, and neoplasia.

Encephalitis can cause seizures, ataxia, cranial nerve dysfunction, circling, and nystagmus.

Avian picornavirus encephalomyelitis can cause enlargement of the globe, cataracts, fixed pupils, and blindness. Tremors, paralysis, and ataxia may also occur.

Clinical signs associated with toxoplasmosis include anorexia, diarrhea, conjunctivitis, blindness, head tilt, circling, and ataxia.

Pituitary adenomas cause somnolence, convulsions, wing flapping, leg twitches, and unconsciousness. Other signs that may occur include ataxia, tremors, inability to perch, polydipsia, polyuria, cere color change, feather abnormalities, obesity, exophthalmos, blindness, lack of pupillary light response, and mydriasis.

Clinical signs associated with lead toxicosis may include lethargy, anorexia, weakness, regurgitation, diarrhea, ataxia, head tilt, blindness, circling, paresis, paralysis, head tremors, convulsions, weight loss, and death.

Organochlorine (DDT and DDE) toxicosis is rare in pet birds. Clinical signs consist of convulsions, blindness, and ataxia.

Clinical signs of hepatic encephalopathy usually occur shortly after eating. Signs include depression, ataxia, decreased proprioception, and seizures.

Algorithm for Blindness

See Figure 5–6.

Diagnostic Plan for Blindness

Stabilize severely ill birds before performing diagnostic tests, and provide supportive care as needed during the diagnostic evaluation (see Chapter 1).

Selection of appropriate diagnostic tests is based on consideration of the signalment and history of the bird and the findings of the physical and ophthalmic examinations. Use the history to rule out exposure to toxins, toxoplasmosis, and trauma. The physical examination is used to determine if eyelid, corneal, or lens lesions are causing the blindness and to check for signs of involvement of other body systems (e.g., neurologic or gastrointestinal).

Retinal causes can be differentiated from central blindness with an electroretinogram.

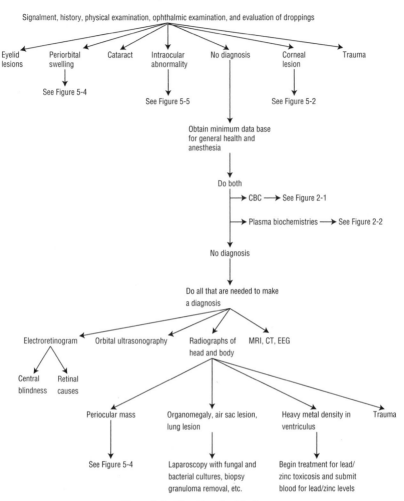

Figure 5–6. Algorithm for blindness.

Hematology is useful in supporting infectious, inflammatory, and some toxic diagnoses. Perform a CBC if septic or systemic disease is suspected, when a bird is unresponsive to treatment, or to help determine the general health of the bird. Changes in the hemogram commonly seen in blind birds are detailed below.

Nonregenerative anemias may occur with chronic inflammatory diseases, including chlamydiosis, aspergillosis, mycobacteriosis, neoplasia, mycotoxicosis, and lead toxicosis.

Nonregenerative anemias with decreased plasma protein may be seen with acute blood loss resulting from trauma or coagulopathies as a result of liver disease (e.g., mycotoxicosis, hepatic lipidosis). If blood loss is not continuous, as may occur with trauma, a regenerative anemia will develop within several days. This will be characterized by the appearance of polychromasia and anisocytosis.

Regenerative anemias with normal plasma protein may occur with lead toxicosis or mycotoxicosis. Lead toxicosis may cause an exaggerated response with more polychromasia and rubricytes than would be expected for the degree of anemia present. Basophilic stippling and cytoplasmic vacuolization may sometimes be seen with lead toxicosis. Hypochromasia can be associated with lead toxicosis.

Leukocytosis and heterophilia may be caused by stress, neoplasia, or inflammatory diseases (e.g., bacteria, chlamydiosis, fungi). Differential diagnoses to consider in blind birds with a WBC count in excess of 40,000/μl include chlamydiosis, mycobacteriosis, and aspergillosis. Monocytosis may occur with chlamydiosis, mycobacteriosis, aspergillosis, and chronic bacterial infections.

Leukopenia may be associated with an overwhelming bacterial, fungal, chlamydial, or viral septicemia and endotoxemia.

Plasma biochemistry tests are important in the diagnosis of metabolic disease and to evaluate the general health of the bird. The most useful biochemistries for blind birds include AST, plasma protein, bile acids, CK, and glucose. Bile acid concentrations may be useful to evaluate liver function. With impaired function, bile acids may increase. An elevation in AST is usually the result of liver or muscle damage. The AST may be elevated in blind birds as a result of liver damage caused by chlamydiosis, hepatic lipidosis, mycotoxicosis, hemochromatosis, toxoplasmosis, reovirus infection, or hepatitis caused by bacterial infections (including mycobacteriosis).

An unexplained persistent elevation of AST or bile acids is an indication for liver biopsy. Liver biopsy is used to determine the etiology of hepatopathies. Diagnosis of hepatic lipidosis, hemochromatosis, and mycotoxicosis is aided with liver biopsy. Indications for liver biopsy include radiographic evidence of hepatomegaly or microhepatia or abnormal hepatic biochemistry tests (e.g., AST, bile acid, albumin). Histologic evaluation of liver parenchyma is required to determine the etiology of many hepatopathies. Hepatopathies resulting in blindness that may be differentiated with liver biopsy and histopathology include hepatitis, hepatic lipidosis, hemochromatosis, and mycotoxicosis. Toxoplasmosis may be identified if the liver is also involved. The technique to perform the procedure is described in Chapter 14.

Hepatic lipidosis is indicated histologically by fatty infiltration of hepatocytes. Impression smears made from biopsies of affected livers contain enlarged hepatocytes that contain round, cytoplasmic vacuoles, and lipid material in the background. Histopathologic changes that occur with hemochromatosis include the abnormal storage of iron in the liver. Mycotoxicosis may produce changes that mimic other diseases or may be altered because of secondary infections resulting from immunosuppression.

Orbital ultrasonography is useful in larger birds to view orbital or ocular lesions. Radiology is useful for diagnosing periorbital and systemic disease, hepatomegaly, and trauma. Metal densities in the ventriculus may indicate lead toxicosis; however, toxicosis may be present without this radiographic sign. Radiographic abnormalities in blind birds include trauma lesions, periocular masses, organomegaly, and metallic densities in the gastrointestinal tract. Fractures of the skull or scleral ossicles indicate head trauma. Fractures elsewhere in the body may indicate trauma.

Evaluation of the hepatic silhouette may reveal hepatomegaly or microhepatia.

Hepatomegaly in a blind bird can be consistent with hepatic lipidosis, hemochromatosis, mycotoxicosis, chlamydiosis, toxoplasmosis, or bacterial infections.

Ascites, which may accompany hemochromatosis and other abdominal abnormalities, causes an overall loss of organ detail of the ventrodorsal view. On the lateral view, ascites will cause loss of detail in the celomic cavity, with the lung, intestinal gas, and grit in the ventriculus often being the only identifiable features.

Magnetic resonance imaging, computed tomography, and electroencephalography are useful for diagnosis of atherosclerosis, cerebrovascular accidents, ischemic infarction, and neoplasia (e.g., pituitary tumors).

It is difficult to obtain cerebrospinal fluid on a tap without blood contamination.

Cultures, titers, blood lead levels, special stains, and virus tests may be required for a definitive diagnosis. Selection of tests is based on clinical signs.

Samples for chlamydial testing are discussed in Chapter 9. Plasma protein electrophoresis is useful for detection and identification of various illnesses (e.g., chlamydiosis, mycobacteriosis, aspergillosis, and some kidney and liver problems).

Serologic testing for aspergillosis is available for pet birds. False-negative results occur. Aspergillosis can sometimes be demonstrated with a fungal culture. Useful samples to culture include swabs of suspect lesions, sinus aspirates, tracheal washes, and swabs of the choana, if respiratory signs are also present. Samples should be sent to a laboratory familiar with avian aspergillosis. False-negative results occur. False-positive results occur if the sample is contaminated with *Aspergillus* from the environment.

Acid-fast staining can be used to identify acid-fast *Mycobacterium*, which affects the digestive tract in most birds. Feces or biopsy samples may reveal acid-fast organisms.

Whole blood, with lithium heparin used for the anticoagulant, is the sample of choice for determining blood lead concentrations. Whole blood lead levels greater than 0.2 ppm are suggestive of lead toxicosis, and levels greater than 0.5 ppm are diagnostic of lead toxicosis.

Various tests are available for diagnosis of viral infections (see Chapter 12). A suspicion of infection is based on signalment, history, and clinical signs. Concurrent signs are usually present with viral infections.

Diagnosis of avian picornavirus encephalomyelitis is based on histology postmortem. Histologic changes include neuronal degeneration with lymphocytic perivascular cuffing and gliosis in the brain and spinal cord.

Treatment for Blindness

Provide supportive care as needed (see Chapter 1).

Hematomas resolve without treatment.

Lens luxations are a surgical emergency requiring immediate referral.

Treatment of bacterial CNS infections is usually ineffective in birds with CNS signs and blindness. Attempted therapy may be initiated with cefotaxime or chloramphenicol, both of which may penetrate the CNS in effective concentrations.

If uveitis is present, treat the primary cause. Corticosteroids are used topically. If hepatic encephalopathy is present, treat the underlying cause of hepatic failure. Symptomatic relief with lactulose, vitamin supplementation, neomycin sulfate, and a low protein, high carbohydrate, high-quality protein diet may improve clinical signs while the underlying hepatopathy is being treated.

Treatment of malignant tumors is usually unrewarding. Various combinations of surgery, chemotherapy, and radiation therapy have been used. If the tumor can be surgically removed, surgery is usually the treatment of choice.

Cataracts may cause blindness. Most pet birds do well with limited or no vision, except passerines. Some raptors will survive in the wild with vision in only one eye (e.g., owls); others cannot catch prey.

Treatment of cerebrovascular accidents or infarction includes intravenous dexamethasone, a stress-free environment (dark and quiet), and control of seizures, if present, with diazepam.

Management of viral infections includes symptomatic therapy and prevention of secondary bacterial infection and contagion. Chlorhexidine in the drinking water is used to decrease spread in flock situations. Vaccines are available to decrease spread of avian picornavirus encephalomyelitis.

Treat other disorders according to their primary causes.

References and Additional Reading

Bauck L. Three treatment protocols for cockatiel conjunctivitis. *Proc Assoc Avian Vet* 1989;92–96.

Campbell TW. Cytology in avian diagnostics. In Kirk RW (ed): *Current Veterinary Therapy IX, Small Animal Practice.* Philadelphia, WB Saunders, 1986, pp 725–731.

Campbell TW. *Avian Hematology and Cytology,* ed 2. Ames, Iowa State University Press, 1995.

Clipsham R. Noninfectious diseases of pediatric psittacines. *Semin Avian Exot Pet Med* 1992;1(1):22–33.

Greenacre CB, Watson E, Ritchie BW. Choanal atresia in an African grey parrot (*Psittacus erithacus erithacus*) and an umbrella cockatoo (*Cacatua alba*). *J Assoc Avian Vet* 1993;7(1):19–22.

Jenkins JR. Avian metabolic chemistries. *Semin Avian Exot Pet Med* 1994;3(1):25–32.

Karpinski LG. Ophthalmology. In Harrison GJ, Harrison LR (eds): *Clinical Avian Med Surg.* Philadelphia, WB Saunders, 1986, pp 278-281.

Karpinski LG, Clubb SL. Clinical aspects of ophthalmology in caged birds. In Kirk RW (ed): *Current Veterinary Therapy IX, Small Animal Practice.* Philadelphia, WB Saunders, 1986, pp 616–621.

Kern TJ. Disorders of the special senses. In Altman RB, Clubb SL, Dorrestein GM, Quesenberry K (eds): *Avian Medicine and Surgery.* Philadelphia, WB Saunders, 1997, pp 563–589.

Kern TJ, Paul-Murphy J, Murphy CJ, et al. Disorders of the third eyelid in birds: 17 cases. *J Avian Med Surg* 1996;10(1):12–18.

King AS, McLelland J. Special sense organs. In *Birds: Their Structure and Function,* ed 2. London, Bailliere Tindall, 1984, pp 284-314.

Krautwald ME, Neumann W, Rink P. Ophthalmological procedures and differentiated diagnostics in psittacine birds. *Proc Assoc Avian Vet* 1989;82–91.

LaBonde J. Pet avian toxicology. *Proc Assoc Avian Vet* 1988;159–174.

Lawton M. Avian anterior segment disease. *Proc Assoc Avian Vet* 1993;223–227.

Murphy CJ. Ocular lesions in birds of prey. In Fowler ME (ed): *Zoo and Wild Animal Medicine, Current Therapy 3*. Philadelphia, WB Saunders, 1993, pp 211–221.

Murphy CJ. Ocular lesions in birds of prey. *Proc N Am Vet Conf* 1995;562–563.

Murphy J. Psittacine fatty liver syndrome. *Proc Assoc Avian Vet* 1992;78–82.

Parrott T. Hepatopathy and neurological abnormalities in an umbrella cockatoo after vaccination with Pacheco's killed virus vaccine. *Proc Assoc Avian Vet* 1992;140.

Porter SL. Vehicular trauma in owls. *Proc Assoc Avian Vet* 1990;164–170.

Ritchie BW, Harrison GJ, Harrison LR (eds): *Avian Medicine: Principles and Application*. Lake Worth, FL, Wingers Publishing, 1994.

Romagnano A. Unilateral conjunctival cysts in an African grey parrot. *Proc Assoc Avian Vet* 1995;357–358.

Rosskopf WJ, Woerpel RW, Asterino R. Successful treatment of avian tuberculosis in pet psittacines. *Proc Assoc Avian Vet* 1991;238–250.

VanDerHeyden N. Evaluation and interpretation of the avian hemogram. *Semin Avian Exot Pet Med* 1994;3(1):5–13.

Williams D. Ophthalmology. In Ritchie BW, Harrison GJ, Harrison LR (eds): *Avian Medicine: Principles and Application*. Lake Worth, FL, Wingers Publishing, 1994, pp 673-694.

Williams DL. A wing guided by an eye. *Proc N Am Vet Conf* 1993;715–716.

Williams M, Smith PJ, Loerzel SM, et al. Evaluation of the efficacy of vecuronium bromide as a mydriatic in several differrent species of aquatic birds. *Proc Assoc Avian Vet* 1996;113–117

Chapter 6

Neurologic Signs

Clinical signs associated with neurologic disease are common in pet birds. This chapter presents a diagnostic approach for neurologic signs commonly seen in pet birds. The chapter is divided into four sections, with signs grouped according to the diagnostic approach required to diagnose the cause of the illness. Each section begins with general information and definition of terms followed by a list of differential diagnoses. This is followed by appropriate signalment information. Common causes of the clinical sign are presented for each group of pet birds. Pertinent information on which species and ages of birds may be affected by the diseases in the differential diagnosis is also given. The history section is useful to explore important historical information that may help narrow differential diagnoses. The physical examination section guides interpretation of the physical findings. An algorithm is included in each section to provide a quick reference for recommended tests. The diagnostic plan suggests useful tests. Consult Chapter 12 for techniques of sample collection and assistance with test interpretation. Once a diagnosis is made, specific treatments may be found in Chapter 9. General treatments for neurologic problems follow appropriate sections of the chapter. Consult the formulary in Chapter 17 for drug dosages.

Visual deficits are discussed in Chapter 5. Proventricular dilatation syndrome (PDS) is discussed in Chapters 4 and 9.

Clinical signs of neurologic disease include seizures, tremors, ataxia, paralysis, head tilt, circling, nystagmus, and visual deficits. Weight loss, ataxia, vomiting, and the passing of undigested food in the droppings can be associated with proventricular dilatation syndrome. Diseases of the peripheral nervous system (PNS) or central nervous system (CNS) may produce neurologic signs.

THE NEUROLOGIC EXAMINATION

The purpose of a systematic neurologic examination is to determine the extent of the problem and whether the lesion is focal or diffuse, and if focal, to localize the lesion. A complete neurologic examination includes evaluation of mentation, posture, and movement; functional assessment of the cranial nerves; palpation for determination of the degree of muscle tone, strength, and atrophy; evaluation of proprioception deficits and spinal reflexes; and sensory evaluation.

The mental status of the bird is evaluated based on level of consciousness and behavior. Consciousness is evaluated by the bird's awareness of its surroundings and ability to perform its normal activities. Consciousness is recorded as alert, depressed, stuporous, or comatose. Depression may be caused by systemic problems or be associated with diffuse disease of the cerebral cortex or reticular formation. Stupor and coma indicate a central lesion. Behavioral changes include aggression, disorientation, fear, and withdrawal. Behavior disorders may be caused by CNS disease, pain, or discomfort or be related to training or the environment.

Assessment of the posture includes orientation of the head, trunk, and legs. A head tilt, rolling of the body, or wide-based stance may indicate a central or peripheral vestibular lesion or a lesion of the cerebellum. Movement is evaluated and ataxia, circling, paralysis, and dysmetria noted.

Cranial nerve function assessment may help to localize lesions. Cranial nerve I (CN I) is difficult to assess. Olfaction may be tested by response to noxious odors such as alcohol.

Observe the posture of the head. A head tilt may be the result of central or peripheral vestibular disorders. The palpebral reflex and menace response can be performed. The palpebral reflex tests two divisions of CN V. The menace response tests CN II and CN V; however, absence of this response does not indicate dysfunction. The pupils are observed for anisocoria, and the pupillary light reflex is evaluated. Anisocoria indicates dysfunction of CN III or sympathetic dysfunction. The pupillary light reflex evaluates CN II and CN III. A consensual response is often absent in normal birds. Birds have some voluntary control of pupillary constriction because of skeletal muscles in the iris. Birds will constrict and dilate their pupils when excited. The eyes are observed for strabismus (symmetry in the palpebral fissure) and nystagmus. Strabismus indicates vestibular dysfunction or a dysfunction of CN III, CN IV, or CN VI. Abnormal nystagmus indicates vestibular dysfunction (central or peripheral). The head is moved from side to side, then dorsally and ventrally to elicit physiologic nystagmus. Loss of this normal physiologic nystagmus may occur with CN VIII dysfunction or with brain stem lesions. Horner's syndrome (ptosis, protrusion of nictitating membrane, and inconsistently miosis) may occur with central, cervical sympathetic tract, or brachial plexus lesions. Open and close the bird's mouth to assess tone of the muscles of mastication. Decreased beak strength may indicate predominantly loss of CN V, with possible CN VII dysfunction. Sensory perception of the face may be evaluated by touching or tapping the areas of the face with a finger or hemostat, testing CN V. Observe movement of the tongue and its ability to manipulate objects. Paralysis indicates CN XII dysfunction. Atrophy of the tongue begins to be apparent 1 week after loss of the nerve supply. Examine the oropharynx and larynx for symmetry, and elicit a gag or swallowing response by inserting a tongue depressor into the pharynx. Asymmetry and lack of gag or swallowing response indicates a dysfunction of CN IX or CN X. Atony of the crop or dysphagia may also be caused by CN IX or X dysfunction and possibly by CN XII. Deafness indicates a dysfunction of CN VIII.

Palpation of muscle tone, strength, and size is important to assess function and use of associated muscles. Atrophy may indicate peripheral disease or disuse.

Loss of proprioception is indicated by the bird knuckling over and resting weight on the dorsum of the foot.

Assessment of spinal reflexes is difficult in birds. The wing withdrawal reflex requires intact peripheral nerves, but does not require an intact cervical spinal cord. Hyperreflexia caused by a cervical spinal cord lesion is difficult to distinguish from normal reflex activity. The leg withdrawal reflex and vent tone also require intact peripheral nerves but do not require an intact spinal cord. The crossed extensor reflex is indicated by an extension of the opposite limb when the withdrawal reflex is initiated. It is abnormal and is the result of a lesion in descending pathways (i.e., spinal cord or brain stem lesion).

A cervical spinal cord lesion results in weakness of the wings and legs, normal to exaggerated wing and leg withdrawal reflexes and vent tone, and loss of pain perception in the wings and legs, with normal cranial nerve function. Thoracolumbar spinal cord lesions result in weakness of the legs, diminished or exaggerated leg withdrawal reflexes and vent tone, and loss of pain perception in the legs, with normal wing withdrawal reflexes, pain perception, and cranial nerve function. Lumbosacral spinal cord lesions may result in normal or absent leg withdrawal reflexes; hypertonic or absent vent tone, with intact leg and wing withdrawal reflexes; and normal cranial nerve function.

Sensory evaluation is performed at the end of the neurologic exam, because painful stimuli may alter the bird's attitude, making reflexes more difficult to evaluate. Pain perception must be differentiated from reflex activity. Wing and leg withdrawal reflexes can be present without pain perception from the extremity with spinal lesions. Pain perception is indicated by an attempt to escape or bite, turning the head, or vocalization.

Neurologic responses of pediatric patients are difficult to interpret. Compare responses to a normal chick of the same species and age, if possible. Differences in rates of development occur between species. The most useful tests for pediatric neurologic evaluation include the menace response, withdrawal reflex, sensory response, and the ability to perch, vocalize, and use the wings to balance.

A neurologic examination report form is useful to record results of the neurologic examination (Fig. 6–1).

SEIZURES

Seizures are commonly seen in birds. Seizures can result from disorders of the brain that cause spontaneous depolarization of cerebral neurons. Such disorders may be caused by a primary lesion in the brain (e.g., neoplastic, infectious, or traumatic) or may be secondary to extracranial causes (e.g., metabolic or toxic). Seizures have three components. The actual seizure is called the ictus. The ictus in birds can have various manifestations. The typical avian ictus consists of a short period of disorientation and ataxia, followed by loss of the ability to grip or perch, falling to the floor of the cage. The bird may become rigid or begin spastic motor activity, vocalize, and pass droppings. The length of the ictus is variable, usually lasting several seconds. The aura is the phase immediately preceding the ictus, which may be manifested as a period of altered behavior. The postictal phase follows the ictus and lasts for a variable period of time (seconds to hours). During the postictal phase, birds may be lethargic, confused, disoriented, or restless. The character and length of the aura and the postictal phase do not correspond to the severity or cause of the seizure.

Signalment:

History:

Physical examination:

Neurological examination

   Observation

Mentation	alert		depressed		stuporous		comatose	
Behavior	aggression		disorientation		fear		withdrawal	
Posture	normal		head tilt		rolling		wide stance	
Movement	ataxia		circling		paralysis		dysmetria	

   Cranial nerves

KEY: 3 = exaggerated, 2 = normal, 1 = diminished, 0 = absent		
L	R	
		Olfaction (CNI)
		Hearing (CN VIII)
		Palpebral reflex (CN V)
		Menace reflex (CN II, V)
		Pupils resting (CN III, sympathetic)
		Pupillary light reflex (CN II, III)
		Strabismus (vestibular, CN III, IV, VI)
		Nystagmus, resting (vestibular)
		Loss of physiologic nystagmus (CN VIII, brain stem)
		Muscles of mastication (CN V, VII)
		Sensory (CN V)
		Tongue (CN XII)
		Anisocoria (CNIII, sympathetic)
		Gag swallow reflex (CN IX, X)

   Comments:

   Palpation:

   Spinal reflexes and proprioception

L	R	
		Proprioception
		Wing withdrawal
		Leg withdrawal
		Crossed extensor
		Vent response

   Sensation (locate and describe abnormal):

Figure 6–1. Neurologic examination report form.

Differential Diagnoses for Seizures

1. Infectious
   a. Bacterial: any organism that causes encephalitis, meningitis, CNS abscesses, or CNS granulomas (*Clostridium* spp., *Salmonella, Mycobacterium, Mycoplasma, Pasteurella multocida, Staphylococcus, Streptococcus,* other)
   b. Chlamydial: *Chlamydia psittaci*
   c. Viral: Pacheco's disease, duck viral enteritis, duck viral hepatitis
   d. Fungal: *Aspergillus*

2. Metabolic: °hypocalcemia, °liver disease (hepatic lipidosis, mycotoxicosis, hemochromatosis, bacterial hepatitis, viral hepatitis, and Pacheco's vaccine–induced hepatopathy), hypoglycemia, heat stress
3. Nutritional: calcium, phosphorus, or °vitamin D_3 imbalances; °vitamin E or selenium deficiency; pyridoxine deficiency (vitamin B_6); thiamine deficiency (vitamin B_1)
4. Toxic: °lead, °zinc, mycotoxin, °insecticides (organophosphate, carbamate, organochlorine), polytetrafluoroethylene (Teflon) (PTFE), toxic plants (crown vetch), salt poisoning
5. Physical: °trauma, °cerebrovascular accident, hydrocephalus, heatstroke, °emboli (yolk, parasites), atherosclerosis
6. Neoplastic: astrocytoma, choroid plexus tumor, glioblastoma multiforme, hemangiocytoma, Schwannoma, undifferentiated sarcoma
7. Iatrogenic: dimetridazole, amphotericin B, ivermectin
8. Other: °idiopathic epilepsy, behavioral head shaking

Signalment

Common causes of seizures in Amazon parrots include trauma, liver disease resulting from hepatic lipidosis or mycotoxin, lead and zinc toxicoses, and hypocalcemia. Epilepsy is a common cause of seizures in red-lored Amazon parrots. Hypocalcemia is suggested to cause seizures in African gray parrots. Seizures in budgies are often the result of cerebrovascular accidents, hepatic lipidosis, or nutritional imbalances and deficiencies. Common causes of seizures in canaries and finches include yolk emboli, hepatic lipidosis, and terminal PTFE toxicosis. Epilepsy, heatstroke, and yolk emboli are common causes of seizures in lovebirds. Common causes of seizures in cockatiels include trauma, lead and zinc toxicoses, yolk emboli, and liver disease. Raptors often have seizures caused by hypoglycemia and trauma. Seizures in mynahs are commonly caused by epilepsy or hemochromatosis.

Nutritional deficiencies are common in young birds. Young and growing birds have smaller body stores of vitamin E and calcium, and they require increased amounts of calcium for rapid growth.

Behavioral head shaking that occurs in some African gray parrots when they are excited should not be mistaken for a seizure. Dimetridazole toxicosis occurs in budgies, goslings, pigeons, and ducks. Pacheco's disease affects only psittacines, and seizures are a rare clinical sign associated with the disease.

History

A complete history may reveal trauma, iatrogenic toxicosis, nutritional deficiencies or imbalances, or exposure to toxins or infectious diseases. Isolated birds and those in closed collections are commonly ill because of toxicoses, trauma,

---

°Common causes.

nutritional deficiencies and imbalances, metabolic problems, reproductive disorders, neoplasia, and chronic infections such as chlamydiosis and mycobacteriosis.

Birds recently exposed to other birds may become ill as a result of infectious diseases, including viral, chlamydial, and bacterial infections, or as a result of problems occurring in isolated birds. Some diseases have carrier states. Conures can be carriers of Pacheco's disease, which can cause illness and death in exposed psittacines. Group contact also increases stress, predisposing to disease.

Significant dietary information for birds with seizures includes type of diet, supplements, intake, and freshness. Onset of signs after food intake may indicate hepatic encephalopathy. Diets that contain low calcium, high phosphorus, or low vitamin D content or that are contaminated with mycotoxin can result in abnormalities that cause seizures in birds.

Mycotoxins are metabolic byproducts of molds. They are undetectable by sight, smell, or taste. Ingestion of a toxic dose of mycotoxin can result in death in a few days. Chronic exposure can cause liver disease, leading to hepatic encephalopathy and associated seizures.

The calcium content of the diet is important. Secondary nutritional hyperparathyroidism will develop if calcium use exceeds absorption from the intestines over a prolonged period of time. Blood calcium levels usually remain normal until calcium stores are depleted. Fractures are commonly the first symptom, but seizures can occur if hypocalcemia develops. Increased use of calcium occurs with heavy egg production. Decreased calcium absorption commonly occurs as a result of a calcium-deficient diet. Seed diets are low in calcium and high in phosphorus and fat. The high-fat content of a seed diet may also interfere with calcium absorption. Meat is low in calcium and high in phosphorus. Raptors fed only day-old chicks, meat, or pinky mice may develop calcium deficiency.

A hypocalcemic syndrome occurs in African gray parrots and less commonly in Amazon parrots, lovebirds, and mynahs. Affected hypocalcemic birds do not mobilize calcium from body stores. Predisposed birds may develop hypocalcemia while eating diets containing calcium considered adequate for other birds.

Seed diets may be deficient in vitamin E and selenium. Birds on high-fat diets such as seeds are more likely to show signs of vitamin E deficiency than are birds on diets low in fat. Thiamine deficiency is uncommon in birds on a seed diet or formulated diet because seeds and grains generally contain sufficient thiamine. Thiamine deficiency is seen in carnivorous birds fed only meat or day-old chicks and in fish-eating birds fed fish containing thiaminase. Signs of vitamin B_6 deficiency rarely occur unless dietary protein levels are high.

Important environmental factors in birds with seizures include access to potential toxins, overheating, and flight capabilities. Birds allowed out of their cages are more susceptible to trauma. Free-flight episodes are conducive to collisions with windows, walls, and ceiling fans, leading to head trauma.

A history of exposure or access to a potential toxin is significant in a bird with seizures. Toxins that may cause seizures include lead, zinc, mycotoxin, crown vetch, chocolate, salt, tobacco, PTFE, and organophosphate, carbamate, and organochlorine insecticides. Some sources of lead are listed in Table 9–3. Sources of zinc include pennies minted since 1982, Monopoly game pieces, and galvanized wire, containers, dishes, and hardware cloth. Ornamental dough and sea sand are common sources of salt ingested by pet birds, causing salt toxicosis. Polytetrafluoroethylene fumes are produced when some nonstick surfaces overheat (e.g., Teflon). Common items include nonstick cookware, drip pans, irons, ironing board covers, heat lamps, and carpet and upholstery sprays.

A history of dimetridazole, amphotericin B, or ivermectin administration is consistent with an iatrogenic toxicosis.

Egg laying or nesting behavior before a seizure can be consistent with egg yolk peritonitis or embolus.

The duration of the illness is important. Note the owner's description of the clinical signs and the course of the disease. Note previous illnesses, including signs, treatment, and response to treatment.

Physical Examination

Complete physical and neurologic examinations are important to identify other neurologic and physical abnormalities in birds with seizures. The neurologic examination is discussed in a previous section. When clinical signs of involvement of other systems occur, consult appropriate sections of the text for assistance in making a diagnosis. Common findings in birds with seizures are discussed below.

Blood in the mouth, ears, or eyes indicates head trauma. Look at the skin at the top of the head; meningeal hematomas may be visualized through the calvarium in some cases. Fractures or bruises located anywhere in the body indicate that trauma has occurred and that head trauma may have occurred. Part the feathers and moisten the skin with alcohol to allow better visualization of the skin for evidence of bruising or wounds. This technique is useful on the head, legs, wings, skull, and spine.

Evaluation of the droppings of birds with seizures often provides insight to the cause of the seizures. Polyuria (increased water content of the droppings) may be caused by stress, Pacheco's disease, lead or zinc toxicosis, or amphotericin B administration. Hematuria may be an indication of lead or zinc toxicosis, especially in Amazon parrots and African gray parrots, or Pacheco's disease. Biliverdinuria (green-colored urates) indicates liver disease, which may occur from lead or zinc toxicoses, hepatic lipidosis, Pacheco's disease, or hemochromatosis. Diarrhea may be seen with tobacco, chocolate, lead or zinc toxicoses, Pacheco's disease, or liver disease. Dark-colored feces have been reported with chocolate toxicosis.

Edema of the skin is consistent with thiamine deficiency, and ventral edema may occur with vitamin E or selenium deficiency.

Clinical signs associated with Pacheco's disease include diarrhea, biliverdinuria, sinusitis, conjunctivitis, and convulsions or tremors. Clinical signs and severity of disease vary with species susceptibility.

Seizures may occur in conjunction with gastrointestinal signs with bacterial infections, chlamydiosis, Pacheco's disease, duck viral enteritis, duck viral hepatitis, hepatic disease, lead and zinc toxicoses, salt toxicosis, insecticide toxicosis, calcium, phosphorus, or vitamin D_3 imbalance, amphotericin B administration, and trauma.

Seizures may occur in conjunction with respiratory signs with bacterial infections, chlamydiosis, Pacheco's disease, aspergillosis, liver disease, heat stress, trauma, and zinc and PTFE toxicosis.

Algorithm for Seizures

See Figure 6–2.

Diagnostic Approach for Seizures

Diazepam injections are used to stop seizure activity. Stabilize severely ill birds before performing diagnostic tests, and provide supportive care as needed (see Chapter 1).

Remove perches, swings, and toys from the cages of birds with seizures.

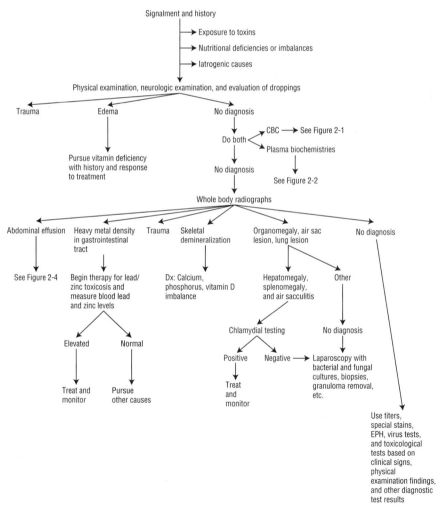

Figure 6–2. Algorithm for seizures.

Hospitalized patients require cages with soft bedding and without perches. Use shallow food and water bowls, and consider spreading food on the floor of the cage if the bird has difficulty maneuvering to get food.

Selection of appropriate diagnostic tests is based on consideration of the signalment and history of the bird and the findings of the physical and neurologic examinations.

Nutritional and iatrogenic causes must be sought for the history. Exposure to possible toxins may be noted historically. Evidence of trauma may be noted or an enlarged liver may be palpated on physical examination.

Vitamin E or selenium deficiency is suspected based on diet history and clinical signs, including tremors, ataxia, incoordination, abnormal head movements, reluctance to walk, and recumbency. Response to vitamin E and selenium administration allows a presumed diagnosis.

A diagnosis of thiamine deficiency is based on appropriate clinical signs, including anorexia, opisthotonos, seizures, or death, and on the response to thiamine administration.

A diagnosis of mycotoxicosis is based on clinical signs, postmortem examination, and detecting high quantities of the toxin in the food or gastrointestinal contents. It is often difficult to diagnose because the clinical signs are not specific, and often the food source has been consumed before the onset of clinical signs. Liver biopsy and histology may indicate mycotoxic insult may have occurred.

The diagnoses of heatstroke and chocolate and salt toxicoses are based on clinical signs and a history of exposure.

A complete blood count (CBC) and plasma biochemistries are the next step in evaluating a bird with seizures. A CBC is useful in supporting infectious, nutritional, inflammatory, and some toxic diagnoses. Perform a CBC if systemic disease is suspected, when a bird is unresponsive to treatment, or to help determine the general health of the bird. Changes in the hemogram commonly seen in birds with seizures are detailed below.

Nonregenerative anemias may occur with chronic inflammatory diseases, including chlamydiosis, mycobacteriosis, egg yolk peritonitis, neoplasia, mycotoxicosis, and lead and zinc toxicoses. Nonregenerative anemias with decreased plasma protein may be seen with acute blood loss resulting from trauma or coagulopathies resulting from liver disease (e.g., mycotoxicosis or hepatic lipidosis). If blood loss is not continuous, which may occur with trauma, a regenerative anemia will develop within several days. This will be characterized by the appearance of polychromasia and anisocytosis.

Regenerative anemias with normal plasma protein may occur with lead or zinc toxicoses or mycotoxicosis. Lead or zinc toxicoses may cause an exaggerated response, with more polychromasia and rubricytes than would be expected for the degree of anemia present. Hypochromasia can be associated with lead or zinc toxicoses.

Leukocytosis and heterophilia may be caused by stress, neoplasia, or inflammatory diseases (e.g., bacteria, fungi, or egg yolk peritonitis). Leukocytosis often accompanies the hypocalcemia in African gray parrots affected with the hypocalcemic syndrome. Heterophilia and lymphopenia may be seen with vitamin B_6 deficiency. Differential diagnoses to consider in a bird with seizures with a white blood cell (WBC) count in excess of 40,000/µl include egg yolk peritonitis or embolus, chlamydiosis, aspergillosis, and mycobacteriosis. Monocytosis may occur with chlamydiosis, mycobacteriosis, and bacterial granulomas. Leukopenia may be associated with Pacheco's disease.

Plasma biochemistry tests are important in the diagnosis of metabolic diseases. Important plasma biochemistries to evaluate in a bird with seizures include aspartate aminotransferase (AST or SGOT), bile acids, glucose, calcium, phosphorus, uric acid, creatine kinase (CK), albumin, and total protein. Blood calcium levels below 6.0 mg/dl may precipitate hypocalcemic seizures in birds. Calcium must be interpreted along with total protein concentrations.

Blood glucose values less than 150 mg/dl indicate hypoglycemia. Hypoglycemic seizures usually occur when blood glucose levels fall below 100 mg/dl.

Bile acid concentrations may be useful to evaluate liver function. With impaired liver function, bile acids may increase.

An elevation in AST is usually the result of liver or muscle damage. The AST may be elevated in birds with seizures from liver damage caused by Pacheco's disease or chlamydiosis. Muscle damage caused by trauma or irritating intramuscular injections also cause an elevation in AST. Creatine kinase activity increases with muscle damage and may be used to differentiate an increase in AST caused by liver disease from an increase caused by muscle damage. If evidence of liver disease is present, rule out chlamydiosis. If chlamydiosis is not the cause of the liver disease, a liver biopsy may be necessary for a definitive diagnosis.

An elevation of uric acid often accompanies lead and zinc toxicoses.

Radiology is useful in diagnosing lead and zinc toxicoses, trauma, and nutritional secondary hyperparathyroidism, and it provides information on liver size and systemic disease. Radiographic abnormalities in a bird with seizures may include trauma lesions, organomegaly, abdominal effusions, skeletal demineralization, or heavy metal densities in the ventriculus. Fractures of the skull or scleral ossicles indicate head trauma. Fractures elsewhere in the body may indicate trauma or a calcium, phosphorus, or vitamin D imbalance.

Evaluation of the hepatic silhouette may reveal hepatomegaly or microhepatia. Radiographic evidence of hepatomegaly in the ventrodorsal view includes loss of the hourglass silhouette between the heart and liver, compression of the abdominal air sacs, and extension of the liver lateral to a line drawn from the coracoid to the acetabulum. On the lateral view, hepatomegaly is indicated by the cranial displacement of the heart, dorsal elevation of the proventriculus, and caudodorsal displacement of the ventriculus. Hepatomegaly may be the result of hepatic lipidosis, hemochromatosis, mycotoxicosis, Pacheco's disease, mycobacteriosis, or chlamydiosis.

Ascites and peritonitis cause an overall loss of organ detail on the ventrodorsal view. This loss of detail may be difficult to distinguish from hepatomegaly. On the lateral view, ascites and peritonitis will cause loss of detail in the celomic cavity, with the lung, intestinal gas, and grit in the ventriculus often being the only identifiable features. Abdominocentesis or treatment with furosemide for several days will increase visualization of organs. Both ascites and hepatomegaly may be present with hemochromatosis or egg yolk peritonitis.

Thickening of the caudal thoracic and abdominal air sacs on lateral radiographs and diffuse increased opacity of these air sacs on ventrodorsal views indicate airsacculitis. Splenomegaly, hepatomegaly, and airsacculitis support a diagnosis of chlamydiosis.

Skeletal demineralization may be observed with calcium, phosphorus, and vitamin D_3 imbalances. Skeletal demineralization is not observed in birds with seizures with hypocalcemic syndrome (e.g., African gray parrots).

Plasma protein electrophoresis (EPH) is useful in identifying many disease states (e.g., chlamydiosis, aspergillosis, mycobacteriosis, peritonitis, liver disease, or renal disease).

Cholinesterase assays, cultures, titers, and lead and zinc blood levels are used to rule in or out specific diseases. Lead blood levels are measured on whole blood, with lithium heparin used for the anticoagulant. Whole blood lead levels greater than 0.2 ppm are suggestive of lead toxicosis, and levels greater than 0.5 ppm are diagnostic of lead toxicosis. Serum zinc levels greater than 200 μg/dl (2 ppm) are diagnostic of zinc toxicosis and are often above 1000 μg/dl (10 ppm).

Cholinesterase assay is used when organophosphate toxicosis is suspected. Cholinesterase levels less than 1000 IU/l in avian plasma are considered diagnostic.

Diagnosis of chlamydiosis can be difficult. No single test or combination of tests can detect *Chlamydia* infection in all infected or carrier birds and not result in false-positive results in uninfected birds. Antigen tests are useful in-house tests in birds showing clinical signs of infection. False-negative and -positive results occur. Serology is useful in birds large enough to provide a blood sample adequate for evaluation (50 g or larger birds). False-negative titers can occur early in the disease before antibody production and in some species of birds (e.g., cockatiels). Low titers may be difficult to interpret. The laboratory performing the titer will aid in interpretation of titer results. Chlamydial culture of nasal or ocular discharges or feces may provide a diagnosis if shedding of the organism is occurring at the time of sampling. Obtain culture samples before beginning antibiotic therapy. False-negative cultures occur (see Chapter 9). Plasma protein electropheresis is useful for chlamydial diagnosis.

Serologic testing for aspergillosis is available for pet birds. A rare CNS fungal granuloma may produce adequate antibodies for a positive diagnosis. False-negative results occur.

Abdominocentesis is performed in birds with physical or radiographic evidence of abdominal effusion (e.g., distension due to egg-related peritonitis). Removal of the effusion will decrease compression of the abdominal air sacs and will provide a sample for evaluation of the effusion. To perform an abdominal tap, the cranial abdomen is surgically prepared. A 21- to 25-gauge needle is inserted just distal to the point of the sternum on the ventral midline. The needle is directed to the right side of the abdomen to avoid the ventriculus (see Chapter 12). Remove only the volume needed for fluid evaluation and to relieve dyspnea.

Little or no fluid can be collected from the abdomen of normal birds. Normal fluid contains few cells. An occasional mesothelial cell and macrophage is normal. Egg-related peritonitis can produce an effusion that grossly appears reddish brown and opaque. The effusion is an exudate, highly cellular (greater than 5,000/mm^3), with a specific gravity greater than 1.020 and a protein content greater than 3.0 g/dl. The cell population may contain heterophils, macrophages, and lymphocytes.

Other abdominal effusions are discussed in Chapter 12.

Electroencephalography, computed tomography (CT), and magnetic resonance imaging (MRI) are useful tests for diagnosing some brain lesions. These tests require specialized equipment that may be available at referral centers. An electroencephalogram (EEG) is useful for evaluation of cerebral disease and monitoring healing of CNS lesions or injuries. An EEG can be used to determine if the cerebral disease is focal or diffuse, acute or chronic, or inflammatory or degenerative. Both MRI and CT are useful for imaging lesions that may not be visible with plain radiographs (e.g., tumors or hydrocephalus).

Aviaries or flock situations benefit from complete necropsy examinations.

Treatment of Seizures

Diazepam injections are used to stop seizure activity. Treat the underlying cause of the seizures. Phenobarbital is used for long-term control of epilepsy. Check blood phenobarbital concentration 1 month after beginning therapy to evaluate the dosage.

Treatment of head trauma includes intravenous dexamethasone, stress-free environment (dark and quiet), and fluid replacement if hemorrhage has occurred. One-half to two-thirds the normal volume of fluids may be given if hemorrhage has occurred. Mannitol may be beneficial if the bird does not respond to initial therapy. The prognosis is guarded to poor.

Response to intramuscular or oral administration of thiamine is rapid when a deficiency is present. Correct the diet to prevent recurrences.

Muscular dystrophy as a result of vitamin E or selenium deficiency may respond to vitamin E and selenium supplementation and antiprotozoal therapy, but encephalomalacia rarely responds to therapy.

Treat the underlying cause of hepatic failure, when present. Symptomatic relief with lactulose, vitamin supplementation, neomycin sulfate, and a low-protein, high-carbohydrate, high-quality protein diet may improve clinical signs while the underlying hepatopathy is being treated.

Parenteral administration of calcium gluconate will control seizural activity when hypocalcemia is the cause. Do not use corticosteroids in these patients. Place the bird on a proper diet and begin oral calcium and vitamin supplementation. Lifelong calcium and vitamin supplementation may be required even with a good diet. Evaluate serum calcium concentrations in 2 months and periodically thereafter to assess effectiveness of treatment.

Intravenous 50% dextrose is given for acute relief of clinical signs of hypoglycemia. Treat the underlying cause.

Treatment of cerebral vascular accidents includes intravenous dexamethasone, a stress-free environment (dark and quiet), and control of seizures as needed. Treatment for emboli consists of intravenous dexamethasone, a stress-free environment, control of seizures, and treatment of egg-related peritonitis if present (see Chapter 15).

Heatstroke is treated by reducing the body temperature, which is accomplished by wetting the feathers to the skin with cool water and placing the feet and legs in cool water. Flunixin meglumine may be used to reduce hyperthermia in addition to cooling with water. If the hyperthermia is severe, low doses of intravenous or intraosseous fluids and dexamethasone are administered. Control seizures with diazepam as needed. Mannitol may help control cerebral edema, if present.

Provide supportive care for birds suffering from toxicosis. Treatment of tobacco toxicosis consists of absorbent (activated charcoal) and laxative therapy (mineral oil), and supportive care. Chocolate toxicosis is treated with administration of a gastrointestinal protectant (e.g., bismuth subsalicylate), cathartic (mineral oil), and supportive care. Treatment for salt poisoning includes the use of diuretics and sodium-poor intravenous or intraosseous fluids (D_5W or 2½% dextrose in 0.45% saline). Intravenous dexamethasone is suggested for treatment of ivermectin toxicosis. With levamisole toxicosis, surviving birds usually recover without treatment.

Treatment for bacterial CNS infections is usually ineffective in birds with CNS signs. Attempted therapy may be initiated with cefotaxime or chloramphenicol, both of which may penetrate the CNS in effective concentrations.

Treat other disorders according to their primary causes.

ATAXIA

Ataxia is the loss of coordination without paresis, spasticity, or involuntary movement. It is recognized clinically by a broad-based stance and uncoordinated movements of the head, body, legs, or wings. Other neurologic signs often accompany ataxia in birds. Ataxia is the result of disorders of the proprioceptive system, cerebellum, or vestibular system.

Musculoskeletal abnormalities may result in ataxia, mimicking neurologic clinical signs. Consult Chapter 7 for additional information on musculoskeletal problems, if present.

Differential Diagnoses for Ataxia

1. Infectious
   a. Bacterial: any organism that causes encephalitis, CNS abscesses, CNS granulomas, or otitis interna
   b. Chlamydial: *Chlamydia psittaci*
   c. Viral: polyomavirus (budgerigar fledgling disease), paramyxovirus 1 (PMV 1) (including Newcastle disease), avian picornavirus encephalomyelitis, reovirus, togaviruses (eastern and western equine encephalomyelitis), duck viral enteritis, adenovirus
   d. Fungal: *Aspergillus, Cryptococcus*
   e. Parasitic: *Baylisascaris, Toxoplasma, Sarcocystis*
   f. Other: proventricular dilatation syndrome (macaw wasting disease, neuropathic gastric dilatation [NGD])
2. Metabolic: °hypocalcemia, °liver disease (hepatic lipidosis, mycotoxicosis, hemochromatosis, bacterial hepatitis, viral hepatitis, and Pacheco's vaccine–induced hepatopathy)
3. Nutritional: vitamin E or selenium deficiency, thiamine deficiency (vitamin B_1)
4. Toxic: °lead, °zinc, °insecticides, PTFE, salt

°Common causes.

5. Physical: °head trauma, atherosclerosis, °gout
6. Neoplastic
7. Iatrogenic: levamisole, dimetridazole
8. Other: conure bleeding syndrome

Signalment

Common causes of ataxia in large psittacines include lead and zinc toxicoses, trauma, and liver disease resulting from hepatic lipidosis and mycotoxicosis. Hypocalcemia is a common cause of ataxia in African gray parrots. Cockatiels are commonly ataxic as a result of head trauma, lead or zinc toxicoses, and insecticide toxicosis. Ataxic budgies are often ill because of hepatic lipidosis, polyomavirus infection, or trauma. A common cause of ataxia in canaries and finches is insecticide toxicosis. Ataxic mynahs are often ill from hemochromatosis. Common causes of ataxia in raptors include trauma and hypoglycemia.

Young birds are commonly ill as a result of nutritional deficiencies. Young and growing birds have smaller body stores of vitamin E and calcium and require increased amounts of calcium for rapid growth.

Neurologic signs associated with PMV 1 occur more commonly in older birds and birds with chronic infections. Avian picornavirus encephalomyelitis occurs in pigeons and gallinaceous birds. Reovirus is commonly seen in imported birds and primarily affects African gray parrots, cockatoos, and other Old World psittacines. Pet birds affected by togavirus encephalitis include finches and pigeons. Ducks, emus, turkeys, pheasants, and some cranes may also develop clinical signs as a result of togavirus infection. *Baylisascaris* infection has been documented in cockatiels, gallinaceous birds, ratites, and passerines. *Sarcocystis* is primarily a disease of Old World psittacines (cockatoos) and nestlings of New World species (macaws).

Clinical signs of polyomavirus in budgies begin to appear at 10 to 15 days of age. Signs in larger psittacines are common at weaning. Older psittacines may be susceptible to infection during epornitics.

History

A complete history may reveal trauma, iatrogenic toxicosis, nutritional deficiencies or imbalances, or exposure to toxins or infectious diseases. Infectious diseases are seen most frequently in birds recently exposed to other birds. Isolated birds and those in closed collections are commonly ill as a result of toxicoses, trauma, metabolic problems, nutritional deficiencies and imbalances, neoplasia, and chronic diseases.

Significant dietary information for ataxic birds includes type of diet, supplements, intake, and freshness. Onset of signs after food intake may indicate hepatic encephalopathy. Diets that are contaminated with mycotoxin can cause liver disease that results in ataxia.

°Common causes.

Mycotoxins are metabolic byproducts of molds. They are undetectable by sight, smell, or taste. Ingestion of a toxic dose of mycotoxin can result in death in a few days. Chronic exposure can cause liver disease, leading to hepatic encephalopathy and associated ataxia.

Seed diets are high in fat and may be deficient in vitamin E and selenium. Birds on high-fat diets are more likely to show signs of vitamin E deficiency than are birds on diets low in fat. Thiamine deficiency is uncommon in birds on a seed or formulated diet because seeds and grains generally contain sufficient thiamine. Thiamine deficiency is seen in carnivorous birds fed only meat or day-old chicks and in fish-eating birds fed fish containing thiaminase.

A hypocalcemic syndrome occurs in African gray parrots and less commonly in Amazon parrots, lovebirds, and mynahs. Affected hypocalcemic birds do not mobilize calcium from body stores. Predisposed birds may develop hypocalcemia while eating diets containing calcium considered adequate for other birds.

Important historical environmental factors in ataxic birds include access to potential toxins and flight capabilities. Birds allowed out of their cages are more susceptible to trauma. Free-flight episodes are conducive to collisions with windows, walls, and ceiling fans, leading to head trauma and fractures.

A history of exposure or access to a potential toxin is significant in an ataxic bird. Toxins that may cause ataxia include lead, zinc, mycotoxin, salt, PTFE, and organophosphate, carbamate, and organochlorine insecticides. Some sources of lead are listed in Table 9–3. Sources of zinc include pennies minted since 1982, Monopoly game pieces, and galvanized wire, containers, dishes, and hardware cloth. Ornamental dough and sea sand are common sources of salt ingested by pet birds, causing salt toxicosis. Polytetrafluoroethylene fumes are produced when some nonstick surfaces overheat (e.g., Teflon). Common items include nonstick cookware, drip pans, irons, ironing board covers, and heat lamps. Organophosphate toxicosis may be acute or delayed; therefore, signs may appear immediately or 7 to 10 days after exposure. A history of levamisole or dimetridazole administration is significant in an ataxic bird.

Access to cat feces, raccoon feces, opossum feces, or cockroaches can be significant. Psittacine birds can serve as the intermediate host for *Sarcocystis*. Infection occurs when birds ingest the feces of an infected opossum that contain sporocysts or ingest cockroaches that have eaten infected opossum feces. Neurologic signs develop as a result of the presence of schizonts in the brain. Toxoplasmosis is acquired through the ingestion of oocysts in the feces of infected cats, coprophagic arthropods, or food or water supplies contaminated with infected feces. Cerebrospinal nematodiasis is caused by the raccoon ascarid *Baylisascaris*. The larva migrate through the tissues when infective eggs are ingested by the bird.

The duration of the illness is important. Note the owner's description of the clinical signs and the course of the disease. Note previous illnesses, including signs, treatment, and response to treatment.

Physical Examination

A complete physical examination and neurologic examination are important to identify other neurologic and physical abnormalities in ataxic birds. The neurologic examination is discussed in the beginning of this chapter. Other common findings in ataxic birds associated with trauma and evaluation of droppings are similar to birds with seizures and are discussed in the previous section. Musculoskeletal abnormalities may cause ataxia, mimicking neurologic signs.

Gout may cause gait abnormalities mimicking neurologic disease. A stiff gait with ataxia and weakness may occur before subcutaneous uric acid deposits (tophi) are visible through the skin of joints and legs.

Otitis interna may occur as a result of otitis externa or media and may be visualized with an otoscope or endoscope through the external ear canal.

Clinical signs of organophosphate toxicosis include ataxia, prolapsed nictitans, inability to fly, and seizures. Signs of delayed organophosphate toxicosis include weakness, ataxia, decreased proprioception, and paralysis and occur 7 to 10 days after exposure to the insecticide.

Ventral edema may occur with vitamin E or selenium deficiency, and edema of the skin may occur with thiamine deficiency.

Polyomavirus (budgerigar fledgling disease) may affect feather formation as well as cause ataxia. Budgies infected as neonates develop normally until 10 to 15 days old. Then they may die with no premonitory signs, or they may develop abdominal distention; subcutaneous hemorrhage; tremors of the head, neck, and limbs; ataxia; and reduced formation of down and contour feathers. Survivors may develop symmetrical feather abnormalities, including dystrophic primary and tail feathers, lack of down feathers on the back and abdomen, and lack of filoplumes on the head and neck. These feather abnormalities are not observed in larger psittacines infected with polyomavirus.

Large psittacines infected with polyomavirus may die peracutely or develop depression, anorexia, delayed crop emptying, regurgitation, diarrhea, dyspnea, weight loss, and subcutaneous hemorrhages. Ataxia, tremors, and paralysis may also occur.

Birds with PDS may be seen with CNS signs alone or in conjunction with gastrointestinal signs and wasting.

Birds with PMV 1 may be seen with ataxia, torticollis, tremors, leg paralysis, conjunctivitis, and occasionally dyspnea and diarrhea. Finches may be asymptomatic carriers or may have conjunctivitis, pseudomembranous formation of the larynx, and neurologic signs, or they may die before they are seen.

Clinical signs associated with avian picornavirus encephalomyelitis include depression, ataxia, paresis or paralysis, and fine head and neck tremors.

Clinical signs associated with reovirus include dyspnea, diarrhea, ataxia, and sometimes a bloody brown nasal discharge.

Western and eastern equine encephalitis can cause paresis, paralysis, ataxia, tremors, depression, dyspnea, and death. Diarrhea may be present. Birds may die peracutely or acutely.

Ducks with duck viral enteritis may have photophobia, ataxia, seizures, penile prolapse, lethargy, hemorrhagic diarrhea, and serosanguinous nasal discharge.

Ataxia in conjunction with gastrointestinal signs can occur in birds with bacterial and chlamydial infections, polyomavirus in large psittacines, PMV 1, reovirus, western and eastern equine encephalitis, duck viral enteritis, PDS, conure bleeding syndrome, liver disease, gout, and lead, zinc, insecticide, and levamisole toxicoses.

Respiratory signs may accompany ataxia in birds with bacterial and chlamydial infections, polyomavirus in budgies and large psittacines, PMV 1, reovirus, western and eastern equine encephalitis, duck viral enteritis, conure bleeding syndrome, and insecticide, PTFE, and levamisole toxicoses.

Feather abnormalities may occur in conjunction with ataxia with polyomavirus in budgies and liver disease.

Algorithm for Ataxia

See Figure 6–3.

Diagnostic Approach for Ataxia

Selection of appropriate diagnostic tests are based on consideration of the signalment and history of the bird and the findings of the physical and neurologic examinations. See the section on the diagnostic approach for seizures for interpretation of the following tests: plasma biochemistry tests, hematology, lead and zinc blood levels, cholinesterase assay, radiography, chlamydiosis diagnosis, EEG, MRI, CT, vitamin E/selenium and thiamine deficiencies, mycotoxicosis, salt toxicosis, and heatstroke. Interpretation of additional tests follows.

A liver biopsy is indicated with persistent elevation of AST or bile acids or with hepatomegaly unrelated to chlamydiosis.

Additional plasma biochemistry interpretations follow. Togavirus infection may cause an increase in AST, lactate dehydrogenase (LDH), and uric acid. The

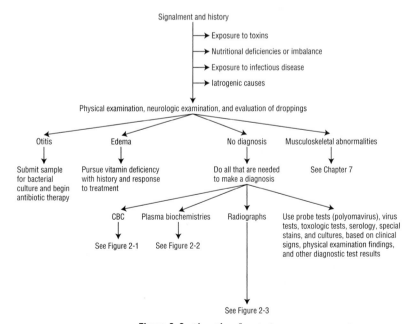

Figure 6–3. Algorithm for ataxia.

WBC count is usually normal. Uric acid is usually elevated with gout. An increase of AST, LDH, and alkaline phosphatase is common with polyomavirus infection.

If PDS is suspected based on radiology (i.e., distended proventriculus), a crop or ventricular biopsy may be performed for a definitive diagnosis. A negative biopsy result does not rule out PDS. Perform less-invasive techniques before biopsy to help rule out other common problems.

Signs of *Baylisascaris* infection are the result of visceral larval migration, with larvae entering the CNS. Infective eggs from the raccoon ascarid are ingested by the bird. The larvae penetrate the intestinal wall and migrate through tissues. No diagnostic stages of the parasite are released into the environment. This parasite is normally diagnosed histologically at necropsy.

Diagnosis of toxoplasmosis is based on necropsy findings and histology. Necropsy findings include congestion and consolidation of the lungs, hepatomegaly, vasculitis, and necrotic foci in the lungs, liver, and heart.

Diagnosis of *Sarcocystis* infection is based on necropsy findings and histology. Necropsy findings include pulmonary congestion, pulmonary hemorrhage, splenomegaly, and hepatomegaly.

Diagnosis of *Cryptococcus* infection is usually made postmortem. An impression smear of gelatinous material may reveal the encapsulated fungal organism. This gelatinous material may be obtained from affected sinuses antemortem with some systemic infections. *Cryptococcus neoformans* is an oval to round yeast with a mucopolysaccharide capsule (see Chapter 12). Yeast cells stain basophilic with Wright's or Diff-Quik stain. The *Cryptococcus* capsule portion of the yeast does not stain but does form a clear halo around the yeast.

The signs of delayed organophosphate toxicosis are caused by organophosphate ester-induced neuropathy, not associated with inhibition of acetylcholine as seen in acute toxicosis. Cholinesterase assay will not detect this delayed toxicosis. Diagnosis is based on exposure and clinical signs.

A variety of tests are available to aid in the diagnosis of viral infections (see Chapter 12). A suspicion of viral infection is based on signalment, history, and clinical signs.

Diagnosis of PMV 1 is based on isolation of the virus from cloacal swabs in live birds. Postmortem cases may be diagnosed through isolation of the virus from the brain or organs.

Diagnosis of avian picornavirus encephalomyelitis is based on postmortem histology. Histologic changes include neuronal degeneration, with lymphocytic perivascular cuffing and gliosis in the brain and spinal cord.

Viral-specific DNA probes are useful for detecting polyomavirus shedders. A cloacal swab is the best antemortem sample in larger psittacine birds. Subclinical carriers that intermittently shed polyomavirus occur and may give a false-negative result. A swab of the cut surface of the spleen, liver, and kidney (on one swab) is the best sample to submit for postmortem confirmation of polyomavirus infection.

Cloacal swabs and samples from affected organs may be used for virus isolation and culture for identification of reovirus infection. Viral antigen may be detected by immunofluorescence in affected tissue.

Western and eastern equine encephalitis virus may be isolated from a homogenate of blood, liver, spleen, and brain.

Hemorrhagic bands may be noted on the small intestine at necropsy in ducks with duck viral enteritis.

Treatment of Ataxia

Keep ataxic birds in cages without perches or swings and provide soft bedding. Use shallow food and water bowls and consider spreading food on the floor of the cage if the bird has difficulty maneuvering to get food.

See the section on treatment of seizures for treatments for head trauma, hypocalcemia, vitamin E/selenium deficiency, thiamine deficiency, salt toxicosis, bacterial CNS infections, and neoplasia.

Treat other disorders according to their primary causes.

PARALYSIS OR PARESIS

Clinical signs associated with paralysis or paresis include wing droop or the inability to perch. Paralysis or paresis indicates that there is loss or decrease in motor function in a part of the body. Lesions in the cerebrum, brain stem, spinal cord, or peripheral nerves may cause motor deficits. Trauma to peripheral or spinal nerves is a significant cause of movement disorders involving one leg or one wing and often results from skeletal fractures or luxations. With cerebral and brain stem lesions, the paresis is upper motor neuron (UMN) in the affected part and is associated with increased tone, loss of voluntary motor activity, weakness, and normal or increased spinal reflexes. With lesions of the PNS, the signs are lower motor neuron (LMN) in the affected part and are associated with loss of voluntary and reflex activity, weakness, and muscle atrophy. A weak grip or a lack of the ability to grip and perch can be the result of a central or peripheral lesion.

Pain or musculoskeletal abnormalities can mimic neurologic deficits. Perform a complete physical examination to assist in ruling out musculoskeletal causes such as fractures, gout, etc.

Differential Diagnoses of Paralysis or Paresis

1. Infectious
   a. Bacterial: any organism that causes neuritis, myelitis, meningitis, or encephalitis (including *Escherichia coli, Klebsiella, Listeria, Salmonella, Staphylococcus, Mycobacterium,* other)
   b. Chlamydial: *Chlamydia psittaci*
   c. Viral: reovirus, PMV 1 and PMV 3 (including Newcastle disease), avian picornavirus encephalomyelitis, togaviruses (eastern and western equine encephalitis), Marek's disease virus, polyomavirus
   d. Fungal: *Aspergillus*
   e. Parasitic: *Sarcocystis*
   f. Other: proventricular dilatation syndrome

2. Nutritional: vitamin E, selenium, thiamine (vitamin B_1), or riboflavin (vitamin B_2) deficiencies
3. Toxic: lead, zinc, delayed organophosphate toxicosis, °botulism
4. Physical: head trauma, spinal trauma, °peripheral nerve trauma, °musculoskeletal trauma, brachial plexus avulsion, pelvic plexus avulsion, °egg binding/internal trauma with egg laying, atherosclerosis, cerebral vascular accidents, gout, °abdominal mass (renal adenocarcinoma, embryonal nephroma, ovarian adenocarcinoma, granulosa cell tumor, nephritis)
5. Neoplasia: °renal tumors, °gonadal tumors, pituitary tumors
6. Iatrogenic: Pacheco's vaccine reaction, aminoglycoside toxicosis

Signalment

Paresis affecting one or both legs is more common than are wing problems. Common causes of leg paresis include fractures, soft tissue trauma, renal or gonadal tumors, and trauma associated with egg laying. Less common causes include lead or zinc toxicosis, nerve trauma, infection, vertebral trauma, neoplasia, and secondary nutritional hyperparathyroidism.

Common causes of wing paralysis include fractures and soft tissue trauma. Less common causes include lead or zinc toxicoses, nerve trauma, infection, or vertebral trauma.

Trauma, renal tumors, and gonadal tumors are common causes of unilateral or bilateral leg paralysis, especially in budgies.

Dystocia is most frequent in budgies, canaries, finches, cockatiels, and lovebirds. Botulism is uncommon in companion birds, but common in waterfowl. Neuromuscular synaptic dysfunction associated with aminoglycoside toxicosis is most common in cockatiels. Marek's disease affects primarily gallinaceous birds, but it has been reported in owls, ducks, swans, and a kestrel. Avian picornavirus encephalomyelitis is primarily a disease of chickens, but it also occurs in pheasants, quail, waterfowl, and turkeys. Canaries are particularly susceptible to *Listeria* infection.

Nutritional deficiencies are more common in young birds. Young and growing birds have smaller body stores of vitamin E and calcium, and they require increased amounts of calcium for rapid growth. Paralysis associated with riboflavin deficiency has been reported in young chicks, young waterfowl, an eagle, and ratites.

Vascular accidents are most common in older budgies.

History

A complete history may reveal trauma, nutritional deficiencies or imbalances, exposure to toxins or infectious diseases, or recent vaccination with Pacheco's disease vaccination. Isolated birds and those in closed collections are commonly

---

°Common causes.

ill because of trauma, toxicoses, nutritional deficiencies, reproductive disorders, neoplasia, or chronic disease. Birds recently exposed to other birds may become ill as a result of infectious diseases, including viral and bacterial infections, or as a result of problems occurring in isolated birds.

The diet history may reveal possible problems. Seed diets are high in fat and may be deficient in vitamin E and selenium. Birds on high-fat diets are more likely to show signs of vitamin E deficiency than are birds on diets low in fat. Thiamine deficiency is uncommon in birds on a seed diet or formulated diets because seeds and grains generally contain sufficient thiamine. Thiamine deficiency is seen in carnivorous birds fed only meat or day-old chicks and in fish-eating birds fed fish containing thiaminase.

The calcium content of the diet is important in paretic birds. Secondary nutritional hyperparathyroidism will develop if calcium use exceeds absorption from the intestines over a prolonged period of time. Blood calcium levels usually remain normal until calcium stores are depleted. Paresis associated with fractures is common. Increased use of calcium occurs with heavy egg production. Decreased calcium absorption commonly occurs as a result of a calcium-deficient diet. Seed diets are low in calcium and high in phosphorus and fat. The high-fat content of a seed diet may also interfere with calcium absorption. Meat is low in calcium and high in phosphorus. Raptors fed only day-old chicks, meat, or pinky mice may develop calcium deficiency.

Important historical environmental factors in paretic birds include access to potential toxins and flight capabilities. Birds allowed flight out of their cages are more susceptible to trauma. Free-flight episodes are conducive to collisions with windows, walls, and ceiling fans, leading to trauma.

Access or exposure to potential toxins is significant in a paretic bird. Toxins that may cause paresis include lead, zinc, botulism toxin, and organophosphate insecticides. The neuropathy associated with organophosphate exposure is delayed 7 to 21 days after exposure. Intoxication with botulism toxins occurs after ingestion of contaminated food such as decaying organic matter or toxin-laden maggots. Some sources of lead are listed in Table 9–3. Sources of zinc include pennies minted since 1982, Monopoly game pieces, and galvanized wire, containers, dishes, and hardware cloth.

A recent history of egg binding or dystocia is consistent with an associated paralysis.

Recent vaccination for Pacheco's disease or treatment with aminoglycoside antibiotics support associated dysfunction.

The duration of the paresis is important. Note the owner's description of the clinical signs and the course of the disease. Note previous illnesses, including signs, treatment, and response to treatment.

Physical Examination

Complete physical and neurologic examinations are important to identify neurologic and physical abnormalities in paretic birds. The neurologic examination is discussed in the beginning of this chapter. Other common findings in paretic birds are discussed below.

Paresis of the leg is indicated by an inability to grip with the foot. Birds with leg paresis will often curl the toes and are not able to perch with the affected foot. Paresis of the wing is indicated by a wing droop; one wing stays extended more than the other and is held in a lower position.

Blood in the mouth, ears, or eyes indicates head trauma. Look at the skin at the top of the head; meningeal hematomas may be visualized through the calvarium in some cases. Fractures or bruises anywhere on the body indicate trauma. Part the feathers and moisten the skin with alcohol to allow better visualization of the skin for evidence of bruising or wounds. This technique is useful on the legs, wings, skull, and spine.

Abdominal palpation may reveal organomegaly, retained egg, or other abdominal mass. The maximal distance from the keel to pubic bone in budgies is 4 to 5 mm. An increase in this distance is common with abdominal masses. Renal and gonadal tumors may affect nerves supplying the legs.

Evidence of dystocia on the physical examination includes depression, persistent wagging of the tail, straining movements of the abdomen, and an abnormally wide stance. Droppings may be absent or large and wet. Canaries often have drooped wings. The egg is usually palpable if paresis is present from the egg pressing on the nerves supplying the legs as they course through the pelvic region.

Hematuria may be an indication of lead or zinc toxicosis, especially in Amazon parrots.

Assess cloacal tone, grasping strength of the feet, and ability to move the tail. Look for muscle atrophy.

Botulism toxin causes a peripheral neuropathy. Leg paresis is usually the earliest clinical sign, characterized by the bird sitting on its sternum with legs extended caudally. Leg paresis is followed by wing paresis. Loss of control of the neck and head occurs in the terminal stages, resulting in the term *limber neck disease.*

Gout may cause gait abnormalities mimicking neurologic disease. A stiff gait with ataxia and weakness may occur before subcutaneous uric acid deposits (tophi) are visible through the skin of joints and legs.

Nestling budgies with riboflavin deficiency may walk on their toes.

Ventral edema may occur with vitamin E or selenium deficiency; skin edema may occur with thiamine deficiency.

Clinical signs of delayed organophosphate toxicosis include an inability to fly, ataxia, prolapsed nictitans, and convulsions.

Polyomavirus (budgerigar fledgling disease) may affect feather formation as well as cause paralysis and ataxia. Budgies infected as neonates develop normally until 10 to 15 days old. Then they may die with no premonitory signs or they may develop abdominal distension; subcutaneous hemorrhage; tremors of the head, neck, and limbs; ataxia; and reduced formation of down and contour feathers. Survivors may develop symmetrical feather abnormalities, including dystrophic primary and tail feathers, lack of down feathers on the back and abdomen, and lack of filoplumes on the head and neck. These feather abnormalities are not observed in larger psittacines infected with polyomavirus.

Large psittacines infected with polyomavirus may die peracutely or develop depression, anorexia, delayed crop emptying, regurgitation, diarrhea, dyspnea, weight loss, and subcutaneous hemorrhages. Ataxia, tremors, and paralysis may also occur.

Birds with PMV 1 may have ataxia, torticollis, tremors, leg paralysis, conjunctivitis, and occasionally dyspnea and diarrhea. Finches may be asymptomatic carriers or may have conjunctivitis or pseudomembranous formation of the larynx, and neurologic signs, or they may die before they are seen.

Birds with PDS may have CNS signs alone or in conjunction with wasting, abdominal distention, and gastrointestinal signs (e.g., passing undigested food or vomiting).

Clinical signs associated with avian picornavirus encephalomyelitis include depression, ataxia, paresis, paralysis, and fine head and neck tremors.

Clinical signs associated with reovirus include labored breathing, diarrhea, ataxia, and sometimes a bloody, brown nasal discharge.

Western and eastern equine encephalitis virus can cause paresis, paralysis, ataxia, tremors, depression, dyspnea, and death. Diarrhea may be present. Birds may die peracutely or acutely.

Birds with Marek's disease may have paralysis caused by lymphocytic proliferation in peripheral nerves. Tumors may also be associated with infection.

Paralysis may occur with gastrointestinal signs in birds with bacterial and chlamydial infections, reovirus, PMV, western and eastern equine encephalitis, polyomavirus in large psittacines, *Sarcocystis*, PDS, egg binding, gout, and lead, zinc, and aminoglycoside toxicoses.

Respiratory signs may occur with paralysis in birds with bacterial and chlamydial infections, reovirus, PMV, western and eastern equine encephalitis, polyomavirus in budgies and large psittacines, aspergillosis, *Sarcocystis*, egg binding, abdominal masses, and zinc toxicosis.

Feather abnormalities may occur with paralysis with polyomavirus infection in budgies.

Algorithm for Paralysis or Paresis

See Figure 6–4.

Diagnostic Approach for Paralysis or Paresis

Stabilize critically ill birds before performing diagnostic tests, and provide supportive care as needed (see Chapter 1).

Selection of appropriate diagnostic tests are based on consideration of the signalment and history of the bird and the findings of the physical and neurologic examinations. Radiographs are useful to detect fractures or lytic lesions of the long bones, shoulder girdle, or spine; coxofemoral luxations; intra-abdominal masses; hepatomegaly; egg binding; and heavy metal densities in the gastrointestinal tract. Lesions associated with systemic diseases may be noted radiographically. A CBC and plasma biochemistries rarely provide a diagnosis, but they are useful in supporting infectious, toxic, and systemic diseases. Lead and zinc blood levels, cultures, and titers are used to rule in or out specific diseases. For some brain and spinal cord lesions, EEG, CT, and MRI are useful tests. These tests require specialized equipment and expertise that may be available at referral centers.

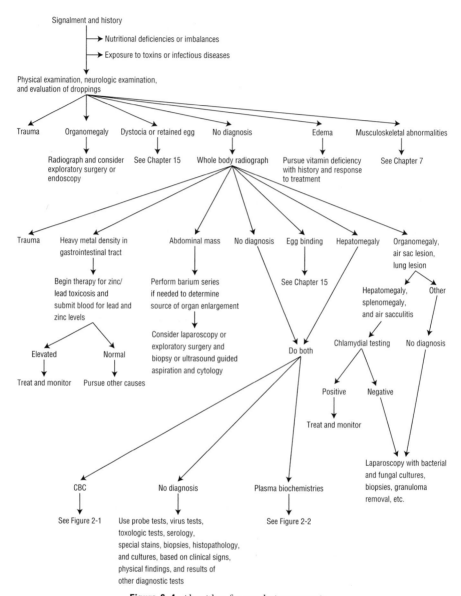

Figure 6–4. Algorithm for paralysis or paresis.

See the section on diagnostic approach for seizures for test interpretation for hematology, lead and zinc blood levels, radiography, chlamydial testing, EEG, MRI, CT, and vitamin E/selenium deficiency. Interpretation of additional tests follows.

Togavirus infection may cause an increase in AST, LDH, and uric acid. The WBC count is usually normal. Uric acid is usually elevated with articular gout.

Diagnosis of *Sarcocystis* infection is based on necropsy findings and histology. Necropsy findings include pulmonary congestion, pulmonary hemorrhage, splenomegaly, and hepatomegaly. The lung is the tissue of choice for histologic examination. Histologic findings include diffuse interstitial and exudative pneumonia, reticuloendothelial cell hyperplasia, and schizonts or merozoites in the capillary endothelium.

Tests available for diagnosis of viral infections are discussed in Chapter 12. A suspicion of viral infection is based on signalment, history, and clinical signs.

Diagnosis of PMV 1 is based on isolation of the virus from cloacal swabs in live birds. Postmortem cases may be diagnosed through isolation of the virus from the brain or organs.

Diagnosis of avian picornavirus encephalomyelitis is based on postmortem histology. Histologic changes include neuronal degeneration with lymphocytic perivascular cuffing and gliosis in the brain and spinal cord.

Viral-specific DNA probes are useful for detecting polyomavirus shedders. A cloacal swab is the best antemortem sample in larger psittacine birds. Subclinical carriers that intermittently shed polyomavirus occur, and they may give a false-negative result. A swab of the cut surface of the spleen, liver, and kidney (on one swab) is the best sample to submit for postmortem confirmation of polyomavirus infection.

Cloacal swabs and samples from affected organs may be used for virus isolation and culture for identification of reovirus infection. Viral antigen may be detected by immunofluorescence in affected tissue.

Western and eastern equine encephalitis virus may be isolated from a homogenate of blood, liver, spleen, and brain.

Enlarged peripheral nerves are common on postmortem examination of birds with Marek's disease.

If PDS is suspected based on radiology (i.e., distended proventriculus), a crop or ventricular biopsy may be performed for a definitive diagnosis. A negative biopsy result does not rule out PDS. Perform less-invasive techniques before biopsy to help rule out other common problems.

Treatment

Treat the underlying cause. The prognosis is difficult to assess with most avian neurologic injuries. Birds may regain neurologic function days to months after neurologic damage. Paralysis associated with fractures of the leg is usually reversible.

See the section on treatment of seizures for treatment of paralysis associated with bacterial CNS infections; vitamin E, selenium, and thiamine deficiencies; head trauma; cerebrovascular accidents; and neoplasia. See Chapter 7 for treatment of fractures.

Splint paretic toes in the proper perching position to avoid knuckling to prevent damage to the dorsal surface of the toes.

Treatment of malignant abdominal tumors is often unrewarding. Various combinations of surgery and chemotherapy have been used. If the tumor can be surgically removed, surgery is usually the treatment of choice. Dexamethasone may reduce clinical signs in cases of advanced or inoperable neoplasia.

Treat other disorders according to their primary cause (see Chapter 9).

HEAD TILT, CIRCLING, OR NYSTAGMUS

Head tilt, circling, or nystagmus can be caused by central or peripheral vestibular disease. A head tilt indicates an abnormality in the vestibular system. Vestibular lesions may be peripheral (middle or inner ear) or central (brain stem). Peripheral lesions cause a head tilt toward the side of the lesion, and the bird usually falls, drifts, or circles toward the side of the lesion. Central lesions may cause a head tilt, drifting, or circling in the opposite direction. A head tilt with paresis or proprioceptive deficits indicates a central vestibular lesion. Nystagmus may be caused by central or peripheral vestibular disease. Peripheral vestibular disease may occur with facial (CN VII) and sympathetic nerve deficits. Dysfunction of other cranial nerves associated with a head tilt indicates a central vestibular lesion.

Middle-ear lesions usually cause a head tilt with no other signs. Inner-ear disease usually produce a head tilt with falling, circling, nystagmus, strabismus, or asymmetric ataxia. The head tilt is ipsilateral to the lesion.

Differential Diagnoses for Head Tilt, Circling, or Nystagmus

1. Infectious
    a. Bacterial: any organism that causes °otitis media, °otitis interna, or encephalitis
    b. Viral: any organism that causes encephalitis (paramyxovirus, avian picornavirus encephalomyelitis, eastern and western equine encephalitis, other)
    c. Fungal: *Aspergillus, Cryptococcus*
    d. Parasitic: toxoplasmosis, schistosomiasis, *Sarcocystis*
    e. Other: proventricular dilatation syndrome
2. Nutritional: vitamin E/selenium deficiency
3. Toxic: °lead, aminoglycoside antibiotics
4. Physical: °trauma, neoplasia

Signalment

Common causes of head tilt, circling, and nystagmus in psittacines include otitis media or otitis interna, lead toxicosis, and trauma. Trauma is a common cause of the clinical signs in raptors.

Vitamin E or selenium deficiency is most common in young birds. Toxoplasmosis primarily affects gallinaceous and passerine birds. Schistosomiasis affects ducks, geese, and swans. *Sarcocystis* is primarily a disease of Old World psittacines (cockatoos) and nestlings of New World species (macaws).

°Common causes.

History

A complete history may reveal trauma, nutritional deficiencies, or possible exposure to toxins or infectious diseases. Isolated birds and those in closed collections are commonly ill because of toxicoses, trauma, nutritional deficiencies, neoplasia, and chronic diseases. Birds recently exposed to other birds may become ill as a result of infectious diseases or as a result of problems occurring in isolated birds.

Significant historic dietary information for birds showing vestibular signs includes an all-seed diet. Seed diets are high in fat and may be deficient in vitamin E and selenium. Birds on high-fat diets are more likely to show signs of vitamin E deficiency than are birds on diets low in fat.

Important historical environmental factors in birds with head tilt, circling, or nystagmus include access to potential toxins or cat feces, opossum feces, or cockroaches and flight capabilities. Birds allowed out of their cages are more susceptible to trauma. Free-flight episodes are conducive to collisions with windows, walls, and ceiling fans, leading to head trauma.

Toxicoses that can result in vestibular signs include lead toxicosis and aminoglycoside therapy. Some sources of lead are listed in Table 9–3. Aminoglycoside antibiotics can cause degeneration within the vestibular and auditory nerves. Signs can be unilateral or bilateral. Ototoxicity is more common with high doses, prolonged therapy, or impaired renal function.

Psittacine birds can serve as the intermediate host for *Sarcocystis*. Infection occurs when birds ingest the feces of an infected opossum that contains sporocysts or ingest cockroaches that have eaten infected opossum feces. Neurologic signs develop as a result of the presence of schizonts in the brain. Toxoplasmosis is acquired through the ingestion of oocysts in the feces of infected cats.

The duration of the illness is important. Note the owner's description of the clinical signs and the course of the disease. Note previous illnesses, including signs, treatment, and response to treatment.

Physical Examination

Complete physical and neurologic examinations are important to identify other neurologic and physical abnormalities. The neurologic examination is discussed in the beginning of this chapter. Other common findings in birds with head tilt, circling, or nystagmus are discussed below.

Horner's syndrome (miosis, ptosis, protrusion of the nictitating membrane) may be seen with central lesions or with a lesion in the cervical sympathetic tract or the brachial plexus.

Asymmetric ataxia without postural deficits or nystagmus that does not change with different positions of the head indicate peripheral vestibular system disease. Head tilt or nystagmus with any sign of brain stem dysfunction indicates a central vestibular lesion. Deficits in postural reactions, paresis, or loss of proprioception with a head tilt or nystagmus indicate a central vestibular lesion. Postural reactions are the complex responses that maintain the bird in a normal, upright position.

Loss of physiologic nystagmus may occur with lesions to CN VIII or vestibular pathways. Signs of loss of function of CN VIII include head tilt, deafness, nystagmus, and rolling of the body.

Blood in the mouth, ears, or eyes indicates head trauma. Look at the skin at the top of the head; meningeal hematomas may be visualized through the calvarium in some cases. Fractures or bruises anywhere on the body indicate trauma. Part the feathers and moisten the skin with alcohol to allow better visualization of the skin for evidence of bruising or wounds. This technique is useful on the legs, wings, skull, and spine.

Hematuria may be an indication of lead toxicosis, especially in Amazon parrots.

Assess cloacal tone, grasping strength of the feet, and ability to move the tail. Look for muscle atrophy.

Otitis media or otitis interna may occur as a result of otitis externa. Inflammation of the inner ear may cause a head tilt and circling toward the side of the lesion. Infection can progress to affect other cranial nerves and the midbrain. The ear canal and tympanic membrane can be examined using an otoscope or endoscope. The external ear canal is short and directed ventrally and caudally from the external acoustic meatus to the tympanic membrane. The normal canal is smooth and pale and may contain a small amount of debris. The normal tympanic membrane projects outward, and the extracollumellar cartilage may be visualized through the membrane. Erythema, swelling, or exudate of the outer ear may indicate bacterial otitis externa. Extension to middle and inner ear may occur. Evaluate the tympanic membrane for rupture, thickening, and fluid within the middle ear.

Ventral edema may occur with vitamin E or selenium deficiency, and skin edema may occur with thiamine deficiency.

Clinical signs associated with toxoplasmosis include anorexia, diarrhea, blindness, conjunctivitis, head tilt, circling, and ataxia. Head tilt, circling, weakness, and extension of the head and neck may indicate schistosomiasis in swans, ducks, or geese. *Sarcocystis* infections are usually peracute. Clinical signs that may occur before death include dyspnea, yellow-pigmented urates, lethargy, and neurologic signs.

Birds with PDS may have CNS signs alone or in conjunction with wasting, abdominal distention, or gastrointestinal signs (e.g., passing undigested food or vomiting).

Gastrointestinal signs may occur with head tilt, circling, or nystagmus with bacterial and *Sarcocystis* infections, PDS, and lead and aminoglycoside toxicoses.

Respiratory signs may occur with head tilt, circling, or nystagmus with bacterial or *Sarcocystis* infections, toxoplasmosis, or trauma.

Algorithm for Head Tilt, Circling, or Nystagmus

See Figure 6–5.

Diagnostic Approach for Head Tilt, Circling, or Nystagmus

Stabilize critically ill birds before performing diagnostic tests and provide supportive care as needed (see Chapter 1).

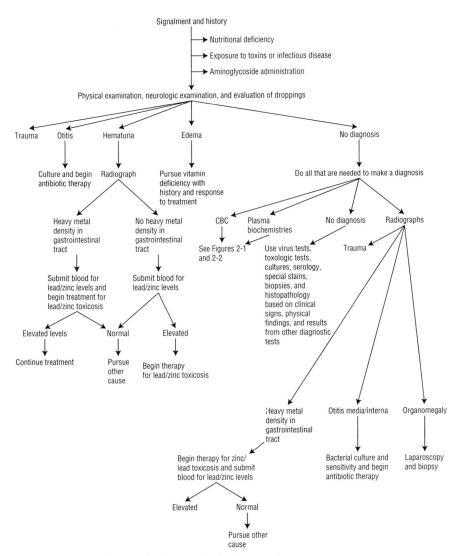

Figure 6–5. Algorithm for head tilt, circling, or nystagmus.

Selection of appropriate diagnostic tests is based on consideration of the signalment and history of the bird and the findings of the physical and neurologic examinations.

Exudates from the external ear canal are cultured, and sensitivity of the organism is determined so that an appropriate antibiotic is chosen for treatment.

A CBC and plasma biochemistries rarely provide a diagnosis, but they are useful in supporting diagnosis of infectious, toxic, and systemic diseases. Perform a CBC if systemic disease is suspected, when a bird is unresponsive to treatment, or to help determine the general health of the bird. Changes in the hemogram commonly seen in birds with head tilt, circling, or nystagmus are detailed below.

Nonregenerative anemias are usually normocytic and normochromic, but hypochromasia, anisocytosis, and poikilocytosis frequently occur in birds. Nonregenerative anemias may occur with chronic inflammatory diseases such as lead toxicosis. Nonregenerative anemias with decreased plasma protein may be seen with acute blood loss caused by trauma. If blood loss is not continuous, which may occur with trauma, a regenerative anemia will develop within several days. This will be characterized by the appearance of polychromasia and anisocytosis.

Regenerative anemias with normal plasma protein may occur with lead toxicosis. Lead toxicosis may cause an exaggerated response with more polychromasia and rubricytes than would be expected for the degree of anemia present. Basophilic stippling and cytoplasmic vacuolization may be seen with lead toxicosis. Hypochromasia can be associated with lead toxicosis.

Leukocytosis and heterophilia may be caused by stress, neoplasia, and inflammatory diseases (e.g., bacterial encephalitis).

Perform plasma biochemistry tests when systemic disease is suspected, if a bird is unresponsive to treatment, or to help determine the general health of the bird. Useful plasma biochemistries include AST, uric acid, LDH, and glucose. An elevation of uric acid usually accompanies lead and zinc toxicoses. An elevation of LDH and AST enzyme activities may occur in birds infected with *Sarcocystis*.

Radiology is useful in diagnosing otitis media, trauma, PDS, and heavy metal densities in the gastrointestinal tract. Lesions associated with systemic diseases may be noted radiographically. Radiographic abnormalities in a bird with head tilt, circling, or nystagmus may include trauma lesions, organomegaly, or metal densities in the proventriculus. Fractures of the skull or scleral ossicles indicate head trauma. Fractures elsewhere in the body may indicate trauma.

Evaluation of the hepatic silhouette may reveal hepatomegaly. Hepatomegaly and an increase in lung field density resulting from congestion and consolidation of the lungs occur with toxoplasmosis and *Sarcocystis* infection. Splenomegaly also occurs with *Sarcocystis* infection.

If PDS is suspected based on radiology (i.e., distended proventriculus), a crop or ventricular biopsy may be performed for a definitive diagnosis. A negative biopsy result does not rule out PDS. Perform less-invasive techniques before biopsy to help rule out other common problems.

Blood lead levels, cultures, and titers are used to rule in or out specific diseases. For some brain and spinal cord lesions, EEG, CT, and MRI are useful tests. These tests require specialized equipment and expertise that may be available at referral centers.

See the section on diagnostic approach for seizures for test interpretation of blood lead level, EEG, MRI, CT, vitamin E or selenium deficiency, trauma, and neoplasia. Interpretation of additional tests follows.

A diagnosis of toxoplasmosis is based on necropsy findings and histology. Necropsy findings include congestion and consolidation of the lungs, hepatomegaly, vasculitis, and necrotic foci in the lungs, liver, and heart.

A diagnosis of *Sarcocystis* infection is based on necropsy findings and histology. Necropsy findings include pulmonary congestion, pulmonary hemorrhage, splenomegaly, and hepatomegaly. The lung is the tissue of choice for histologic examination. Histologic findings include diffuse interstitial and exudative pneumonia, reticuloendothelial cell hyperplasia, and schizonts or merozoites in the capillary endothelium.

A diagnosis of schistosomiasis is based on presence of *Dendritobilhargia* in arteries at necropsy.

Treatment for Head Tilt, Circling, or Nystagmus

Provide supportive care as needed (see Chapter 1). Use shallow food and water bowls and consider spreading food on the floor of the cage if the bird has difficulty maneuvering to get food. Tube feed as needed.

Once a diagnosis is made, treat the underlying cause. Specific treatments are found in Chapter 9.

Medical treatment of otitis media or otitis interna includes long-term systemic antibiotic therapy based on culture and sensitivity results. Therapy is initiated with later-generation beta-lactams (piperacillin, cefotaxime) or fluoroquinolones (enrofloxacin) until sensitivity can be determined.

Neurologic deficits that result from chronic otitis interna may be permanent. Some birds are able to compensate for their vestibular deficits.

Aminoglycoside ototoxicity is treated by reducing the dose or preferably by replacing the aminoglycoside with a nontoxic antibiotic. Vestibular signs usually improve when the ototoxic antibiotic is discontinued. Deafness may be permanent.

Treatment of head trauma includes intravenous dexamethasone, stress-free environment (dark and quiet), and fluid replacement if hemorrhage has occurred. One-half to two-thirds the normal volume of fluids may be given if hemorrhage has occurred. Mannitol may be beneficial if the bird does not respond to initial therapy. The prognosis is guarded to poor.

Muscular dystrophy caused by vitamin E or selenium deficiency may respond to vitamin E and selenium supplementation and antiprotozoal therapy, but encephalomalacia rarely responds to therapy.

Symptomatic therapy for CNS neoplasia includes dexamethasone to decrease cerebrospinal fluid production, and phenobarbital to control seizures, if needed.

Treatment of bacterial CNS infection is usually ineffective in birds with CNS signs. Attempted therapy may be initiated with cefotaxime or chloramphenicol, pending sensitivity determination.

Treat other disorders according to their primary causes.

References and Additional Reading

Bennett RA. Neurology. In Ritchie BW, Harrison GJ, Harrison LR (eds): *Avian Medicine: Principles and Application.* Lake Worth, FL, Wingers Publishing, 1994, pp 723–747.

Clubb SL. Viscerotropic velogenic Newcastle disease in pet birds. In Kirk RW (ed): *Current Veterinary Therapy VIII, Small Animal Practice.* Philadelphia, WB Saunders, 1983, pp 628–630.

Cray C, Bossart G, Harris D. Plasma protein electrophoresis: Principles and diagnosis of infectious disease. *Proc Assoc Avian Vet* 1995;55–59.

Cross GM. Newcastle disease. *Vet Clin North Am Small Anim Pract* 1991;21(6):1231–1239.

Dorrestein GM. Physiology of the brain and special senses. In Altman RB, Clubb SL, Dorrestein GM, Quesenberry K (eds): *Avian Medicine and Surgery.* Philadelphia, WB Saunders, 1997, pp 459–460.

Greenacre CB, Latimer KS, Ritchie WB. Leg paresis in a black palm cockatoo caused by aspergillosis. *J Zoo Wild Med* 1992;23(1).

Hochleithner M. Convulsions in African gray parrots (*Psittacus erithacus*). *Proc Assoc Avian Vet* 1989;78–81.

Jenkins JR. Avian metabolic chemistries. *Semin Avian Exot Pet Med* 1994;3(1):25–32.

Jones MP, Orosz SE. Overview of avian neurology and neurological diseases. *Semin Avian Exot Pet Med* 1996;5(3):150–164.

King AS, McLelland J. Nervous system. In *Birds, Their Structure and Function,* ed 2. London, Bailliere Tindall, 1984, pp 237–283.

Klappenbach KM. Cerebral spinal fluid analysis in psittacines. *Proc Assoc Avian Vet* 1995;39–41.

LaBonde J. Pet avian toxicology. *Proc Assoc Avian Vet* 1988;159–174.

Leach MW, Higgins RJ, Lowenstine LJ, et al. Paramyxovirus infection in a moluccan cockatoo (*Cacatua moluccensis*) with neurologic signs. *J Assoc Avian Vet* 1988;2(2):87–90.

Lyman R. Neurologic examination. In Harrison GJ, Harrison LR (eds): *Clinical Avian Medicine and Surgery.* Philadelphia, WB Saunders, 1986, pp 282–285.

Murphy J. Psittacine fatty liver syndrome. *Proc Assoc Avian Vet* 1992;78–82.

Oliver JE, Lorenz MD. *Handbook of Veterinary Neurology,* ed 2. Philadelphia, WB Saunders, 1993.

Orosz SE. Anatomy of the central nervous system. In Altman RB, Clubb SL, Dorrestein GM, Quesenberry K (eds): *Avian Medicine and Surgery.* Philadelphia, WB Saunders, 1997, pp 454–459.

Orosz SE. Principles of avian clinical neuroanatomy. *Semin Avian Exot Pet Med* 1996;5(3):127–139.

Orosz SE. A review of avian neuroanatomy and neurology. *Proc Avian Acad Series* June 1994;91–108.

Ottinger MA. Aging in the avian brain: Neuroendocrine considerations. *Semin Avian Exot Pet Med* 1996;5(3):172–177.

Parrott T. Hepatopathy and neurological abnormalities in an umbrella cockatoo after vaccination with Pacheco's killed virus vaccine. *Proc Assoc Avian Vet* 1992;140.

Paul-Murphy J. Avian neurology. *Proc Assoc Avian Vet* 1992;420–432.

Porter SL. Vehicular trauma in owls. *Proc Assoc Avian Vet* 1990;164–170.

Quesenberry K. Avian neurologic disorders. In Birchard SJ, Sherdig RG (eds): *Saunders Manual of Small Animal Practice.* Philadelphia, WB Saunders, 1994, pp 1312–1316.

Quesenberry KE. Neurologic disorders in caged birds: A retrospective review of cases. *Proc Assoc Avian Vet* 1988;175–176.

Ritchie BW, Harrison GJ, Harrison LR (eds): *Avian Medicine: Principles and Application.* Lake Worth, FL, Wingers Publishing, 1994.

Romagnano A, Shiroma JT, Heard DJ, et al. Magnetic resonance imaging of the avian brain and abdominal cavity. *Proc Assoc Avian Vet* 1995;307–309.

Rosenthal K. Disorders of the avian nervous system. In Altman RB, Clubb SL, Dorrestein GM, Quesenberry K (eds): *Avian Medicine and Surgery.* Philadelphia, WB Saunders, 1997, pp 461–474.

Rosenthal K, Stefanacci J, Quesenberry K, et al. Computerized tomography in 10 cases of avian intracranial disease. *Proc Assoc Avian Vet* 1995;305.

Rosskopf WJ, Woerpel RW. Epilepsy in peach-faced and pied peach-faced lovebirds. *Proc Assoc Avian Vet* 1988;225–229.

Rosskopf WJ, Woerpel RW. An unusual case of spinal aspergillosis in a Mexican red headed Amazon parrot (*Amazona viridigenalis*). *Proc Assoc Avian Vet* 1995;351–355.

Rosskopf WJ, Woerpel RW. Successful treatment of a convulsive disorder in an umbrella cockatoo: A case report. *Proceedings of the First International Conference of Zoo Avian Medicine*, 1987, pp 267–271.

Rupiper DJ. Treatment of toxicosis affecting CNS in pigeons. *J Assoc Avian Vet* 1993;7(2):99.

Shivaprasad HL. Diseases of the nervous system in pet birds: A review and report of diseases rarely documented. *Proc Assoc Avian Vet* 1993;213–222.

Sims MH. Clinical electrodiagnostic evaluation in exotic animal medicine. *Semin Avian Exot Pet Med* 1996;5(3):140–149.

VanDerHeyden N. Velogenic viscerotropic Newcastle disease in three Amazon chicks. *Proc Assoc Avian Vet* 1992;158–161.

VanDerHeyden N. Evaluation and interpretation of the avian hemogram. *Semin Avian Exot Pet Med* 1994;3(1):5–13.

Young LA, Citino SB, Seccareccia V, et al. Eastern equine encephalomyelitis in an exotic avian collection. *Proc Assoc Avian Vet* 1996;163–165.

Chapter 7

Musculoskeletal Signs

Musculoskeletal abnormalities are common in pet birds, especially fractures, developmental abnormalities, and soft tissue injuries. Because birds have little subcutaneous tissue along much of the wings and legs, fractures often result in open and contaminated fractures. Infectious and metabolic problems are also fairly common in pet birds.

Signs of abnormalities of the musculoskeletal system of the leg include limping, lameness, swollen joints, and leg deformities. Signs of abnormalities of the musculoskeletal system of the wing include wing drooping, fractures, and swollen joints.

This chapter presents a diagnostic approach for musculoskeletal signs commonly seen in pet birds. The chapter is divided into leg signs, wing signs, swollen joints, and management of fractures. Sections associated with signs begin with general information and definitions of terms, followed by a list of differential diagnoses. This is followed by appropriate signalment information. Common causes of the clinical sign are presented for each group of pet birds. The history section can be used to explore important historical information. The physical examination section guides interpretation of the physical findings. An algorithm is included in each section to provide a quick reference for recommended tests. The diagnostic plan suggests useful tests. Consult Chapter 12 for techniques of sample collection and for assistance with test interpretation. Once a diagnosis is made, general treatments are discussed at the end of each section. Treatments for specific diseases are found in Chapter 9. Consult the formulary in Chapter 17 for drug dosages. See Appendix VI for general skeletal anatomy. The treatment of various fractures is discussed at the end of the chapter, including fracture repair techniques, splint applications, and bandage applications.

LIMPING, LAMENESS, OR LEG DEFORMITIES

Limping and lameness can be the result of neurologic or musculoskeletal abnormalities. Neurologic abnormalities often mimic musculoskeletal signs. Careful observation of the leg for willful movement will help in determining if the problem is neurologic or musculoskeletal. Observe for response to pain, movement, swelling, skin lesions, etc. Lack of movement or response to pain indicates a neurologic problem. Swelling of the foot, leg, or joints of the leg or the presence of skin lesions can indicate musculoskeletal abnormalities. Neurologic causes of lameness, limping, paralysis, and paresis are discussed in Chapter 6. Skin lesions associated with the foot and leg are discussed in Chapter 8.

Musculoskeletal-associated limping or lameness is often the result of an injury; however, arthritis, tenosynovitis, osteomyelitis, and cellulitis do occur. Arthritis results in a swollen joint and is discussed later in this chapter.

Leg deformities are common. Developmental and traumatic causes are common.

Differential Diagnoses for Limping, Lameness, or Leg Deformities

1. Infectious
   a. Bacterial: gram-negative, gram-positive (including *Mycobacterium*, others)
   b. Fungal: *Aspergillus*
2. Metabolic: °gout
3. Nutritional: °calcium deficiency, °calcium/phosphorus imbalance, vitamin D deficiency
4. Toxic: °lead, zinc
5. Physical: °trauma, °improper substrate material
6. Neoplastic
7. °Developmental
8. Genetic

Signalment

Common causes of limping or lameness in large psittacines include trauma, lead toxicosis, gout, and neurologic causes. Small psittacines are most commonly lame or limping as a result of trauma, gout, lead toxicosis, zinc toxicosis, or neurologic disease. Raptors are commonly lame or limping as a result of trauma or neurologic disease.

Common causes of limping or lameness in young birds include nutritional diseases (homemade formulas), fractures, and bone deformities. Leg deformities in young birds may be associated with calcium deficiency, calcium/phosphorus imbalance, vitamin D deficiency, improper substrate material, congenital defects, trauma, and developmental malpositioning in the egg.

Common causes of leg deformities in adult birds include trauma-induced fractures or fractures associated with weakened bones as a result of calcium deficiency, calcium/phosphorus imbalances, or vitamin D deficiency.

History

Isolated birds and those in collections with no recently added new birds are commonly ill as a result of trauma, toxicoses, nutritional deficiencies, neoplasia, or management-related causes (e.g., improper substrate materials). Chronic

---

°Common causes.

diseases may also occur in isolated birds (e.g., mycobacteriosis or aspergillosis). In birds recently exposed to other birds, infectious causes must be considered in addition to those conditions occurring in solitary birds.

Significant dietary history includes type of diet and vitamin supplementation. Seed diets are low in calcium and high in phosphorus and fat. Secondary nutritional hyperparathyroidism will develop if calcium utilization exceeds absorption from the intestines over a prolonged period of time. Blood calcium levels usually remain normal until calcium stores in bone are depleted. Fractures commonly result when the cortex of the bone thins from calcium depletion. The high fat content of a seed diet may also interfere with calcium absorption. Meat is low in calcium and high in phosphorus. Raptors fed only meat, day-old chicks, or pinky mice may develop calcium deficiency. Vitamin D–deficient diets, especially in conjunction with calcium-deficient foods, may result in decreased bone density.

Important environmental factors include flight capabilities, access to potential toxins, exposure to natural sunlight, and management practices. Birds allowed flight out of their cages are more susceptible to trauma. Free-flight episodes are conducive to collisions with windows, walls, and ceiling fans, leading to trauma and fractures. Sunlight is important in the activation of vitamin D_3. Growing birds placed on slick or slippery surfaces may develop leg deformities because of the lack of traction. Some sources of lead are listed in Table 9–3. Sources of zinc include pennies minted since 1982, Monopoly game pieces, hardware cloth, and galvanized materials.

The duration of the illness is important. Note the owner's description of the clinical signs and the course of the disease. Note previous illnesses, including signs, treatment, and response to treatment.

Physical Examination

Limping and lameness of neurologic origin may appear as a musculoskeletal abnormality. If a lesion or deformity is not observed with physical examination, a neurologic examination should be performed (see Chapter 6).

A complete physical examination is important to identify the extent of the problem and the involvement of other body systems. Observe for trauma, abdominal swelling, neurologic deficits, etc. If abnormalities are present, consult appropriate chapters to assist in making a diagnosis. Common findings of birds with lameness, limping, or leg deformity are discussed below.

Observe the bird in the cage. Look for weight bearing on both legs and ability to grasp with the feet. Check the cage for blood and smooth perches of different diameter. Check the nest or cage substrate material to see if the surface is too smooth for the nestling to get the necessary traction to hold the feet under the body. Observe fresh droppings for polyuria, hematuria, or biliverdinuria, indicating possible lead or zinc toxicoses, kidney disease, or liver disease.

Catch the bird, taking care not to cause further injury. Inspect the leg for bruises, swollen joints, swelling along the bones, deformity, crepitation, or obvious fractures. Determine if the bird can grasp with the affected foot. If a joint is swollen, check for heat, pain, and erythema. Look for evidence of trauma elsewhere. Moisten the skin with alcohol and part the feathers to get better visualization if needed. Check for subcutaneous emphysema. With ruptured air sacs or fractures of pneumatic bones (e.g., humerus, femur, etc.), air may leak from damaged bone into subcutaneous areas.

Splay leg is a common leg deformity where one or both legs splay laterally at the hip (Fig. 7–1).

Pain may limit use and appear as a neurologic problem. Damage to nerves may occur with musculoskeletal injuries. Check for neurologic deficits.

Gastrointestinal signs (e.g., diarrhea, polyuria) may be noted in conjunction with lameness, limping, or leg deformities with bacterial and fungal diseases, proventricular dilatation syndrome (PDS), renal disease, trauma from egg laying, lead toxicosis, zinc toxicosis, and gout.

Algorithm for Limping, Lameness, or Leg Deformities

See Figure 7–2.

Diagnostic Plan for Limping, Lameness, or Leg Deformities

Stabilize severely ill birds before performing stressful diagnostic tests, and provide supportive care as needed during the diagnostic evaluation (see Chapter 1).

Dietary causes must be sought from the history. History and physical examination may allow a diagnosis of trauma or fractures. Radiology is required to determine the extent of the problem. Nutritional deficiencies may cause weakened bones, resulting in fractures.

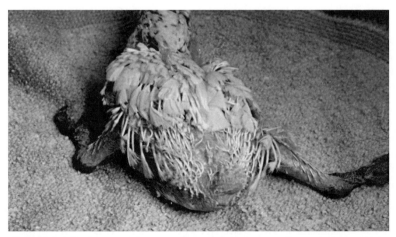

Figure 7–1. Splay leg in a Moluccan cockatoo. (Photo courtesy of Brian L. Speer, DVM, ABVP-avian.)

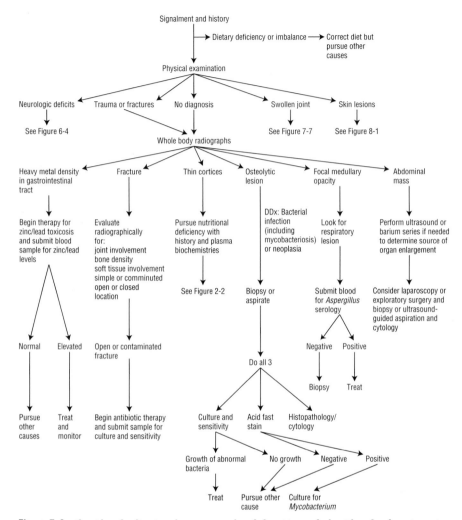

Figure 7–2. Algorithm for limping, lameness, or leg deformities and algorithm for drooping wing or fractures.

Swollen joints are aspirated, and the sample is evaluated cytologically. Consult the section on diagnostic plan for swollen joints for cytologic evaluation.

Radiology is the next step in evaluating a lame or limping bird. Obvious fractures will be noted. All fractures are radiographed and evaluated for location, joint involvement, bone density, soft tissue involvement, simple or comminuted, and open or closed. With recently incurred fractures, the bone segments will be distinct, sharp, and well defined. Soft tissue swelling is usually present. Older fractures and healing fractures will show endosteal filling and indistinct fracture fragments. When a fracture is suspected, but cannot be identified radiographically, repeat radiographs in 10 to 14 days. An endosteal response will be apparent with fractures at that time. In birds, there is minimal periosteal response in stable healing fractures.

Thin cortices, with or without fractures, can be the result of nutritional deficiencies.

Osteolytic lesions may be the result of osteomyelitis or neoplasia. Mycobacteriosis is a common cause of lytic lesions in birds. A single area of punctate radiolucency of bone can indicate mycobacteriosis. Aspiration or biopsy may be used for acid-fast staining to identify mycobacteria. Submit a sample for bacterial culture and sensitivity testing for other bacteria. Pododermatitis is a common avenue of localized bone invasion by bacteria.

A focal increase in medullary opacity may be caused by granuloma formation. Aspergillosis is a common cause of granulomas in bones of birds. Respiratory lesions are often also present (airsacculitis or focal granulomas of the air sac or lung).

Generalized increased endosteal bone opacity or polyostotic hyperostosis may be caused by egg laying or inappropriate gonadal activity (e.g., ovarian cysts). This does not result in lameness and would be an incidental finding when radiographing a lame or limping patient. Ultrasonography of the gonads may be indicated if recent egg laying has not occurred (see Chapter 15).

Treatment for Limping, Lameness, or Leg Deformities

Once a diagnosis is made, treat the underlying cause. Provide supportive care as needed (see Chapter 1). Treatment of leg fractures and dislocations are discussed at the end of this chapter. Treatments of specific diseases are discussed in Chapter 9.

Correct dietary deficiencies if present. The loss of bone density leaves the bone fragile and difficult to work with when nutritional deficiencies have caused thin cortices and fractures. Pinning may result in further damage to the fragile bone.

Pediatric patients with leg deformities are radiographed. Valgus (lateral deviation) and varus (medial deviation) of the hips, knees, hocks, and metatarsus may be evident. Radiology helps determine the degree of correction needed. Nutritional deficiencies, trauma, or placing the birds on an inappropriate surface are common causes of orthopedic problems in young birds. Correct dietary deficiencies. Many leg deformities of the hips, femur, and tibiotarsus in young birds can be treated using deep nesting cups padded with absorbent toweling that holds the legs under the body of the bird and hobbles between the legs at the distal femur, the tibiotarsus, and tarsometatarsus (Fig. 7–3). Do not place a constricting bandage around the leg because the young bird's rapid growth rate may cause vascular impairment. Severe leg defects require splinting or corrective surgery (Clipsham, 1992, 1991, 1989; Bennett, 1995; Greenacre, Aron, and Ritchie, 1994). Circulation and growth of young birds must be considered when applying braces to the legs of young birds.

WING DROOPING OR FRACTURES

Wing drooping is noted when one or more joints of the wing extend more than normal. When one wing is affected, often the affected wing will be held

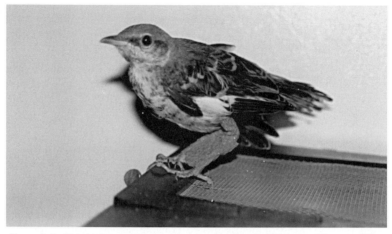

Figure 7–3. This bird is hobbled to correct splay leg. Hobbles may be successful in correcting leg deformities in young birds. Use a padded deep nesting cup in conjunction with the hobbles.

lower than the other. The long wing feathers may rest on the perch or extend more ventral than normal. The long wing feathers may be held dorsally, and the proximal wing may droop ventrally.

Wing drooping may be the result of musculoskeletal abnormalities or neurologic problems. Neurologic problems are discussed in Chapter 6. Neurologic abnormalities often mimic musculoskeletal signs. Careful observation of the extremity for willful movement will help in determining if the problem is neurologic or musculoskeletal. Observe for response to pain, movement, swelling, skin lesions, etc. Consult Chapter 6 for assistance with diagnosis of neurologic causes of wing drooping.

Differential Diagnoses for Wing Drooping or Fractures

1. Infectious
   a. Bacterial: gram-negative, gram-positive (including *Mycobacterium*, other)
   b. Fungal: *Aspergillus*
2. Metabolic: gout
3. Nutritional: calcium deficiency, calcium/phosphorus imbalance, vitamin D deficiency, excess protein
4. Toxic: °lead, zinc
5. Physical: °trauma, brachial plexus avulsion
6. Neoplastic

°Common causes.

Signalment

The most common cause of wing drooping or fractures in birds is trauma. Nutritional deficiencies must be considered as a predisposing cause of fractures. Lead toxicosis and neurologic disease are also common causes of wing drooping. In young birds, nutritional diseases are common.

History

Isolated birds and those in collections with no recently added new birds are commonly ill because of trauma, toxicoses, nutritional deficiencies, neoplasia, and gout. Chronic bacterial and fungal diseases (mycobacteriosis or aspergillosis) are also seen.

Birds recently exposed to other birds are commonly ill as a result of those illnesses occurring in isolated birds or infectious diseases. Mycobacteriosis can be a flock problem.

Significant dietary history includes type of diet and vitamin supplementation. Baby birds being hand fed homemade diets are susceptible to nutritional deficiencies. Secondary nutritional hyperparathyroidism will develop if calcium utilization exceeds absorption from the intestines over a prolonged period of time. Blood calcium levels usually remain normal until calcium stores in the bones are depleted. Fractures commonly result when the cortex of the bones thin from calcium depletion. Seed diets are low in calcium and high in phosphorus and fat. The high fat content of a seed diet may also interfere with calcium absorption. Meat is low in calcium and high in phosphorus. Raptors fed only meat, day-old chicks, or pinky mice may develop calcium deficiency. Vitamin D–deficient diets, especially in conjunction with calcium-deficient foods, may result in decreased bone density with lack of exposure to natural sunlight. Excess protein in the diet or a calcium-deficient diet may cause rotation of the distal wing of waterfowl, resulting in "airplane wing" (Fig. 7–4). Other factors that may be involved in the development of this condition include rapid growth, genetic, improper incubation, hatching problems, trauma, and inadequate exercise.

Important environmental factors include exposure to infectious diseases, access to potential toxins, and flight capabilities. Birds allowed flight out of their cages are more susceptible to trauma. Free-flight episodes are conducive to collisions with windows, walls, and ceiling fans, leading to trauma and fractures. Animal bites may result in fractures or neurologic damage. Some sources of lead are listed in Table 9–3. Sources of zinc include pennies minted since 1982, Monopoly game pieces, hardware cloth, and galvanized materials.

The duration of the illness is important. Note the owner's description of the clinical signs and the course of the disease. Note previous illnesses, including signs, treatment, and response to treatment.

Physical Examination

Wing drooping of neurologic origin may appear as a musculoskeletal abnormality or generalized weakness. If a lesion or deformity is not observed with physical examination, a neurologic examination is performed (see Chapter 6).

A complete physical examination is important to identify the extent of the

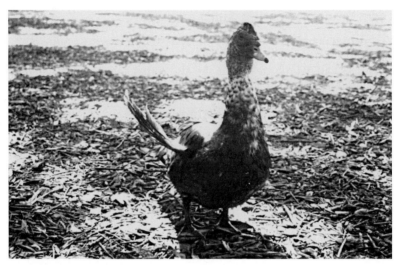

Figure 7–4. A duck with rotation of the distal wing, resulting in "airplane wing."

problem and to identify involvement of other body systems. The humerus is pneumatic (contain air spaces) and communicates with air sacs. The ulna is the larger bone of the distal wing. Observe for trauma, swellings, neurologic deficits, abnormal droppings, etc. If abnormalities are present, consult appropriate sections of the text to assist in making a diagnosis. Common findings in birds with wing drooping or fractures are discussed below.

Observe the bird in the cage. Look at respiration rate, position of the wings, and general attitude. The injury often involves the ulna, radius, or both, or distally when the wing is held resting on the perch (Fig. 7–5). When the wing feathers are held off the perch but the wing is drooping, the injury is often from the mid ulna to the mid humerus. When the proximal wing droops and the long distal wing feathers are held dorsally, the injury often involves the mid humerus to shoulder joint. Check the cage for blood. Observe fresh droppings for polyuria, hematuria, or biliverdinuria, which indicate possible lead or zinc toxicoses, kidney disease, or liver disease.

Catch the bird, taking care not to cause further injury. Inspect the wing for swelling, blood, fractures, or hematomas. If a joint is swollen, check for pain, erythema, and heat. Look for evidence of trauma elsewhere. Moisten the skin with alcohol and part the feathers to get better visualization, if needed. With fractures of pneumatic bones or ruptured air sacs, air may leak from damaged bone into subcutaneous tissue, resulting in subcutaneous emphysema.

Pain may limit use of the wing and appear as a neurologic problem. Damage to nerves may occur with musculoskeletal injuries. Check for neurologic deficits. If neurologic deficits exist, consult Chapter 6 for additional aid in determining the etiology.

Gastrointestinal signs may occur with wing drooping or fractures with bacterial or fungal diseases, gout, and lead and zinc toxicoses. Respiratory signs may occur with musculoskeletal causes of wing drooping or fractures with aspergillosis, trauma, mycobacteriosis, or other bacterial infections.

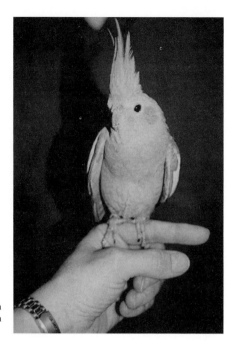

Figure 7–5. When the wing is held resting on the perch, as with this cockatiel, the injury often involves the ulna and/or radius, or distally.

Algorithm for Wing Drooping or Fractures

See Figure 7–2.

Diagnostic Plan for Wing Drooping or Fractures

Stabilize severely ill birds before performing stressful diagnostic tests, and provide supportive care as needed during the diagnostic evaluation (see Chapter 1).

Dietary factors must be sought from the history. History and physical examination may allow a diagnosis of trauma or fractures. Radiology is required to determine the extent of the problem. Consider nutritional deficiencies as a possible cause of weakened bones, resulting in fractures.

Swollen joints are aspirated, and the sample is evaluated cytologically. Consult the section on diagnostic plan for swollen joints for cytologic evaluation.

Radiology is the next step in evaluating a bird with a drooping wing or fracture. All fractures are radiographed and evaluated for location, joint involvement, bone density, soft tissue involvement, simple or comminuted, and open or closed.

With recently incurred fractures, the bone segments will be distinct, sharp, and well defined. Soft tissue swelling is usually present. Older fractures and healing fractures will show endosteal filling and indistinct fracture fragments. When a fracture is suspected, but cannot be identified radiographically, repeat radiographs in 10 to 14 days. An endosteal response will be apparent with fractures at that time. In birds, there is minimal periosteal response in stable healing fractures. Chronic fractures show indistinct fracture fragments and endosteal filling.

Thin cortices, with or without fractures, can be the result of nutritional deficiencies.

Osteolytic lesions may be the result of osteomyelitis or neoplasia. Mycobacteriosis is a common cause of lytic lesions in birds. A single area of punctate radiolucency of bone can indicate mycobacteriosis. Aspiration or biopsy may be used for acid-fast staining to identify mycobacteria. Submit a sample for bacterial culture and sensitivity testing for other bacteria. Pododermatitis is a common avenue of localized bone invasion by bacteria.

A focal increase in medullary opacity may be the result of granuloma formation. Aspergillosis is a common cause of granulomas in bones of birds. Respiratory lesions are often also present (airsacculitis or focal granulomas of the air sac or lung).

A generalized increase in endosteal bone opacity or polyostotic hyperostosis may be caused by egg laying or inappropriate gonadal activity (e.g., ovarian cysts). This does not result in fractures or wing drooping and would be an incidental finding when radiographing a bird with a wing droop. Ultrasonography of the abdomen to visualize the gonads is indicated with polyostotic hyperostosis if recent egg laying has not occurred (see Chapter 15).

A heavy metal density object may be noted in the ventriculus, consistent with lead and zinc toxicoses.

Treatment for Wing Drooping or Fractures

Once a diagnosis is made, treat the underlying cause. Provide supportive care as needed (see Chapter 1). Treatment of wing fractures and dislocations are discussed at the end of this chapter. Treatment of specific diseases are found in Chapter 9.

Correct dietary deficiencies if present. The loss of bone density leaves the bone fragile and difficult to work with when nutritional deficiencies result in thin cortices and fractures. Pinning may result in further damage to the fragile bone.

SWOLLEN JOINT OR JOINTS

Swollen joints may occur alone or in conjunction with other musculoskeletal abnormalities.

Differential Diagnoses for Swollen Joints

1. Infectious
   a. Bacterial: °gram-negative, °gram-positive (*Staphylococcus, Streptococcus, Mycobacterium,* other)
   b. Fungal: *Aspergillus*

°Common causes.

2. Metabolic: °gout
3. Nutritional: deficiencies (zinc, manganese, biotin, pantothenic acid, folic acid), high mineral diet
4. Physical: °trauma, obesity
5. Neoplastic

Signalment

Common causes of swollen joints in psittacines include trauma, bacterial infections, and gout. Raptors are commonly affected by trauma and bacterial infections.

Perosis most commonly occurs in young gallinaceous birds, cranes, and ratites. Raptors, cockatiels, and rosellas may also be affected.

History

Isolated birds and those in collections with no recently added new birds are commonly ill because of gout, nutritional deficiencies, or neoplasia. Chronic bacterial and fungal diseases (mycobacteriosis or aspergillosis) and bacterial infections are also seen.

Birds recently exposed to other birds are commonly ill as a result of those problems occurring in isolated birds or infectious diseases. Mycobacteriosis can be a flock problem.

Significant dietary history includes type of diet and vitamin supplementation. High dietary levels of protein, calcium, or vitamin D_3 may interfere with the ability of the kidney to adequately excrete uric acid, resulting in gout. Deficiency of manganese, biotin, pantothenic acid, or folic acid may contribute to slipped tendon of the hock (perosis). Obesity or high mineral diets may also predispose birds to this condition. Zinc deficiency may contribute to enlargement of the hock without perosis.

Important environmental factors include exposure to infectious diseases and flight capabilities. Infectious diseases, such as mycobacteriosis, may be spread through direct contact with infected birds in the aviary or with wild birds as well as by exposure to the organism in the soil, etc. Birds allowed flight out of their cages are more susceptible to trauma. Free-flight episodes are conducive to collisions with windows, walls, and ceiling fans, leading to trauma and fractures.

The duration of the illness is important. Note the owner's description of the clinical signs and the course of the disease. Note previous illnesses, including signs, treatment, and response to treatment.

Physical Examination

A complete physical examination is important to identify the extent of the problem and to identify involvement of other body systems. If abnormalities are

---

°Common causes.

present, consult appropriate chapters to assist in making a diagnosis. Common findings of birds with a swollen joint or joints are discussed below.

Observe the bird in the cage. Look for weight bearing on both legs and the ability to grasp with the feet. Check the cage for blood. Evaluate the droppings.

Catch the bird, taking care not to cause further injury. Inspect the legs and wings for bruises, fractures, swelling, or deformity. Observe the swollen joint for pain, erythema, heat, or laceration. Look for evidence of trauma elsewhere.

Articular gout usually affects multiple joints. White uric acid deposits (tophi) may be visible in joints through the skin (Fig. 7–6). Deposits may also be noted along tendons.

Gastrointestinal signs may occur with swollen joints with bacterial and fungal diseases, gout, and trauma. Respiratory signs may accompany swollen joints with bacterial and fungal diseases and trauma. Neurologic signs may be present with swollen joints with trauma and deficiencies in pantothenic acid, biotin, or manganese. Dermatologic abnormalities may be present with swollen joints with bacterial and fungal infections, gout, trauma, and deficiencies in pantothenic acid, biotin, or zinc.

Algorithm for Swollen Joints

See Figure 7–7.

Diagnostic Plan for Swollen Joints

Stabilize severely ill birds before performing stressful diagnostic tests, and provide supportive care as needed during the diagnostic evaluation (see Chapter 1).

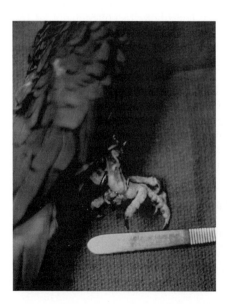

Figure 7–6. Swollen joints as a result of gout in an Amazon parrot. (Photo courtesy of Stephen Fronefield, DVM.)

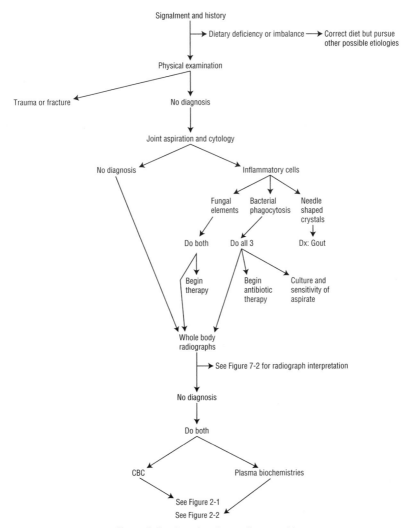

Figure 7–7. Algorithm for swollen joint(s).

Dietary causes must be sought from the history. When dietary causes are suspected, correct the diet while exploring other possible etiologies.

History and physical examination may allow a diagnosis of trauma or fractures. Radiology is required to determine the extent of the problem.

Swollen joints are aspirated, and the sample is evaluated cytologically. Cytology of a normal joint sample may contain macrophages, a few leukocytes, and synovial lining cells with a granular background with Wright's stain. An increase in heterophils and vacuolated macrophages is abnormal. An increase in heterophils and loss of the granular appearance may be seen with inflammation (e.g., trauma or infection). Bacterial phagocytosis by leukocytes indicates a septic condition. Needle-shaped crystals are indicative of gout. Inflammatory cells are usually present with articular gout.

Radiograph swollen joints of possible bacterial or fungal etiology. Radiology will help determine the extent of the problem as well as the prognosis. Trauma will usually have some soft tissue swelling with or without fractures. With recently incurred fractures, the bone segments will be distinct, sharp, and well defined. Soft tissue swelling is usually present. Older fractures and healing fractures will show endosteal filling and indistinct fracture fragments. When a fracture is suspected, but cannot be identified radiographically, repeat radiographs in 10 to 14 days. An endosteal response will be apparent with fractures at that time. In birds, there is minimal periosteal response in fracture healing.

Osteolytic lesions may be the result of osteomyelitis or neoplasia. Mycobacteriosis is a common cause of lytic lesions in birds. Pododermatitis is a common avenue of localized bone invasion by other bacteria. A single area of punctate radiolucency of bone can indicate mycobacteriosis. Aspiration or biopsy may be used for acid-fast staining to identify mycobacteria. Submit a sample for bacterial culture and sensitivity testing for other bacteria.

A focal increase in medullary opacity may result from granuloma formation. Aspergillosis is a common cause of granulomas in bones of birds. Respiratory lesions are often also present (focal granulomas of the air sac or lung or airsacculitis).

If the problem is not obvious, a complete blood count (CBC) and plasma biochemistries are performed. A CBC is useful in supporting infectious and inflammatory diagnoses. If the white blood cell (WBC) count is in excess of 40,000/μl, rule out mycobacteriosis and aspergillosis with EPH, cytology, biopsy, and acid-fast staining. Plasma biochemistries are important in the diagnosis of metabolic diseases. Useful biochemistry tests for birds with swollen joints includes uric acid, total protein, and creatine kinase (CK). Dehydration, renal disease, or gout may result in an elevated uric acid. An elevation of CK may occur with muscle damage. Total protein is useful in the evaluation of hydration status.

Treatment for Swollen Joints

Once a diagnosis is made, treat the underlying cause. Provide supportive care as needed (see Chapter 1). Treatment of specific diseases is found in Chapter 9.

WING AND LEG FRACTURE AND DISLOCATION REPAIR

Stabilize the bird before permanent fracture repair. A temporary bandage is used to immobilize the fractured bone to reduce further damage while the bird is being stabilized. Provide supportive care as needed, including intravenous or intraosseous fluids, antibiotics, and warmth (80° to 88° F).

Lower the perches to a few inches above the floor of the cage. Place food and water where they are easily accessible.

Open or contaminated fractures are cultured. A broad-spectrum antibiotic (e.g., trimethoprim/sulfamethoxazole, enrofloxacin, or cephalexin) is begun pending culture results. The wound is cleaned and debrided. Open fractures have a poorer prognosis for healing.

Injuries to a leg require treatment that results in a rapid return of weight bearing to that leg to prevent pododermatitis (bumblefoot) in the unaffected foot. Pododermatitis may occur when one foot bears most of the weight of the bird for an extended period of time.

The rate of fracture healing is dependent on blood supply, amount of displacement, degree of motion at the fracture site, and presence of infection. The method of repair is determined by multiple factors. Some fractures respond well to bandaging, whereas others require surgical repair to increase stability and likelihood of return of adequate function. Avian fractures heal rapidly. Healing occurs primarily by forming an endosteal callus, with little periosteal callous formation in stable fractures. Intramedullary (IM) pins may disrupt endosteal callous formation, but they are often successfully used in avian fracture stabilization. Avian bone is brittle, often resulting in comminuted and open fractures. Many avian bones are too straight to avoid penetration of joints with IM pinning. Penetration of articular surfaces must be avoided.

Factors that must be considered when determining the type of fracture repair include goal of repair, site of fracture, size of the bird, acute or chronic, simple or comminuted, presence of an open fracture or infection, concomitant problems, age of the bird, and knowledge and ability of the veterinarian. Return of normal or near normal function is required for birds to survive in the wild. Breeding birds require return of function necessary for courtship and breeding. Caged pet birds may not need return of flight capabilities or perfect conformation. The location, bone affected, and involvement of other bones affect the choice of repair. Fractures near joints often result in a decrease in function. Coaptation splints are more successful with fractures in small birds. Acute fractures have a better prognosis than chronic fractures. Simple fractures heal more readily and with fewer complications than comminuted fractures. Comminuted fractures often require external fixation. Open fractures and those with bacterial contamination have a much poorer prognosis. Necrosis of bone occurs. Avoid placement of implants in infected sites. External fixators are well suited for most contaminated fractures. Consider concomitant problems such as the common occurrence of aspergillosis and bumblefoot associated with the stress of the fracture and captivity in raptors. Also consider the age of the bird. Young birds heal quickly, but they also outgrow coaptation splints rapidly. Damage to growing bones may result in deformity. Surgical repair of fractures requires knowledge of the anatomy and techniques useful in the repair of fractures. Detailed surgical anatomy is beyond the scope of this book; consult the references for additional information (Bennett, 1997, 1995, 1992; Martin, 1994; Orosz, 1994, 1992; Hess, 1994; Howard, 1994).

Nonsurgical management of fractures may include cage rest, splints, and bandages. Many fractures respond well to coaptation when complete return to normal function is not required. Bandages and splints must be carefully monitored for tissue abrasions, swelling, and slipping. Bandages and splints must be well padded to prevent pressure necrosis. Wooden splints, aluminum rods, or lightweight cast materials (such as Orthoplast, VTP, or Vet-lite) can be used for reinforcement materials (Table 7–1).

Surgical management is often required for complete return of function after

TABLE 7–1. Animal Care Products Available for Use in Fractures

Orthoplast: Johnson & Johnson Medical, Arlington, TX 76004-3130; (817) 456-3141; (800) 433-5170
Vet-lite, formerly Hexcelite: Hexcel Medical Company, Dublin, CA 94566; (510) 847-9500
Veterinary Thermoplastic: VTP, IMEX Veterinary Inc, Longview, TX 75604; (800) 828-4639
Vetwrap: 3M Animal Care Products, St. Paul, MN 55144-1000; (612) 733-1110; (800) 848-0829
SAM Splint: Seaberg Company Inc, South Beach, OR 97366; (541) 967-4726; (800) 818-4726

fracture healing. Surgical repair of fractures may include external fixators, IM pins, plates, or combinations of these. Advantages of surgical repair of fractures include increased stability, increased probability of return of normal function, and often faster healing. Disadvantages include increased expense, more labor intensive initially, requires knowledge of associated anatomy and repair techniques, external fixators are heavy and cumbersome, and IM pins may decrease intramedullary callus formation. The integrity of nerves, blood vessels, tendons, and joints must be preserved.

External fixators often provide the stabilization necessary in birds that require a complete return of function. Type I fixators, half-pin splints, consist of pins penetrating one skin surface and both cortices of the bone (Fig. 7–8). Connecting bars are placed on one side of the limb. Type II fixators, full-pin splints, consist of pins passing through both skin surfaces and both cortices and connecting bars on both sides of the limb in one plane (Fig. 7–9). Type II fixators are more stable than type I fixators. When type I fixators must be used, as in proximal humerus and femur fractures, the use of positive-profile threaded pins provides

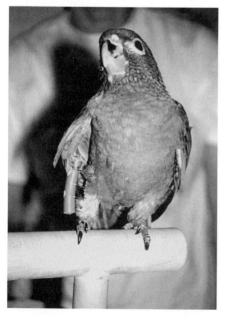

Figure 7–8. An applied type I fixator. (Photo courtesy of Brian L. Speer, DVM, ABVP-avian.)

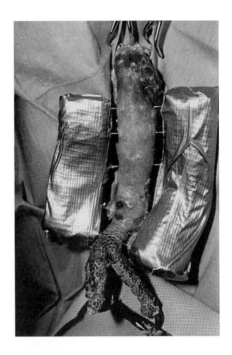

Figure 7–9. An applied type II fixator. (Photo courtesy of Laurel Degernes, DVM, ABVP-avian.)

increased stability. Open, contaminated, and comminuted fractures and corrective osteotomies maintain a better prognosis with external fixator use. External fixators are placed through small skin incisions, not through the primary incision or open wound. Avoid large muscle masses. Pre-drill holes to decrease wobble and increase pin purchase. A minimum of two pins are placed in each bone segment. Place pins perpendicular to the bone with type II fixators, and at 30- to 50-degree angles to the long axis of the bone for type I fixators. Place the most proximal and distal pins through the bone first. Connect the connecting bar to these pins with the interior clamps attached. Use the interior clamps as a drill guide for placement of the remaining stabilizing pins. Polymethylmethacrylate, cast material, or dental acrylic may be used to stabilize the pins to the connecting bar. Bend the tips of the pins parallel to the long axis of the bone to increase stabilization, carefully avoiding force to the fracture site or joints or loosening of the stabilizing pins. Alternatively, stabilizing pins can be placed through a clear plastic tube or straw that is then filled with polymethylmethacrylate. Hypodermic needles can be used as stabilizing pins in small birds. These needles are attached to a stabilizing bar (e.g., toothpick) with cyanoacrylate glue or epoxy. Apply a collar to prevent pin removal by the bird.

Intramedullary pins may be used to neutralize bending forces and provide fracture alignment. Intramedullary pins do not neutralize rotational or shear forces. Do not penetrate articular surfaces. Bones are often too straight to avoid penetration of joints. Joint, tendon, or ligament damage may result in decreased function. Intramedullary pins may impair intramedullary callus formation. Intramedullary pins may be useful for stabilizing some fractures when postsurgical function is not important. Single pins should fill one-half to two-thirds of the medullary cavity. Long bone fractures stabilized with IM pins may require additional immobilization with bandages or splints for 10 to 21 days. A decrease in the range of motion occurs when joints are immobilized along with IM pinning. Polypropylene welding rods and polymethylmethacrylate have been successfully used to stabilize long bone fractures using a shuttle technique (Redig, Howard, and Talbot, 1993; Kuzma and Hunter, 1989; Lind, Gushwa, and Vanek, 1988). The Doyle technique is a combination of intramedullary pinning with external fixation (Martin and Ritchie, 1994).

FRACTURES OR DISLOCATIONS OF THE LEG

Dislocation of the Coxofemoral Joint

Closed reduction is attempted. Open reduction may be required to replace the femoral head in a normal position. Nonabsorbable supporting sutures are placed from the trochanter to the dorsal iliac crest, and from the trochanter to the cranial acetabular rim. A spica splint is applied for further immobilization of the coxofemoral joint for several weeks. Excisional orthoplasty has been successfully used as a salvage procedure for end-stage diseases of the coxofemoral joint.

Fractures of the Femur

Nondisplaced fractures in small birds and waterfowl usually heal with cage rest. Further stability may be accomplished with taping the femur to the body over the synsacrum, then over the open foot, across the abdomen, and up the other side of the body. Intramedullary pins or type I external fixators with or without IM pinning are commonly used for femoral fractures in larger birds. Single or stacked pins are retrograded out the trochanter and normograded into the condyles using a lateral approach. Plates, shuttle pins, or the Doyle method may also be used to stabilize femoral fractures. A poor prognosis is associated with comminuted fractures. Proximal comminuted fractures may respond best to cage rest. Type I fixators alone may be used on distal comminuted fractures. Reinforced Robert Jones bandages may provide the necessary stabilization in simple distal femur fractures in larger birds.

Fractures of the Tibiotarsus

Tape splints may be used in birds up to 200 g. A modified Schroeder-Thomas splint may be used to provide more stabilization of fractures of the distal one-third of the tibiotarsus. Type II external fixators are used on the lateral and medial aspects of the leg to stabilize metaphyseal fractures. Intramedullary pins may be used in conjunction with other methods of stabilization in closed fractures. Pins are normograded out the hock and retrograded into the proximal tibiotarsus, or placed exiting the stifle, using a medial approach. Also, the pin may be introduced from the tibial crest and normograded down the proximal and then distal segments. Plates may be used in midshaft closed fractures.

Comminuted or contaminated fractures are immobilized with type II external fixators.

Fractures of the Tarsometatarsus

A tape splint or Robert Jones bandage combined with a ball bandage is useful in immobilizing fractures of the tarsometatarsus in birds smaller than 500 g. A modified Schroeder-Thomas splint may be used in larger birds. Type II external fixators (medial and lateral orientation) generally work well for this area. If IM pins must be used, they are introduced through the fracture into the proximal segment and retrograded out the proximal condyle, then normograded into the distal segment, using a lateral approach. Contaminated fractures are repaired with external fixators.

Fractures of the Toes

Fractures of the toes may be immobilized by taping two toes together, a ball bandage, reinforced padded splints, splinting the entire foot with a padded molded reinforcement on the plantar surface, or external fixators.

FRACTURES OR DISLOCATION OF THE WING

Fractures of the Coracoid, Clavicle, or Scapula

Minimally displaced fractures may be stabilized by a wing-body wrap. Markedly displaced coracoid fractures may require IM pinning (Howard and Redig, 1993; Orosz, Ensley, and Haynes, 1992; Ritchie, Harrison, and Harrison, 1994).

Fractures of the Humerus

External fixators combined with shuttle pins or IM pins are used in birds where a return to normal function is required (e.g., wild birds intended for release). Polymethylmethacrylate bone cement may increase stability of the fracture site. Most simple proximal and distal fractures of the humerus in other birds respond well to applying both a figure-of-eight bandage and wing-body wrap. Midshaft fractures of the humerus are usually displaced and require surgical repair. Intramedullary pins or type I external fixators with or without IM pins may be used to stabilize the fracture site. The connecting bar is placed on the dorsolateral aspect of the humerus. External fixators are used with contaminated fractures of the humerus.

Dislocations of the Elbow

Acute luxations are nonsurgically reduced, and the joint is immobilized with a figure-of-eight bandage for 7 to 10 days.

Fractures of the Ulna and Radius

When a full return of function is required, IM pins or external fixators are used to repair all but minimally displaced radial fractures. Full return of function may not be achieved, but this technique is most likely to achieve the needed results. In birds in which a complete return of function is not important, most closed radial or ulnar fractures heal with a figure-of-eight bandage. Some loss of range of motion of the elbow and carpus is likely to occur. When both the ulna and radius are fractured, IM pins or external fixators are optimal to stabilize the fracture site. Type II external fixators, IM pins, shuttle pins, plates, or a combination of these methods may be used with closed fractures. A figure-of-eight bandage may be required for further stability postsurgically, but a decrease in the range of motion of the elbow and carpus can be expected.

Fractures of the Carpometacarpus

Most closed minimally displaced fractures of the carpometacarpus heal with a figure-of-eight bandage. Small, lightweight external fixators and IM pins may be used for increased stabilization. If IM pins are used, they are placed through the fracture site and normograded distally, then retrograded proximally into the proximal fragment, taking care to not penetrate the carpal joint. Open or contaminated fractures are stabilized with external fixators.

SPLINTS AND BANDAGES

Bandages and splints are used in the management of some fracture repairs, dislocations, soft tissue trauma, and after some surgical repairs of fractures. Anesthesia is required during the application of the bandage or splint. Splints are well padded with soft, nonadhesive materials. Wire, wood, plastic, or lightweight cast material may be used to reinforce splints. Self-adherent bandage materials (e.g., Vetwrap) is used for the outer layer (see Table 7–1).

Bandages for stabilization of fractures are usually left on for 3 to 5 weeks. Prolonged bandaging can cause joint stiffness, muscle atrophy, bony changes, and occasionally sloughed flight feathers. Weekly bandage changes with controlled physical therapy under anesthesia will help maintain joint mobility. Physical therapy consists of careful flexion and extension of bandaged joints.

Tape Splint

The feathers are plucked from the site of the bandage. Position the leg in a normal position and apply porous bandage tape or masking tape to each side of the leg. Incorporate the joint above and below the fracture. Use hemostats to compress the tape for a tight fit. Multiple layers of tape can be applied to increase support (Fig. 7–10). Tissue glue may be applied to the tape for added support. Malleable foam-covered splinting material (e.g., SAM Splint) may be incorporated into the splint (see Table 7–1).

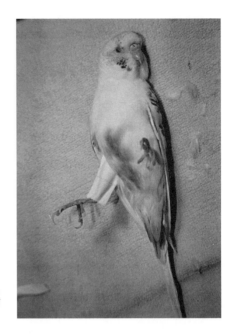

Figure 7–10. An applied tape splint on a budgie with a fractured tibiotarsus. (Photo courtesy of Brian L. Speer, DVM, ABVP-avian.)

Robert Jones Splint

Cast padding is wrapped from the top of the foot to the proximal thigh. A layer of conforming gauze is applied over the padding with leg slightly flexed. Additional splinting material is added if further reinforcement is needed, and then tape or self-adherent bandaging material is used to cover the bandage. Malleable foam-covered splinting material (e.g., SAM Splint) may be incorporated into the splint for added support (see Table 7–1). Monitor the toes for swelling or discoloration, which indicates the need to remove the bandage.

Modified Schroeder-Thomas Splint

Wire is used to mold a splint that positions the leg with slight flexion at the hock joint and is slightly longer than the leg with the toes extended. The wires are bent away from the body, then ventrally, just distal to the loop, so that the leg is held in a normal position (Fig. 7–11,A). A light bandage of gauze and tape is applied to the leg, and the wire splint is placed on the leg (Fig. 7–11,B). The leg is suspended within the splint by alternating taping the leg to the cranial and caudal aspects of the splint (Fig. 7–11,C). The splint is then covered with a self-adherent bandaging material (Fig. 7–11,D).

Spica Splint

The splint is molded to extend from the foot, up the leg, over the lateral thigh, and over the synsacrum (Fig. 7–12,A). The splint can be formed with orthopedic cast material or other lightweight material. Heavy padding is applied

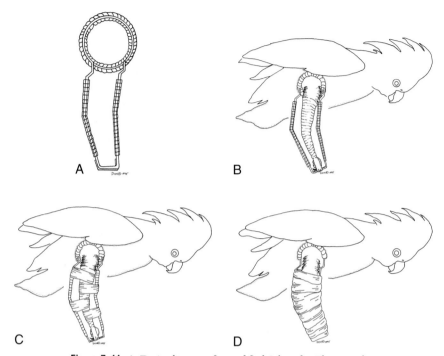

Figure 7–11. A–D, Application of a modified Schroeder-Thomas splint.

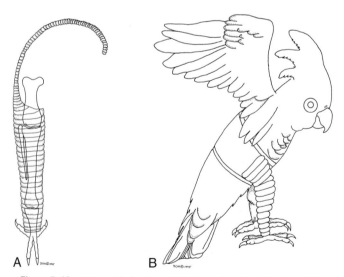

Figure 7–12. A, A molded spica splint. **B,** Application of a spica splint.

around the leg and over the hip to prevent pressure necrosis, and the splint is applied with self-adherent bandaging material (Fig. 7–12,B). Do not restrict respiration or block the vent (Fig. 7–13).

Figure-of-Eight Bandage

The wing is folded in a normal position (Fig. 7–14,A). Rolled cotton padding or gauze is applied in a figure-of-eight fashion, wrapping the gauze around the caudal humerus at the axilla, cranially and laterally over the lateral proximal carpometacarpus, ventrally and medially toward the shoulder, and over the lateral distal carpometacarpus, and under the wing to the axilla (Fig. 7–14,B). Repeat as needed for support. The cotton or gauze bandage is covered with a self-adhesive bandage. When a figure-of-eight bandage is applied correctly, the wing is held in a normal position and is symmetrical to the normal wing. The feathers of the wing remain uncrossed, and the primary feathers remain lateral to the secondary feathers.

Wing Body Wrap

The figure-of-eight bandaged wing is adhered to the body with a self-adhering tape in a normal flexed position. The body wrap is applied halfway between the cranial and caudal edges of the keel. The legs are extended while the tape is applied (Fig. 7–15, A and B). The wrap is applied tight enough to prevent wing motion but not compromise respiration. Do not cover the vent.

Ball Bandage

Gauze sponges are stacked and placed in the grasp of the foot, and the foot and distal tarsometatarsus is wrapped with conforming gauze (Fig. 7–16). An outer layer of tape or self-adherent bandaging material is applied.

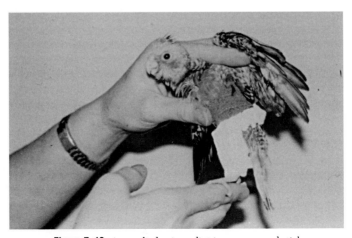

Figure 7–13. An applied spica splint in a young cockatiel.

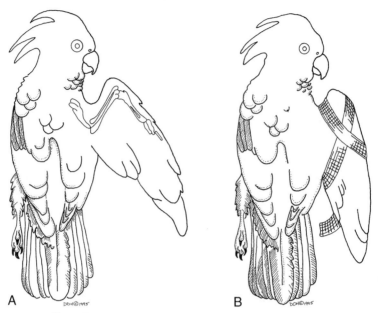

Figure 7–14. A and **B,** Application of a figure-of-eight bandage.

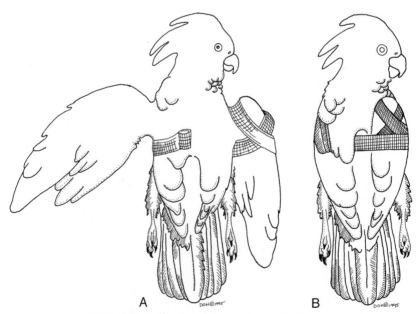

Figure 7–15. A and **B,** Application of a wing body wrap.

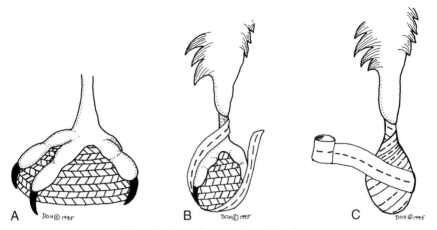

Figure 7–16. Application of a ball bandage.

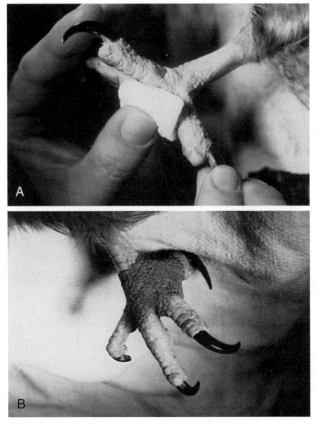

Figure 7–17. A and **B,** An interdigitating bandage. (Photo courtesy of Jonathan X. Di Cesare.)

Interdigitating Bandage

Gauze is placed on the metatarsal pad and is held in place with cotton padding. The bandage is then covered with self-adherent bandaging material (Fig. 7–17).

References and Additional Reading

Ackermann J, Porter S. Femoral head ostectomy in a red-shouldered hawk (*Buteo lineatus*). *J Avian Med Surg* 1995;9(2):127–130.

Altman R. Fractures of the extremities of birds. In Kirk RW (ed): *Current Veterinary Therapy VI*. Philadelphia, WB Saunders, 1977.

Bauck L. Nutritional problems in pet birds. *Semin Avian Exot Pet Med* 1995;4(1):3–14.

Bennett RA. Bandaging techniques in birds. *Proc N Am Vet Conf Proc* 1993;703–704.

Bennett RA. Orthopedic surgery. In Altman RB, Clubb SL, Dorrestein GM, Quesenberry K (eds): *Avian Medicine and Surgery*. Philadelphia, WB Saunders, 1997, pp 733–766.

Bennett RA. Review of orthopedic surgery. *Proc Assoc Avian Vet* 1995;291–296.

Bennett RA, Kuzma AB. Fracture management in birds. *J Zoo Wild Med* 1992;23(1):5–38.

Bush M. External fixation to repair long bone fractures in larger birds. In Kirk RW (ed): *Current Veterinary Therapy VIII, Small Animal Practice*. Philadelphia, WB Saunders, 1983, pp 630–633.

Campbell TW. Cytology of synovial fluid. In *Avian Hematology and Cytology*, ed 2. Ames, Iowa State University Press, 1995, pp 71–73.

Campbell TW, Rudd RG. Excision arthroplasty in a toco toucan (*Rhamphastos toco toco*) for correction of an osteoarthritis of the right coxofemoral joint. *Proceedings of the First Conference of Zoological and Avian Medicine* 1987; pp 227–278.

Cannon CA. Nonsurgical fracture repair. *Proc Assoc Avian Vet* 1995;491–498.

Clipsham R. Pediatric leg repair. *J Assoc Avian Vet* 1989;3(3):131.

Clipsham R. Noninfectious diseases of pediatric psittacines. *Semin Avian Exot Pet Med* 1992;1(1):22–33.

Clipsham RC. Correction of pediatric leg disorders. *Proc Assoc Avian Vet* 1991;200–204.

Cooney J, Mueller L. Postoperative management of the avian orthopedic patient. *Semin Avian Exot Pet Med* 1994;3(2):100–107.

Degernes LA. Trauma medicine. In Ritchie BW, Harrison GJ, Harrison LR (eds): *Avian Medicine: Principles and Application*. Lake Worth, FL, Wingers Publishing, 1994, pp 417–433.

Ekstrom DD. Avian gout. *Proc Assoc Avian Vet* 1989;130–138.

Flammer K. Pediatric medicine of psittacine birds. In *Avian Medicine*. TG Hungerford Refresher Course for Veterinarians, Proc 178, Sydney, Australia, 1991, pp 421–428.

Greenacre CB, Aron DN, Ritchie BW. Dome osteotomy for successful correction of angular limb deformities. *Proc Assoc Avian Vet* 1994;39–43.

Hess RE. Management of orthopedic problems of the avian pelvic limb. *Semin Avian Exot Pet Med* 1994;3(2):63–72.

Howard DJ, Redig PT. Analysis of avian fracture repairs: Implications for captive and wild birds. *Proc Assoc Avian Vet* 1993;78–82.

Howard DJ, Redig PT. Orthopedics of the wing. *Semin Avian Exot Pet Med* 1994;3(2):51–62.

King AS, McLelland J. Skeletomuscular system. In *Birds: Their Structure and Function*, ed 2. London, Bailliere Tindall, 1984, pp 43–78.

Kostka V, Drautwald ME, Tellhelm B, et al. A contribution to radiologic examination of bone alterations in psittacines, birds of prey and pigeons. *Proc Assoc Avian Vet* 1988;37–59.

Kuzma AB, Hunter B. Avian fracture repair using intramedullary bone cement and plate fixation. *Proc Assoc Avian Vet* 1989;177–181.

Lind PJ, Degernes LA, Olson DE, et al. Bone cement/polypropylene rod orthopedic technique. *J Assoc Avian Vet* 1989;3(4):203–205.

Lind PJ, Gushwa DA, Vanek JA. Fracture repair in two owls using polypropylene rods and acrylic bone cement. *AAV Today* 1988;2(3):128–132.

Martin HD, Bruecker KA, Remple JD, et al. Elbow luxations in raptors: A review of eight cases. In Redig PT, Cooper JE, Remple JD, Homer DB (eds): *Raptor Biomedicine.* Minneapolis, University of Minnesota Press, 1993.

Martin HD, Kabler R, Sealing L. The avian coxofemoral joint, a review of regional anatomy and report of an open-reduction technique for repair of a coxofemoral luxation. *J Assoc Avian Vet* 1989;1(1):22–30.

Martin H, Ritchie BW. Orthopedic surgical techniques. In Ritchie BW, Harrison GJ, Harrison LR (eds): *Avian Medicine: Principles and Application.* Lake Worth, FL, Wingers Publishing, 1994, pp 1137–1169.

McCluggage DM. Applications of splints, bandages, and collars. In Kirk RW, Bonagura JD (eds): *Current Veterinary Therapy XI, Small Animal Practice.* Philadelphia, WB Saunders, 1992, pp 1163–1170.

MacCoy DM. Excision arthroplasty for management of coxofemoral luxations in pet birds. *J Am Vet Med Assoc* 1989;194(1):95–97.

Meij BP, Hazewinkel HAW, Westerhof I. Treatment of fractures and angular limb deformities of the tibiotarsus in birds by type II external skeletal fixation. *J Avian Med Surg* 1996;10(3):153–162.

Orosz SE. Surgical anatomy of the avian carpometacarpus. *J Assoc Avian Vet* 1994;8(4):179–183.

Orosz SE, Ensley PK, Haynes CJ. *Avian Surgical Anatomy, Thoracic and Pelvic Limbs.* Philadelphia, WB Saunders, 1992.

Parrott T. Pododermatitis in three Amazon parrots, and treatment with l-thyroxine. *Proc Assoc Avian Vet* 1991;263–264.

Porter SL. Vehicular trauma in owls. *Proc Assoc Avian Vet* 1990;164–170.

Redig PT. Basic orthopedic surgical techniques. In Harrison GJ, Harrison LR (eds): *Clinical Avian Medicine and Surgery.* Philadelphia, WB Saunders, 1986, pp 596–598.

Redig PT. Evaluation and nonsurgical management of fractures. In Harrison GJ, Harrison LR (eds): *Clinical Avian Medicine and Surgery.* Philadelphia, WB Saunders, 1986, pp 380–394.

Redig PT, Brown PA, Gordon JJ. Classification of fractures of avian long bones. *Proc Assoc Avian Vet* 1996; 33–38.

Redig PT, Howard D, Talbot B. Of pins, wires, bone cement and hexacelite for the repair of avian fractures. *Proc Assoc Avian Vet Pract Labs* 1993;45–50.

Ritchie BW, Harrison GJ, Harrison LR (eds): *Avian Medicine: Principles and Application.* Lake Worth, FL, Wingers Publishing, 1994.

Rosenthal K, Hillyer E, Mathiessen D. Stifle luxation repair in a Moluccan cockatoo and a barn owl. *J Assoc Avian Vet* 1992;6(4):235–238 and 1994;8(4):173–178.

Rupiper DJ. Application of visible light curing composite splints to fractured avian legs. *J Assoc Avian Vet* 1993;7(3):147–149.

Tanzella DJ. Ulnar ostectomy in a pale-headed rosella (*Platycercus adscitus*) with multiple injuries. *J Assoc Avian Vet* 1993;7(3):153–155.

Wheler CL, Machin KL, Lew LJ. Use of antibiotic-impregnated polymethylmethacrylate beads in the treatment of chronic osteomyelitis and cellulitis in a juvenile bald eagle (*Haliaeetus leucocephalus*). *Proc Assoc Avian Vet* 1996; 187–194.

Woltmon JR. The use of cerclage wire for immobilization of the metacarpal-phalangeal joint after tenectomy and arthrodesis. *Proc Assoc Avian Vet* 1992;221–222.

Yeisley CL. Surgical correction of valgus carpal deformities in waterfowl. *Proc Assoc Avian Vet* 1993;161–163.

Chapter 8

Dermatologic Signs

Skin, feather, beak, and feet lesions are fairly common in pet birds. Both local and systemic diseases may cause abnormalities of the integument. Nutritional and environmental factors may also affect these structures.

Abnormalities of the skin, feathers, beak, and feet include any irregularity in the color, shape, or contour of the area. Skin lesions include erythema, edema, ulceration, thickening, bleeding, exudation, laceration, hyperkeratosis, and masses. Abnormalities of the feathers include broken, malformed, dirty, missing, abnormally colored feathers, stress marks, or feather picking. Abnormalities of the beak include overgrown upper or lower beak, overgrown side of the beak, crossed upper and lower beaks (scissors beak), shortened upper beak, and areas of swelling, grooves, or necrosis. Feet abnormalities include swelling, erythema, ulceration, thickening, constrictions, masses, or other proliferative lesions.

This chapter presents a diagnostic approach for dermatologic signs commonly seen in pet birds. The chapter is divided into common clinical signs. Each section begins with general information and definitions of terms, followed by a list of differential diagnoses. This is followed by appropriate signalment information. Common causes of the clinical sign are presented for each group of pet birds. The history section explores important historical information. The physical examination section guides interpretation of the physical findings. An algorithm is included in each section to provide a quick reference for recommended tests. The diagnostic plan suggests useful tests. Consult Chapter 12 as needed for techniques of sample collection and for assistance with test interpretation. Once a diagnosis is made, general treatments conclude each sign. Treatments of specific diseases are discussed in Chapter 9. Consult the formulary in Chapter 17 for drug dosages. Neurologic and musculoskeletal problems of the feet are discussed in Chapters 6 and 7.

SKIN LESIONS

Avian skin consists of the epidermis, dermis, and subcutaneous tissue. It is thin and delicate and lacks glands except for the uropygial gland and glands around the eyes, ears, and vent. The uropygial gland is absent in many pigeons, Amazon parrots, and some other psittacines. It is located dorsally at the base of the tail. Secretions from the uropygial gland are spread over the feathers during preening, keeping the feathers, beak, and scales waterproof and supple. The secretions may also suppress the growth of microorganisms. The uropygial gland can be affected by abscesses, impaction, and neoplasia.

Abnormalities of the skin include erythema, edema, ulceration, thickening, bleeding, exudation, laceration, hyperkeratosis, and masses. Skin lesions involving the feet will be discussed later in this chapter.

Differential Diagnoses for Skin Lesions

1. Infectious
   a. Bacterial: °gram-negative, °gram-positive (*Mycobacterium, Staphyloccus, Streptococcus, Pseudomonas,* other)
   b. Viral: herpesvirus, Marek's disease, °polyomavirus, °poxvirus
   c. Fungal: °*Aspergillus, Candida,* dermatophytes
   d. Parasitic: *Giardia,* lice, °mites (feather, *Knemidokoptes, Dermanyssus,* other)
2. Metabolic: liver disease, nephritis, diabetes mellitus
3. Nutritional: general malnutrition, deficiency (°vitamin A, vitamin E/selenium, biotin, pantothenic acid, riboflavin, zinc)
4. Toxic: cleaning solutions, trichotecene, chemical irritation
5. Physical: °crop burn, °feather cyst, °trauma, frostbite, °leg-band necrosis, subcutaneous foreign body, bee sting, insect bite (fly, mosquito, gnat, flea), tumor (°lipoma, xanthoma, papilloma, folliculoma)
6. Trauma: °hematoma, °laceration, °animal bite, burn, °cagemate bite, °self-mutilation
7. Allergic: food, other
8. °Behavioral
9. Neoplastic
10. Endocrine: hypothyroid, other
11. Genetic: °feather cysts

Signalment

Common causes of skin lesions in large psittacines include general malnutrition, vitamin A deficiency, bacterial infections, crop burns, trauma, polyomavirus, poxvirus, and behavioral and psychotic causes. Small psittacines are commonly affected by *Knemidokoptes,* lipomas, trauma, general malnutrition, vitamin A deficiency, animal bites, polyomavirus, and bacterial infections. Common causes in passerines include feather cysts, poxvirus, *Knemidokoptes* mites, malnutrition, and bacterial infections. Skin lesions in raptors are commonly the result of malnutrition, bacterial infections, poxvirus, or trauma. Poxvirus, bacterial infections, and neoplasia are common in pigeons and doves.

Common causes of skin lesions in young birds include nutritional deficiencies, trauma, crop burns, bacterial infections, polyomavirus, and poxvirus.

Polyomavirus affects psittacines. Herpesvirus causes skin problems in cockatoos and Mallard ducks. *Knemidokoptes* mites are primarily a problem in budgies, cockatiels, canaries, and finches, but other birds can be affected. *Giardia* can

---

°Common causes.

cause dry skin and feather picking in cockatiels and budgies. Feather cysts are common in canaries, but they also occur in other birds.

History

Isolated birds and those in collections with no recently added new birds are commonly ill because of nutritional deficiencies, trauma, neoplasia, toxicoses, genetic, metabolic, allergic, and management-related problems (faulty hand-feeding practices, leg-band necrosis, exposure to irritants). Bacterial infections are common. Chronic bacterial, viral, and parasitic infections (mycobacteriosis, polyomavirus, aspergillosis, *Giardia, Knemidokoptes* mites) are also seen.

Birds recently exposed to other birds are commonly ill as a result of infectious diseases, including bacterial, viral, and parasitic diseases. This is the result of stress and exposure to infectious disease. Polyomavirus, poxvirus, mycobacteriosis, bacterial infections, and many parasitic diseases are common in flock environments. Illnesses that occur in isolated birds also occur in those in flock environments.

Infectious and toxic etiologies are suspected when multiple birds are affected.

Significant dietary history includes type of diet, freshness, and vitamin supplementation. Seed diets are high in fat and may be deficient in vitamin E and selenium. Vitamin A deficiency and lipomas are common in birds on an all-seed diet. Birds on high-fat diets are more likely to show signs of vitamin E deficiency than are birds on diets low in fat. Biotin, pantothenic acid, riboflavin, and zinc are rare deficiencies in pet birds.

Baby birds being hand fed are susceptible to crop burns.

Grains heavily damaged by insects are more likely to contain trichothecene.

Liver-associated dermatopathy can be the result of poor diet. Hepatic lipidosis, mycotoxicosis, and hemochromatosis may cause picking at the skin.

Important environmental factors include exposure to infectious diseases, changes in the environment, access to potential toxins, flight capabilities, management practices, sanitation, and exposure to wild birds or disease vectors. Ask what type of cleaner is used to clean the cage. Animal bites are common.

The duration of the illness is important. Note the owner's description of the clinical signs and the course of the disease. Note previous illnesses, including signs, treatment, and response to treatment.

Physical Examination

A complete physical examination is important to identify the extent of the problem and to identify involvement of other body systems. Observe for trauma, abdominal swelling, feather abnormalities, respiratory signs, and neurologic signs. If abnormalities are present, consult appropriate chapters to assist in making a diagnosis. Common findings of birds with skin lesions are discussed below.

Inspect the cage. Note the diet, character of the droppings, and evidence of bleeding or vomiting.

When birds are molting, the feather sheath is preened off the developing feather, producing white flakes. This is normal.

Erythema of the skin without ulceration or swelling can be the result of contact dermatitis, trauma, early crop burn, dermatophytes, ectoparasites, or burns.

Crop burns may be noted as skin lesions just cranial to the thoracic inlet. Erythema or edema of the area over the affected portion of the crop is usually the first sign. The feathers over the burn often fall out. The skin becomes leathery and black with time (see Fig. 4–3). The necrotic tissue may slough, and food and fluid may leak onto the chest.

Ulcerative skin lesions may be the result of bacterial infection, mycobacteriosis, trauma, severe burns, leg-band necrosis, foreign body, vitamin E/selenium deficiency, or exposure to toxins. Tumors, hernias, diabetes, nephritis, hepatitis, and giardiasis may result in ulcerative lesions.

Proliferative lesions may be the result of vitamin A deficiency, poxvirus infection, papillomas, *Knemidokoptes* mites, *Myialges* mites, foreign body, mycobacteriosis, feather cyst, neoplasia, or benign tumor. *Knemidokoptes* infection results in characteristic crusty, honeycombed proliferations around the beak, cere, eyes, or vent, or on the feet and legs. *Myialges* mites may cause crusting and flaking, usually on the top of the head.

Cutaneous and subcutaneous lumps may be caused by tumors, insect bites, mycobacteriosis, bacterial infection, foreign body, feather cyst, xanthoma, bone deformities, fractures, or uropygial gland abscess, tumor, or impaction.

Edema may occur with septicemia, insect bites, leg-band necrosis, irritation, vitamin E/selenium deficiency, liver disease, or Marek's disease.

Pruritus may be caused by ectoparasites, liver disease, or allergy.

Subcutaneous hemorrhages may be seen with polyomavirus, trauma, and septicemia.

Neurologic signs may accompany skin lesions with polyomavirus, Marek's disease, trauma, vitamin E/selenium deficiency, and liver disease.

Gastrointestinal signs such as diarrhea, regurgitation, delayed crop emptying, or polyuria may be noted in conjunction with skin lesions with polyomavirus, liver disease, poxvirus, giardiasis, crop burns, food allergy, malnutrition, vitamin A deficiency, diabetes, nephritis, and trichothecene exposure.

Respiratory signs may accompany skin lesions with polyomavirus, poxvirus, mycobacteriosis, aspergillosis, lipomas, trauma, animal bites, liver disease, malnutrition, and vitamin A deficiency.

Algorithm for Skin Lesions

See Figure 8–1.

Diagnostic Plan for Skin Lesions

Provide supportive care as needed during the diagnostic evaluation (see Chapter 1).

Dietary causes must be sought from the history. Malnutrition and nutritional deficiencies are common in birds with skin problems. Correct the diet while exploring other possible etiologies.

Perform a fecal examination and direct smear for intestinal parasites. Use

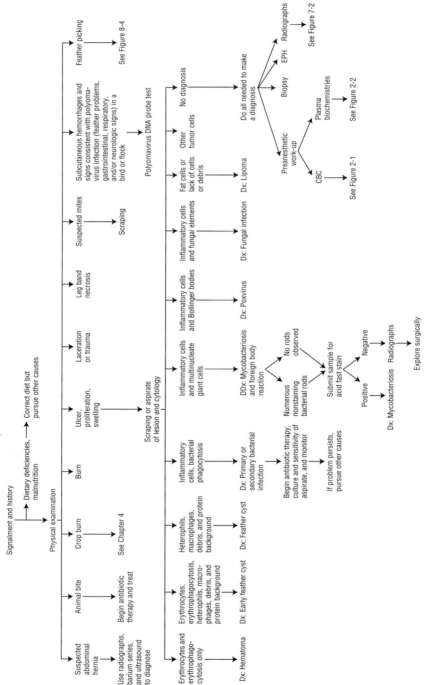

Figure 8-1. Algorithm for skin lesions.

fresh feces to observe for the motile trophozoite of *Giardia*. If the bird is a cockatiel or budgie and there are the typical clinical signs associated with giardiasis (feather pulling with screaming), a pooled fecal sample is submitted for a trichrome stain or an enzyme-linked immunosorbent assay (ELISA) antigen test. A trial treatment for this parasite may provide a presumptive diagnosis.

Lacerations, trauma, leg-band necrosis, crop burns, other burns, exposure to toxins, and animal bites can be diagnosed with history and physical examination findings. Hernias are suspected based on physical examination findings. Typical feather cysts and *Knemidokoptes* infections can usually be recognized also. A scraping of the honeycomb proliferations will reveal the mites for the diagnosis of *Knemidokoptes* (see Fig. 12–26). Scrapings of crusts on the top of the head may reveal *Myialges* mites, if present.

Ulcers, proliferations, and swellings can be scraped or aspirated. Gram's stain is used to identify bacteria and candidiasis. Wright's stain is used for cytologic evaluation. Erythrocytes, possibly with erythrophagocytosis, are indicative of a hematoma. Early feather cysts may also contain erythrocytes and erythrophago-cytosis. Debris, heterophils, macrophages, and a protein (blue) background will also be present in aspirates from feather cysts. Heterophils, bacteria, and macrophages indicate a bacterial or foreign body origin. Bacterial infections may be primary or secondary. Imprints or scrapings of xanthomas contain highly vacuolated macrophages, multinucleated giant cells, and cholesterol crystals. These crystals may dissolve in the fixative of some stains such as Diff-Quik. Bollinger bodies (large eosinophilic intracytoplasmic inclusion bodies) may be seen with poxvirus infection. *Aspergillus* is characterized by septate hyphae that branch. Hyphae may stain poorly or basophilic with Wright's or Diff-Quik stain. *Mycobacterium* bacteria may be observed as bacterial rods that fail to stain with Wright's or Diff-Quik stain; acid-fast staining is required to demonstrate the organism. The presence of fat cells or lack of cells or debris is consistent with a diagnosis of lipoma. Tumor cells may be identified.

Submit a sample for culture with suspected bacterial infections. The best sample for cultures is an aspirate after surgical preparation (scrub) and drying. Small numbers of *Streptococcus* and *Staphylococcus* may be normal.

Biopsy lesions of uncertain etiology. Granulomas, poxvirus lesions, fungal lesions, papillomas, and other benign and malignant tumors may be identified with histopathology.

If a diagnosis cannot be made based on cytology, hematology and plasma biochemistry tests are the next step if these tests have not been performed prior to anesthesia for biopsy sample collection. A CBC (complete blood count) is useful in supporting infectious and inflammatory diagnoses. If the white blood cell (WBC) count is in excess of $40,000/\mu l$, rule out mycobacteriosis and aspergillosis with cytology, biopsy, EPH, serology, and acid-fast staining.

Plasma biochemistries are important in the diagnosis of metabolic diseases. Important biochemistry tests for birds with skin lesions include aspartate aminotransferase (AST), uric acid, albumin, total protein, and glucose. Lactate dehydrogenase (LDH), creatine kinase (CK), and bile acids may also be useful to evaluate the liver. Hepatitis may cause an increase in AST, LDH, and bile acids. Elevation of uric acid levels may occur with kidney disease or dehydration. Moderate increases in glucose are consistent with diabetes.

Radiology may be necessary to diagnose abdominal hernias. Radiology also allows evaluation of liver and kidney size and other celomic structures.

If polyomavirus is suspected based on clinical signs or flock involvement, a DNA probe for polyomavirus is performed.

Thyroid hormone level and a thyroid stimulation test are performed if hypothyroidism is suspected based on clinical signs (obesity, lack of feather regrowth, lack of molting).

Self-mutilation may be the result of an underlying problem. Psychogenic self-mutilation is diagnosed when other causes are ruled out.

Treatment for Skin Lesions

Treat the underlying cause. Correct any dietary problems. Administer parenteral multivitamins and trace minerals if the bird is not eating a commercial pelleted diet. Place the bird on a pelleted diet supplemented with fruits and vegetables.

Base selection of antibiotics on sensitivity results.

A collar or a bandage may be used temporarily if needed to prevent chewing and further destruction of the affected site. Treatment of self-mutilation may include temporary collaring and treatments used for feather picking.

Animal bites and suspected animal bites are treated immediately with systemic antibiotics. Penicillins (e.g., piperacillin) are the antibiotics of choice. Septicemia develops rapidly if left untreated. Clean, debride, and flush wounds. Do not close puncture wounds. Large wounds may require partial closure.

Lipomas and xanthomas may respond to correction of the diet. Surgically remove and debride granulomas, tumors, cysts, and foreign bodies.

FEATHER LOSS, FEATHER PICKING, OR FEATHER ABNORMALITIES

The feathers of birds provide insulation, waterproofing, and flight capabilities. They grow in tracts (pterylae) with featherless areas between tracts (apteria). These featherless areas appear as bare skin and are normal. Feathers grow from follicles similar to hair follicles.

Birds may molt continuously or two to three times per year. Molting is influenced by light exposure and controlled by hormones. During molting, birds preen more to remove the feather shaft from the newly erupted feather. White flaking associated with this feather shaft material is normal. Growing feathers contain a vascular shaft that appears dark.

Abnormalities of the feathers include broken, malformed, dirty, missing, or abnormally colored feathers or stress marks. Stress marks are translucent or dark lines across the feather. The normal feather is smooth and flat, with unfrayed edges.

It is important to determine if a feather abnormality occurs during development or if it was injured after normal growth. To determine when the abnormality is occurring, an abnormal feather may be pulled. The pulled feather is used for diagnostic tests (see below). Observe regrowth of the new feather during the subsequent 3 weeks. If the feather does not regrow, a systemic or follicular abnormality is suspected. If the feather regrows but is abnormal, a follicular, metabolic, or systemic problem is suspected. If the feather regrows normally, self-inflicted or cagemate-inflicted injury or cage trauma is suspected.

Feather picking and self-mutilation are common problems in pet birds and require diagnostic tests to determine the etiology. A diagnosis is extremely important for treatment to be effective. Behavioral or psychotic feather pickers are difficult to treat effectively.

Differential Diagnoses for Feather Loss, Feather Picking, or Feather Abnormalities

1. Infectious
   a. Bacterial: °gram-negative, °gram-positive (*Mycobacterium, Staphyloccus, Streptococcus, Pseudomonas,* other)
   b. Viral: adenovirus, herpesvirus, parvovirus-like virus, °polyomavirus, °psittacine beak and feather disease (PBFD)
   c. Fungal: *Aspergillus, Candida,* dermatophytes, other
   d. Parasitic: ascarids, °cestodes (tapeworms), °*Giardia,* lice, °mites (*Knemidokoptes, Myialges,* other)
   e. Chlamydial
2. Metabolic: liver disease, nephritis, airsacculitis
3. Nutritional: °general malnutrition, deficiencies (°vitamin A, choline, riboflavin, lysine, folic acid, iron, carotenoids)
4. Toxic: arsenic
5. Physical: °poor wing trim, oil contamination, glue traps, tumor (xanthoma, lipoma, other)
6. Trauma: °broken blood feather, other
7. Allergic: food, cooking fumes, tobacco smoke, contact with conifers
8. Behavioral: °boredom, °frustration, breeding behavior, °stress, °overpreening (self or cagemate), °reproductive frustration, brooding behavior, °attention getting, °psychosis, undesired contact with strangers or family pets, anxiety, lack of sleep
9. Neoplastic
10. Endocrine: hypothyroid, hyperadrenocorticism, °testosterone responsive baldness
11. Genetic: °baldness
12. Environmental: low humidity, crowding, dominance, change, territorial
13. Iatrogenic: praziquantel, fenbendazole

Signalment

Common causes of feather abnormalities, loss, and picking in large psittacines include broken blood feathers, bacterial infection, polyomavirus, PBFD, malnu-

---

°Common causes.

trition, liver disease, boredom, and frustration. Small psittacines commonly have feather problems as a result of malnutrition, broken blood feathers, giardiasis, frustration, feather cysts, polyomavirus, and PBFD. Lutino cockatiels often have a larger-than-normal bare area caudal to the crest on the top of the head that is permanent. Feather abnormalities in passerines are commonly the result of cagemate overpreening, aggression, bacterial infection, malnutrition, male baldness, dermatophytes, and mites. Raptors are often affected by malnutrition and trauma.

Common causes of feather abnormalities in young birds include nutritional diseases (homemade formulas), bacterial infections, and polyomavirus.

Polyomavirus and PBFD affect only psittacines. Signs associated with polyomavirus are most common around weaning age. Although older birds may develop lesions, PBFD usually affects only young birds up to 3 years of age. Adenovirus and parvovirus-like virus cause feather abnormalities in waterfowl. An adenovirus causes a folliculitis in lovebirds. *Giardia* commonly causes feather picking with screaming and flaky skin in cockatiels and budgies.

History

Isolated birds and those in collections with no recently added new birds are commonly ill because of nutritional deficiencies, neoplasia, trauma, and metabolic, behavioral, endocrine, genetic, and management-related problems (too small a cage, low humidity, crowding). Bacterial infections are common. Chronic bacterial, viral, and fungal diseases (mycobacteriosis, PBFD, polyomavirus, aspergillosis) are also seen.

Birds recently exposed to other birds are commonly ill as a result of infectious diseases, including bacterial, viral, and parasitic diseases. This is the result of stress and exposure to infectious disease. Polyomavirus, PBFD, mycobacteriosis, and many parasitic diseases are common in flock environments. Illnesses that occur in isolated birds also occur in individuals in flock environments.

Infectious and toxic etiologies are suspected when multiple birds are affected.

The dietary history may reveal possible problems. Note the type of diet and vitamin supplementation. Poor diets may contribute to liver disease (hepatic lipidosis, hemochromatosis, mycotoxicosis). General malnutrition and vitamin A deficiency from a seed diet may cause feather abnormalities. Abnormal pigmentation of feathers may result from dietary deficiencies of lysine, folic acid, iron, choline, or riboflavin. Lack of bright colors may result from lack of dietary carotenoids.

Important environmental factors include exposure to infectious diseases, change of environment, too small of a cage, access to potential toxins, and management-related practices (humidity, crowding, sanitation).

Iatrogenic causes of feather abnormalities include administration of praziquantel or fenbendazole.

The duration of the illness is important. Note the owner's description of the clinical signs and the course of the disease. Note previous illnesses, including signs, treatment, and response to treatment.

Physical Examination

A complete physical examination is important to identify the extent of the problem and to identify involvement of other body systems. Observe for trauma, abdominal swelling, skin lesions, oropharyngeal lesions, and gastrointestinal, neurologic, and respiratory signs. If abnormalities are present, consult appropriate chapters to assist in making a diagnosis. Areas of feather loss are noted in the record for comparison during subsequent visits. Common findings of birds with feather abnormalities are discussed below.

Determine if there is lack of feather growth, abnormal feather development, or feather destruction.

A lack of feather growth will result in bare areas where feathers should be (feather tracts). Malnutrition-associated feather loss occurs. Lutino cockatiels may be affected by a genetic baldness caudal to the crest. Scarring, with destruction of feather follicles, can result in areas lacking feathers. Some birds may seasonally develop a brood patch, a bare area on the ventral body and lower leg. Feather loss around the eyes may be the result of chronic conjunctivitis and ocular discharge (see Fig. 5–1). An allergic syndrome has been reported in lories and hyacinth macaws of feather loss on the neck associated with contact with conifers. *Knemidokoptes* mites can cause feather loss along with the typical honeycomb lesions around the cere, beak, eyes, and vent, or on the feet. *Myialges* mites can cause feather loss with crusting, usually on the top of the head. If there is lack of feather regrowth or lack of molting, the presence of obesity or lipomas may indicate hypothyroidism. Hypothyroidism may also cause abnormal feather development. Hypothyroidism is rare. An increase in fat deposition may also occur with prolonged corticosteroid administration.

Folliculitis and polyfolliculitis may occur as a result of bacterial or viral disease (PBFD or other disease). Areas lacking feathers occur with later stage PBFD because of inactive follicles. Other feather abnormalities, with or without beak abnormalities, may be present (see below).

Abnormal feather development includes stress marks, bleeding growing feathers, abnormal color, retained sheath, and abnormal shape. Causes include trauma or follicular, metabolic, or systemic problems.

A broken or injured pin feather (growing feather) will bleed profusely from the break in the vascular shaft. This is usually the result of trauma or injury. Developing feathers may also break or bleed because of PBFD or polyomavirus infection.

Stress marks appear as translucent lines perpendicular to the feather shaft. These can be caused by stress, malnutrition, disease, or an injection of corticosteroids during the development of the feather.

Color abnormalities may be the result of nutritional deficiencies, hepatopathy, or PBFD. Abnormally white feathers (achromia) may be the result of choline deficiency in cockatiels or lysine, folic acid, or iron deficiency in fowl. Black discoloration of normally green feathers in Amazon parrots may be caused by a vitamin deficiency or liver disease. Abnormal yellow feathers in Amazon parrots and macaws may occur with nutritional deficiencies or liver disease.

Retained feather sheaths can be the result of PBFD, low humidity (neonates), or a suspected viral infection associated with a polyfolliculitis syndrome in budgies and lovebirds.

Abnormally shaped feathers include any variation from the normal shape of the feather. Malnutrition and trauma are common causes of feather abnormalities. The tail feathers are especially prone to breaking and trauma when the bird is kept in too small of a cage. Hypothyroidism is a rare cause of misshapen feathers. Lipomas and obesity will usually accompany hypothyroidism. Finches and pigeons may develop abnormal feathers after administration of praziquantel or fenbendazole.

Viral-induced feather abnormalities are common. Polyomavirus and PBFD can cause abnormally shaped feathers. Lovebirds and budgies may develop abnormally shaped feathers as a result of a suspected unidentified viral infection.

Polyomavirus causes symmetrical feather abnormalities in young budgies. Less commonly, poor feather formation has been associated with chronic polyomavirus infection in larger psittacines. Feather abnormalities caused by polyomavirus infection include abnormally shaped primary (long distal wing feathers) and tail feathers, lack of down feathers (small, fluffy feathers) on the back and abdomen, and lack of filoplumes (hairlike feathers) on the head and neck. Developing primary and secondary feathers (long proximal wing feathers) may break or fall out, resulting in bleeding. Subcutaneous hemorrhages and neurologic signs may occur. Feather lesions usually resolve after several months in budgies.

Young birds are most often affected by PBFD, but older birds may develop lesions. Lesions are usually symmetrical. The course of the disease can be peracute, acute, or chronic. In the acute presentation, young or fledgling birds have depression and abnormal developing feathers and may show crop stasis and diarrhea. Feather abnormalities include necrosis, fractures, bending, bleeding, and premature shedding of diseased feathers. Chronic infection results in progressive abnormal developing feathers with each molt. Abnormalities include retention of feather sheaths; hemorrhage in the pulp cavity; fracture of the feather where it emerges from the skin; short, clubbed, deformed, curled, circumferential constrictions of the feather shaft; and stress marks. Abnormal feathers usually appear on the flanks and legs first, and then on the head and other parts of the body. The long wing and tail feathers are usually last to become abnormal. In cockatoos, the down feathers are often the first to be affected. The beak may be affected, growing excessively long or containing transverse or longitudinal fractures or areas of necrosis. A shiny beak in cockatoos may be an early sign of infection. Oral ulcers may be present. Nails are occasionally affected by deformities, fractures, necrosis, or sloughing. Lesions of PBFD are progressive.

French molt is used to describe various conditions causing abnormal feather development. Affected birds are often called runners, creepers, or hoppers because they cannot fly. Etiologies include polyomavirus infection, PBFD, parasites, and genetic and environmental influences.

Feather destruction may occur as a result of self-destruction, cagemate picking, or damage from a cage that is too small. Damage from a small cage involves primarily the tail feathers. With cagemate overpreening, the feathers on the head are often involved. Self–feather picking will result in damage or loss of feathers only in areas that the bird is able to reach. The head will have normal feathers.

Cagemates will pick other birds because of boredom, frustration, reproductive frustration, overcrowding, stress, and dominance and to defend their territory. Sick or weak birds may be attacked by other birds in a group environment.

Self–feather picking is a common and frustrating problem in pet birds. Etiologies include infectious (bacterial, viral, fungal, parasitic), metabolic, nutritional, toxic (arsenic), poor wing trim, tumors, neoplasia, sexual frustration, and behavioral causes. Look for involvement of other systems (e.g., diarrhea, polyuria, dyspnea, neurologic signs, and other gastrointestinal signs). Feather picking may become habitual. Picking may continue after the inciting cause is gone. A common time of onset of feather picking in Amazon parrots and African gray parrots is just before sexual maturity, at 1½ to 3 years of age. Amazon parrots and macaws often begin picking the contour feathers of the chest at 5 to 10 years of age (Fig. 8–2). Some cases become severe, and the bird may begin to mutilate the skin (Fig. 8–3). With sexual frustration, courtship behaviors may be present, including feeding, mounting, and masturbation.

Scratching along with feather picking or self-mutilation may indicate pruritus.

Neurologic signs may accompany feather problems with polyomavirus, bacterial, chlamydial, mycobacterial, and fungal infections, liver disease, and kidney disease.

Gastrointestinal signs (e.g., diarrhea, polyuria) may be noted in conjunction with feather abnormalities, feather loss, or feather picking with polyomavirus, bacterial, mycobacterial, fungal, and parasitic infections, PBFD, liver disease, kidney disease, malnutrition, fenbendazole and praziquantel administration, arsenic toxicosis, food allergy, stress, oil contamination, oral lesions, and beak abnormalities.

Ophthalmic signs and feather abnormalities or loss may occur with vitamin A deficiency, *Knemidokoptes,* and hepatopathies.

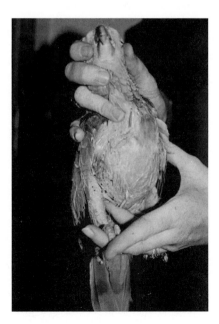

Figure 8–2. The chest is a common site of feather picking, as in this Amazon parrot.

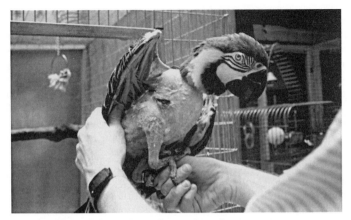

Figure 8–3. Feather picking and mutilation in a macaw.

Respiratory signs may occur with feather abnormalities, loss, or picking with bacterial, chlamydial, mycobacterial, or fungal infections, malnutrition, vitamin A deficiency, airsacculitis, liver disease, kidney disease, and *Knemidokoptes*.

Algorithms for Feather Loss, Feather Picking, or Feather Abnormalities

See Figures 8–4, 8–5, 8–6, and 8–7.

Diagnostic Plan for Feather Problems

A diagnosis of behavioral or psychologically induced mutilation is made only if no etiology can be determined with diagnostic testing.

Poor diet, low humidity, lack of natural sunlight, and a small cage are common causes of feather problems. When behavioral problems are suspected, modify the environment. Correct these conditions while exploring other possible etiologies. A temporary collar can be applied to prevent mutilation in severe cases. Hospitalize the bird initially after applying the collar to observe for self-trauma and injury caused by discomfort of the collar.

Upon initial examination, it may not be evident whether the abnormality is a lack of feather growth, abnormal feathers, or feather destruction. Remove a few abnormal feathers on the initial visit. Use these feathers for initial diagnostic tests and observe the regrowth of these feathers during the next 3 weeks. Examine the feather microscopically for parasites, and perform cytology on the feather pulp. A slide can be made by squashing the proximal end of an affected developing feather between two slides. Examine the slide for bacteria, fungal elements, inflammatory cells, and inclusion bodies. If bacteria or inflammatory cells are present, submit a sample for bacterial or fungal cultures and sensitivity testing. If inclusion bodies are present, submit samples for polyomavirus and

PBFD probe tests. All birds with abnormally shaped feathers without an obvious cause should be tested for polyomavirus and PBFD with DNA probe tests.

If the red mite *(Dermanyssus)* is suspected, the owner can place a white cloth over the cage at night. In the morning, the cloth is inspected for the presence of red mites.

A detailed diagnostic approach is given below for lack of feather growth, abnormal feathers, and feather destruction.

Lack of Feather Growth

History and physical examination is used to diagnose scarring, the presence of a brood patch, chronic ocular discharge, conifer contact allergy, and genetic balding in lutino cockatiels. Malnutrition, *Knemidokoptes,* and endocrine abnormalities are suspected based on physical examination findings. Consider the diet.

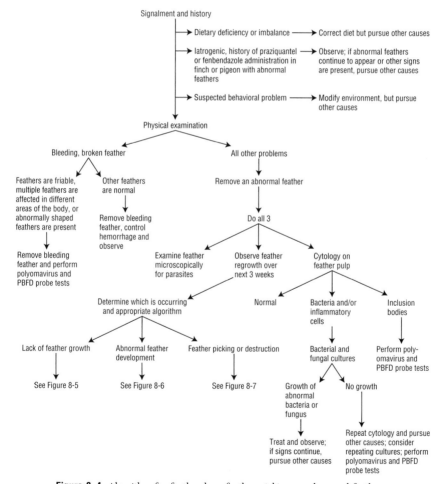

Figure 8–4. Algorithm for feather loss, feather picking, or abnormal feathers.

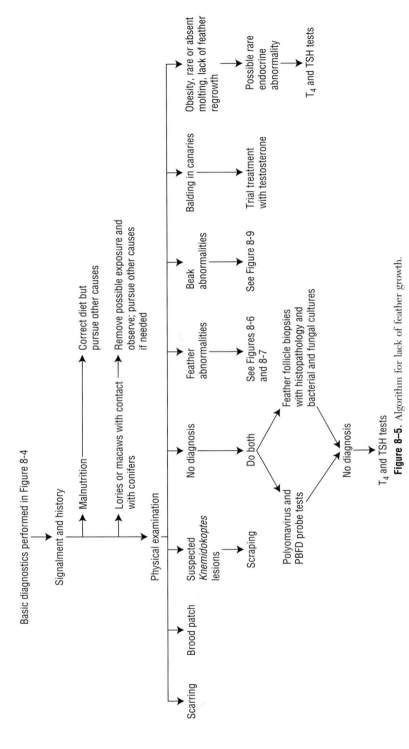

Figure 8–5. Algorithm for lack of feather growth.

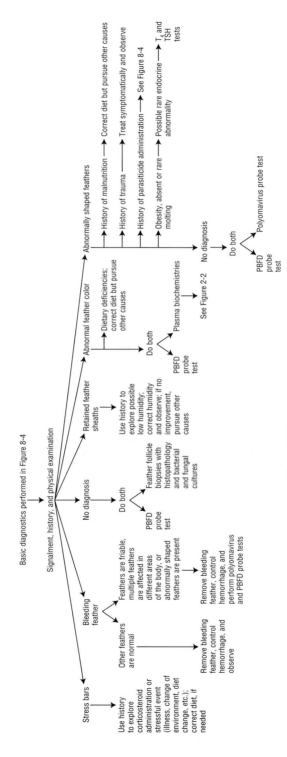

Figure 8–6. Algorithm for abnormal feathers.

241

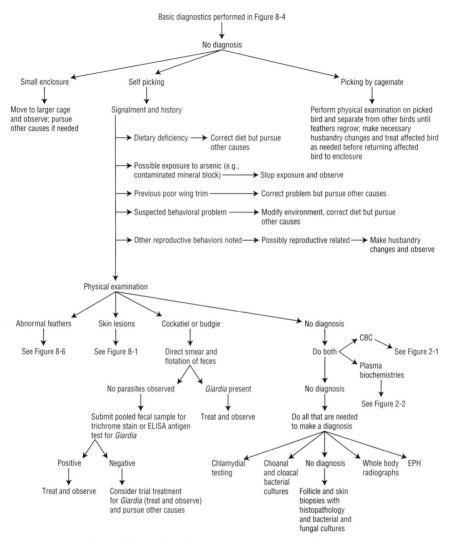

Figure 8–7. Algorithm for feather destruction or feather picking.

Skin scrapings are done for a definitive diagnosis of *Knemidokoptes* presence. Obesity, lipomas, lack of feather regrowth, and lack of molting suggests hypothyroidism. Measurement of thyroxine and thyroid-stimulating hormone (TSH) testing must be performed for a definitive diagnosis. Balding in canaries may respond to a trial of testosterone administration. Adverse effects may result from use of testosterone in birds with liver disease; use caution in these birds.

Birds with viral diseases usually have concurrent feather or beak abnormalities present when areas lacking feathers are found. For definitive diagnosis of PBFD and polyomavirus, DNA probes are available.

Feather follicle biopsy is performed if a diagnosis is not obvious. Folliculitis or polyfolliculitis caused by bacterial or viral diseases (PBFD or other) may be diagnosed histologically. Suspected cases of PBFD or polyomavirus are definitively diagnosed with DNA probe tests.

Abnormal Feather Development

History and physical examination are important in the diagnosis of the etiology of stress bars, bleeding pin feathers, abnormal feather color, and retained feather sheaths. A thorough review of the history may reveal malnutrition, an injection of corticosteroids, previous or current signs of disease, or other stress in a bird with stress bars. No treatment is needed for stress bars, but correct the diet or determine underlying cause.

Bleeding pin feathers may be the result of trauma, polyomavirus, or PBFD. If abnormal feathers are present, submit a sample for DNA probe testing for polyomavirus and PBFD. Bleeding pin feathers must be removed. Wing feathers are commonly affected and are attached to the periosteum. The feather is pulled with forceps while the bone is held firmly to prevent fractures. Pressure applied to the follicle will control hemorrhage. Do not use clotting powders in feather follicles.

Abnormal coloration of feathers may be the result of malnutrition, nutritional deficiencies, hepatopathy, hypothyroidism, or PBFD. Use the history to evaluate the diet. Correct the diet, but pursue other causes. Plasma biochemistries are performed to look for liver disease. Appropriate biochemistries include AST, albumin, total protein, LDH, and CK. If liver disease is suspected based on clinical signs or abnormal plasma biochemistries, analysis of bile acids is performed. Definitive diagnosis of the etiology of liver disease, if present, often requires a liver biopsy. In addition to plasma biochemistries, a PBFD DNA probe is submitted. Thyroxine and TSH tests are performed if hypothyroidism is suspected.

Retained feather sheaths may be the result of low humidity, polyfolliculitis, PBFD, or other virus. Low humidity can be diagnosed historically. Cytology of the feather pulp may reveal an etiologic agent. Examine the slide for bacteria, fungal elements, inflammatory cells, and inclusion bodies. If bacteria or inflammatory cells are present, submit a sample for bacterial culture and sensitivity testing. Other feather abnormalities are usually present if PBFD is the cause, but a DNA probe is performed even when other signs are lacking to rule out the disease.

If a diagnosis is still not apparent, a feather follicle biopsy is taken and submitted for culture and histopathology. Lovebirds and budgies may be affected with a polyfolliculitis that appears with multiple short quills with retained sheaths. This may be caused by PBFD or another agent.

Abnormally shaped feathers may be caused by malnutrition, trauma, hypothyroidism, parasiticide administration, polyomavirus, or PBFD. History and physical examination usually reveal nutritional deficiencies, parasiticide administration (finches and pigeons), and traumatic injuries. Hypothyroidism usually occurs with concurrent obesity, lipomas, and absent or rare molting. Thyroxine and TSH testing is required for a definitive diagnosis of hypothyroidism.

Viral-induced feather abnormalities are common. All birds with abnormally shaped feathers without obvious cause are tested for polyomavirus and PBFD with DNA probe tests.

Lovebirds and budgies may develop abnormally shaped feathers as a result of a suspected unidentified viral infection.

In flock situations, a complete necropsy is important in the control of disease. The best sample to submit for polyomavirus detection on postmortem examination is a swab of the cut surface of the spleen, liver, and kidney (on the same swab).

Feather Destruction or Feather Picking

Feather destruction may be the result of being kept in too small an enclosure, cagemate picking, or self-picking. Broken and dirty tail feathers are usually the result of cage trauma. The tail feathers are broken and frayed from brushing against the sides or bottom of the enclosure. Clinical judgment of adequacy of cage size and observation of the bird in the cage are used to diagnose this problem.

Feather destruction in areas where the bird cannot reach is usually the result of picking by a cagemate. Causes include boredom, frustration, reproductive frustration, territorial, overcrowding, stress, and dominance of the picking cage mate. Sick birds are sometimes picked on by other birds in the enclosure. Perform a thorough physical examination on the picked bird, looking for evidence of illness. Separate the picked bird until feathers regrow. Make necessary husbandry changes before returning the affected bird to the enclosure.

Self-picking is a common problem. Determining the cause and controlling the problem are often frustrating, time consuming, and difficult. Causes of feather picking, from most common to least common, include behavioral, malnutrition, underlying disease, folliculitis, endocrine imbalance, and feather or skin parasites. When behavioral problems are suspected, modify the environment. Make dietary changes as needed. Correct these conditions while exploring other possible etiologies. A temporary collar can be applied to allow feather regrowth, break the cycle, and prevent mutilation. A diagnosis of behavioral feather picking is made only when other causes are ruled out with extensive testing.

History and physical examination are used to diagnose nutritional and toxic (arsenic) causes, tumors, and previous poor wing trims. Reproductive frustration may be the cause when other reproductive behaviors are noted (feeding, mounting, masturbation). Metabolic disease may be suspected based on physical examination findings (biliverdinuria, polyuria, respiratory signs, etc.). Some birds begin to pick when a wing trim leaves frayed edges or rough ends on the feathers. This picking may become a habit, and the bird will continue to overpreen or pick feathers after normal feathers have replaced the previously damaged wing feathers.

Birds may pick feathers over or around cutaneous and subcutaneous tumors. Ulcers, proliferations, and swellings are scraped or aspirated. Wright's stain is used for cytologic evaluation. Erythrocytes, possibly with erythrophagocytosis, are indicative of a hematoma. Early feather cysts may also contain erythrocytes and erythrophagocytosis. Debris, heterophils, macrophages, and a protein (blue) background will also be present in aspirates from feather cysts. Heterophils, bacteria, and macrophages indicate a bacterial or foreign body origin. Bacterial infections may be primary or secondary. Submit a sample for culture with suspected bacterial infections. Small numbers of *Streptococcus* and *Staphylococcus* may be normal. Imprints or scrapings of xanthomas contain highly vacuolated macrophages, multinucleated giant cells, and cholesterol crystals. These crystals may dissolve in the fixative of some stains such as Diff-Quik. Bollinger bodies are large eosinophilic cytoplasmic inclusion bodies that may be seen with poxvirus infection. *Aspergillus* is characterized by septate branching hyphae. Hyphae may stain poorly or basophilic with Wright's or Diff-Quik stain. *Mycobacterium* bacteria may be observed as bacterial rods that fail to stain with Wright's or Diff-Quik stain. Acid-fast staining is required to demonstrate the organism. The presence of fat cells or lack of cells or debris is consistent with a diagnosis of lipoma. Tumor cells may be identified. Cutaneous neoplasms found in birds include fibrosarcoma, lymphosarcoma, and other less common neoplasms. Biopsy lesions of uncertain etiology. Granulomas, poxvirus lesions, fungal lesions, papillomas, and other benign and malignant tumors may be identified with histopathology.

Gram's stain is used to identify bacteria and candidiasis.

Perform a fecal flotation and direct smear to look for parasites, especially in picking cockatiels and budgies. Use fresh feces when looking for *Giardia* trophozoites. Pooled feces may be submitted for trichrome staining or an antigen detection test.

Examine an affected feather microscopically for parasites and perform cytology on the pulp, if not done previously. A slide can be made by squashing the proximal end of a developing feather between two slides. Examine the slide for bacteria, fungal elements, inflammatory cells, and inclusion bodies. Submit a sample of feather pulp for bacterial and fungal cultures.

If a diagnosis is not obvious, a CBC and plasma biochemistries are performed. Electrophoresis can be used to determine if inflammatory disease is present. A CBC is useful for diagnosis of inflammatory or infectious diseases. Useful plasma biochemistries include AST, LDH, CK, uric acid, and total protein. Bile acids are submitted if liver disease is suspected.

Cloacal and choanal bacterial cultures and chlamydial tests are performed if a diagnosis is still not clear.

If abnormal feathers are present, submit viral-specific DNA probes for polyomavirus and PBFD.

Radiology is useful to evaluate organ size and position and to observe for abnormalities not obvious on the physical examination.

If a diagnosis still has not been made, a follicle and skin biopsy is taken. Samples are submitted for histopathology. Electron microscopy may be useful to look for viruses.

If no etiologic agent or other cause can be diagnosed, a behavioral problem may be the cause.

Treatment for Feather Loss, Feather Picking, or Feather Abnormalities

Once a diagnosis is made, treat the underlying cause. Specific treatments are found in Chapter 9.

Control of picking when caused by behavioral problems is difficult. Increased interaction with family members and television or radio noise when left alone may decrease picking. Develop a regular schedule of interaction between the owner and the bird. Planned interaction between the owner and the bird at regular specific times each day may allow the bird to expect scheduled interaction. This will sometimes decrease feather picking. New toys or frequent moving of the cage may cause a decrease or increase in picking. Provide some foods that require an effort to eat (e.g., corn on the cob). Daily misting with water may encourage normal preening. In appropriate climates, moving the cage outside may provide positive stimulation. The addition of another bird may provide companionship and reduce picking. New birds must be quarantined and tested for infectious diseases before introduction into the household. The feather picking bird may teach the new bird to feather pick. If stress is suspected as a cause of picking (e.g., a high-strung bird), provide a quiet environment and a hide box, and partially cover the cage. Cover the cage completely at night.

If increased interaction and stimulation fail, chemotherapeutic agents can be tried. Haloperidol may be effective in some cases. Other drugs that have been reported to be effective in some cases include fluoxetine hydrochloride, naltrexone hydrochloride, thyroxine, hydroxyzine hydrochloride, diphenhydramine, and medroxyprogesterone acetate. Chemotherapeutic agents may have undesirable side effects. As a last resort, a tube or Elizabethan collar may be applied. Hospitalize the bird for 8 to 12 hours to observe the reaction to the collar. Observe for ability to eat, excitability, and listlessness.

Areas of mutilation are cultured, cleaned, and treated sparingly with topical prednisone. The lesion may be sealed with Nexaband (Table 8–1). A collar may be needed to prevent further mutilation.

Treatment of sexual frustration may include decreasing the amount of exposure to light (change the photoperiod), removing the nest box, or pairing with a mate. Pharmacologic agents (medroxyprogesterone acetate) may have serious side effects.

BEAK ABNORMALITIES

The beak consists of the bones of the upper and lower jaws (the premaxilla and nasal above, and the mandible below) and their keratinized sheaths (rhamphotheca). The rate of replacement of the rhamphotheca varies. In large parrots, the upper rhamphotheca is completely replaced in about 6 months. In toucans, the upper rhamphotheca grows about 0.5 cm in 2 years. Caged birds may be classified as hardbills (e.g., psittacines) or softbills (e.g., mynahs).

TABLE 8–1. Animal Care Products for Use in Dermatologic Disorders

---

Nexaband: Tri-point Medical, Raleigh, NC (919) 876-7800
Collodion Flexible: Humco Labs, Texarkana, TX (800) 866-3967
Preparation: H: Whitehall Labs Inc, New York, NY (800) 322-3129
Dermaheal: Bristol Meyer, Princeton, NJ (800) 332-2056
DuoDerm: Bristol Meyer, Princeton, NJ (800) 332-2056

Abnormalities of the beak include overgrown upper or lower beak, overgrown side of the beak, crossed upper and lower beaks (scissors beak), shortened upper beak (prognathism, when the tip of the upper beak does not extend over the lower beak), and areas of swelling, grooves, or necrosis.

Differential Diagnoses for Beak Abnormalities

1. Infectious
   a. Bacterial: °gram-negative, gram-positive
   b. Viral: polyomavirus-like virus (finches), °poxvirus, °PBFD
   c. Fungal: °*Aspergillus, Candida*
   d. Parasitic: °*Knemidokoptes, Trichomonas*
2. Metabolic: °liver disease
3. Nutritional: vitamin D deficiency, calcium deficiency, calcium/phosphorus imbalance
4. Toxic: trichothecene
5. Physical: lack of use
6. °Trauma: puncture, laceration, split, avulsion, fracture
7. Allergic: tobacco smoke
8. Behavioral: °mate-induced trauma
9. Neoplastic
10. Developmental: °prognathism, °scissors beak

Signalment

Common causes of beak abnormalities in large psittacines include developmental causes, PBFD, *Aspergillus,* and trauma. Mate-induced trauma is common in cockatoos, especially early in the breeding season. Common causes in small psittacines include *Knemidokoptes,* gram-negative bacterial infection, liver disease, trauma, and developmental causes. Passerines are commonly affected by *Knemidokoptes,* gram-negative and gram-positive bacteria, poxvirus, and trauma. Common causes of beak abnormalities in raptors include trauma, poxvirus, *Aspergillus,* and bacterial infections.

Common causes of beak abnormalities in young birds include nutritional diseases (homemade formulas), gram-negative bacteria, *Candida,* trauma, and developmental abnormalities (scissors beak, prognathism).

Although PBFD occurs in many species of psittacines, it is most common in cockatoos. *Aspergillus*-associated beak lesions are common in African gray parrots.

History

Isolated birds and those in collections with no recently added new birds are most commonly ill because of developmental abnormalities, liver disease,

---

°Common causes.

Aspergillus, trauma, toxicoses, nutritional deficiencies, and neoplasia. Bacterial infections are also seen. Chronic bacterial, viral, and fungal infections (mycobacteriosis, PBFD, aspergillosis) occur.

Birds recently exposed to other birds are commonly ill as a result of infectious diseases, including bacterial, viral, and parasitic diseases. This is the result of stress and exposure to infectious disease. Mycobacteriosis, PBFD, *Knemidokoptes,* and poxvirus are common in flock environments. Illnesses that occur in isolated birds also occur in birds in flock environments.

Significant dietary history includes type of diet, freshness, vitamin supplementation, and techniques associated with the preparation of hand-feeding diets. Diets that contain low calcium, high phosphorus, or low vitamin D content may result in an abnormally pliable beak (rubber beak). Seed diets are low in calcium and high in phosphorus and fat. The high fat content of a seed diet may also interfere with calcium absorption. Meat is low in calcium and high in phosphorus. Raptors fed only day-old chicks, meat, or pinky mice may develop calcium deficiency.

Liver-associated beak abnormalities can be the result of poor diet. Hepatic lipidosis, mycotoxicosis, and hemochromatosis may cause liver failure. High-fat diets (e.g., seed diets) and unbalanced diets (biotin, choline, and methionine deficient) may lead to hepatic lipidosis.

Poor hand-feeding techniques may lead to beak abnormalities. Deviation of the beak may possibly occur when a bird is fed continually on one side of the beak; there are other developmental causes as well. Hand-fed birds are often affected by candidiasis and bacterial infections associated with improper handling of formula. Using previously heated and reheated food is a common cause that should be avoided. Fresh food should be mixed for each feeding and leftover food discarded.

Important environmental factors include exposure to infectious diseases, exposure to tobacco smoke, flight capabilities, presence of a cagemate, sanitation, and exposure to wild birds or disease vectors.

The duration of the illness is important. Note the owner's description of the clinical signs and the course of the disease. Note previous illnesses, including signs, treatment, and response to treatment.

Physical Examination

A complete physical examination is important to identify the extent of the problem and to identify involvement of other body systems. Other concurrent problems may be noted. Observe for trauma, respiratory signs, feather abnormalities, oral lesions, etc. If abnormalities are present, consult appropriate chapters to assist in making a diagnosis. Common findings in birds with beak abnormalities are discussed below.

Inspect the cage. Look for evidence of trauma (e.g., blood) or vomiting, and look at the diet being eaten. Lack of beak use with a soft diet and toys may result in an overgrown beak in hardbills. Evaluate the feces. Look for diarrhea, polyuria, abnormally colored urates, etc.

Observe the bird in the cage.

Examine the bird. Increased pliability of the beak may be the result of calcium or vitamin D deficiency or a calcium/phosphorus imbalance. Color changes in the beaks of toucans and lorikeets may be the result of malnutrition or systemic disease. A shiny beak in birds that normally have abundant powder down (e.g., cockatoos) may be an early indication of PBFD. Note lesions on the outside of the beak. Brown hypertrophy of the cere is seen in some older female budgies. Keratin layers build up on the cere and develop a horn-looking structure. The layers of keratin may be softened with lotion and peeled or scraped off. Scissors beak may be observed as crossed upper and lower beaks (Fig. 8–8). Beak overgrowth may be the result of lack of use, developmental abnormalities, liver disease (especially in budgies), *Knemidokoptes* (budgies), or a polyomavirus-like virus (finches). Affected finches may have a long and tubular lower beak. Traumatic lesions are usually obvious if recently incurred. Old traumatic lesions, necrosis, *Aspergillus* infection, bacterial infection, and PBFD lesions may appear as sunken, irregular abnormalities in the beak. Proliferative growths around the margins of the beak may be the result of poxvirus infection, *Knemidokoptes*, or bacterial infection. Necrotic lesions at the commissure of the beak may be caused by poxvirus, trichothecene toxicosis, or *Trichomonas* (cockatiels). Inspect the oral cavity for ulcers, plaques, or other abnormalities. White plaques and excessive mucus in the mouth may be the result of vitamin A deficiency, *Candida, Trichomonas,* trichothecene toxicosis, or bacterial infection. Necrosis caused by PBFD usually starts as a brown necrotic area inside the upper beak.

Search the body for evidence of other dermatologic lesions. *Knemidokoptes* and poxvirus lesions may occur on other unfeathered areas such as around the eyes and vent or on the feet. Observe for feather abnormalities that may occur with PBFD.

Palpate the abdomen for hepatomegaly or other abnormalities. Palpate the skeleton for calluses from previous fractures caused by calcium deficiency.

Neurologic signs may accompany beak lesions with trauma, liver disease, trichothecene toxicosis, and calcium or vitamin D deficiency.

Gastrointestinal signs (e.g., diarrhea, polyuria) may be noted in conjunction with beak abnormalities with bacterial infections, poxvirus, PBFD, aspergillosis, candidiasis, trichomoniasis, and liver disease.

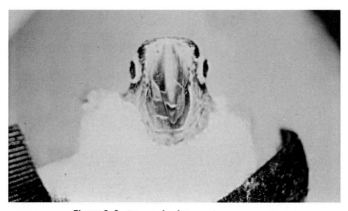

Figure 8–8. Scissors beak in an Amazon parrot.

Respiratory signs may occur in conjunction with beak abnormalities as a result of bacterial infections (especially sinusitis), poxvirus, PBFD, aspergillosis, candidiasis, liver disease, trauma, and chronic cigarette smoke exposure. *Knemidokoptes* mite proliferations may cause dyspnea if the lesions obstruct the nostrils.

Ophthalmic signs may occur in conjunction with beak abnormalities with *Knemidokoptes*, poxvirus, bacterial infections, candidiasis, aspergillosis, and trauma.

Algorithm for Beak Abnormalities

See Figure 8–9.

Diagnostic Plan for Beak Abnormalities

Diagnostic plans are provided for sunken or lytic areas in the beak, proliferative growths at beak margins, necrotic lesions at the commissure of the beak, beak overgrowth, scissors beak, and trauma. Oral plaques are discussed in Chapter 4.

Sunken or lytic areas in the beak may be the result of previous trauma, sinusitis, necrosis, bacterial infection, aspergillosis, or PBFD. Use the history to rule out trauma. If trauma is not the cause and a defect in the beak originates at the nostril (see Fig. 3–2), perform a sinus aspirate and evaluate it cytologically. If an adequate sample cannot be obtained with a sinus aspiration, perform a sinus flush and collect a sample. Cytology of a normal sinus contains few cells and no intracellular bacteria. A few extracellular bacteria and an occasional squamous epithelial cell with associated bacteria may be present in a cytologic sample from a normal infraorbital sinus.

Inflammatory cells indicate sinusitis. The number and type of inflammatory cells depend on the cause. Intracytoplasmic bacteria in leukocytes may be seen with primary bacterial sinusitis or may be secondary to vitamin A deficiency, neoplasia, allergy, fungal infection, or a foreign body. Bacterial cocci in chains suggests *Streptococcus* sinusitis. Aspirates containing intracytoplasmic bacteria, high numbers of extracellular bacteria, or inflammatory cells should be cultured. Treat sinusitis as described in Chapter 3.

Fungal elements may be identified. *Aspergillus* is characterized by branching septate hyphae (see Fig. 12–29). Hyphae may stain poorly or basophilic with Wright's or Diff-Quik stain. Methylene blue stain may be used to better visualize hyphae. Basophilic staining of fungal spores or conidiophores may be seen. *Candida* is identified by the presence of many oval budding yeasts (see Fig. 12–20). Sinus aspirates containing primarily eosinophils suggest an allergic response. Aspirates may contain inflammatory cells without an etiologic agent being apparent.

Submit samples for bacterial and fungal cultures.

If the lesion appears lytic, cytology is performed on a scraping of the affected area. Assess the sample using the above guidelines.

Hematology and plasma biochemistries are performed if a diagnosis cannot be made with cytology. An elevated WBC count may occur with inflammatory or infectious diseases. If the WBC count is in excess of 40,000/μl, rule out aspergillosis with cytology, radiology, and fungal cultures. An ELISA test for aspergillosis is available, but false-negatives can occur.

Psittacine beak and feather disease can cause beak, feather, and nail abnormalities. Necrotic beak lesions may be present without other abnormalities. Secondary bacterial and fungal infections are common. Submit samples for PBFD probe testing on all psittacines with necrotic beak lesions.

Proliferative growths at beak margins may be caused by poxvirus, *Knemidokoptes,* or bacterial infection. Evaluate skin scrapings for the presence of *Knemidokoptes* mites. Cytology of a scraping of proliferative lesions may include inflammatory cells if bacterial infection or poxvirus infection are the cause. Phagocytized bacteria indicates a septic inflammatory lesion. Submit a sample for bacterial culture and sensitivity testing. Poxvirus lesions contain squamous epithelial cells that contain large cytoplasmic vacuoles (Bollinger bodies) that push the nucleus to the cell margin. The vacuoles may contain small, pale eosinophilic inclusions. An inflammatory response is often present because of secondary bacterial infection.

Necrotic lesions at the commissure of the beak may be the result of poxvirus infection, trichothecene toxicosis, or trichomoniasis. Trichothecene toxicosis is suspected based on history and clinical signs (beak lesions, poor feathering, constrictive lesions of the digits, or contact dermatitis if litter is contaminated). Lesions associated with trichomoniasis occur in cockatiels. Scrapings and wet mount may allow visualization of the motile parasite. Cytology of a scraping of the lesion may reveal Bollinger bodies if the cause is poxvirus (see previous paragraph).

Beak overgrowth and scissors beak may be the result of lack of use, lack of hard chewing material, developmental abnormalities, or liver disease. Developmental abnormalities may be noted within the first week after hatching or may develop as the chick grows. If abnormalities are noted in a young chick before the beak hardens, manual manipulation may correct mild problems. Prosthetics made with acrylics, applied early, are very effective. With mild deviation of the upper beak, manually correct the position of the beak at every feeding and feed from the other side. Trim the lower beak at an angle such that the upper beak slides over to the side opposite the curvature. See Clipsham, 1997, and Clipsham, 1994, for application of an acrylic prosthesis. In young birds, when the upper beak is shortened and the tip of the upper beak does not extend over the lower beak, the upper beak is pulled over the lower beak at least four times each day (using gauze in larger birds). Grind the lower beak if it is uneven. See Clipsham, 1997, and Clipsham, 1994, for prosthetic application in older birds and those unresponsive to physical therapy. Scissors beak in adult birds requires continued grooming with periodic grinding of the beak to maintain the beak to enable the bird to eat.

Severe *Knemidokoptes* lesions can cause beak overgrowth in budgies. Periodic beak trims may be required.

Lack of use or lack of adequate hard material to chew is diagnosed with history and physical examination. If the diagnosis is not obvious, hematology and plasma biochemistries are used to identify infectious or inflammatory diseases and liver or other metabolic problems.

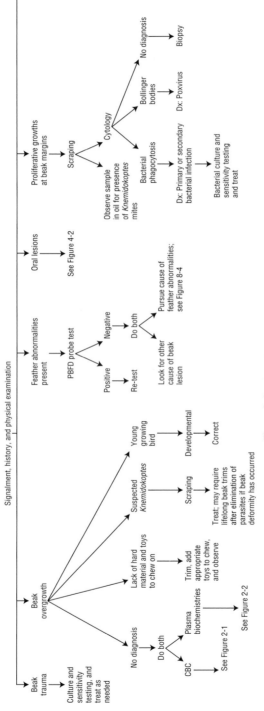

Figure 8–9. Algorithm for beak abnormalities.

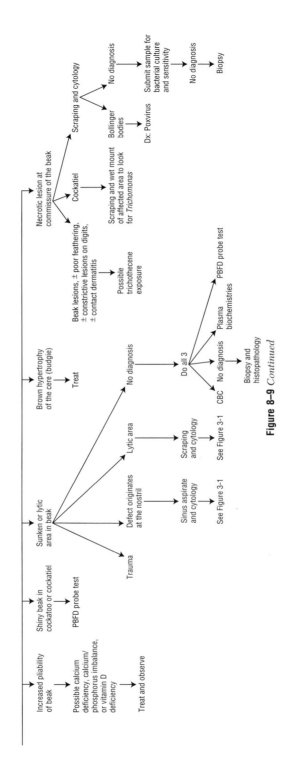

Figure 8–9 *Continued*

Periodic beak trimming may be required after treatment of the underlying cause.

Beak trauma may consist of a cracked upper beak tip, split lower beak, puncture of the keratinized sheath, or avulsion. If the tip of the upper beak is cracked, remove the tip by grinding or trim it with nail clippers. Control hemorrhage with styptic powder. If the lower beak is cracked the entire length of the beak, temporary repair with wire and dental acrylics will temporarily hold the pieces together. There is no permanent cure. Birds can eat with this problem, but occasional trimming of the lower beak segments may be necessary.

Puncture wounds to the beak are cultured (bacterial and fungal) and debrided. Debride irregular and necrotic areas under anesthesia. Once infection is controlled, the defect can be patched with acrylic compounds.

Damage to the base of the beak may require surgical reattachment, wiring the beak to bones of the skull. Damage to the germinal layer at the base of the beak may result in a permanent defect.

Avulsion of the entire upper or lower beak is not reversible. Avulsion of the proximal third of the beak is usually not reversible. Forced feeding may allow time for the beak to scar over, and the bird may adjust to a soft diet. Avulsion of the distal third of the beak is treated like a puncture wound. Regeneration of the beak may occur, but the beak may never appear normal.

For further information on repair of traumatic beak lesions, consult Clipsham, 1997; Altman, 1997; and Clipsham, 1994.

FEET OR LEG LESIONS

The feet and part of the legs of birds are covered by scales. Clinical signs of abnormalities of the feet and legs include swelling, erythema, ulceration, thickening, constrictions, masses, or other proliferative lesions. Refer to neurologic and musculoskeletal sections for neurologic abnormalities, swollen joints, or other musculoskeletal signs.

Differential Diagnoses for Feet or Leg Lesions

1. Infectious
   a. Bacterial: °gram-negative, °gram-positive (*Mycobacterium, Pseudomonas, Staphylococcus, Streptococcus,* other)
   b. Viral: herpesvirus (cockatoos and mallard ducks), papilloma, PBFD, °poxvirus
   c. Fungal: *Aspergillus,* other
   d. Parasitic: subcutaneous filarial nematodes, °*Knemidokoptes*
2. Metabolic: °gout
3. Nutritional: °general malnutrition, deficiencies (°vitamin A, biotin, calcium, vitamin D$_3$) calcium/phosphorus imbalance
4. Toxic: trichothecene, cleaning solutions, ergot poisoning

°Common causes.

5. Physical: °abrasion, °constricting fibers, frostbite, bite wound, amputation, °self-mutilation, °leg-band necrosis, insect bites (fly, mosquito, gnat, ant)
6. Trauma: °fracture, °laceration, burn, °bite wounds
7. Allergic: tobacco smoke
8. Behavioral: °self-mutilation
9. Neoplastic
10. Other: °Amazon foot skin necrosis syndrome, °constricted toe syndrome, aging

Signalment

Common causes of foot and leg lesions in large psittacines include bacterial infection, leg-band necrosis, malnutrition, nutritional deficiencies, trauma, constricted toe syndrome, and self-mutilation. Small psittacines are commonly affected by gout, bacterial infections, malnutrition, nutritional deficiencies, trauma, and *Knemidokoptes* mites. Foot and leg lesions in passerines are commonly the result of poxvirus, insect bites, strangulating fibers, *Knemidokoptes* mites, aging, and malnutrition. Common causes of leg and foot lesions in raptors include bacterial infection and trauma.

Common causes of lesions in young birds include bacterial infections, poxvirus, nutritional deficiencies, insect bites, and fractures.

History

Isolated birds and those in collections with no recently added new birds are commonly ill because of nutritional deficiencies, exposure to toxins, trauma, self-mutilation, leg-band necrosis, insect bites, and allergies. Chronic bacterial, viral, and fungal diseases (mycobacteriosis, PBFD, aspergillosis) occur. Gram-negative bacterial infections are also seen.

Birds recently exposed to other birds are commonly ill as a result of infectious diseases, including bacterial, viral, and parasitic diseases. This is the result of stress and exposure to infectious disease. Mycobacteriosis, poxvirus, and PBFD are common in flock environments. Illnesses that occur in isolated birds also occur in birds in flock environments.

Significant dietary history includes type of diet, freshness, changes in diet, vitamin supplementation, and treats. Malnutrition, vitamin A deficiency, and calcium deficiency may occur with seed diets. Calcium deficiency may cause loss of bone density, resulting in fractures. Meat is low in calcium and high in phosphorus. Raptors fed only day-old chicks, pinky mice, or meat may develop calcium deficiency. High dietary calcium and protein may contribute to gout. Malposition of the digits in neonates may be caused by malnutrition. Molded foods may contain toxins leading to ergot poisoning.

Important environmental factors include exposure to infectious diseases, access to potential toxins, flight capabilities, management practices, sanitation, and

---

°Common causes.

exposure to wild birds or insects. Fibers from cloth placed in a cage can encircle and constrict the blood supply to the toe. This is common in small passerines. Cleaning solutions and litter contaminated by trichothecene toxin may cause a contact dermatitis. Trauma may occur when birds are allowed free flight or have cagemates, or if they are allowed to perch on cages containing birds. Toes are often amputated when a bird perches on a cage inhabited by an aggressive bird. Management practices that may lead to feet or leg lesions include placement of leg bands, exposure to freezing temperatures leading to frostbite, and exposure to tobacco smoke or contact with heavy smokers. Poxvirus can be spread by mosquitoes or other biting arthropods or by contact with damaged epithelial surfaces. Birds with lesions should be isolated from the flock and placed in a mosquito-proof environment. Ants may attack neonates in nest boxes. Other insect bites may cause skin lesions.

The duration of the illness is important. Note the owner's description of the clinical signs and the course of the disease. Note previous illnesses, including signs, treatment, and response to treatment.

Physical Examination

A complete physical examination is important to identify the extent of the problem and to identify involvement of other body systems. Observe for trauma, respiratory signs, neurologic signs, etc. If abnormalities are present, consult appropriate chapters to assist in making a diagnosis. Common findings of birds with feet and leg abnormalities are discussed below.

Inspect the cage. Perches should be clean and of varying sizes. Feces or vomitus on perches may lead to bacterial infections. Sandpaper perches may lead to trauma, callus formation, and infection of the plantar surfaces of the foot.

During the examination, look for abnormally shaped feathers, swellings, erosions, ulcers, and proliferative lesions on the feet and legs. Proliferative lesions may be the result of bacterial infection, poxvirus, *Knemidokoptes,* vitamin A deficiency, papillomas, or other tumors. Proliferations on the feet of passerines are commonly the result of aging, *Knemidokoptes,* and abrasions. Subcutaneous swellings may result from bacterial infections (including mycobacterial), fungal infection, filarial nematodes, gout, granulomas, callus formation from an old fracture, or insect bites. Swelling of the toes or feet may occur with vascular constriction (leg band, threads), frostbite, burns, and trauma. Constrictions of the toes occur with constricting fibers, constricted toe syndrome, and ergot poisoning. Initially, the segment distal to the constriction swells. Later, the distal portion of the toe may become devitalized, leathery, and dark. Erosions or ulcers may be the result of bacterial infection, fungal infection, self-mutilation, or trauma. Swelling and ulceration on the plantar surface of the foot (commonly called pododermatitis or bumblefoot) may be the result of trauma, bacterial infection, or malnutrition (Fig. 8–10). Erythema may result from exposure to harsh cleaning solutions, trichothecene contact, frostbite, or burns. Necrosis may occur with bacterial infections, PBFD, fungal infections, tumors, burns, frostbite, constricting leg band, self-mutilation, lacerations, and Amazon foot skin necrosis syndrome. Broken nails may be the result of trauma or PBFD.

Other dermatologic abnormalities may be present with PBFD, poxvirus,

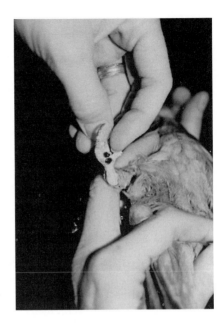

Figure 8–10. Pododermatitis in an African gray parrot.

Knemidokoptes, malnutrition, nutritional deficiencies, exposure to toxins, and tobacco smoke exposure.

Neurologic signs may accompany feet and leg lesions with PBFD, gout, calcium deficiency, and trauma.

Gastrointestinal signs may be noted in conjunction with feet or leg lesions with PBFD, gout, malnutrition, and vitamin A deficiency.

Respiratory signs may occur in conjunction with feet or leg lesions with PBFD, poxvirus, malnutrition, vitamin A deficiency, fractures, trauma, chronic exposure to cigarette smoke, and if the nares are occluded with *Knemidokoptes* proliferations.

Algorithm for Feet or Leg Lesions

See Figure 8–11.

Diagnostic Plan for Feet or Leg Lesions

Malnutrition commonly contributes to dermatologic problems. If a poor diet is currently offered, improve the diet (change to a commercial pelleted food) but continue to look for other causes. Expose the bird to natural sunlight and daily misting. Stop exposure to tobacco smoke and contact with heavy smokers. If the owner smokes, he or she should limit smoking to outdoors and wash hands and arms before handling the bird.

Dietary causes must be sought from the history. A complete history and

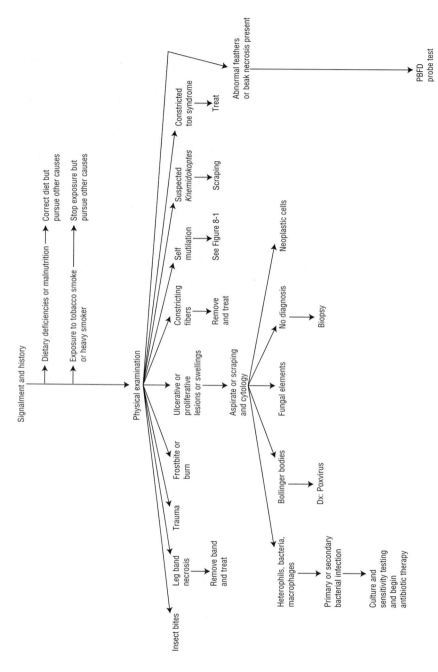

Figure 8–11. Algorithm for feet or leg lesions.

physical examination may allow a diagnosis of frostbite, burns, self-mutilation, insect bites, and trauma.

Honeycomb proliferative lesions typical of *Knemidokoptes* mites are scraped and placed in oil for microscopic evaluation. Constricted toe syndrome and necrosis of the leg as a result of the leg band are diagnosed on physical examination.

Ulcerative or proliferative lesions or swellings are aspirated or scraped and evaluated cytologically. Heterophils, bacteria, and macrophages indicate a bacterial or foreign body origin. Bacterial infections may be primary or secondary. Submit a sample for culture and sensitivity with suspected bacterial infections. Small numbers of *Streptococcus* and *Staphylococcus* may be normal. Bollinger bodies (eosinophilic intracytoplasmic inclusion bodies) may be seen with poxvirus infection. *Aspergillus* is characterized by septate branching hyphae. Hyphae may stain poorly or basophilic with Wright's or Diff-Quik stain. *Mycobacterium* bacteria may be observed as bacterial rods that fail to stain with Wright's or Diff-Quik stain. Acid-fast staining is required to demonstrate the organism. Tumor cells may be identified. Cutaneous neoplasms found in birds include fibrosarcoma, lymphosarcoma, and other less common neoplasms.

Bacterial infections involving the plantar surface of the feet (pododermatitis) are serious. Submit a sample for bacterial and fungal cultures and sensitivity testing. Radiograph all affected feet, with the digits extended. Osteomyelitis is common and results in a graver prognosis.

Biopsy lesions of uncertain etiology. Granulomas, poxvirus lesions, fungal lesions, papillomas, and other benign and malignant tumors may be identified with histopathology.

Cytologic samples from joint swellings with inflammatory cells indicate inflammatory disease (e.g., trauma, bacterial infection, gout). Bacterial phagocytosis by leukocytes indicates a septic lesion. Submit a sample for culture and sensitivity testing. Monosodium urate crystals, present with articular gout, appear needle shaped. They may appear birefringent under polarized light. With Wright's stain they may stain eosinophilic. Inflammatory cells are often present.

If abnormal feathers or beak necrosis are present with nail necrosis or broken nails, submit a blood sample for PBFD probe testing.

Treatment for Feet or Leg Lesions

Once a diagnosis is made, treat the underlying cause. Provide supportive care as needed (see Chapter 1). Treatments of specific diseases are found in Chapter 9.

Subcutaneous nematodes are surgically removed.

Toe constrictions are observed with magnification. In passerines, an encircling fiber is usually the cause. Fibers are removed with the aid of magnification. Constricted toe syndrome of large psittacines is treated surgically, see Chapter 14. Treatment of ergot poisoning in flocks may include antifungal therapy to decrease losses.

With leg-band necrosis or constriction, the band is removed by cutting or twisting the band, taking care to avoid cutting the skin or fracturing bones. Twisting of an incomplete band may be accomplished with pliers (see Fig. 1–10).

Steady firm pressure is required. Clean the wound. If severe, the wound is cultured and treated with systemic antibiotics.

Treatment of pododermatitis (bumblefoot) varies with the severity of the condition. To inspect the foot adequately and evaluate the severity of the problem, the bird is anesthetized and the foot is scrubbed with a surgical scrub. Mild changes of slight thinning or erythema are treated by softening the feet with a bovine udder balm or a lanolin-based lotion to prevent the formation of hyperkeratosis; painting reddened or thinning areas with a tissue glue, Collodion Flexible (see Table 8–1), camphor spirits, tincture of benzoin, or fingernail polish; and correcting the housing and perches. Preparation H promotes healing (see Table 8–1). Monitor weekly.

More severe lesions characterized by hyperkeratosis are treated by correcting perching surfaces and enclosure sanitation, applying udder balm or a lanolin-based lotion to affected areas for several weeks, and supplementing with vitamin A. If slight swelling or epithelial degeneration has occurred, treat with a preparation of DMSO, an anti-inflammatory agent, and an antibiotic (5 ml dimethyl sulfoxide, 4 mg dexamethasone, 1 g piperacillin in 3 ml saline; refrigerate and mix fresh solution weekly). Place a ball or interdigitating bandage on the affected foot or feet for 1 to 3 days.

Severe pododermatitis with necrosis, abscessation, and swelling requires intensive treatment. Radiograph the foot and evaluate for osteomyelitis. If osteomyelitis is present, there is a poorer prognosis. Remove devitalized tissue by excision or scraping. Culture the defect and irrigate the lesion with dilute povidone-iodine in saline (1:100). Begin parenteral antibiotics. Enrofloxacin, piperacillin, or carbenicillin are used to initiate antibiotic therapy. Substitute a different antibiotic for these only if sensitivity testing indicates a resistance to these three drugs. Swab swollen and inflamed areas with the DMSO/anti-inflammatory/antibiotic combination listed above. Sterile iodine-soaked gauze is placed in the defect if swelling is severe or if abundant exudate is present. Sterile gauze sponges are placed over the wound, and a ball bandage is applied. Confine the bird to an appropriately sized cage with a padded bottom and no perches. Change the flooring daily.

Clean and bandage the foot once or twice daily for 2 to 4 days, until most fluctuant areas of swelling are gone. Clean with sterile, cotton-tipped applicators. Systemic antibiotics can usually be discontinued in 7 to 10 days. Discontinue treatment with the DMSO/anti-inflammatory/antibiotic when swelling decreases. Discontinue the iodine-soaked sponges when exudation stops. At this point, a hydroactive wound dressing (e.g., Dermaheal or DuoDerm [see Table 8–1]) is used to enhance wound healing and prevent secondary infection. Changing of the bandages can be done every to 2 to 5 days, as needed. When all swelling has subsided and healthy granulation tissue is covering the defect, treatment can be limited to a ball bandage. Treatment usually requires 6 to 8 weeks. Full recovery takes about 4 to 6 months.

Monitor the unaffected foot. Occasionally, a ball bandage must be applied to prevent development of pododermatitis caused by increased weight bearing. Keep bandages dry. Water is provided by gavage or by saturation of the food. With raptors, food must be cut into bite-sized pieces.

Soft, padded perches are used to prevent recurrences.

References and Additional Reading

Altman RB. Beak repair, acrylics. In Altman RB, Clubb SL, Dorrestein GM, Quesenberry K (eds): *Avian Medicine and Surgery.* Philadelphia, WB Saunders, 1997, pp 787–799.

Bauck L. Diseases of the foot in cage and aviary birds. *Proc First Intl Conf Zoo Avian Med* 1987;109–115.

Bauck L. Radical surgery for the treatment of feather cysts in the canary. *J Assoc Avian Vet* 1987;1(5):200–201.

Bauck L. Avian dermatology. In Altman RB, Clubb SL, Dorrestein GM, Quesenberry K (eds): *Avian Medicine and Surgery.* Philadelphia, WB Saunders, 1997, pp 548–562.

Bond MW. Avian pediatrics. *Proc Assoc Avian Vet* 1991;153–160.

Bond MW. Sample collection and interpretation of results of nucleic acid probes for psittacine beak and feather disease. *J Assoc Avian Vet* 1993;7(1):10–11.

Brown R. Sinus, articular, and subcutaneous *Mycobacterium tuberculosis* infection in a juvenile red-lored Amazon parrot. *Proc Assoc Avian Vet* 1990;305–308.

Burgmann PM. Common psittacine dermatologic diseases. *Semin Avian Exot Pet Med* 1995;4(4):169–183.

Campbell TW. *Avian Hematology and Cytology*, ed 2. Ames, Iowa, Iowa State University Press, 1995.

Clipsham R. Beak repair, rhamphorthotics. In Altman RB, Clubb SL, Dorrestein GM, Quesenberry K (eds): *Avian Medicine and Surgery.* Philadelphia, WB Saunders, 1997, pp 773–786.

Clipsham R. Surgical beak restoration and correction. *Proc Assoc Avian Vet* 1989;164–176.

Clipsham R. Surgical correction of beaks: Practical lab. *Proc Assoc Avian Vet* 1990;325–333.

Clipsham R. Noninfectious diseases of pediatric psittacines. *Semin Avian Exot Pet Med* 1992;1(1):22–33.

Clipsham R. Rhamphorthotics and surgical corrections of maxillofacial defects. *Semin Avian Exot Pet Med* 1994;3(2):92–99.

Clipsham R. Scissors beak correction. *J Assoc Avian Vet* 1989;3(4):188–189.

Dahlhausen B, Radabaugh S. Update on psittacine beak and feather disease and avian polyomavirus testing. *Proc Assoc Avian Vet* 1993;5–7.

Davis C. Behavior modification counseling: An alliance between the veterinarian and behavior consultant. *Semin Avian Exot Pet Med* 1995;4(1):39–42.

Davis C. Parrot psychology and behavior problems. *Vet Clin North Am* 1991;21(6):1281–1288.

Degernes L. Wound management in avian patients. *J Assoc Avian Vet* 1989;3(3):130–131.

Degernes LA. Soft tissue wound management in avian patients. *Proc Assoc Avian Vet* 1992;476–483.

Degernes LA, Redig PT. Soft tissue wound management in avian patients. *Proc Assoc Avian Vet* 1990;182–190.

Dorrestein GM. Physiology of avian dermatology. In Altman RB, Clubb SL, Dorrestein GM, Quesenberry K (eds): *Avian Medicine and Surgery.* Philadelphia, WB Saunders, 1997, pp 545–547.

Drew ML, Ramsay E. Dermatitis associated with *Mycobacterium* spp. in a blue-fronted Amazon parrot. *Proc Assoc Avian Vet* 1991;252–254.

England TS, Renning AN, Bowbeer GRN. Use of human orthodontic hardware in the correction of a beak deformity due to parental trauma. *Proc Assoc Avian Vet* 1991;267–268.

Flammer K. Diseases of the integument of caged and aviary birds. In *Avian Medicine.* TG Hungerford Refresher Course for Veterinarians, Proceedings 178. Sydney, Australia, 1991, pp 431–440.

Galvin C. The feather picking bird. In Kirk R (ed): *Current Veterinary Therapy VIII, Small Animal Practice,* Philadelphia, WB Saunders, 1983, pp 646–651.

Gould J. Avian dermatology. *Proc Am Animal Hosp Assoc* 1992;294–298.

Graham DL. The avian integument: Its structure and selected diseases. *Proc Assoc Avian Vet* 1985;33–52.

Greenacre CB, Latimer KS, Niagro FD, et al. Psittacine beak and feather disease in a scarlet macaw (*Ara macao*). *J Assoc Avian Vet* 1992;6(2):95–98.

Harrison GJ. Disorders of the integument. In Harrison GJ, Harrison LR (eds): *Clinical Avian Medicine and Surgery.* Philadelphia, WB Saunders, 1986, pp 509–424.

Hess RE. The use of dental acrylic shoes for the treatment of bumblefoot. *Proc Assoc Avian Vet* 1993;135–137.

Hillyer EV. Avian dermatology. In Birchard SJ, Sherding RG (eds): *Saunders Manual of Small Animal Practice.* Philadelphia, WB Saunders, 1994, pp 1271–1281.

Hillyer EV, Quesenberry KE, Baer K. Basic avian dermatology. *Proc Assoc Avian Vet* 1989;101–121.

Hochleithner M, Hochleithner C. Surgical treatment of ulcerative lesions caused by automutilation of the sternum in psittacine birds. *J Avian Med Surg* 1996;10(2):84–88.

Hoefer HL, Liu SK, Kiehn TE, et al. Systemic *Mycobacterium tuberculosis* in a green winged macaw. *Proc Assoc Avian Vet* 1996;167–168.

Hudelson S, Hudelson P. Dermatology of raptors: A review. *Semin Avian Exot Pet Med* 1995;4(4):184–194.

Johnson-Delaney C. Feather picking: Diagnosis and treatment. *J Assoc Avian Vet* 1992;6(2):82–83.

King AS, McLelland J. Integument. In *Birds: Their Structure and Function,* ed 2. London, Bailliere Tindall, 1984, pp 23–42.

King WW, Tully TN. Management of a large cutaneous defect in a moluccan cockatoo. *Proc Assoc Avian Vet* 1993;142–145.

Lamberski N. A diagnostic approach to feather picking. *Semin Avian Exot Pet Med* 1995;4(4):184–194.

Latimer KS, Niagro FD, Canpagnoli RP, et al. Diagnosis of concurrent avian polyomavirus and psittacine beak and feather disease virus infections using DNA probes. *J Assoc Avian Vet* 1993;7(3):141–146.

Latimer KS, Rakich PM, Niagro FD, et al. An updated review of psittacine beak and feather disease. *J Assoc Avian Vet* 1991;5(4):211–220.

Lennox AM, VanDerHeyden N. Haloperidol for use in treatment of psittacine self-mutilation and feather plucking. *Proc Assoc Avian Vet* 1993;119–120.

McCluggage DM. Surgery of the integument: Selected topics. *Semin Avian Exot Pet Med* 1993;2(2):76–82.

Morris PJ, Weigel JP. Methacrylate beak prosthesis in a marabou stork (*Leptoptilos crumeniferus*). *J Assoc Avian Vet* 1990;4(2):103–107.

Oglesbee BL, McDonald S, Warthen K. Avian digestive system disorders. In Birchard SJ, Sherding RG (eds): *Saunders Manual of Small Animal Practice.* Philadelphia, WB Saunders, 1994, pp 1290–1301.

Oglesbee BL, Oglesbee MJ. Feather dystrophy in a cockatiel (*Nymphicus hollandicus*). *J Assoc Avian Vet* 1994;8(1):16–21.

Oppenheimer J. Feather picking: Systematic approach. *Proc Assoc Avian Vet* 1991;314–315.

Orosz SE. Avian dermatology. *Proc N Am Vet Cont* 1995;564–565.

Orosz S. Anatomy of the integument. In Altman RB, Clubb SL, Dorrestein GM, Quesenberry K (eds): *Avian Medicine and Surgery.* Philadelphia, WB Saunders, 1997, pp 540–545.

Parrott T. Pododermatitis in three Amazon parrots and treatment with l-thyroxine. *Proc Assoc Avian Vet* 1991;263–264.

Parsons B, Wissman MA. Acrylic beak repair techniques. *Proc Assoc Avian Vet* 1995;503–504.

Pass DA. Normal anatomy of the avian skin and feathers. *Semin Avian Exot Pet Med* 1995;4(4):152–160.

Perry RA. Pruritic polyfolliculosis and dermatitis in budgerigars (*Melopsittacus undulatus*) and African lovebirds (*Agapornis* spp.). *Proc Assoc Avian Vet* 1991;32–37.

Perry RA, Gill J, Cross GM. Disorders of the avian integument. *Vet Clin North Am Small Anim Pract* 1991;21:1307–1327.

Rae M. Endocrine disease in pet birds. *Semin Avian Exot Pet Med* 1995;4(1):32–38.

Raidal SR. Viral skin diseases of birds. *Semin Avian Exot Pet Med* 1995;4(2):72–82.

Ramsay EC, Grindlinger H. Use of clomipramine in the treatment of obsessive behavior in psittacine birds. *J Assoc Avian Vet* 1994;8(1):9–15.

Reavill DR, Schmidt RE, Fudge AM. Avian skin and feather disorders: A retrospective study. *Proc Assoc Avian Vet* 1990;248–253.

Redig PT. Bumblefoot treatment in raptors. In Fowler ME (ed): *Zoo and Wild Animal Medicine, Current Therapy 3*. Philadelphia, WB Saunders, 1993, pp 181–188.

Remington KH. *Myialges (metamicrolichus) nudus* in a lilac-crowned Amazon (*Amazona finschi*). *Proc Assoc Avian Vet* 1990;312–313.

Ritchie BW, Harrison GJ, Harrison LR (eds): *Avian Medicine: Principles and Application*. Lake Worth, FL, Wingers Publishing, 1994.

Rosenthal K. Differential diagnosis of feather-picking in a pet bird. *Proc Assoc Avian Vet* 1993;108–112.

Rosskopf WJ, Woerpel RW. The psittacine mutilation syndrome: Management, incidence, possible etiology and therapy. *Proc Assoc Avian Vet* 1990;301–304.

Sawyer BA. Bumblefoot in raptors. In Kirk RW (ed): *Current Veterinary Therapy VIII, Small Animal Practice*. Philadelphia, WB Saunders, 1983, pp 614–616.

Schmidt RE. Avian skin diseases: A pathologist's perspective. *Proc First Intl Conf Zoo Avian Medicine* 1987;117–123.

Schmidt RE. Use of biopsies in the differential diagnosis of feather picking and avian skin disease. *Proc Assoc Avian Vet* 1993;113–115.

Tully TN, Morris JM, Veazey RS, et al. Liposarcomas in a monk parakeet (*Myiopsitta monachus*). *J Assoc Avian Vet* 1994;8(3):120–124.

Turner R. Trexan (naltrexone hydrochloride) use in feather picking in avian species. *Proc Assoc Avian Vet* 1993;116–118.

VanDerHeyden N. Clinical manifestations of mycobacteriosis in pet birds. *Semin Avian Exot Pet Med* 1997;6(1):18–24.

Wilson L. Non-medical approach to the behavioral feather plucker. *Proc Assoc Avian Vet* 1996;3–9.

Chapter 9

Common Diseases and Treatments

This chapter provides general information on illnesses common in pet birds. Etiology, signalment, history, clinical signs, physical examination findings, necropsy findings, treatment, and prevention are discussed for common infectious, metabolic, endocrine, and nutritional diseases and toxicoses. Because it is beyond the scope of this book to provide an exhaustive discussion of all diseases and illnesses, consult previous chapters and the References and Additional Readings for further information.

INFECTIOUS DISEASES

Infectious diseases are caused by invasion and multiplication of microorganisms in body tissues. Bacteria, *Chlamydia*, *Mycoplasma*, viruses, fungi, and parasites are common causes of infectious diseases in pet birds.

Bacteria

Primary or secondary bacterial infections are common in birds. Isolated bacteria may be normal flora, primary pathogens, opportunistic or secondary pathogens, or transient. Consult Chapter 12 for guidelines for interpretation of culture results to help determine if an organism is a primary pathogen, secondary invader, normal flora, or transient. Treat birds that have clinical signs. Monitor birds with abnormal bacterial flora without clinical signs.

Normal flora of the choana and cloaca is predominantly gram-positive and includes *Bacillus*, *Corynebacterium*, *Lactobacillus*, non–beta-hemolytic *Streptococcus*, and *Staphylococcus* (excluding *S. aureus*). The conjunctiva is usually sterile, but *Staphylococcus epidermidis*, alpha-hemolytic *Streptococcus*, and *Corynebacterium* are frequently isolated from normal birds. The trachea and air sacs are usually sterile, but small numbers of *Streptococcus* and other bacteria are occasionally found in normal birds. Small numbers of *Streptococcus* and *Staphylococcus* may be normal when culturing the skin. The liver, spleen, kidneys, and lungs should be sterile, but occasionally very small numbers of *Bacillus*, *Corynebacterium*, *Streptococcus*, or *Staphylococcus* are found in normal birds.

Gram-Negative Bacteria

BORRELIA ANSERINA. *Borrelia* may infect geese, ducks, turkeys, chickens, pheasants, grouse, partridges, pigeons, crows, magpies, house sparrows, starlings, and African gray parrots. Ticks are the main vectors for the transmission of the disease, but mosquitos, other biting insects, and bird-to-bird transmission by excreta can contribute. The incubation period is 4 to 8 days. Chicks are especially susceptible (1 to 3 weeks of age). Adult birds may be infected.

Clinical signs in acute cases include anorexia, depression, yellowish diarrhea, lethargy, ataxia, and paralysis. Signs of chronic disease include anemia, paralysis, and dyspnea. Hepatomegaly with hemorrhages and necrotic foci, mucoid hemorrhagic enteritis, serofibrinous pericarditis, and swollen kidneys may be noted at necropsy. The liver size may be small or normal in pheasants infected with *Borrelia*.

Diagnosis may be made by observing the motile organism in blood with dark-field microscopy or on Giemsa-stained blood smears. *Borrelia* is difficult to culture. Antibodies may be demonstrated in the blood of infected birds 4 to 30 days after infection.

CAMPYLOBACTER. *Campylobacter* has a wide host range, including finches and canaries, but few infections have been reported in psittacines. Asymptomatic infections occur. Clinical signs are common in birds with parasites.

Campylobacter causes subacute to chronic hepatitis. Clinical signs associated with *Campylobacter* infection include lethargy, anorexia, diarrhea, yellow-stained feces, and emaciation. Heterophilia is common. Catarrhal or hemorrhagic enteritis may also occur. On necropsy, the liver is pale, greenish, and enlarged.

Diagnosis is based on isolation of *Campylobacter* from infected tissues or feces; transport media are necessary for survival of the organism.

In vitro susceptibility does not always correlate with response to treatment. Erythromycin or tetracyclines may be tried. Recurrent infections are common.

CITROBACTER. *Citrobacter* is a common pathogen in weaver finches, waxbills, and ostrich chicks. It is most often reported in finches and is uncommon in psittacines. *Citrobacter amalonaticus* is frequently cultured for normal psittacines.

Clinical signs of *Citrobacter* include diarrhea and depression or death with no antemortem signs. Necropsy findings include petechiae on the heart, musculature, and parenchyma.

Diagnosis is based on culture of the organism from affected tissues.

Treatment is based on culture and sensitivity results. Neomycin may be effective for intestinal infections. Find and treat or remove carrier birds.

ESCHERICHIA COLI. The virulence of *E. coli* varies from extreme to nonpathogenic. Mammalian and human virulence factors are not applicable in birds. Each serotype contains virulent and avirulent strains, and all lysine decarboxylase–negative strains are virulent in birds. Avian strains of *E. coli* produce few exotoxins except enterotoxins. These enterotoxins cause diarrhea.

Clinical signs associated with *E. coli* depend on the portal of entry. Clinical signs of septicemia include lethargy, anorexia, ruffled feathers, diarrhea, and polyuria. Central nervous system (CNS) signs, ocular lesions, and serofibrinous arthritis occasionally occur. Catarrhal enteritis is common. On necropsy, fibrinous polyserositis may be noted.

Clinical signs of localized enteritis include diarrhea, dehydration, and cachexia. Pseudomembranous or ulcerative enteritis may be noted on necropsy.

Escherichia coli can cause granulomas, especially in chickens, turkeys, peafowl, and partridges. Clinical signs include diarrhea, polyuria, and chronic weight loss. Granulomatous dermatitis occasionally occurs. On necropsy, varying sizes of granulomas (grayish foci) may be noted in the liver, intestinal subserosa, spleen, and kidneys. Use acid-fast staining to differentiate from mycobacterial granulomas.

Rhinitis, pneumonia, salpingitis, and oophoritis can be the result of *E. coli* infection.

Diagnosis is based on culturing the organism from affected tissues.

Treatment usually requires parenteral antibiotics based on culture and sensitivity results. Consider the ability of the antibiotic to penetrate the affected tissues or granulomas. Oral antibiotics may be effective in treating infections limited to the intestinal mucosa. Provide supportive care. Long-term avian lactobacilli administration may be of benefit.

HAEMOPHILUS SPECIES. *Haemophilus paragallinarum* infection causes coryza in chickens. Other *Haemophilus* species have been isolated from birds with coryza, but the pathogenicity is questionable. *Haemophilus* has rarely been described in pet birds.

Clinical signs associated with *Haemophilus* infection include catarrhal to fibrinous rhinitis, conjunctivitis, or sinusitis. On necropsy, catarrhal to fibrinous rhinitis, bronchopneumonia, and airsacculitis may be observed.

KLEBSIELLA PNEUMONIAE AND K. OXYTOCA. *Klebsiella* can cause systemic or local infections. Kidney infections are common. The lungs may be chronically infected, resulting in respiratory signs. Encephalomyelitis occasionally occurs. Local infections can involve the sinuses, skin, oral cavity, or crop.

Diagnosis and treatment are based on culture of the organism and sensitivity testing.

PASTEURELLA. *Pasteurella multocida* is the etiologic agent of fowl cholera and is a common cause of septicemia after cat bites in pet birds. Fowl cholera in waterfowl can cause rapid death in large numbers of birds with few clinical signs. *Pasteurella gallinarum* can cause chronic respiratory infections in birds. *Pasteurella pneumotropica* can cause pneumonia in aviary birds and pigeons.

Pasteurella is shed from the respiratory tract. Transmission occurs through direct contact with contaminated aerosols or through mechanical vectors (e.g., blood-sucking mites). Rodents and carrier birds are common sources.

Virulent strains result in septicemia and death. Clinical signs include diarrhea, cyanosis, dyspnea, and death. Less virulent strains result in chronic respiratory infections or septicemia with organ colonization. Clinical signs include sinusitis, conjunctivitis, otitis media, arthritis, CNS signs, and granulomatous dermatitis. On necropsy, acute cases may lack lesions or show petechiae or ecchymoses of parenchymal organs. Prominent lesions associated with fowl cholera include multifocal liver necrosis and hemorrhages in multiple organs. Abnormalities associated with chronic infections include exudative serositis, catarrhal or fibrinous rhinitis, pneumonia, sinusitis, blepharoconjunctivitis, and tracheitis. Septicemia may result in arthritis, osteomyelitis, or otitis media. Granulomas may be observed in the liver, spleen, or skin.

Diagnosis is based on culture of the organism. Treatment includes antibiotics and hyperimmune serum. Treatment of septicemic birds is usually unsuccessful because of irreversible damage to parenchymal organs. Good hygiene, wild bird control, and rodent control are important in preventing infections. Vaccines from strains from individual facilities may be successful in long-term control. Control of fowl cholera includes carcass removal and removal of birds from contaminated sites.

PSEUDOMONAS. Pseudomonas aeruginosa is a common avian pathogen. Waterfowl, free-ranging birds, and penguins are especially susceptible. Contaminated water is a common source, including water hoses and automatic watering system pipes.

Clinical signs of septicemia include dehydration, diarrhea, and dyspnea. Upper respiratory tract infections can result in rhinitis, sinusitis, and laryngitis. Skin infections may be edematous or necrotizing. On necropsy, hemorrhages and necrosis in the liver, spleen, and kidney and enteritis may be noted.

Diagnosis is based on culture of the organism. Treatment consists of susceptible antibiotic therapy and supportive care. *Pseudomonas aeruginosa* is often resistant to many commonly used antibiotics. A combination of amikacin and piperacillin or enrofloxacin may be effective. Base selection of antibiotic on sensitivity testing. Provide supportive care. Control consists of good hygiene with clean water bowls, food bowls, and water pipes. Chlorhexidine is not an effective disinfectant against *Pseudomonas.* Quaternary ammonia, bleach, aldehydes, iodophors, and phenols are effective when properly used.

SALMONELLA. Common sources of *Salmonella* infection include other birds, rodents, flies, and other vectors. Oral ingestion is the most common route of infection, but aerogenous transmission from contaminated dust from feces or feathers and egg transmission occurs. *Salmonella* is zoonotic but avian strains rarely affect humans.

Disease syndromes range from acute to chronic. Multiple organ systems are often involved. Clinical signs of acute disease include lethargy, anorexia, polydipsia, and diarrhea. Clinical signs associated with subacute to chronic infections include dyspnea, CNS signs, or arthritis. Dermatitis, conjunctivitis, iridocyclitis, and panophthalmia may occur. Peracute disease with high flock mortality may occur with *Salmonella* outbreaks in lories and penguins. Chronic disease with granulomatous dermatitis, arthritis, and tenovaginitis is typical with infections in African gray parrots. Tangares, quetzals, barbets, terns, and sparrows commonly have respiratory signs and myocardial lesions. Geese and ducks commonly have CNS signs. Granulomatous ingluvitis may occur with finches. Sudden death is a common presentation in aviary infections. Dehydration, gastroenteritis, hepatomegaly, splenomegaly, bile congestion, nephropathy, and degeneration or necrosis of skeletal muscles may be noted on necropsy. The liver and spleen may contain disseminated small whitish foci. Pericarditis, degeneration or inflammation of the ovary or testis, and liver, spleen, and kidney granulomas are common with chronic infections. Fibrin may fill the cecal lumen.

Diagnosis is based on culture of the organism. Treatment of *Salmonella*-infected birds and carriers is controversial. Select antibiotics based on sensitivity testing, and use drugs with good tissue and cell penetration (e.g., enrofloxacin or chloramphenicol). Clindamycin or a combination of erythromycin and ampicillin are used to treat L forms. Chronic infections and those with CNS signs are usually unresponsive to treatment. Prevent egg transmission by identifying and removing subclinically infected breeders.

YERSINIA. Toucans, toucanets, aracaris, barbets, and turacos are extremely susceptible to *Yersinia pseudotuberculosis*. Finches and ducks are also especially susceptible.

Peracute to chronic infections occur. Peracute disease is characterized by death without clinical signs. On necropsy, hepatomegaly, splenomegaly, and bloody to fibrinous exudate in the body cavity may be noted. Clinical signs associated with acute disease include dehydration, lethargy, diarrhea, and dyspnea. On necropsy, submiliary to miliary, sharply demarcated grayish foci may be noted in the liver, lungs, spleen, and kidneys. Subacute and chronic disease are associated with emaciation, wasting, and flaccid paresis or paralysis. On necropsy, granulomas may be noted in organs and skeletal muscles. Ascites and osteomyelitis may be present. Swollen tarsal joints containing caseous exudate are common in infected ducks.

Diagnosis is based on culture. Place culture swabs or tissues in a cool environment for 2 weeks to increase recovery of the organism.

Parenteral antibiotics are used to treat infections. Chronic cases are difficult to treat because of granuloma formation. To control spread of the disease, treat carriers, use good sanitation procedures, and culture mice before feeding them to toucans or feed only laboratory-raised mice.

Gram-Positive Bacteria

CLOSTRIDIUM. *Clostridium* is part of the normal flora in raptors, ducks, geese, swans, and gallinaceous birds, and it is ubiquitous. Colonization of the intestinal tract appears to depend on decreased gastrointestinal motility. *Clostridium* can cause necrotic enteritis, gangrenous dermatitis, and botulism.

Necrotic enteritis is most common in lorikeets, gallinaceous birds, and ostriches, in primarily young birds. Clinical signs associated with acute disease include diarrhea, polydipsia, and death. Chronic infection may lead to slowed growth, weight loss, and death. On necropsy, diffuse or focal hyperemia, necrosis, or ulceration of the mucosa of the jejunum may be noted. Swelling and necrosis of the liver, spleen, and kidneys are common. Diagnosis is based on identification of characteristic lesions and isolation of the organism.

Gangrenous dermatitis occurs with colonization of damaged skin. A blue-red or almost black discoloration of the skin is characteristic. The skin may also become edematous and painful. Death results from toxemia. On necropsy, emphysema, edema, and hemorrhages in the subcutis, skeletal muscles, and myocardium may be noted. Diagnosis is based on isolation of the organism from affected tissues.

Botulism is usually the result of ingestion of neurotoxins produced by *Clostridium botulinum* in food such as decaying organic matter or maggots that have fed on carcasses containing toxin. Maggots may concentrate the toxin. Clinical signs include an ascending flaccid paralysis. Leg paresis is usually the earliest clinical sign, characterized by the bird sitting on its sternum with legs extended caudally. Leg paresis is followed by wing paresis. Loss of control of the neck and head occurs in the terminal stages, resulting in the term *limber neck disease.* On necropsy, petechial hemorrhage of the cerebellum and focal necrosis and hemorrhage of the central lobe of the cerebrum may be noted. Diagnosis is based on demonstrating the presence of the toxin in serum, liver, or kidney using the mouse protection test. The toxin is heat sensitive, so samples should be preserved by freezing. A commercial antitoxin may be used in the treatment of affected birds.

ENTEROCOCCUS. *Enterococcus* is part of the normal flora of the skin and the mucosal surfaces of the respiratory, digestive, and reproductive tracts. *Enterococcus* is a ubiquitous organism. Infection with *Enterococcus* may be secondary to concomitant infections, immunosuppression, or exposure to a variety of toxins. Septicemia and endocarditis may follow infections in young or immunosuppressed birds. *Enterococcus fecalis* may cause primary respiratory disease in canaries.

Respiratory signs, gastrointestinal signs, omphalitis, paresis, and arthritis can be associated with *Enterococcus* infection. On necropsy, subepicardial and myocardial hemorrhages, serofibrinous polyserositis, congestion of the subcutaneous tissues, serosal membranes, and pericardium, lung congestion, pneumonia, petechiation of the laryngeal and tracheal mucosa, hepatomegaly with green discoloration, catarrhal enteritis, skeletal muscle hemorrhages, and swollen kidneys may be noted in acute cases. Chronic infections may result in arthritis, mucoid exudate, and coagulated or dried exudates in the body cavity, and granulomatous atrioventricular inflammation may be noted.

Diagnosis is based on culture of the organism from affected tissues. Treatment consists of aggressive administration of parenteral antibiotics based on sensitivity testing. Joint and tendon sheath infections may require joint lavage, surgery, and prolonged antibiotic therapy.

ERYSIPELOTHRIX. *Erysipelothrix rhusiopathiae* infections are most common in ducks and geese, but they can occur in other species. *Erysipelothrix rhusiopathiae* is a ubiquitous organism. Infections are most common in the late fall, winter, and early spring in the northern hemisphere. Rodents, pigs, and raw fish are reservoirs.

Erysipelothrix rhusiopathiae infection usually results in peracute death. Lethargy, weakness, anorexia, dyspnea, greenish discolored droppings, nasal discharge, and hyperemia or bruising of the skin may occur. On necropsy, petechiae may be seen in the subcutis, musculature, and intestinal mucosa, and discolored (red to black) and friable liver and spleen may be noted.

Diagnosis is based on culture of the organism. The best samples for culture from fresh tissues are liver or spleen. Treatment includes antibiotic therapy based on sensitivity testing. A bacterin is available, but it may potentiate chronic disease. Hygiene and rodent control are important in control of the disease.

LISTERIA. *Listeria* can infect canaries, psittacines, and other species. *Listeria monocytogenes* is a ubiquitous organism.

Acute disease usually results in bacteremia and death within 1 to 2 days. On necropsy, no lesions may be noted, or a few petechiae may be noted. If clinical signs occur with subacute and chronic infection, blindness, torticollis, tremor, stupor, and paresis or paralysis may be observed. Subacute and chronic infections usually result in a marked monocytosis, ten to twelve times normal. On necropsy, serofibrinous pericarditis and myocardial necrosis may be noted. No gross lesions are usually evident in the brain.

Diagnosis is based on isolation of the organism from affected tissues. Special transport media are required to maintain viability of samples during shipment.

MEGABACTERIA. Megabacteria are large (1 × 09 μm) rods found in the proventriculus of normal and abnormal birds. The organism is difficult to culture. Disease believed to be associated with this organism is most common in budgies, cockatiels, finches, canaries, and lovebirds. It has been reported in young ostriches, chickens, and a cockatoo.

Clinical signs include chronic emaciation over a 12- to 18-month period that may involve intermittent periods of recovery. Digested blood may be present in the feces. Some birds recover spontaneously.

Radiology may reveal proventricular dilatation. An hourglass-like retraction between the proventriculus and ventriculus with contrast radiography is suggestive of megabacteriosis. Gram's staining of feces may reveal the organism in severely affected birds.

On necropsy, proventriculitis or proventricular ulcers with or without hemorrhages may be noted. The organism can be readily seen at low magnification from proventricular scrapings.

The organism is resistant to all antibiotics. Lactobacillus may lower the pH of the gastrointestinal tract and may help.

MYCOBACTERIUM AVIUM. All species of birds may be susceptible to *M. avium*. Mycobacteriosis is especially common in waterfowl, gray-cheek parakeets, and other *Brotogeris* species. Budgies, ring-necked and related parakeets, Amazon parrots, *Pionus* parrots, canaries, and toucans are other pet birds commonly affected. The organism is shed in the feces and urine, contaminating the soil, water, and food sources, resulting in ingestion and infection. *Mycobacterium avium* can survive in the environment for months to years. Aerosol transmission of *M. avium* can occur.

Mycobacterium avium affects the digestive tract in most birds. Pigeons, doves, ducks, geese, and some weaver finches typically develop a respiratory infection. Clinical signs are variable and may include chronic wasting usually associated with a good appetite, diarrhea, polyuria, anemia, lameness, poor feathering, abdominal distention, conjunctival masses, and skin or oropharyngeal granulomas or ulcers. Respiratory signs may occur if the lungs are affected.

On necropsy, the intestinal wall may be thickened, and hepatomegaly, splenomegaly, or granulomas may be observed in the wall of the intestinal tract, liver, spleen, skin, or bone marrow. The liver and spleen may contain necrotic foci.

Diagnosis is based on clinical signs, cytology, hematology, radiology, acid-fast positive rods in tissues or on cytologic preparations, and culture of the organism. Mycobacteriosis is a chronic disease resulting in granuloma formation. Very high white blood cell (WBC) counts are common with *Mycobacterium* infection. Cytology of aspirates or impression smears reveal heterophils, lymphocytes, macrophages or epithelioid cells with ghostlike nonstaining rods, and occasionally giant cells. Radiographs may reveal focal osteolytic disease; endosteal bone densities in the humerus, tibiotarsus, ulna, and occasionally the femur; or hepatomegaly, splenomegaly, or pulmonary granulomas. Intestines may appear thickened and may contain gas. A single area of punctate radiolucency of bone may occur with mycobacteriosis.

Use acid-fast staining to identify acid-fast positive *Mycobacterium*. Biopsy samples (liver or lung) may reveal acid-fast positive organisms. Feces are useful in suspected cases showing clinical signs of mycobacteriosis. Samples from the trachea are useful if the organism is causing a respiratory infection. A negative result does not rule out mycobacteriosis, because the bird must be shedding the organism in numbers high enough to produce a positive result. Submit samples to laboratories familiar with avian mycobacteriosis to decrease false-positive results. Plasma protein electrophoresis (EPH) is useful for diagnosis of mycobacteriosis. Liver biopsy may be the best method for routine diagnosis of mycobacteriosis. Culture is required for definitive diagnosis.

Treatment of *M. avium* infection is controversial. The extent of the zoonotic potential of *M. avium* is unclear. There appears to be minimal zoonotic potential in immunocompetent adult humans, but there may be a significant risk of infection in immunocompromised individuals and children. Infected birds may continuously shed large numbers of the organism in the environment. Euthanasia must be considered in birds definitively diagnosed with *M. avium* through biopsy of affected tissues and histopathology and culture.

Some drug combinations used to treat mycobacteriosis are listed in Table 9–1. An intact immune system may be required in additional to chemotherapy to eliminate the organism. Length of treatment has not been determined in birds. Many birds become asymptomatic within 1 month of initiating therapy, but treatment for at least 1 year is recommended. Biopsy of previously affected organs, hematology, and radiology are performed at 9 months of treatment. Isolate infected birds for the duration of the treatment.

Exposed birds are removed from the contaminated area, quarantined for 2 years, and periodically screened with serology, hematology, and fecal acid-fast staining. Contaminated soil should be removed to a depth of at least 6 inches. Contaminated ponds should be drained and dredged.

STAPHYLOCOCCUS. *Staphylococcus* may occur as part of the normal flora or act as a primary or secondary pathogen.

Staphylococcus aureus may occur as a part of the normal flora of the skin or mucosal surfaces of the respiratory and gastrointestinal tracts. These bacteria may also act as primary or secondary pathogens. The decision to treat should be based on the likelihood of the organism acting as a pathogen (see Chapter 12). Diagnosis is based on culture.

STREPTOCOCCUS. *Streptococcus* is a ubiquitous organism and part of the normal flora of the skin and mucosal surfaces of the respiratory, digestive, and reproductive tracts. This organism may act as a pathogen in immunosupressed birds, occur as a secondary pathogen, or occasionally act as a primary pathogen. Base the decision to treat on the likelihood of the organism acting as a pathogen (see Chapter 12). Diagnosis is based on culture.

TABLE 9–1. Some Drug Combinations Used to Treat Mycobacteriosis

Azithromycin, 43 mg/kg°; ethambutol, 30 mg/kg† (56–85 mg/kg°); rifabutin, 15 mg/kg† (56 mg/kg°) PO SID
Clarithromycin, 85 mg/kg°; ethambutol, 30 mg/kg† (56–85 mg/kg°); rifabutin, 15 mg/kg† (56 mg/kg°) PO SID
Either of the above with a fluoroquinolone, 15 mg/kg PO BID, or aminoglycoside, 15 mg/kg PO BID
Either of the first two with clofazamine, 6 mg/kg† (6–12 mg/kg°)PO BID

SID = once daily; PO = by mouth; BID = twice daily.
°mg/kg = dose based on allometric scaling.
†mg/kg = dose used in literature.

Chlamydia

CHLAMYDIA PSITTACI. *Chlamydia psittaci* is the organism that causes psittacosis in birds and ornithosis in other animals and humans. It is an obligate intracellular bacteria that does not grow on cell-free media. There are many strains of *Chlamydia psittaci*. Virulence and clinical signs depend on the strain and host species. Macaws and Amazon parrots appear more susceptible than cockatoos and African gray parrots. Young birds are generally more susceptible to *Chlamydia* infections than are adults. Carrier states exist. Cockatiels are common carriers. Stress may result in clinical signs or increase shedding of the organism in carriers.

The organism is shed in feces, urine, oropharyngeal mucus, and lacrimal and nasal secretions, and crop milk in pigeons. The organism can survive for long periods in dried feces and secretions. The organism is usually ingested, but vertical transmission also occurs.

Clinical signs of infection depend on the age of the bird, virulence of the strain, and the species of the bird infected. Common clinical signs include diarrhea, anorexia, depression, biliverdinuria, sneezing, mucopurulent nasal discharge, dyspnea, sinusitis, and conjunctivitis. Clinical signs associated with low-grade, chronic infections include poor feathering, wasting, diarrhea, and sometimes conjunctivitis. Central nervous system signs occur occasionally and may include tremors, seizures, opisthotonos, and paralysis. *Chlamydia* can cause a localized infection and conjunctivitis in finches. Conjunctivitis and nasal discharge are characteristic of chlamydiosis in domestic pigeons. Conjunctivitis may be the predominant clinical sign of chlamydiosis in infected ducks and geese.

On necropsy, gross lesions vary. Common lesions include airsacculitis, hepatomegaly, splenomegaly, enteritis, peritonitis, pericarditis, bronchopneumonia, and sinusitis. No gross lesions may be noted in some infected birds.

Diagnosis is based on clinical signs, clinical pathology, radiology, and cytology with the help of culture, serology, and electrophoresis. At this time, there is no single test that will detect infection in all infected or carrier birds and not result in false-positive results in uninfected birds.

A severe leukocytosis is common in *Chlamydia*-infected large psittacines, primarily due to a heterophilia, monocytosis, and basophilia. A normal WBC count may be present with subclinical infections. Small birds usually show only a mild leukocytosis. An anemia may be present, and an elevation of aspartate aminotransferase (AST or SGOT), lactate dehydrogenase (LDH), creatine kinase (CK), and bile acids is common.

Radiology often reveals hepatomegaly, airsacculitis, and splenomegaly.

Cytology is useful in diagnosing chlamydiosis in birds with conjunctivitis or on postmortem samples of the liver, spleen, air sacs, and pericardium. Conjunctival smears of infected birds may contain macrophages with small, round, basophilic intracytoplasmic inclusions (seen with Wright's or Diff-Quik stain) and heterophils, lymphocytes, and plasma cells (Fig. 12–19). On necropsy, impression smears of air sacs and the uncut surfaces of the liver, spleen, and pericardium may contain macrophages with chlamydial inclusions described above. Macchiavellos and Gimenez stains aid in the identification of chlamydial inclusions (Fig. 12–17).

Serology is useful in birds large enough to provide a blood sample adequate for evaluation (40 to 50 g and larger birds). False-negative titers can occur early in the disease before antibody production. Low titers may be difficult to interpret. The laboratory performing the titer will aid in interpretation of titer results. Enzyme-linked immunosorbent assay (ELISA), complement fixation (CF), latex agglutination (LA), and elementary body agglutination (EBA) are serologic tests useful in the diagnosis of chlamydiosis. A positive ELISA titer indicates either an active infection or past infection. False-negative results may occur before antibody production, but the ELISA test can detect infections earlier than can CF and LA tests.

Complement fixation is useful in detecting recently infected birds, but chronic infections may be missed. Paired serum samples collected 2 weeks apart are needed to establish a positive diagnosis. A single serum sample is of value if the titer is sufficiently high. Titers up to 1:8 are considered negative. Titers of 1:16 to 1:32 are suspicious, and titers greater than 1:64 are considered positive. Titers drop slowly and may remain high after successful treatment. False-negative results may occur early in the disease before adequate antibody formation. Young birds, budgies, cockatiels, canaries, and finches may not produce antibody titers high enough to be detected by CF.

Latex agglutination is less sensitive than CF, but it can be used to detect current infections and monitor success of treatment. Latex agglutination titers drop quickly when *Chlamydia* are eliminated from the body. Positive LA titers indicate a current infection. False-negative results are common in budgies, cockatiels, lovebirds, and some young birds and in later stages of the disease.

An EBA titer of 10 or 20 may indicate a low-grade infection or past infection. A titer of 40 may indicate a current infection or recently treated infection. A titer of 80 or more may indicate chlamydial infection. Confirm results with other chlamydial tests or hematology and plasma biochemistries.

Chlamydial antigen may be detected in nasal, ocular, cloacal, and oropharyngeal swabs using the Kodak SureCell Chlamydia test or Clearview Chlamydia test (Table 9–2). Useful samples include choana, naso-ocular discharges, or cloaca. These tests are useful for in-house testing of sick birds. False-negative results occur as a result of intermittent shedding or antibiotic therapy or when insufficient numbers of chlamydial particles are present in the sample. False-positive results can occur when high concentrations of some other bacteria are present. Confirm positive antigen results with another method of testing. Negative results should be interpreted with caution in asymptomatic birds.

Culture is considered the current standard for *Chlamydia* detection. Culturing

---

TABLE 9–2. Products Used for Diagnosis and Treatment of Various Diseases

Kodak SureCell Chlamydia Test: Eastman Kodak Co., Rochester, NY
Clearview Chlamydia Test: Wampole Labs, Cranbury, NJ 08512 (800) 257-9525
Roudybush Proventricular Formula, Kidney Formula, Obesity Formula: Roudybush, Paso Robles, CA (800) 326-1726; FAX (805) 237-9993
Harrison's Low Iron Formula, Adult Lifetime Formula: Harrison's Bird Diets, Omaha, NE (800) 346-0269
Kaytee Softbill Diet: Kaytee Products, Chilton, WI (800) 529-8331
Bird of Paradise Diet: Ziegler Bros. Inc., Gardners, PA (800) 841-6800

requires live organisms, and shedding may be intermittent, resulting in false-negative results. Useful samples include exudates or feces in live animals. Consider collection of multiple samples over several days. Spleen, liver, or air sacs are useful postmortem samples. Samples must be placed in proper transport media and must be taken before administration of antibiotics. The organisms must be viable to be detected by culture.

Electrophoresis may also be useful in establishing a diagnosis of chlamydiosis. Treat all suspected and confirmed cases of *Chlamydia* infections.

Tetracyclines are used to treat chlamydial infections. Doxycycline may be used orally, or specially formulated intramuscular (IM) preparations can be injected. The intravenous (IV) form of doxycycline should not be injected IM or subcutaneously. Feeds medicated with doxycycline and chlortetracycline have been used successfully. Long-term treatment is necessary, and the organism may possibly survive a prolonged course of treatment. During treatment, hygienic practices are important. Decrease exposure to aerosolized feces and feather dander with daily removal of droppings from the cage.

Supportive care may be required, including heat, tube feeding, fluid therapy, and antibiotic therapy for secondary bacterial infections.

Prevention of introduction of chlamydiosis into a collection of birds is difficult. Lack of an accurate screening test for carriers makes detection difficult. Quarantine new birds and perform serologic and antigen screening tests to decrease likelihood of introduction of the disease into aviaries.

Chlamydiosis is a zoonotic disease resulting in flulike symptoms in infected humans, including fever, severe headaches, and shortness of breath, and it may result in death.

Mycoplasma

Pathogenic strains of *Mycoplasma* occur in poultry and waterfowl. The significance of *Mycoplasma* infections in pet birds is unproved. In pet birds, it is usually associated with sinusitis or conjunctivitis in budgies and cockatiels. Infections are most common when birds are overcrowded. Specialized media are required for culture of the organism. Treat with tetracyclines, fluoroquinolones, or macrolides.

Viruses

ADENOVIRUS. Many species of birds are susceptible to adenovirus. Psittacines may die without prior clinical signs, or they may show signs associated with hepatitis, pancreatitis, pneumonia, or enteritis (diarrhea, yellow urates, polyuria, dyspnea, depression, and lethargy); CNS signs; conjunctivitis; and death. On necropsy, the liver may be mottled, discolored, enlarged, and friable.

Electron microscopy may be used to detect the virus in feces or pharyngeal secretions. The virus may be isolated from feces or pharyngeal secretions. Postmortem samples for virus isolation include liver, kidney, intestines, or pancreas.

Treatment includes supportive care and antibiotics to prevent secondary bacterial infections.

AMAZON TRACHEITIS. Amazon parrots, chickens, and the common pheasant are susceptible to the Amazon tracheitis virus. Clinical signs in Amazon parrots include nasal and ocular discharges, dyspnea, and coughing. The disease may be peracute, acute, subacute, or chronic. Pharyngeal swabs are useful for culture of the virus. Treatment includes supportive care and prevention of secondary bacterial infections and contagion.

AVIAN INFLUENZA. Most species of birds are susceptible to avian influenza virus. The disease is called fowl plague in chickens. Clinical signs in psittacines can include lethargy, diarrhea, respiratory signs, CNS signs, and death. Definitive diagnosis is based on demonstration of the organism. Cloacal and tracheal swabs are useful in live birds. Lung, liver, spleen, and brain are the best postmortem samples for isolation of the virus. Treatment is nonspecific and consists of supportive care. Isolate treated birds for 3 to 4 weeks after resolution of clinical signs.

AVIAN PICORNAVIRUS ENCEPHALOMYELITIS. Chickens, pheasants, waterfowl, turkeys, and Japanese quail are susceptible to avian encephalomyelitis. Clinical signs include depression, ataxia, paresis or paralysis, and fine head and neck tremors. Diagnosis is based on antibody detection or postmortem histology. Vaccines are available for use in chickens and turkeys.

AVIAN SARCOMA/LEUKOSIS VIRUS. Avian sarcoma/leukosis virus has been described in many species of birds. Clinical signs vary with the organ or organs affected. This virus induces various types of neoplasia (e.g., fibrosarcoma, mesothelioma, endothelioma, chondroma). It may damage the immune system, resulting in infections. Abdominal distention and dyspnea may be present, caused by abdominal tumors. The liver may be enlarged. Multiple tumors, often involving multiple organs, usually occur with this infection. Lymphoid leukosis is common in chickens. Plasma, serum, or neoplastic tissue is best for demonstrating the presence of avian sarcoma/leukosis virus. Treatment is generally ineffective; prednisolone may prolong survival time. Vaccines are not available.

AVIAN VIRAL SEROSITIS FORM OF EASTERN EQUINE ENCEPHALITIS. Some psittacines are susceptible to avian viral serositis, including macaws, rose-ringed parakeets, and others. The disease appears to be primarily a problem in young birds. Infected birds may die acutely or develop clinical signs, including abdominal distention, ascites, and weight loss, and they may develop respiratory distress.

DUCK VIRAL ENTERITIS (DUCK PLAGUE). Ducks, geese, and swans of all ages are susceptible to duck plague. The incubation period is 3 to 12 days. Clinical signs include depression, nasal discharge, serous to hemorrhagic lacrimation, conjunctivitis, dyspnea, cyanosis, polydipsia, anorexia, vomiting, diarrhea, photophobia, and occasionally CNS signs. Death may occur without clinical signs. On necropsy, annular bands of hemorrhage are common in the intestine. Petechiae may be seen on the surface of the esophagus and intestine, and diphtheritic membranes and hemorrhage may be noted on the mucosa of the oropharynx, esophagus, intestines, and cloaca. Virus isolation is required for definitive diagnosis. Administration of an attenuated-live virus vaccine may reduce mortality during an outbreak.

DUCK VIRAL HEPATITIS. Duck viral hepatitis affects young ducks up to 3 weeks of age. The disease spreads rapidly, with sudden onset of signs and an acute course of the disease. Clinical signs include lethargy, weakness, ataxia, and death.

GOULDIAN FINCH HERPESVIRUS. Gouldian finch herpesvirus affects gouldian finches and possibly other finches and waxbills. Clinical signs include chemosis, swollen eyelids, mild nasal discharge, and severe dyspnea. Histopathology is used for diagnosis. Treatment includes symptomatic therapy.

PIGEON HERPESVIRUS (INCLUSION BODY HEPATITIS VIRUS OF PIGEONS). Pigeons and budgerigars are susceptible to pigeon herpesvirus. Birds of any age can be infected, but squabs 4 to 16 weeks of age are most susceptible. Clinical signs include rhinitis, nasal discharge, conjunctivitis, dyspnea, diarrhea, anorexia, vomiting, and polydipsia. Central nervous system signs may also occur. Ulcers may occur on the mucous membranes of the larynx and oropharynx, cere, and commissure of the beak. On necropsy, no gross lesions may be noted, or small ulcerations may be observed on the mucosa of the upper respiratory tract and occasionally on the crop and intestines. Systemic infections may result in hepatomegaly and splenomegaly. In live birds, swabs from ulcerative lesions may reveal intranuclear inclusion bodies in epithelial cells. Pharyngeal swabs and feces may be used for virus isolation. Antibodies may be detected in infected birds. On necropsy, oropharyngeal swabs, feces, trachea, lungs, and liver may be used to isolate the virus. Carriers may intermittently shed the virus and are difficult to identify. Provide supportive care for treatment.

INFECTIOUS LARYNGOTRACHEITIS. Chickens, pheasants, and peafowl are susceptible to infectious laryngotracheitis. Canaries may also be susceptible to infectious laryngotracheitis in addition to a herpesvirus strain found only in canaries. All ages of birds are susceptible, but the disease is most common in young birds. Clinical signs and severity vary with the virulence of the strain and environmental factors and include anorexia, depression, coughing, sneezing, dyspnea, inspiratory wheeze, expectoration of bloody mucus, ocular and nasal discharge, and sinusitis. On necropsy, tracheal mucosa may be thickened, and hemorrhagic or fibrinous inflammation may be noted. Necrotic debris, casts, or fibrinonecrotic pseudomembranes may be noted in the trachea. Yellow necrotic plaques may be present in the oropharynx. Diagnosis is based on virus isolation, which is most successful early in the disease. Collect samples from a number of birds, especially those with recent infection. Fluorescent antibody staining of smears or sections from the trachea, ELISA, immunodiffusion, and virus neutralization can be used for diagnosis. Intranuclear inclusion bodies in respiratory epithelial cells from tracheal swabs are indicative but not confirmatory of the disease and may not be detected in all infected birds. Treatment includes supportive care. Vaccines are available for chickens.

MAREK'S DISEASE. Marek's disease is primarily a disease of chickens 12 to 24 weeks of age. Clinical signs may include paralysis or signs associated with viral-induced lymphoid tumors in the liver, spleen, kidney, skin, muscle, bone, or gonads. On necropsy, enlarged peripheral nerves are common and visceral tumors may be noted. Heparinized blood is the preferred antemortem sample for virus isolation. Liver, spleen, kidneys, and viral-induced tumors are useful postmortem samples for virus isolation. Acyclovir reduces disease severity. Vaccination, management procedures, and genetics are used to aid in control of the virus in gallinaceous birds.

PACHECO'S DISEASE. Pacheco's disease is a herpesvirus affecting only psittacine birds. New World psittacines appear more susceptible than do Old World psittacines. Most birds showing clinical signs die within 2 days. Infection with less-virulent strains may result in acute deaths in highly susceptible birds, and other birds may show clinical signs for several days to several weeks, including respiratory disease, diarrhea, and polyuria. Nanday and Patagonian conures appear resistant to the disease and may be asymptomatic carriers that intermittently shed the virus. Any bird that recovers from Pacheco's disease infection may be a carrier. Carriers can shed the virus in the feces when stressed. Large concentrations of the virus are shed in feces and respiratory secretions of clinical ill birds. Transmission usually occurs by the oral route, usually through contamination of food and water. Aerosol transmission may occur. The incubation period is approximately 3 to 14 days.

The most common clinical sign is sudden death or death after a very brief illness in birds in excellent body condition. Clinical signs can consist of fluffing, lethargy, depression, anorexia, regurgitation, diarrhea, and biliverdinuria (green urates). Sinusitis, polydipsia, polyuria, conjunctivitis, and CNS signs (tremors, ataxia, opisthotonos, seizures) may also occur.

On necropsy, usually no lesions are noted, but kidney enlargement, hepatomegaly, focal hepatic necrosis and hemorrhage, and splenomegaly may be present. Hemorrhage may be present in the skin, liver, spleen, pancreas, intestinal tract, and body cavity.

Pacheco's disease is suspected based on suggestive clinical signs, necropsy, and the presence of intranuclear inclusion bodies observed histologically in the liver, kidney, or spleen. Inclusions caused by Pacheco's disease virus may appear similar to polyomavirus or adenovirus. Definitive diagnosis is based on virus isolation from liver, kidney, intestine, or feces or by specific immunohistochemical studies, electron microscopy, or viral-specific DNA probes.

Isolate ill birds. Treatment includes supportive care, limiting spread of the disease, and acyclovir. Acyclovir is used to increase survival of infected birds and decrease virus dissemination in an outbreak. Acyclovir may be administered to exposed birds by gavage or in the food (e.g., beans and rice or mash formulation) if they are still eating. Treat for 7 days. Birds with clinical signs are given acyclovir by gavage every 8 hours until they are eating; then it can be added to food. Fluid therapy and nonhepatotoxic antibiotics (e.g., trimethoprim/sulfadiazine or enrofloxacin) to prevent secondary bacterial infections are beneficial.

Control of Pacheco's disease is accomplished through isolating all birds with clinical signs and latently infected birds. Disinfect cages and feces-contaminated surfaces of affected birds. Identify and remove suspected latently infected birds. Birds that are common carriers of the disease (e.g., Nanday and Patagonian conures) should be housed separately from susceptible species. A Pacheco's disease vaccine is available, but granulomas and paralysis after administration of the vaccine have been reported. Cockatoos, blue and gold macaws, and African gray parrots appear to be especially sensitive to the vaccine.

PAPILLOMAVIRUS. Papillomavirus has been detected in skin tumors in finches, canaries, and African gray parrots. Gastrointestinal papillomas are common in psittacine birds, but a viral etiology has not been proved. Skin papillomas appear as wartlike epithelial proliferations on the feet, legs, head, or eyelids. The papillomas common in psittacines occur on mucosal surfaces of the gastrointestinal tract. Cloacal papillomas are common in Amazon parrots, macaws, and hawk-headed parrots. Cloacal papillomas appear as singular or multiple pink to red raised proliferative growths in the cloaca or protruding from the cloaca. Oral papillomas resemble cloacal papillomas. Clinical signs associated with cloacal papillomas include straining to defecate, blood in droppings, malodorous stools, flatulence, and persistent enteric bacterial infections. Oral papillomas may cause dyspnea, wheezing, dysphagia, and persistent oral bacterial infections. Clinical signs associated with crop, esophageal, and proventricular papillomas may include regurgitation, vomiting, and weight loss. Bile duct carcinomas have occurred in some birds affected by cloacal papillomas; clinical signs included decreased activity, weight loss, and anorexia.

Diagnosis is based on physical examination, biopsy, and histopathology. Application of 5% acetic acid (e.g., apple cider vinegar) to suspected lesions cause papillomatous lesions to blanch from red or pink to white. A definitive diagnosis of papillomavirus requires demonstration of the virus particles or antigen in lesions, which may be detected with immunohistochemical techniques or electron microscopy.

Papillomas are treated by cauterization (preferable) or surgical removal. Care must be taken to prevent excessive tissue damage and scarring. Electrosurgery is required for surgical removal to limit blood loss. Silver nitrate sticks may be used to cauterize the lesions. The lesions are exteriorized with a moistened cotton swab, and the lesion is treated by rubbing the silver nitrate stick on the affected area. The area is immediately flushed with fluids to prevent cauterization of unaffected tissues. The procedure is repeated every 2 weeks until complete removal is achieved.

An infectious etiology of gastrointestinal papillomas is suspected. A thorough physical examination may aid in control of spread of the disease. Avoid addition of birds with lesions to a collection.

PARAMYXOVIRUS. Many serotypes of paramyxoviruses affect birds. Paramyxoviruses 1, 2, and 3 are clinically important in pet birds. Paramyxovirus 1 includes the strain that causes Newcastle disease and other strains. Newcastle disease affects many species of birds, but susceptibility and clinical course of the disease is variable between species. All ages of birds are susceptible. The virus is excreted in the feces and respiratory secretions, and oral and respiratory routes of transmission occur. Vertical transmission and infection of embryos through virus-contaminated egg shells occurs. The incubation period for Newcastle disease is typically 4 to 7 days.

Clinical signs vary with the strain and species of bird infected. Common clinical signs include diarrhea, anorexia, nasal and ocular discharges, conjunctivitis, dyspnea, and CNS signs. At necropsy, no gross lesions may be observed, or petechiae on serosal surfaces and mucosa of the larynx, trachea, and proventriculus; necrotizing enteritis; or hyperemia of the brain may be noted.

Definitive diagnosis is based on culturing the virus from feces or respiratory discharges in live birds or from affected organs at necropsy. Serology can also be used for diagnosis of paramyxovirus 1 infections, but titers vary. Inform the United States Department of Agriculture of all birds diagnosed as having Newcastle disease.

There is no treatment for Newcastle disease. Hyperimmune serum can be used to protect exposed birds, but it is ineffective once clinical signs are present.

The main source of Newcastle disease virus infection is smuggled birds. No vaccine is available for psittacine birds.

Paramyxovirus 2 can cause mild upper respiratory tract disease in passerines, and pneumonia, tracheitis, emaciation, and death in psittacines.

Paramyxovirus 3 can cause diarrhea, dyspnea, dysphagia, CNS signs, and death in passerines, and ocular lesions, paralysis, and nasal discharge in psittacines.

POLYOMAVIRUS. Polyomavirus is the virus that causes budgerigar fledgling disease, but it also causes illness in larger psittacines. Infected budgies younger than 15 days of age may die suddenly with no premonitory signs, or they may develop clinical signs, including abdominal distention, subcutaneous hemorrhage, head and neck tremors, ataxia, and symmetrical feather abnormalities. Feather abnormalities include loss of developing primary and secondary feathers, dystrophic primary and tail feathers, lack of down feathers on the back and abdomen, and lack of filoplumes on the head and neck. These feather lesions may appear grossly the same as those resulting from psittacine beak and feather disease (PBFD) or nutritional problems. Many affected birds are unable to fly and are called runners or hoppers. Feather lesions usually resolve after several months. Budgies infected after 14 days of age may show similar clinical signs, but the mortality rate is much lower.

Polyomavirus infection in larger psittacines may result in death without premonitory signs or death after a brief (12 to 24 hours) illness. Clinical signs include anorexia, depression, weight loss, delayed crop emptying, regurgitation, diarrhea, dehydration, subcutaneous hemorrhages, dyspnea, and polyuria. Central nervous system signs may also occur. Feather abnormalities associated with polyomavirus infection are uncommon in larger psittacines. Clinical signs are common at weaning. Most psittacines in excess of 6 months of age do not become ill when exposed to polyomavirus. Lovebirds, eclectus parrots, caiques, and some Australian parakeets may die as a result of polyomavirus infection as young adults or adults.

Hepatomegaly, splenomegaly, subcutaneous hemorrhage, intestinal and subserosal hemorrhage, epicardial and myocardial hemorrhage, pale kidneys, pale skeletal musculature, and feather dystrophy may be noted at the time of necropsy. Ascites and hydropericardium may also be observed.

Polyomavirus may be shed in the feces and feather dust. Transmission can occur through oral or aerogenous routes. Vertical transmission may occur. The incubation period appears to be short (5 to 7 days).

A presumptive diagnosis is based on clinical signs and necropsy findings. A definitive diagnosis is based on viral-specific DNA probes, histopathology, or immunohistochemical staining of tissues. Shedding is intermittent in latently infected carrier birds. A DNA probe test of cloacal swabs will detect infected and carrier birds if the bird is shedding the virus. The best sample to submit for DNA probe testing at necropsy is a swab of the cut surfaces of liver, spleen, and kidney on one swab.

Treatment for polyomavirus infection includes supportive care and vitamin K injections. Control is achieved through removal of carrier birds from the aviary, never introducing birds from other collections into the nursery, using one prefilled feeding syringe per bird for each feeding, and disinfecting syringes before each use. Avoid raising budgies and lovebirds with expensive psittacines because they are a common source of polyomavirus. Never introduce birds from other collections into the nursery; exposure of weanlings may result in a devastating clinical course of disease. All young birds brought into the aviary should be quarantined in separate facilities where strict hygienic practices are used. Using separate disinfected syringes for each chick will decrease spread of the disease. Quaternary ammonium disinfectants containing a detergent or a stabilized chlorine dioxide disinfectant are used to disinfect the syringes after thoroughly cleaning. Bleach diluted 1:10 or 1:20 can be used to disinfect bowls, incubators, and other equipment after cleaning to remove organic material. Chlorhexidine is a poor disinfectant against polyomavirus.

Treat with supportive care. Carrier birds may be difficult to identify, and DNA probe testing will only identify birds shedding the virus. Testing birds at the beginning and end of the breeding season, before selling, and after purchase will identify many of the carrier birds. Carrier birds that intermittently shed the virus have been thought to maintain high antibody titers; therefore, serology may be useful in screening for polyomavirus carriers.

A polyomavirus vaccine is available.

POXVIRUS. Poxvirus is uncommon in pet birds. It is most common in quarantine stations, canaries, pigeons, and wild birds. Pathotypes are adapted to certain species of birds. Amazonpox is most virulent for Amazon parrots and *Pionus* species, but it also affects conures, macaws, caiques, and parakeets. Lovebirdpox is most virulent for lovebirds. Cockatiels, cockatoos, African parrots, lories, lorikeets, and eclectus parrots are rarely affected by poxviruses. Canarypox can cause disease in canaries and the species that can be crossed with them. Psittacines are resistant to poxviruses that affect birds of other avian orders.

Poxvirus is transmitted through mechanical vectors (mosquitos), ingestion, or inhalation or by direct transmission of the virus between birds through wounds. The incubation period is 5 to 10 days.

Clinical signs vary with the virulence and pathotype of the virus strain, mode of transmission, and susceptibility of the host. There are cutaneous, diphtheroid, and septicemic forms of the disease. The cutaneous form, sometimes called dry pox, is the most common form of disease in raptors and passerines (Fig. 9–1). It is rare in psittacines. Signs include papular lesions on unfeathered skin around

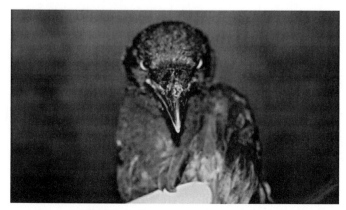

Figure 9–1. Cutaneous poxvirus in a crow.

the eyes, beak, nares, legs, and feet. The lesions progress from macule, papule, pustule, to scab. Periorbital lesions may cause blepharitis, symblepharon, keratitis, uveitis, cataracts, and shrunken globe. Lesions may become secondarily infected with bacteria or fungi. The diphtheroid form, sometimes called wet pox, is the most common form in psittacines. Signs include fibrinous to caseous gray to brown lesions on the mucosa of the tongue, oropharynx, and larynx. Dyspnea may also occur. Cutaneous and diphtheroid forms may occur in the same bird and in flock outbreaks. The septicemic form is most common in canaries and finches. Clinical signs include an acute onset of fluffing, somnolence, cyanosis, and anorexia.

Diagnosis is based on cytology, histopathology, or cultures. Aspirate samples from cutaneous lesions may reveal Bollinger bodies, which are large cytoplasmic vacuoles that push the nucleus to the margin of the cell. Bollinger bodies contain tiny, round, pale inclusions that stain eosinophilic with Wright's stain. Inflammatory cells are common and may be the result of secondary bacterial or fungal infections. Culture is usually necessary for diagnosis of the septicemic form of the disease.

Antibiotics are used to prevent and treat secondary bacterial infections in birds infected with poxvirus. Selection of antibiotics and antifungals for treatment of secondary bacterial and fungal infections is based on culture and sensitivity testing. Vitamin A supplementation may be helpful. Periocular lesions are treated with topical antibiotic ophthalmic ointment. Do not remove scabs, but soften them with hot or cold compresses soaked in nonirritating baby shampoo. The eyes are then rinsed with a merbromin eyewash, prepared by adding 1 ounce of 2% merbromin to 4 ounces of eyewash solution. Follow this with a topical antibiotic ophthalmic ointment. Daily cleaning and opening the lids often decreases scarring. Crusts may be teased apart at the lateral canthus to allow ocular antibiotic ointment administration. The course of the disease usually takes 3 to 4 weeks for an individual bird to recover. Flock outbreaks last 2 to 3 months.

Control in multiple bird households includes isolation of infected birds, mosquito control, and disinfection of surfaces exposed to infected birds. Effective disinfectants include 1% potassium hydroxide (KOH), 2% sodium hydroxide (NaOH), and 5% phenol. Vaccines are available for psittacines, canaries, pigeons, and domestic fowl and may be useful in high-risk populations such as imported birds, birds exposed to imported birds, and birds in areas in which there are high densities of mosquitos. Some deaths have been associated with vaccine administration.

PSITTACINE BEAK AND FEATHER DISEASE VIRUS. Only psittacines are susceptible to PBFD. Young birds appear to be the most susceptible to infection. The peracute and acute forms of the disease are seen primarily in young psittacines. The chronic form may occur at any age.

The virus is shed in feather dust, feces, and crop secretions. Infection occurs by ingestion or inhalation or vertically (egg transmission). The minimum incubation period is 21 to 25 days, and the maximum incubation period is months to years.

Infection with PBFD virus can cause peracute, acute, or chronic disease. The peracute form occurs in neonatal psittacines, resulting in depression, crop stasis, enteritis, pneumonia, and death. The acute form occurs in fledgling birds and is characterized by several days of depression, crop stasis, and diarrhea. Abnormal feathers may develop, including necrosis, fractures, bending, bleeding, or premature shedding of diseased feathers. Few or many feathers may be affected. The chronic form of the disease is characterized by the development of progressive dystrophic feathers. Abnormalities include retention of sheaths, hemorrhage in pulp cavities, fractured feathers, circumferential constrictions, and short, clubbed, deformed, or curled feathers. Abnormalities are progressive, and birds will develop baldness as feather follicles become inactive if they live long enough. In general, the first feathers affected in older birds are the powder down and contour feathers, and then the primary, secondary, tail, and crest feathers. Abnormal coloration may mark dystrophic feathers, especially in African gray parrots (affected feathers may be red instead of gray). Oral and beak lesions may occur, including progressive elongation of the beak, transverse or longitudinal fractures of the beak, oral ulcerations, and palatine necrosis (necrosis in the rostral dorsal mouth). Deformities, fractures, necrosis, and sloughing of the nails occasionally occur.

At necropsy, peracute cases may show severe bursal or thymic necrosis. Acute and chronic infections may result in feather lesions.

Diagnosis is based on viral-specific DNA probes or finding basophilic intracytoplasmic inclusion bodies in feather pulp or follicular epithelium. Feather lesions caused by PBFD, polyomavirus, nutritional deficiencies, endocrine abnormalities, and drug reactions can appear grossly similar. Feather lesions associated with polyomavirus commonly resolve within several molts. Feather lesions from PBFD are progressive from molt to molt. Concurrent infections occur. Basophilic intranuclear inclusion bodies occur in both PBFD and polyomavirus infections. Psittacine beak and feather DNA probes can be used on blood samples or biopsy samples. Whole anticoagulated blood is the recommended blood sample for DNA probe testing (0.2 to 1.0 ml of blood with 20 units of heparin per milliliter of blood). Positive results in birds with feather abnormalities suggests an active infection. Birds that test positive without lesions are retested in 90 days. If birds are positive when retested, they should be considered a carrier. If birds are negative when retested, they probably have eliminated the virus.

There is no effective therapy for PBFD. Provide supportive care and treat secondary bacterial and fungal infections. The disease is progressive, and euthanasia must be considered when painful lesions develop. Most infected birds survive less than 6 months to 1 year after the onset of clinical signs, although some live much longer. Death is usually the result of secondary bacterial, fungal, chlamydial, or other viral infection or from progression of the disease such that euthanasia is requested.

Control is accomplished through removal of infected birds from breeding collections and nurseries. Test all birds for PBFD before admission into the aviary. The virus appears to be quite stable in the environment. Do not expose noninfected birds, especially neonates, to areas that may have been contaminated by feces or feather dust from infected birds. The DNA probe can be used to screen walls, cages, air circulating ducts, and equipment to determine if PBFD virus is contaminating these surfaces.

REOVIRUS. African gray parrots and cockatoos are most commonly affected by reovirus infection, but other psittacines are susceptible. The incubation period is 2 to 15 days. Transmission occurs both horizontally and vertically. Ingestion and inhalation of viral particles can result in infection. Infected birds shed virus in the feces.

Clinical signs in psittacines include emaciation, anorexia, depression, incoordination, dyspnea, and diarrhea. Uveitis can occur. Leg paralysis, paresis, and bloody nasal discharge occasionally occur. Old World psittacines appear highly susceptible and demonstrate more severe clinical signs, often dying within 3 to 4 days after clinical signs develop. New World psittacines appear less susceptible to infection and often survive with supportive care. Anemia, leukopenia, hypoalbuminemia, hyperglobulinemia, and increased AST and LDH may occur.

At necropsy, hepatomegaly with pale yellow mottling and multifocal gray-white foci, splenomegaly, renomegaly with urate deposits, and necrotic foci in the lungs may be observed.

Diagnosis is based on culture. Feces, liver, and spleen are best for viral isolation.

No specific treatment is available for reovirus infection. Old World psittacines often die, and New World species often survive with supportive care.

Chlorhexidine in the drinking water may decrease spread of the disease in flock situations. Prolonged contact with phenols, aldehydes, 70% ethanol, halides, 0.5% iodine solution, and a temperature of 158°F reduce viral infectivity. Adequate quarantine procedures may help prevent flock exposure. A carrier state may exist.

Suspected Viral Diseases

PROVENTRICULAR DILATATION SYNDROME (NEUROPATHIC GASTRIC DILATATION, PSITTACINE DILATATION SYNDROME, MACAW WASTING DISEASE). Macaws are considered the most susceptible to proventricular dilatation syndrome (PDS), but the disease has been described in many other psittacines. All ages of birds are susceptible. The disease has also been known as neuropathic gastric dilation, psittacine dilatation syndrome, and macaw wasting disease.

The route of transmission and incubation period are unknown, as the agent has not been identified.

Clinical signs include depression, progressive weight loss, vomiting, passing undigested or partially digested food in the droppings, abdominal distention, and neurologic signs. Polydypsia and polyuria may occur. Some birds maintain an excellent appetite but continue to lose weight. Diarrhea may occur late in the disease, usually the result of secondary bacterial or fungal enteritis.

Clinical pathology may reveal a leukocytosis (2 to 3 times normal), hypoglycemia, hypoproteinemia, anemia, and elevated CK levels. Radiology is useful to identify proventricular dilatation. Contrast radiology is often required to positively identify proventricular dilatation and delayed gastric emptying.

A presumptive antemortem diagnosis is based on clinical signs, radiology, and ruling out other causes. A definitive diagnosis requires demonstration of typical lesions in biopsy samples. In birds with chronic crop disorders (e.g., regurgitation, pendulous crop, and chronic crop infections) in addition to clinical signs of NGD, crop biopsy is a less-invasive surgical procedure that often provides an adequate sample for histopathological evaluation. False-negative results may occur as a result of missing the lesion, or the crop may not be affected.

Ventricular biopsies may be more likely to allow demonstration of the lesion; although this procedure is more invasive, it may be indicated. The lesion may still be missed because the sample may be collected from unaffected tissue. Proventricular biopsies are not recommended for diagnosis of NGD because of surgical and postsurgical complications of biopsy of the distended, thin-walled organ.

At necropsy, emaciation, cachexia, and a distended proventriculus, ventriculus, or crop may be noted. Proventricular or crop impaction may be noted. Erosions and ulcerations on the proventricular mucosa may be observed. The muscular layer of the ventriculus may appear whitish in color.

Diagnosis is based on histopathology of affected tissues (nerves of the gastrointestinal tract or CNS). Lesions may be focal, so multiple sections of affected tissues may need to be examined to observe the lesion.

Supportive care, feeding of a liquid or soft gruel diet (e.g., Roudybush Proventricular Formula [see Table 9–2]), and control of secondary infections may prolong life. There is no treatment.

Isolate affected birds. Quarantine birds that have contact with confirmed cases for at least 6 months, with cockatiel fledglings or breeding pairs as sentinels. A 6-month quarantine period may be insufficient to detect latently infected birds new to an aviary.

Fungal

CANDIDA. *Candida albicans* is a common cause of gastrointestinal disease in many species of pet birds. Low numbers of the organism are normal in the gastrointestinal tract of birds. An increase in numbers of the organism or invasion into tissues results in candidiasis. Candidiasis affects primarily young birds, but older birds are sometimes affected. It is common in young cockatiels. Candidiasis may occur as a primary or secondary infection. Predisposing causes include delayed crop emptying, prolonged antibiotic use, poor husbandry, debilitation, and vitamin A deficiency. Candidiasis may also occur secondary to other infectious diseases (e.g., poxvirus or trichomoniasis). *Candida* can cause disease of the gastrointestinal tract, skin, feathers, and reproductive tract. It can also cause systemic disease.

Clinical signs associated with an intestinal tract infection depend on the site of infection. The crop is affected most commonly in young birds. Clinical signs of *Candida*-associated ingluvitis (crop infection) include regurgitation, delayed crop emptying, depression, anorexia, and occasionally crop impaction. The crop may contain mucus. Lesions appear as raised white plaques covered by whitish viscous mucus. Chronic infections may appear as areas of multiple raised plaques appearing like terry cloth. Lesions may be present in the crop only, mouth only, proventriculus and ventriculus only, or a combination of sites. Skin lesions, beak abnormalities, tongue necrosis, cloaca and vent infections, foot lesions, and respiratory infections may also be caused by *Candida*. Systemic candidiasis is rare and usually occurs only in severely debilitated birds. Systemic infection is evidenced by the presence of *Candida* in the blood, bone marrow, or parenchymous organs.

Noninvasive candidiasis results in little inflammatory response. Hematology is often unremarkable in cases of candidiasis.

On necropsy, typical lesions previously discussed may be observed.

Diagnosis is based on clinical signs and the finding of large numbers of yeast cells on smears made from lesions or crop aspirates. *Candida* is identified by the presence of many oval budding yeast cells (see Fig. 12–20). Yeast cells stain gram-positive with Gram's stain and basophilic with Wright's or Diff-Quik stains. *Candida* may also be identified with cultures of affected sites.

Chlorhexidine may be mixed with the drinking water to help prevent *Candida* overgrowth in young birds during antibiotic therapy and in other birds when placed on prolonged antibiotics.

Treatment includes antifungal therapy and eliminating predisposing causes. Antifungal therapies available for treatment of candidiasis in birds includes nystatin, ketoconazole, fluconazole, and itraconazole. Nystatin is not absorbed from the gastrointestinal tract and requires contact with the lesion to be effective. It is easily administered mixed with feeding mixtures to hand-fed birds or as a gavage. Fluconazole and ketoconazole are systemic antifungals commonly used for refractory candidiasis.

ASPERGILLUS. Aspergillosis is a common cause of respiratory disease in companion birds. It is frequently diagnosed in blue-fronted Amazon parrots, African gray parrots, mynahs, raptors, and waterfowl. *Aspergillus* is ubiquitous, and healthy birds may not become infected with exposure to high concentrations of spores. Susceptibility to *Aspergillus* infections increases with stress, poor management techniques, antibiotic administration, corticosteroid administration, respiratory irritants, and concomitant disease. *Aspergillus* can cause upper respiratory, lower respiratory, or disseminated infection. The syrinx, caudal thoracic air sacs, and abdominal air sacs are the most commonly affected sites. The periorbital sinus and lungs are also commonly infected. Other sites that may be affected include skin, muscle, gastrointestinal tract, liver, kidney, eye, and brain.

Clinical signs vary with the site of infection and severity of disease. Clinical signs associated with respiratory infection include weight loss, depression, respiratory distress, and occasionally neuromuscular abnormalities. Biliverdinuria is common. Dyspnea or a change in voice may be the first signs of syringeal or tracheal infections. Nasal and sinus infections may be associated with an abnormally shaped nasal opening, a longitudinal groove in the rhamphotheca (upper beak), or necrosis of the rhamphotheca. In acute overwhelming infections, dyspnea or sudden death is observed.

Hematology often reveals a marked leukocytosis with an absolute heterophilia, monocytosis, and lymphopenia. An anemia is often present. Levels of AST, LDH, and CK are usually increased. Radiology may reveal focal densities in the air sacs or lungs, hyperinflation of the abdominal air sacs, or opacity of the air sac membranes.

Aspergillosis is suspected based on signalment, history, physical examination findings, hematology, radiology, and endoscopy. Tracheal endoscopy may reveal a plaque or a thick, white discharge in the trachea. Laparoscopy of the abdominal or caudal thoracic air sacs may reveal diffuse cloudiness, white or yellow plaques, or green pigmented mold. Samples may be obtained by biopsy or tracheal or air sac wash. Samples are evaluated cytologically and cultured on Sabouraud dextrose agar. Fungal elements are identified in cytologic samples by the presence of branching septate hyphae (see Fig. 12–29). Hyphae may stain poorly or basophilic with Wright's or Diff-Quik stain. New methylene blue stain may be used to better visualize hyphae. Basophilic staining conidiophores or spores may be seen when stained with Wright's or Diff-Quik stains. Definitive diagnosis is based on positive culture results when lesions are present, cytology or histopathology of a biopsy sample, tracheal or air sac wash, sinus aspirate, or positive serologic testing (ELISA). False-negative ELISA results occur. *Aspergillus* is a ubiquitous organism, and culture of the organism in the absence of lesions is not diagnostic.

Upper or lower respiratory infections, if detected before dissemination and treated aggressively, may respond to therapy. Accessible discrete lesions are surgically removed. Amphotericin B may be injected into the air sac space or used intratracheally (via the glottis during inspiration). Systemic therapies include oral administration of itraconazole, flucytosine, fluconazole, or intravenous administration of amphotericin B. Amphotericin B is fungicidal and is used to initiate treatment in acutely ill birds. Itraconazole, fluconazole, and flucytosine are fungistatic, usually requiring months of therapy for effective treatment. An autogenous aspergillosis vaccine has been used to augment systemic therapy, and it may reduce morbidity in susceptible populations during an outbreak. Supportive care is provided as needed, which may include oxygen therapy, fluid therapy, tube feeding, supplemental heat, treatment of concurrent bacterial or yeast infections, and treatment of the underlying cause of immunosuppression. Monitor therapy as needed with hematology, plasma biochemistries (AST, uric acid, total protein), radiology, and endoscopy.

Topical or aerosol treatments include amphotericin B, miconazole, clotrimazole, and enilconazole. Topical treatments are used to treat external lesions in conjunction with systemic therapy.

CRYPTOCOCCUS. *Cryptococcus neoformans* is a rare yeast infection of pigeons and psittacine birds. Clinical signs include dyspnea, weight loss, diarrhea, blindness, and paralysis. Hematology often reveals anemia and heterophilia. On necropsy, gelatinous material may be found in long bones, respiratory tract, abdominal cavity, sinuses, and brain. Diagnosis is based on finding the organism in exudates or tracheal washes. *Cryptococcus neoformans* is an oval to round yeast with a mucopolysaccharide capsule. Yeast cells stain basophilic with Wright's or Diff-Quik stains. The capsule portion of the yeast does not stain with Wright's or Diff-Quik stains, forming a clear halo around the yeast. *Cryptococcus* is a zoonotic disease. Amphotericin B or ketoconazole are possible treatments. There is a poor prognosis associated with disseminated *Cryptococcus* infection.

DERMATOPHYTES. Dermatophyte infections of the skin are rare in birds. *Trichophyton* is the most common dermatophyte infection. Psittacine, passerine, and gallinaceous birds may be affected. Clinical signs may include feather loss with thickened, flaky skin; weeping lesions on the head and neck; or white crusts on the comb and wattles. Diagnosis is made with cytology (wet mounts or Gram's stained smears), culture, or biopsy. Antifungal creams are used to treat infections. Treat any underlying problems. *Trichophyton gallinae* is a zoonotic disease.

Parasitic

ASCARIDS. Ascarid infections are common in cockatiels, budgies, and imported macaws. Infections are most common in birds maintained in enclosures with access to the ground. The life cycle is direct, with eggs becoming infective in 2 to 3 weeks. Eggs are hardy in the environment, resistant to disinfectants, but they can be controlled with steam or flaming. Clinical signs of infection include malabsorption, anorexia, weight loss, growth abnormalities, and diarrhea. Heavy parasite infections may result in intussusception, bowel occlusion, or death. Diagnosis is made by observation of typical ascarid eggs on fecal flotation. Treatments include piperazine, pyrantel pamoate, and fenbendazole.

Baylisascaris procyonis is a raccoon ascarid that has been reported to cause cerebrospinal nematodiasis in a variety of birds. Ingested infective eggs penetrate the intestinal wall and migrate through tissues. Central nervous system signs occur when the larvae enter the CNS. Clinical signs include ataxia, depression, torticollis, and death. Diagnosis is usually made with histopathology on necropsy, because no diagnostic stages of the parasite are released into the environment from the bird. Control is achieved by preventing access of raccoons into aviaries.

Heterakis gallinarum is a cecal worm of gallinaceous birds, budgies, passerines, ducks, geese, and other birds. It has a direct life cycle. Clinical signs include weight loss, diarrhea, and anorexia. On necropsy, nodular lesions may be noted in the submucosa of the ceca.

ATOXOPLASMA. *Atoxoplasma* is highly pathogenic in many passerines, especially mynahs, siskins, and canaries. It most commonly causes clinical signs in fledglings. *Atoxoplasma* has a direct life cycle, and sporulated oocysts are commonly ingested in food or water. Oocysts may remain viable for several months in the environment. Clinical signs include diarrhea, decreased appetite, weight loss, and fluffing. An enlarged liver can occasionally be seen as a dark area caudal to the sternum. Pale-staining intracytoplasmic inclusion bodies may be noted in mononuclear cells on hematology or buffy coat smears stained with Giemsa stain. Diagnosis is made by finding 20.1 × 19.2 μm oocysts in the feces with fecal flotation. Impression smears from liver biopsies or liver, spleen, or lungs at necropsy may reveal asexual stages. Clinical signs may occur before oocysts are shed in the feces. There is no effective therapy for atoxoplasmosis. Primaquine has been suggested for suppression of tissue forms. Sulfachlorpyrazine may decrease shedding of oocysts.

BAYLISASCARIS. See Ascarids.

CAPILLARIA. *Capillaria* are common tiny, threadlike worms that can infect most species of pet birds. Infections are most common in macaws, budgies, canaries, pigeons, and gallinaceous birds. *Capillaria* has a direct life cycle. Eggs become infective in 2 weeks and are hardy in the environment. Adults burrow into the mucosa of the esophagus, crop, or small intestine. Clinical signs include depression, anorexia, dysphagia, regurgitation, weight loss, diarrhea, and melena. Diagnosis is made by observation of the double operculated egg on fecal flotation, crop wash, or scrapings of suspect lesions (see Fig. 12–34). At necropsy, adult worms may be observed. Scrape the mucosa and observe closely; magnification is useful. Treatments include mebendazole, fenbendazole, or ivermectin. Resistant strains occur. Put treated birds in clean quarters 48 hours after treatment and steam clean the cage. Repeat treatment in 6 weeks.

CESTODES (TAPEWORMS). Tapeworm infections are most common in finches, African gray parrots, cockatoos, and eclectus parrots, and occasionally in South American psittacines. Tapeworms require intermediate hosts. Infections are uncommon in birds that do not have access to the ground. No clinical signs may be present, or weight loss, debility, and diarrhea may be observed with heavy worm burdens. An eosinophilia may or may not be present on hematology. Diagnosis is made by observing proglottids or whole worms in the feces or at the cloaca. Eggs may not be present during routine fecal exams. Praziquantel is used for treatment of cestode infections.

COCHLOSOMA. *Cochlosoma* are flagellates that cause disease in some finches. Clinical signs and mortality are usually a problem in nestlings 6 to 12 weeks of age, especially in Australian finches (e.g., Gouldians). Bengalese finches may be inapparent carriers. Clinical signs include debility, dehydration, and passing whole seed in droppings. At necropsy, yellow fluid or whole undigested seeds may fill the intestine. Diagnosis is made by demonstration of the organism on direct wet smears of fresh warm droppings or at necropsy with intestinal contents. *Cochlosoma* has a helicoidal anterior ventral sucker and six anterior flagella. Treat with ronidazole or dimetridazole. Clean and disinfect water containers. *Cochlosoma* is sensitive to most common disinfectants.

CRYPTOSPORIDIUM. *Cryptosporidium* are protozoa that may infect the gastrointestinal, respiratory, and urinary tracts of many pet birds. Young birds are most commonly affected. Sporulated oocysts are passed in the feces. Oocysts are usually ingested in food or water. Clinical signs in budgies, ducks, geese, and gallinaceous birds include depression, anorexia, rhinitis, conjunctivitis, sinusitis, tracheitis, airsacculitis, coughing, sneezing, and dyspnea. Diarrhea may occur in Amazon parrots, budgies, macaws, cockatiels, lovebirds, cockatoos, and gallinaceous birds. On necropsy, intestines may contain yellowish fluid and blunting fusion and atrophy of intestinal villi. Diagnosis is made by demonstration of oocysts on fecal flotation or observation of asexual stages in intestinal or respiratory mucosa at necropsy. Diagnosis is hindered by the small size of the organism (4 to 6 μm) and low shedding rate. There is no effective treatment for cryptosporidiosis.

CYTODITES NUDUS (AIR SAC MITE). *Cytodites nudus* infections are most common in canaries, finches, and budgies. See *Sternostoma tracheocolum.*

DERMANYSSUS (RED MITES, ROOST MITES). *Dermanyssus* is a mite that feeds on blood only at night. During the day they live in crevices within the aviary. Clinical signs include restlessness, anemia, pruritus, and poor growth, primarily in young or debilitated birds. The mite is red if it is engorged with blood; otherwise, it is brown. Diagnose by placing a white cloth over the cage at night and observe the cloth for red mites in the morning. Ivermectin or pyrethrin dusting or dipping and cleaning the cage during the day are treatments for mite infestation.

EIMERIA (COCCIDIOSIS). *Eimeria* is usually a problem in young birds, primarily pigeons and parakeets. *Eimeria* has a direct life cycle. Oocysts are passed in the feces and sporulate in the environment, where oocysts may remain viable for several months. Clinical signs include diarrhea and dehydration. Subclinical infection is common. Diagnosis is based on finding oocysts in feces on flotation. Most of the damage occurs before oocysts are produced. Treat with metronidazole.

FEATHER MITES. Feather mites are rare in pet birds. Some are nonpathogenic; others cause skin or feather problems.

GIARDIA. *Giardia* infections are common in budgies, cockatiels, lovebirds, and gray-cheeked parakeets. Infections are rare in other species of birds. High mortality may occur in nestling budgies and cockatiels. Birds with giardiasis may be asymptomatic, or clinical signs may include depression, anorexia, and diarrhea. Dry skin and feather picking may be a sign of giardiasis in cockatiels and budgies. Diagnosis is based on finding cysts or motile trophozoites in fresh warm feces on wet mount with warm saline or lactated Ringer's solution. Scan the field on 100× with a dark field to observe for movement of the trophozoites. Trophozoites have four pairs of flagella, two nuclei, and an adhesive disc. False-negative results are common. Flotation with zinc sulfate may allow detection of cysts. Feces may be collected and preserved with polyvinyl alcohol or formalin for trichrome staining or formalin for antigen detection. Treat with metronidazole.

HAEMOPROTEUS. *Haemoproteus* infections are common in imported cockatoos but also occur in conures, macaws, and African gray parrots. Infections are usually asymptomatic, except in pigeons and quail, unless the bird is stressed or has concurrent disease. Severe infections can cause anemia, splenomegaly, hepatomegaly, and pulmonary edema. Diagnosis is based on finding the organism in red blood cells (RBCs) on stained blood smears. The gametocytes are pigmented with refractile, yellow to brown pigment granules and partially encircle the nucleus, causing little displacement of the RBC nucleus (see Fig. 12–11). The gametocyte occupies more than half of the cytoplasm. Treatment is not recommended in asymptomatic birds. Quinacrine and treatment of the underlying cause of stress or debility are suggested for treatment when clinical signs occur.

ISOSPORA **(COCCIDIOSIS).** *Isospora* infections are most common in passerines, psittacines, and raptors. *Isospora* infections are a common cause of diarrhea in canary nestlings. Infections may be asymptomatic, or clinical signs may include depression, anorexia, diarrhea, melena, and death. Diagnosis is based on finding oocysts in feces on flotation. Most of the damage occurs before oocysts are shed. Treat with metronidazole.

KNEMIDOKOPTES PILAE **(SCALY LEG MITE, SCALY FACE MITE).** *Knemidokoptes pilae* infections are common in budgies, but they also occur in other psittacine and passerine birds. Clinical signs include proliferative lesions around the beak, cere, eyes, and vent, and on the feet and legs. Lesions have a characteristic honeycomb appearance. Diagnosis is based on observation of the mite or eggs in a skin scraping collected from the affected area. Samples are placed in oil and observed microscopically (see Fig. 12–26). Treat with ivermectin.

LEUKOCYTOZOON. *Leukocytozoon* occurs in wild birds and is highly pathogenic in young Anseriform and gallinaceous birds. The organism has low pathogenicity but may cause illness in waterfowl, turkeys, and occasionally young raptors. Transmission is by black flies. Clinical signs include anorexia, hemolytic anemia, hemoglobinuria, depression, and dehydration. Treat with pyrethamine.

LICE. Lice are common on wild birds. Large numbers occur only on birds too debilitated to preen. Clinical signs include restlessness, feather breakage, and occasionally pruritus. Diagnosis is based on observation of the adults or nits (eggs) on feathers. Treat by dusting or spraying with pyrethrin.

MICROFILARIA. Microfilaria occur in a wide variety of birds. Adults are usually undetected and may occur in air sacs, body cavity, eyes, heart, or joints.

Vectors are biting insects (e.g., mosquitos, black flies). The organism is usually nonpathogenic. Adult worms in joints and subcutaneous tissues can cause severe problems and should be removed.

PLASMODIUM (MALARIA). *Plasmodium* infections are most common in canaries, penguins, ducks, falcons, pigeons, and native wild birds. Mosquitos serve as intermediate hosts. Infections may be asymptomatic or result in depression, anorexia, vomiting, and dyspnea. Hemoglobinuria may occur. Anemia, leukocytosis, lymphocytosis, and elevated AST may be noted on clinical pathology. Death usually occurs in 2 to 3 days after onset of signs. Diagnosis is based on observation of the organism in stained peripheral blood films. Gametocytes, trophozoites, and schizonts may occur. The organisms can be found in RBCs, WBCs, and thrombocytes. Gametocytes contain refractile, yellow to brown pigment granules. Mature gametocytes are round to oval, but occupy less than half of the cytoplasm of the RBC (see Fig. 12–12). The nucleus of the RBC may be displaced. Trophozoites are small and round to oval. Schizonts are round to oval and contain dense staining merozoites in RBCs. *Plasmodium* can be differentiated from *Haemoproteus* by the marked displacement of the RBC nucleus by the parasite, the presence of schizonts in peripheral blood, and the occurrence of organism in WBCs and thrombocytes. On necropsy, hepatomegaly, splenomegaly, and cardiac tamponade may be noted. Treat with chloroquine phosphate and primaquine, and control mosquitos.

SARCOCYSTIS FALCATULA. *Sarcocystis falcatula* is a protozoal parasite that can cause sporadic to heavy losses in Old World psittacines (e.g., cockatoos) and nestlings of New World species (e.g., macaws). Opossums are the definitive host of the organism. Infected opossums shed sporocysts in the feces. Birds become infected when they ingest sporocysts in food or water contaminated with infective opossum feces or cockroaches that have eaten infected opossum feces. Infected birds may die without clinical signs, or before death they may have weight loss, anorexia, diarrhea, dyspnea, ataxia, head tilt, paresis, or head tremors. On necropsy, pulmonary edema, splenomegaly, and hepatomegaly are common. Diagnosis is based on finding *Sarcocystis* tissue stages in stained organ preparations at necropsy. Organisms are particularly common in the lungs. Treatment includes pyrimethanamine and trimethoprim-sulfadiazine, along with supportive care. Prevent access to opossums and roaches to prevent infection.

SPIRURIDS (STOMACH WORMS). *Dispharynx* and *Spiroptera* adult worms burrow into the proventriculus of psittacines. *Acuaria* and *Dispharynx* may cause ventricular and proventricular infections in passerines. Clinical signs include emaciation, ulceration, nodule formation, perforation, proventricular enlargement, or abnormal droppings (mucoid droppings, diarrhea, undigested food in droppings). Diagnosis is made by observing embryonated eggs in the feces. Eggs are shed intermittently. On necropsy, mucosal scrapings may reveal the parasite. Treat with oxfendazole or levamisole.

STERNOSTOMA TRACHEOCOLUM (AIR SAC MITE, TRACHEAL MITE). *Sternostoma* infections are common in canaries, finches, budgies, and cockatiels. These parasites live in the trachea, bronchi, sinuses, or air sacs. Clinical signs include weight loss, loss of vocalization, clicking sound, dyspnea, coughing, sneezing, and death. Diagnosis is made by observation of the parasite in the trachea with transillumination of the trachea. The mites appear as dark, pinhead-sized spots, often moving. To improve visualization, wet feathers over the trachea with alcohol. The eggs of the mite may be observed in the feces or in tracheal wash samples. On necropsy, mites appear as black spots in mucus. Treat with ivermectin.

SYNGAMUS TRACHEA (GAPEWORMS). *Syngamus* infections are common in ducks, geese, and gallinaceous birds. Infections are rare in other companion birds. Infections are most common in young birds. The female worm embeds in the tracheal wall, causing irritation, mucus production, and granuloma formation. Clinical signs include coughing, open-mouth breathing, dyspnea, blood at the commisures of the beak, and death. The adult worm may be visualized in the glottal opening or trachea with transillumination of the trachea with the neck extended. Diagnosis is based on observation of the double operculated egg in mucus or feces (see Fig. 12–36). At necropsy, the large red adult parasites may be noted in the trachea. Treat with ivermectin or thiabendazole, or manually remove the parasites. Improve sanitation and management practices to decrease exposure.

TAPEWORMS. See Cestodes.

TOXOPLASMA. Birds may serve as intermediate hosts for *Toxoplasma gondii*. Oocysts are intermittently shed in the feces of infected cats. Clinical signs include anorexia, weight loss, dyspnea, paralysis, blindness, and diarrhea. Diagnosis is based on finding *Toxoplasma* antibodies in the blood or finding tissue stages on histopathology of organs from necropsy.

TREMATODES (FLUKES). Liver flukes are common only in imported Old World species (e.g., cockatoos). These birds were probably infected in their country of origin. Clinical signs include depression, anorexia, weight loss, hepatomegaly, diarrhea, vomiting, and death. A mild anemia and elevated liver enzymes may be noted with clinical pathology. Diagnosis is based on finding eggs on direct fecal exam. Fluke eggs possess an operculum (see Fig. 12–32). A procedure to concentrate fluke eggs is to break up feces in a 1% liquid soap solution in a tube. Fill the tube with the soap solution. Place the tube in a vertical position for 5 minutes, then decant the fluid but not the sediment. Refill the tube and repeat the procedure 3 to 5 times or until the supernatant is clear. Examine the sediment microscopically for fluke eggs. Treatment may be attempted with praziquantel.

TRICHOMONAS (TRICHOMONIASIS, CANKER, FROUNCE). *Trichomonas* infections are common in pigeons and raptors, but they also occur in canaries, finches, budgies, and other pet birds. *Trichomonas* is transmitted through direct contact (e.g., eating infected birds or parental feeding) or through ingestion of contaminated food or water. Infections may be limited to the oropharynx, esophagus, crop, and trachea. Systemic infections may occur when the liver and lungs are invaded. The incubation period is 4 to 14 days. Clinical signs include anorexia, fluffing, diarrhea, dysphagia, vomiting, dyspnea, weight loss, and increased water consumption. The umbilicus may become infected, resulting in lumps under the skin. Infections can be asymptomatic. On physical examination, sticky, creamy white or cheesy deposits may be present in the mouth, nares, and esophagus. Diagnosis is based on finding the motile trophozoite in direct saline smears of oral fluids and in scrapings taken from lesions. The organism is a pear-shaped flagellate with three to five anterior flagella and one posterior flagellum that swims with an irregular motion. Treat with metronidazole and correct sanitation or management problems.

METABOLIC DISEASES

Gout

Gout is the abnormal accumulation of uric acid crystals in or around joints, along tendon sheaths, on visceral serosal surfaces, in the interstitial connective tissue of the liver and kidneys, or in the excretory ducts of the kidneys. Gout is most common in budgies, waterfowl, and gallinaceous birds and fairly common in other psittacines and raptors. It is rare in canaries and pigeons. Gout may occur with impaired renal function, nephrosis, or excessive dietary protein in which the amount of uric acid formed from the catabolization of protein exceeds the capacity of the kidneys to eliminate the substance. Predisposing factors include high-protein diet, overeating, inactivity, decreased blood circulation, decreased water intake, vitamin A deficiency, poor nutrition, kidney disease (e.g., infection or neoplasia), infectious disease, and toxicoses (hypervitaminosis D_3 and others). There are visceral and articular forms of gout that may occur alone or in combination. Articular gout is characterized by the deposition of uric acid crystals within joints and along tendon sheaths, usually in the feet, legs, and wings (see Fig. 7–6). Early clinical signs include restlessness and frequent shifting of weight from foot to foot. Clinical signs include lameness, difficulty perching, sitting on the cage floor, and an unsteady gait. If wings are affected, the wings may droop and the bird may not be able to fly. On physical examination, joints may be swollen, and uric acid deposits (tophi) may be noted as firm white swellings within joints or along tendon sheaths. Diagnosis is based on aspiration of swollen joints and cytologic evaluation. Contents of tophi are opaque, creamy white to beige. On cytology, needle-shaped or amorphous crystals may be noted that are birefringent under polarized light (see Fig. 12–22). Large numbers of inflammatory cells are also usually present.

Visceral gout occurs when there is deposition of uric acid crystals on visceral serosal surfaces. Birds may show nonspecific clinical signs or die acutely. Clinical signs may include poor appetite, lethargy, emaciation, abnormal droppings, and temperament changes. On necropsy, white flecks are observed on serosal surfaces, especially on the liver, pericardial, and epicardial surfaces. Adhesions may be present. Antemortem diagnosis may be obtained with laparoscopy. Uric acid crystals can dissolve if the tissues are preserved in formalin.

Plasma uric acid levels are usually elevated with gout, but elevation of plasma uric acid occurs as a result of other etiologies and is not diagnostic.

The goal of therapy is to prevent or slow further deposition of uric acid crystals and to reduce inflammation. Treat the underlying cause. Allopurinol reduces production of uric acid deposits, but it has no effect on previously formed urate deposits. Colchicine and probenecid have also been used in the treatment of gout. Surgical removal of tophi is not recommended. Administer vitamin A in birds on poor diets with elevated uric acid levels. Aspirin may be used for analgesia. Corticosteroids are contraindicated. Place the bird on a balanced low-protein diet (e.g., Harrison's Adult Lifetime Formula or Roudybush Kidney Formula). Provide broad low perches, and place food and water within easy access.

Hemochromatosis (Iron Storage Disease)

Hemochromatosis results from an excessive amount of iron accumulation in various body tissues, frequently the liver. Excessive iron in the diet may play a role in the development of the disease. An inherited metabolic defect and altered intestinal absorption of iron may contribute to disease. Hemochromatosis is most commonly seen in toucans, mynahs, birds of paradise, and quetzals, and rarely occurs in psittacines. Clinical signs in mynahs include weakness, coughing, dyspnea, and a swollen abdomen, caused by ascites. Toucans may be asymptomatic or depressed for a day before death. Hepatomegaly and ascites are often noted radiographically, with or without cardiomegaly and splenomegaly. Low plasma protein and elevated AST levels are common plasma biochemistry abnormalities. Abdominocentesis usually reveals a yellow transudate or modified transudate. Because of the debilitated state of most affected birds, a presumptive diagnosis is often made based on clinical signs, radiographic abnormalities, and laboratory results. Definitive diagnosis requires liver biopsy.

Treatment includes aspiration of ascitic fluid to relieve dyspnea if present, phlebotomies, and placing the bird on a diet low in iron and vitamin C. Initially, 1 to 2 ml of blood per day is withdrawn until clinical improvement is noted or the lower limit of normal hematocrit is reached, measuring the hematocrit with each phlebotomy. Then blood is withdrawn weekly at the rate of 1% of the birds' body weight in grams. In the easily stressed bird, initial phlebotomies may need to be less frequent and up to 1% of body weight. Phlebotomies are stopped and monitored when the hematocrit falls below normal. Total serum iron, albumin, hematocrit, repeated radiographs, and body weight are useful for monitoring treatment. Normal serum iron is 200 μg/dl. Deferoxamine has been successfully used to remove iron from body stores.

Low-iron pelleted diets include Harrison's Low Iron Formula, Kaytee Softbill diet, and Bird of Paradise Diet (see Table 9–2). Foods low in iron include yogurt, cooked egg whites, boiled potato cubes, corn, wheat starch, apples, bananas, pears, pineapples, plums, figs, berries, papaya, and melons. Avoid foods high in iron such as egg yolk, liver, raisins, red meat, grapes, and dark green vegetables and greens. Avoid citrus fruits, strawberries, tomatoes, and kiwi, and do not supplement with vitamin C. There is a poor prognosis associated with hemochromatosis, even with intensive therapy.

Hepatic Lipidosis (Fatty Liver)

Hepatic lipidosis is the excessive fat deposition and storage in the liver. Suggested causes include nutritional (high fat content of diet, choline deficiency, biotin deficiency), toxic (ethionine, carbon tetrachloride, chloroform, phosphorus, lead, arsenic), and hereditary factors. Inactivity may also contribute to the problem. Hepatic lipidosis is most frequently diagnosed in budgies, cockatiels, Amazon parrots, and cockatoos.

Clinical signs of hepatic lipidosis include anorexia, depression, diarrhea, biliverdinuria, obesity, poor feathering, dyspnea, and abdominal enlargement. Seizures, ataxia, and muscle tremors may also occur if liver function is impaired and results in hepatic encephalopathy. Liver disease is diagnosed based on physical examination, plasma biochemistries (elevated AST, bile acids, LDH, cholesterol, total protein, and albumin), and radiology (hepatomegaly). Definitive diagnosis of the etiology of the hepatic disease often requires liver biopsy. The best approach for biopsy of the liver is the ventral midline approach.

Treatment of hepatic lipidosis includes placing the bird on a low-fat diet. A commercial avian pelleted diet, supplemented with small amounts of fresh fruits and vegetables, is ideal. If signs of hepatic encephalopathy are present, lactulose may be used to reduce blood ammonia levels. Birds affected with hepatic lipidosis often die soon after the onset of clinical signs, before treatment can be effective. Birds in critical condition may need symptomatic therapy, including supplemental heat, fluid therapy, and tube feeding.

Hypocalcemia

Hypocalcemia is most common in young (2- to 5-year-old) African gray parrots, but it also occurs in other psittacines and raptors. The etiology is uncertain; however, affected birds are often on diets deficient in calcium, phosphorus, or vitamin D_3 or diets with an inappropriate Ca:P ratio (e.g., all-seed diet). In raptors and psittacines other than African gray parrots, calcium is mobilized from the bone to maintain normal blood calcium levels. In African gray parrots, skeletal mineralization often appears normal with hypocalcemia. Clinical signs include seizures, ataxia, opisthotonos, weakness, or tetany. Diagnosis is based on low blood calcium levels and response to calcium therapy. Blood calcium levels below 6.0 mg/dl may result in clinical signs. At necropsy, parathyroid gland enlargement may be observed. Parenteral administration of calcium gluconate will control seizures. Do not use corticosteroids in these patients. Place the bird on a proper diet and begin oral calcium and vitamin supplementation. Life-long calcium and vitamin supplementation may be required for African gray parrots, even with a good diet. Evaluate plasma calcium concentrations in 2 months and periodically thereafter to assess effectiveness of treatment.

Hypoglycemia

Hypoglycemia is uncommon except in anorectic neonates and raptors. Blood glucose values less than 150 mg/dl indicate hypoglycemia. Hypoglycemic seizures usually occur when blood glucose levels fall below 100 mg/dl. Intravenous 50% dextrose is given for acute relief of clinical signs. Treat the underlying cause.

Kidney Disease

Kidney disease is fairly common in birds. Renal disease may be acute or chronic. Etiologies of kidney disease in birds include infectious, neoplastic, toxic (hypercalcemia, vitamin D toxicosis, hemoglobin, myoglobin, lead, zinc, mycotoxins, salt, ethylene glycol, carbon tetrachloride, drugs such as aminoglycoside and sulfonamide antibiotics and allopurinol), metabolic (gout, hemochromatosis, amyloidosis), and physical obstruction (vitamin A deficiency, uroliths, tumors, egg binding, fecaliths, uric acid deposits, inflammation, dehydration). Infectious diseases affecting the kidney include bacterial (gram-negative, gram-positive, mycobacterial, chlamydial), viral (polyomavirus, paramyxovirus, Pacheco's disease virus, pigeon herpesvirus, adenovirus, reovirus, leukosis/sarcoma virus), mycotic (aspergillosis), and parasitic (*Isospora, Cryptosporidium, Microsporidium, Encephalitozoon*).

All types of renal disease can have the same clinical signs, including fluffing, lethargy, depression, weakness, polyuria, polydipsia, anorexia, weight loss, and diarrhea. Organomegaly or ascites may result in abdominal distention. Dyspnea may be present. Lameness may be present. Anuria or oliguria may be present if acute renal failure is present. On physical examination, dehydration, a palpable abdominal mass, or articular gout may be noted. In large birds, the caudal kidneys can be palpated with a lubricated gloved finger through the cloaca.

Diagnosis of renal disease is based on physical examination, clinical signs, urinalysis, hematology, plasma biochemistries, electrolytes, radiology, ultrasonography, laparoscopy, and kidney biopsy. To collect urine for a urinalysis, aspirate the fluid portion of the dropping into a syringe from a clean cage bottom covered with wax paper. Avoid urates. Urinary casts indicate renal pathology. Proteinuria, glucosuria without hyperglycemia, hematuria, and cells in the urinary sediment may indicate kidney disease and warrant further investigation. Hematology (hematocrit, WBC count, differential) is useful for detection of dehydration, anemia, and infectious diseases. Plasma biochemistries important in birds suspected to have kidney disease include uric acid, total protein, and albumin. Elevated uric acid levels may occur when glomerular filtration decreases more than 70% to 80%. Etiologies include vitamin A deficiency, dehydration, bacterial and viral infections, toxicoses, severe tissue damage, and starvation. Renal disease may be present with uric acid levels within the normal range. Elevations of uric acid levels may not occur until a large number of renal tubules have been damaged.

Hyperkalemia may occur with renal failure and lead to life-threatening electrocardiac changes. Administration of 10% calcium gluconate IV will not affect plasma potassium concentration, but it may reverse the cardiotoxic effects of severe hyperkalemia. Administration of insulin in birds for hyperkalemia is not recommended because it may result in acute hypoglycemia, CNS swelling, and death.

Radiology is useful in assessing the size, location, and radiopacity of the kidneys. Kidneys are best seen with a lateral radiograph, appearing as bean-shaped structures posterior to the last rib. Renal enlargement is noted as obliteration of the air space around the kidneys (psittacines), ventral displacement of abdominal viscera beneath the kidneys, or enlargement of the kidney or a portion of a kidney. An increase in the radiopacity of the kidney may occur with dehydration, renal gout, or incomplete renal clearance of urate crystals. Ultrasonography is useful for determining the size, location, and density of the kidney.

Laparoscopy allows visualization of the kidneys and ureters, location, color, size, and shape. Normal kidneys are dark red-brown and evenly colored. Abnormalities that may be noted with laparoscopy include renomegaly, aspergillosis, visceral or renal gout, suspected neoplasia, hemochromatosis, and cysts. A renal biopsy may be required to make a definitive diagnosis. Indications for renal biopsy include renomegaly, consistently elevated uric acid levels, increasing elevated uric acid levels, or unexplained persistent polyuria. Renal biopsy is contraindicated if coagulopathies exist (see next section). The best approach for biopsy of the middle and cranial lobes is the lateral approach through the caudal thoracic air sac. The caudal lobe is best approached via the caudal abdominal air sac. Entry is just caudal to the pubis and ventral to the ischium.

Treat the underlying cause of renal disease. Symptomatic therapy (fluid therapy, tube feeding, and heat supplementation) should be provided as needed.

Restrict fluid intake in anuric or oliguric birds to fluid loss (about 20 ml/kg/day). Monitor daily with weight determination and clinical signs of dehydration or over hydration. Administer furosemide. Feed a low-protein diet containing all essential amino acids, or feed a diet with calories from fat and carbohydrates and absent in protein, sodium, and potassium.

Polyuric birds in acute renal failure require monitoring of hydration and electrolytes to prevent dehydration, hypokalemia, and hyponatremia. Administer daily fluid therapy with lactated Ringer's solution. Administer nonnephrotoxic antibiotics (e.g., piperacillin and cefotaxime). Administer vitamin A to birds on poor diets with elevated uric acid levels.

Liver Disease

Liver disease is common in birds. Liver disease may be acute or chronic. Etiologies of liver disease in birds include infectious diseases, fibrosis, hepatic lipidosis, hemochromatosis, toxicoses, amyloidosis, neoplasia, circulatory disturbances, and mineralization. Infectious causes of liver disease include bacterial (gram-negative, gram-positive, mycobacterial, and chlamydial), viral (adenovirus, polyomavirus, Pacheco's disease, reovirus, paramyxovirus, avian serositis form of eastern equine encephalitis, coronavirus, duck virus hepatitis virus), and parasitic (coccidiosis, *Atoxoplasma, Trichomonas, Histomonas, Leucocytozoon, Toxoplasma, Microsporidium, Plasmodium,* trematodes). Infectious diseases, hepatic lipidosis, and hemochromatosis are discussed elsewhere in this chapter.

Liver disease is most common in cockatiels, Amazon parrots, mynahs, and budgies. Clinical signs include depression, anorexia, fluffing, polyuria, polydipsia, biliverdinuria (dark yellow or green pigmented urates), regurgitation, dehydration, and abdominal swelling. Dyspnea may be present. On physical examination, an enlarged liver may be palpated caudal to the sternum or, in neonates and small passerines, may be observed through the skin. Ascites may be present. Neurologic signs may be present if hepatic encephalopathy is present.

Diagnosis of liver disease is based on physical examination, clinical signs, hematology, plasma biochemistries, radiology, ultrasonography, laparoscopy, and liver biopsy. Hematology (hematocrit, WBC count, differential) is useful for detection of dehydration, anemia, and infectious diseases. Plasma biochemistries important in birds suspected to have liver disease include AST, bile acids, albumin, total protein, and CK. Elevated activities of AST are usually the result of liver or muscle damage and indicate recent cell damage but not necessarily impaired liver function. Liver pathology can be present with normal AST levels. Creatine kinase activity increases with muscle damage and can be used to differentiate an increase in AST caused by liver disease from an increase caused by muscle damage. Bile acids are used to evaluate liver function. Elevation in bile acids indicate hepatic dysfunction and may be present with normal AST levels. Low albumin levels and low protein levels are common with impaired liver function, but they may occur as a result of other factors (see Chapter 12).

Examine the feces for fluke eggs, especially in cockatoos.

Indications of liver disease radiographically include an enlarged hepatic silhouette or microhepatia. An enlargement of the hepatic silhouette can occur as a result of either liver or proventricular enlargement. Contrast studies (i.e., barium series) may be required to differentiate the enlarged organ. Radiology helps determine the presence of abnormal liver size, but it does not aid in the determination of the cause of the liver abnormality. Ultrasonography is useful in determining liver size and providing information on structural aspects of the liver. Abscesses, large metastatic lesions, and cysts may be detected.

Liver biopsy is required to determine the etiology of liver disease. Indications for liver biopsy include persistent elevation of bile acids for 2 weeks or more or when bile acid levels remain elevated after completion of therapy for systemic disease (e.g., chlamydiosis, aspergillosis). Evaluate clotting ability before performing liver biopsy. Prolonged bleeding times after blood collection or thrombocytopenia are contraindications to biopsy. Administration of vitamin K_1 before surgery in cases of liver disease may decrease the incidence of life-threatening hemorrhage. Liver biopsy is best accomplished laparoscopically through a ventral midline approach just caudal to the sternum. Laparotomy and liver tissue excision with scissors can be performed.

Treat the underlying cause of liver disease. Symptomatic therapy (fluid therapy, tube feeding, and heat supplementation) should be provided as needed. If signs of hepatic encephalopathy are present, lactulose may be used to reduce blood ammonia levels.

ENDOCRINE DISEASES

Diabetes Mellitus

Diabetes mellitus is most common in budgies, cockatiels, and toucans. It has been reported in Amazon parrots, raptors, and other birds. Causes of diabetes in birds may be different than in mammals. Hypoinsulinemia is probably not the cause in birds other than raptors. Clinical signs include depression, polyuria, polydipsia, and weight loss despite a good appetite. Blood glucose levels commonly range from 600 to 2,000 mg/dl in diabetic birds. Definitive diagnosis requires finding persistently elevated blood glucose levels (>800 mg/dl). Glucosuria without hyperglycemia does not indicate diabetes mellitus. Normal urine can contain negative to trace amounts of glucose. Successful treatment may not be possible. Place the bird on a low-carbohydrate diet. Placing toucans on a formulated diet (e.g., Harrison's Low Iron Formula or Kaytee Softbill Diet [see Table 9–2]) may lower blood glucose levels. Insulin therapy is hindered by the highly variable dose needed for individual birds, the development of insulin resistance, and the development of pancreatic atrophy and pancreatic insufficiency. A suggested initial dose of regular insulin is 0.1 to 0.2 U/kg. Stable birds may be started on longer-acting NPH or ultralente insulin. Dosages range from 0.067 to 3.3 U/kg IM every 12 to 24 hours. A blood glucose curve should be obtained. Blood glucose levels should be determined initially, then every 2 to 3 hours for 12 to 24 hours. The dose is adjusted based on blood glucose levels. Frequency of administration varies from twice daily to once every several days. Monitor for hypoglycemia. Treat hypoglycemia with oral or injectable dextrose or oral corn syrup. Birds treated with insulin may improve clinically (gain weight). Hyperglycemia and glycosuria often persist. Somatostatin has been reported to aid in the treatment of avian diabetes mellitus.

Hypothyroidism

Hypothyroidism is rare in pet birds. Hypothyroid birds may have feather abnormalities (fringed, elongated, loss of barbules, abnormal color), obesity, lipoma formation, absent or rare molting, or growth retardation. Diagnosis requires a thyroid-stimulating hormone (TSH) response test. The suggested dose for TSH in psittacines is 1 IU/kg IM. Blood should be withdrawn for serum T_4 concentrations prior to TSH administration and 6 hours after TSH administration. In normal birds, serum T_4 levels increase at least double. Hypothyroidism is suspected in birds in which T_4 levels fail to double after administration of TSH. Plasma thyroxine concentrations may decrease as a result of abnormalities from factors other than inadequate thyroid function. Hypothyroidism cannot be diagnosed by a positive response to thyroxine administration.

Treat documented hypothyroidism with thyroxine supplementation.

NUTRITIONAL DISEASES

Obesity

Obesity is the most common nutritional disease in pet birds. Excessive weight gain occurs when energy intake exceeds energy expenditure for a long period of time. Common causes in pet birds include feeding high-oil seeds (sunflower, safflower, hemp, rape, Niger), feeding excess quantities of high-energy or high-fat foods (peanuts or sweets), lack of exercise, and increased food intake from boredom. Obesity is most common in budgies, Amazon parrots, and rose-breasted and sulfur-crested cockatoos. Clinical signs include subcutaneous fat deposits or lipomas. Lipomas and subcutaneous fat deposits are most common over the sternum or abdomen. Dyspnea or exercise intolerance may be present.

Treatment includes placing the bird on a proper diet and increasing exercise. The ideal diet is a commercial avian pelleted diet supplemented with up to 20% fresh vegetables and fruit. A complete balanced diet with reduced calories (e.g., Roudybush Obesity Formula) or complete balanced adult diet may be used. Limiting access to food to 10 minutes morning and evening may decrease calories consumed, especially if the bird eats as a result of boredom. Increase exercise by providing a larger cage with interactive toys (e.g., ladders or swings), allowing supervised exercise out of the cage, and placing food and water bowls at different ends of the cage. Supervised exercise out of the cage can involve climbing and interaction with the owner. Flight in dyspneic birds is not recommended because excessive body fat often decreases air sac capacity. Do not administer thyroxine in the absence of documentation of hypothyroidism with thyroxine and TSH stimulation tests. Lipomas may be surgically removed in stable patients that have not responded to dietary changes and increased exercise. Lipomas may be vascular; use radiosurgery.

Calcium or Phosphorus Deficiency, Calcium/Phosphorus Imbalance, Vitamin D₃ Deficiency, Nutritional Secondary Hyperparathyroidism, Renal Secondary Hyperparathyroidism (Metabolic Bone Disease, Rickets)

Calcium, phosphorus, and vitamin D_3 imbalances are common in birds and can result in metabolic bone disease: osteomalacia in adult birds and rickets in growing birds. Calcium or phosphorus deficiency, calcium/phosphorus imbalance, vitamin D_3 deficiency, and nutritional secondary hyperparathyroidism are diet related. These imbalances occur commonly as a result of feeding an all-seed diet or all-meat diet. Most vegetables and fruits are deficient in calcium. An adequate calcium to phosphorus ratio ranges from 1:1 to 2:1. Hens laying large numbers of eggs require more calcium. Vitamin D_3 deficiency can occur if dietary levels are deficient and the bird lacks exposure to natural sunlight or another source of ultraviolet light. Renal secondary hyperparathyroidism possibly occurs in birds and may result from chronic renal disease.

Osteomalacia is common in adult pet birds and results in thinning and demineralization of bone, often resulting in fractures. Clinical signs include fractures, bending of long bones, or skeletal deformities. The beak may become pliable (rubber beak). Affected birds are often polyuric and polydypsic and may lay abnormal eggs or become egg bound. At necropsy, cortices of the bones are thin and the parathyroid glands enlarged.

Rickets occurs in growing birds and results in deformities of the skeleton and pliable bones. The proximal tibiotarsus, heads of the ribs, costochondral junctions of the ribs, and the beak are most commonly affected. Clinical signs include bendable bones, skeletal deformities, and pliable beak. Dyspnea may occur. On necropsy, enlarged parathyroid glands may be noted in birds with calcium or vitamin D_3 deficiencies but not phosphorus deficiency or excessive calcium intake. Fractures and pliable bones and beak may be noted.

Diagnosis is based on dietary history, clinical signs, physical examination, clinical pathology, and radiology. Important plasma biochemistries to perform in birds suspected of having metabolic bone disease include alkaline phosphatase (AP) and calcium levels. Birds with metabolic bone disease will have elevated AP activities. Plasma calcium levels usually remain normal until the end stage is reached, resulting in hypocalcemic convulsions and tetany.

Treatment for metabolic bone disease that is not the result of chronic renal failure involves correcting the underlying nutritional deficiency, most commonly a calcium deficiency. Initially treat with an injectable calcium supplement (e.g., calcium gluconate, calcium glubionate, or calcium lactate/glycerophosphate). A commercial formulated diet is recommended. Sources of dietary calcium include commercial formulated diet, cuttle bone, broccoli, dark green leafy vegetables, milk products, and egg shells (dried in the oven or microwave).

Goiter (Thyroid Hyperplasia)

Goiter is an enlargement in the thyroid gland as a result of a dietary iodine deficiency. Budgies and pigeons are most commonly affected. In budgies, goiter is the result of feeding an iodine-deficient diet usually of seed grown in iodine-deficient soil. Clinical signs in budgies include wheezing, chirp on expiration, crop distention, delayed crop emptying, or regurgitation. The enlarged thyroid glands are usually not palpable because they are intrathoracic and usually do not distend beyond the thoracic inlet even with enlargement. The normal size of the thyroid gland in budgies is about 2 mm. Goitrous glands may enlarge to 10 to 20 mm and may be cystic. Diagnosis is based on dietary history, physical examination, radiology, and response to iodine supplementation. A dorsal or ventral displacement of the trachea may be visible radiographically.

In pigeons, goiter is the result of feeding an iodine-deficient diet usually of soybeans and maize that may increase iodine demand. Clinical signs in pigeons include lethargy, obesity, myxedema of the face (puffy facial skin), abnormal feathering (long, narrow tail and wing feathers or structural defects in contour feathers), irregular or absent molting, and decreased fertility, reduced hatchability, and reduced viability of squabs. On physical examination, an enlarged thyroid gland may be palpable at the thoracic inlet. Diagnosis is based on dietary history, physical examination, and response to treatment.

Treat goiter in budgies with iodine. Use sodium iodide in dyspneic birds. If improvement is not seen within 3 days of initiating treatment, re-evaluate the diagnosis. Prevent goiter and maintain the status of treated birds by placing the birds on a complete formulated diet.

Vitamin A Deficiency

Vitamin A deficiency is common in pet birds, especially those on a seed-based diet. Vitamin A deficiency results in squamous metaplasia of mucous membranes in the respiratory, gastrointestinal, and urogenital tracts and in hyperkeratosis of epithelial surfaces. Squamous metaplasia may result in blockage of salivary ducts, resulting in swellings around the choana, larynx, under the tongue, or between the mandibles under the chin; the accumulation of white caseous discharge in the sinuses (often accompanied by a secondary bacterial infection); thickening and sloughing of part of the lining of the syrinx, resulting in possible tracheal obstruction; xerophthalmia; kidney damage; and gout (if occlusion of the ureters occurs). Hyperkeratosis is common on the metatarsal and digital pads of the feet, resulting in thickening, and predisposes birds to pododermatitis. The normal scale pattern may be lost, and the area may appear smooth, lacking scale definition. Hypovitaminosis A may result in reduced egg production, egg binding, pitted egg shells, decreased sperm motility, reduced sperm counts, and increased numbers of abnormal sperm.

Clinical signs that may occur with vitamin A deficiency include swollen sinuses, swellings around the eyes, nasal discharge, polyuria, polydipsia, anorexia, and dyspnea. On physical examination, caseous masses (keratin cysts) may be noted around the choana, larynx, under the tongue, between the mandibles under the chin, around the eyes, or in sinuses; the margins of the choana may be swollen, and associated papillae may be blunted or absent; small white pustules or large caseous masses may be observed in the mouth, esophagus, crop, or nasal passages; a nasal discharge may be present; and xerophthalmia may be noted. Xerophthalmia is abnormal dryness and thickening of the conjunctiva and cornea.

Diagnosis of vitamin A deficiency is based on diet history, clinical signs, and physical examination. Cytology of caseous masses reveals debris and desquamated cornified epithelial cells that are abnormal in appearance (see Chapter 12). The presence of inflammatory cells may indicate a secondary bacterial infection. Biopsy of caseous masses may reveal hyperkeratosis or squamous metaplasia.

Treat vitamin A deficiency with parenteral vitamin A weekly, then oral supplementation once improvement is noted (typically 2 to 3 weeks). Correct the diet. Keratin cysts are debrided and cultured. Treat with antibiotics based on culture and sensitivity results.

Prevent vitamin A deficiency by placing birds on a complete and balanced diet, preferably a complete formulated diet. Formulated diets may be supplemented with up to 20% vegetables and fruits and no seed or vitamin supplements.

TOXICOSES

Aflatoxin

See Mycotoxins.

Botulism (Limberneck Disease)

Botulism is common in waterfowl and rare in pet birds. Toxicosis associated with botulism toxins occurs after ingestion of contaminated food such as decaying organic matter or maggots that have fed on carcasses containing toxin. Ingestion of botulism toxin results in a peripheral neuropathy. Leg paralysis is usually the earliest clinical sign, characterized by the bird sitting on its sternum with legs extended caudally. Leg paralysis is followed by wing paralysis. Loss of control of the neck and head occur in the terminal stages, resulting in the term *limberneck disease*. Death is caused by respiratory paralysis. Petechiae and edema may also occur.

Diagnosis requires demonstration of the toxin in serum, liver, or kidney using mouse animal models. Freeze samples to be tested, because these toxins degrade at room temperature.

Most birds with severe clinical signs die. Some birds recover with supportive care. A commercial antitoxin may be used in affected birds.

Carbamate

See Insecticides.

Cholecalciferol Rodenticide

See Vitamin D.

Insecticides

Insecticide toxicosis is common in pet birds. Clinical signs can include weakness, anorexia, diarrhea, ataxia, tremors, paralysis, seizures, dyspnea, and death. Diagnosis is based on history of possible exposure, clinical signs, and cholinesterase assay (organophosphate and carbamate toxicoses). Cholinesterase levels less than 1000 IU/l in avian plasma are considered diagnostic. Postmortem diagnosis may be made based on insecticide residues found in tissues or gastrointestinal contents. Rapid metabolism of insecticides may result in false-negative results. Freeze samples for analysis.

Signs of delayed organophosphate toxicosis (weakness, ataxia, decreased proprioception, and paralysis) occur 7 to 10 days after exposure to the insecticide. The signs are the result of an organophosphate ester-induced neuropathy, not associated with inhibition of acetylcholine as in acute toxicosis. Cholinesterase assay will not detect this delayed toxicosis. Diagnosis is based on exposure and clinical signs.

Administer atropine and pralidoxime chloride (2-PAM) for organophosphate toxicosis treatment. The 2-PAM may only be effective if administered within 24 to 36 hours of exposure. Administer atropine for control of signs of carbamate toxicosis. Dexamethasone may be beneficial if shock or pulmonary edema are present. Give supportive care as needed. Treat delayed organophosphate toxicosis symptomatically; 2-PAM and atropine are of no benefit.

Lead

Lead toxicosis is very common in pet birds and waterfowl. It is most common in psittacines as a result of their tendency to chew and destroy materials. Some sources of lead are listed in Table 9–3. Clinical signs of lead toxicosis include depression, weakness, anorexia, regurgitation, polyuria, diarrhea, emaciation, CNS signs, and death. Central nervous system signs may include wing droop, leg paralysis, ataxia, blindness, head tilt, circling, head tremors, and seizures. Hematuria may be observed in Amazon parrots and African gray parrots. Some birds may show no clinical signs; others may only show wasting. In waterfowl, toxicosis may appear more chronic and may show clinical signs similar to botulism.

Lead toxicosis may cause abnormalities in the hemogram and plasma biochemistries. Affected birds may show a regenerative anemia with normal plasma

Table 9–3. Some Sources of Lead

Lead fishing weights
Lead curtain weights
Lead shot
Lead-based paint
Foil from some champagne and wine bottles
Plaster impregnated with lead
Lead putty
Lead solder
Linoleum
Mirror backs
Stained glass window solder
Tiffany lamps
Costume jewelry
Hardware cloth
Galvanized wire
Some welds on wrought-iron cages
Bird toys with lead weights
Bells with lead clappers
Improperly glazed ceramics
Batteries
Contaminated feed and bone meal

protein levels. Lead toxicosis may cause an exaggerated response with more polychromasia and rubricytes than would be expected for the degree of anemia present. Hypochromasia may occur. Elevations of AST, CK, and LDH often occur in birds with lead toxicosis.

Radiology may show metallic densities in the ventriculus. Lead toxicosis may be present without abnormal radiographic signs (i.e., lack of metallic densities in the gastrointestinal tract).

Definitive diagnosis is based on elevated blood lead levels. Lead blood levels are measured on whole blood, with lithium heparin used for the anticoagulant, not ethylenediamine tetracetic acid (EDTA). Whole blood lead levels greater than 0.2 ppm (20 μg/dl) are suggestive of lead toxicosis, and levels greater than 0.5 ppm (50 μg/dl) are diagnostic of lead toxicosis.

Chelation therapy, supportive care, and sometimes foreign body removal are required in the treatment of lead toxicosis. If seizures are present, diazepam is administered intramuscularly two to three times daily as needed. Chelation therapy is accomplished with edetate calcium disodium or calcium disodium versenate (CaEDTA), D-penicillamine, or dimercaprol (BAL). Calcium EDTA is most commonly used. Chelation therapy is begun with intramuscular injections. Oral chelation therapy may be used in addition to the injections or after resolution of clinical signs with metal still present in the ventriculus. Duration of treatment is determined by the drug used, route of administration, response to therapy, and continued presence of lead in the ventriculus. Peanut butter, mineral oil, or bulk laxatives may aid in the passage of small particles of metal out of the gastrointestinal tract. Large metal pieces can be removed endoscopically, surgically, or by gastric lavage. Patients must be stable and of sufficient size to tolerate the procedures.

Mycotoxins

Mycotoxins are metabolic byproducts of some fungi. Moldy or previously moldy foods may contain mycotoxins. Grains, peanuts, breads, meats, and cheeses are some of the foods on which these molds can grow. Mycotoxins are undetectable by sight, smell, or taste. Clinically significant mycotoxins include aflatoxin, ochratoxin, deoxynivalenol, trichothecene, oosporein, and citrinin. Clinical signs are often vague and may mimic other diseases. Clinical signs can include depression, anorexia, hemorrhage, polyuria, hematochezia, erosive lesions, paralysis, constrictive lesions of the digits, and poor feathering. Ingestion may result in liver or kidney disease or immunosuppression with signs related to failure of these organ systems. Contact dermatitis has been noted with exposure to trichothecene toxin. Diagnosis of mycotoxicosis is based on finding the toxin in food or gastrointestinal contents. Diagnosis is complicated by the fact that the food may have already been consumed and is no longer available for testing.

Organochlorine (Lindane)

See Insecticides.

Organophosphate

See Insecticides.

Polytetrafluoroethylene (Teflon Toxicosis)

Toxic gas may be produced when nonstick surfaces are heated. This toxicosis is very common in pet birds. Affected birds usually collapse suddenly, but clinical signs that may occur include depression, dyspnea, wheezing, ataxia, weakness, and seizures. On postmortem examination, hemorrhage and congestion of the lungs are usually noted. Birds usually die before therapy can be administered. If exposure to this toxic gas is suspected, instruct the owner to provide immediate fresh air and bring the bird to the hospital. Administer oxygen, intratracheal and systemic prednisolone, sodium succinate or dexamethasone, broad-spectrum antibiotics (e.g., enrofloxacin or cefotaxime), and fluid therapy, and place the bird in a warm environment.

Salt

Excessive ingestion of salt may result in depression, polydipsia, polyuria, ataxia, tremors, opisthotonos, seizures, and death. Common sources include ornamental cookie dough or sea sand for grit or nestbox substrate. Treatment includes the use of diuretics and sodium-poor intravenous or intraosseous fluids (D5W or 2½% dextrose in 0.45% saline).

Tobacco

Ingestion of tobacco can result in hyperexcitability, vomiting, diarrhea, seizures, and death. More common exposure to tobacco is through inhalation of secondary smoke or contact with surfaces contaminated with tobacco (e.g., fingers, arms, and clothes of smokers). Clinical signs may include sneezing, nasal discharge, sinusitis, coughing, and feet or cheek skin patch irritation and scabbing. Diagnosis is based on clinical signs and response to treatment. Treatment involves placing the birds in a smoke-free environment. People who smoke should wash hands and arms before contact with sensitive birds. Tobacco toxicosis is treated with administration of activated charcoal and mineral oil and supportive care.

Trichothecene

See Mycotoxins.

Vitamin D

Vitamin D toxicosis can result in hypercalcemia and mineralization of the kidneys, liver, stomach, intestines, heart, and blood vessels. Macaws and African gray parrots appear to be most sensitive to vitamin D toxicosis. Sources of vitamin D include excessive vitamin administration by the owner, commercial pelleted diet supplemented with vitamins, iatrogenic, and cholecalciferol rodenticide ingestion. Vitamin D_3 toxicosis is most common in handfed neonates fed a homemade formula (especially macaws). Clinical signs include lethargy, anorexia, polyuria, and diarrhea. Diagnosis is based on dietary history, possible exposure to rodenticide, clinical signs, blood calcium levels, and radiology. Nephrocalcinosis may be noted radiograpically.

Treat acute rodenticide toxicoses with activated charcoal; administer fluids, furosemide, calcitonin, and prednisolone; provide a low-calcium diet; and avoid exposure to sunlight. Treatment may be prolonged. Monitor calcium, phosphorus, and uric acid weekly.

Prevent nutritionally related vitamin D toxicosis by feeding a complete formulated diet.

Warfarin

Clinical signs of warfarin-containing rodenticide toxicosis include depression, anorexia, petechiation, epistaxis, melena, hematochezia, hematoma formation, and hemorrhage. Treat with vitamin K_1.

Zinc (New Wire Disease)

Zinc toxicosis is most common in psittacines. Sources of zinc include pennies minted since 1982; Monopoly game pieces; galvanized wire, mesh, nails, containers, and dishes; hardware cloth; staples; fertilizers; some paints; zinc oxide; and zinc shampoo. Hardware cloth can be scrubbed with a brush and vinegar or allowed to age exposed to outdoor conditions to decrease toxicity, but it may still result in toxicosis if the wire is chewed and the particles are ingested. Clinical signs of zinc toxicosis include weakness, depression, polydipsia, polyuria, vomiting, diarrhea, weight loss, cyanosis, and seizures. Radiology may show metallic densities in the ventriculus. Zinc toxicosis may be present without abnormal radiographic signs (i.e., lack of metallic densities in the gastrointestinal tract).

Definitive diagnosis is based on elevated blood zinc levels. Zinc blood levels are measured on serum. Use glass or all-plastic syringes and tubes. Rubber stoppers on serum tubes and grommets on some plastic syringes can result in zinc contamination. Serum tubes with royal blue stoppers are best for sample handling and are free of zinc. Serum zinc levels greater than 2 ppm (200μg/dl) are suggestive of zinc toxicosis. Levels above 10 ppm (1000 μg/dl) are common with zinc toxicosis.

Treatment of zinc toxicosis is the same as for lead toxicosis.

References and Additional Readings

Anderson NL. Candida/megabacteria proventriculitis in a lesser sulphur-crested cockatoo *(Cacatua sulphurea sulphurea). J Assoc Avian Vet* 1993;7(4):197–201.

Aguilar RF, Redig PT. Diagnosis and treatment of avian aspergillosis. In Bonagura JD, Kirk RW (eds): *Current Veterinary Therapy XII, Small Animal Practice*. Philadelphia, WB Saunders, 1995, pp 1294–1299.

Aranaz A, Liebana E, Mateos A, Dominguez L. Laboratory diagnosis of avian mycobacteriosis. *Semin Avian Exot Pet Med* 1997;6(1):9–17.

Bauck L. Mycoses. In Ritchie BW, Harrison GJ, Harrison LR (eds): *Avian Medicine: Principles and Application*. Lake Worth, FL, Wingers Publishing, 1994, pp 997–1006.

Bauck L. Nutritional problems in pet birds. *Semin Avian Exot Pet Med* 1995;4(1):3–8.

Brown MB, Ewing ML. Mycoplasmal infections. In Altman RB, Clubb SL, Dorrestein GM, Quesenberry K (eds): *Avian Medicine and Surgery*. Philadelphia, WB Saunders, 1997, pp 380–383.

Candeletta SC, Homer BL, Garner MM, et al. Diabetes mellitus associated with chronic lymphocytic pancreatitis in an African grey parrot *(Psittacus erithacus erithacus). J Assoc Avian Vet* 1993;7(1):39–43.

Carpenter JW, Gentz EJ. Zoonotic diseases of avian origin. In Altman RB, Clubb SL, Dorrestein GM, Quesenberry K (eds): *Avian Medicine and Surgery*. Philadelphia, WB Saunders, 1997, pp 350–363.

Clipsham R. Avian pathogenic flagellated enteric protozoa. *Semin Avian Exot Pet Med* 1995;4(3):112–125.

Clubb SL, Cray C, Greiner E, et al. Cryptosporidiosis in a psittacine nursery. *Proc Assoc Avian Vet* 1996;177–185.

Clyde VL, Patton S. Diagnosis, treatment, and control of common parasites in companion and aviary birds. *Semin Avian Exot Pet Med* 1996;5(2):75–84.

Cornelissen H, Ducatelle R, Roels S. Successful treatment of a channel-billed toucan *(Ramphastos vitellinus)* with iron storage disease by chelation therapy: Sequential monitoring of the liver during the treatment period by quantitative chemical and image analyses. *J Avian Med Surg* 1995;9(2):131–137.

Cross GM. Viral diseases. *Semin Avian Exot Pet Med* 1995;4(2).

Curtis-Velasco M. Eastern equine encephalomyelitis virus in a lady gouldian finch. *J Assoc Avian Vet* 1992;6(4):227–228.

Degernes LA. Toxicities in waterfowl. *Semin Avian Exot Pet Med* 1995;4(1):15–22.

Doolen M. Crop biopsy: A low risk diagnosis for neuropathic gastric dilatation. *Proc Assoc Avian Vet* 1994;193–196.

Dorrestein GM. Bacteriology. In Altman RB, Clubb SL, Dorrestein GM, Quesenberry K (eds): *Avian Medicine and Surgery.* Philadelphia, WB Saunders, 1997, pp 255–280.

Dumonceaux G, Harrison GJ. Toxins. In Ritchie BW, Harrison GJ, Harrison LR (eds): *Avian Medicine: Principles and Application.* Lake Worth, FL, Wingers Publishing, 1994, pp 1030–1052.

Ensley P. Parasitic diseases of cage birds. In Kirk RW (ed): *Current Veterinary Therapy VIII, Small Animal Practice.* Philadelphia, WB Saunders, 1983, pp 641–646.

Flammer K. Chlamydia. In Altman RB, Clubb SL, Dorrestein GM, Quesenberry K (eds): *Avian Medicine and Surgery.* Philadelphia, WB Saunders, 1997, pp 364–379.

Fowler ME. Plant poisoning in pet birds and reptiles. In Kirk RW (ed): *Current Veterinary Therapy IX, Small Animal Practice.* Philadelphia, WB Saunders, 1986, pp 737–743.

Gaskin JM, Homer BL, Eskelund KH. Preliminary findings in avian viral serositis: A newly recognized syndrome of psittacine birds. *J Assoc Avian Vet* 1991;5(1):27–34.

Gerlach H. Bacteriology. In Ritchie BW, Harrison GJ, Harrison LR (eds): *Avian Medicine: Principles and Application.* Lake Worth, FL, Wingers Publishing, 1994, pp 949–983.

Gerlach H. Chlamydia. In Ritchie BW, Harrison GJ, Harrison LR (eds): *Avian Medicine: Principles and Application.* Lake Worth, FL, Wingers Publishing, 1994, pp 984–996.

Gerlach H. Mycoplasma. In Ritchie BW, Harrison GJ, Harrison LR (eds): *Avian Medicine: Principles and Application.* Lake Worth, FL, Wingers Publishing, 1994, pp 1053–1063.

Gerlach H. Viruses. In Ritchie BW, Harrison GJ, Harrison LR (eds): *Avian Medicine: Principles and Application.* Lake Worth, FL, Wingers Publishing, 1994, pp 862–948.

Gould WJ. Liver disease in psittacines. In Kirk RW, Bonagura JD (eds): *Current Veterinary Therapy XI, Small Animal Practice.* Philadelphia, WB Saunders, 1992, pp 1145–1150.

Gregory CR, Latimer KS, Niagro FD, et al. A review of proventricular dilatation syndrome. *J Assoc Avian Vet* 1994;8(2):69–75.

Greiner EC. Parasitology. In Altman RB, Clubb SL, Dorrestein GM, Quesenberry K (eds): *Avian Medicine and Surgery.* Philadelphia, WB Saunders, 1997, pp 332–349.

Greiner EC, Ritchie BW. Parasites. In Ritchie BW, Harrison GJ, Harrison LR (eds): *Avian Medicine: Principles and Application.* Lake Worth, FL, Wingers Publishing, 1994, pp 1007–1029.

Grimes JE. Evaluation and interpretation of serologic responses in psittacine bird chlamydiosis and suggested complementary diagnostic procedures. *J Avian Med Surg* 1996;10(2):75–83.

Harms CA, Hoskinson JJ, Bruyette DS, et al. An experimental model of hypothyroidism in psittacine birds. *Proc Assoc Avian Vet* 1993;250–253.

Harris JM. Zoonotic diseases of birds. *Vet Clin North Am, Small Anim Pract* 1991; 1289–1298.

Hillyer EV, Moroff S, Hoefer H, et al. Bile duct carcinoma in two out of ten amazon parrots with cloacal papillomas. *J Assoc Avian Vet* 1991;5(2):91–95.

Hoop RK. Public health implications of exotic pet mycobacteriosis. *Semin Avian Exot Pet Med* 1997;6(1):3–8.

LaBonde J. Toxicity in pet avian patients. *Semin Avian Exot Pet Med* 1995;4(1):23–31.

LaBonde J. Avian toxicology. *Vet Clin North Am, Small Anim Pract* 1991;1329–1342.

LaBonde J. Household poisonings in caged birds. In Bonagura JD, Kirk RW (eds): *Current Veterinary Therapy XII, Small Animal Practice.* Philadelphia, WB Saunders, 1995, pp 1299–1303.

Latimer KS, Niagro FD, Campagnoli R, et al. Diagnosis of concurrent avian polyomavirus and psittacine beak and feather disease virus infections using DNA probes. *J Assoc Avian Vet* 1993;7(3):141–146.

Latimer KS, Niagro FD, Rakich PM, et al. Comparison of DNA dot-blot hybridization, immunoperoxidase staining, and routine histopathology in the diagnosis of psittacine beak and feather disease in paraffin-embedded cutaneous tissues. *J Assoc Avian Vet* 1992;6(3):165–168.

Ley DH, Flammer K, Cowen P, et al. Performance characteristics of diagnostic tests for avian chlamydiosis. *J Assoc Avian Vet* 1993;7(4):203–207.

Lloyd M. Heavy metal ingestion: Medical management and gastroscopic foreign body removal. *J Assoc Avian Vet* 1992;6(1):25–29.

Macwhirter P. Malnutrition. In Ritchie BW, Harrison GJ, Harrison LR (eds): *Avian Medicine: Principles and Application.* Lake Worth, FL, Wingers Publishing, 1994, pp 842–861.

McDonald SE. Lead poisoning in psittacine birds. In Kirk RW (ed): *Current Veterinary Therapy IX, Small Animal Practice.* Philadelphia, WB Saunders, 1986, pp 713–718.

Mehren KG. Gout. In Kirk RW (ed): *Current Veterinary Therapy VIII, Small Animal Practice.* Philadelphia, WB Saunders, 1983, pp 635–637.

Meier JE. Salmonellosis and other bacterial enteritides in birds. In Kirk RW (ed): *Current Veterinary Therapy VIII, Small Animal Practice.* Philadelphia, WB Saunders, 1983, pp 637–640.

Morris PJ, Avgeris SE, Baumgartner RE. Hemochromatosis in a greater hill mynah: Case report and review of the literature. *J Assoc Avian Vet* 1989;3(2):87–92.

Oglesbee BL. Mycotic diseases. In Altman RB, Clubb SL, Dorrestein GM, Quesenberry K (eds): *Avian Medicine and Surgery.* Philadelphia, WB Saunders, 1997, pp 323–331.

Oglesbee BL, Bishop CL. Avian infectious diseases. In Birchard SJ, Sherding RG (eds): *Saunders Manual of Small Animal Practice.* Philadelphia, WB Saunders, 1994, pp 1257–1270.

Page CD, Haddad K. Coccidial infections in birds. *Semin Avian Exot Pet Med* 1995;4(3):138–144.

Phalen DN. Viruses. In Altman RB, Clubb SL, Dorrestein GM, Quesenberry K (eds): *Avian Medicine and Surgery.* Philadelphia, WB Saunders, 1997, pp 281–322.

Rae M. Endocrine disease in pet birds. *Semin Avian Exot Pet Med* 1995;4(1):15–22.

Rae M. Hemoprotozoa of caged and aviary birds. *Semin Avian Exot Pet Med* 1995;4(3):131–137.

Ritchie BW. *Avian Viruses.* Lake Worth, FL, Wingers Publishing, 1995.

Ritchie BW, Harrison GJ, Harrison LR (eds). *Avian Medicine: Principles and Application.* Lake Worth, FL, Wingers Publishing, 1994.

Ritchie BW, Latimer KS. Avian polyomavirus. In Bonagura JD, Kirk RW (eds): *Current Veterinary Therapy XII, Small Animal Practice.* Philadelphia, WB Saunders, 1995, pp 1284–1288.

Ritchie BW, Latimer KS. Psittacine beak and feather disease virus. In Bonagura JD, Kirk RW (eds): *Current Veterinary Therapy XII, Small Animal Practice.* Philadelphia, WB Saunders, 1995, pp 1288–1294.

Ritchie BW, Niagro FD, Latimer KS, et al. Avian polyomavirus: An overview. *J Assoc Avian Vet* 1991;5(3):147–153.

Ritchie BW, Niagro FD, Lukert PD, et al. A review of psittacine beak and feather disease: Characteristics of the PBFD virus. *J Assoc Avian Vet* 1989;3(3):143–149.

Romagnano A, Grindem CB, Degernes L, et al. Treatment of a hyacinth macaw with zinc toxicity. *J Avian Med Surg* 1995;9(3):185–189.

Rosenthal K, Stamoulis M. Diagnosis of congestive heart failure in an Indian hill mynah (*Gracula religiosa*). *J Assoc Avian Vet* 1993;7(1):27–30.

Rosskopf WJ, Woerpel RW. Pet avian conditions and syndromes of the most frequently presented species seen in practice. *Vet Clin North Am Small Anim Pract* 1991; 1189–1211.

Smith SA. Parasites of birds of prey: Their diagnosis and treatment. *Semin Avian Exot Pet Med* 1996;5(2):97–105.

Spenser EL. Common infectious diseases of psittacine birds seen in practice. *Vet Clin North Am Small Anim Pract* 1991;1213–1230.

Stadler CK, Carpenter JW. Parasites of backyard game birds. *Semin Avian Exot Pet Med* 1996;5(2):85–96.

Suedmeyer WK. Diagnosis and clinical progression of three cases of proventricular dilatation syndrome. *J Assoc Avian Vet* 1992;6(3):159–163.

Tudor DC. *Pigeon Health and Disease.* Ames, Iowa, Iowa State University Press, 1991.

Tully TN. Chlamydiosis. *Semin Avian Exot Pet Med* 1993;2(4).

Turrel JM, McMillan MC, Paul-Murphy J. Diagnosis and treatment of tumors of companion birds I. *AAV Today* 1987;1(3):109–116.

Turrel JM, McMillan MC, Paul-Murphy J. Diagnosis and treatment of tumors of companion birds II. *AAV Today* 1987;1(4):159–165.

VanDerHeyden N. Clinical manifestations of mycobacteriosis in pet birds. *Semin Avian Exot Pet Med* 1997;6(1):18–24.

VanDerHeyden N. New strategies in the treatment of avian mycobacteriosis. *Semin Avian Exot Pet Med* 1997;6(1):25–33.

Worell A. Further investigations in ramphastids concerning hemochromatosis. *Proc Assoc Avian Vet* 1993;98–107.

Worell A. Management and medicine of toucans. *Proc Assoc Avian Vet* 1988;253–262.

Worell A. Phlebotomy for treatment of hemochromatosis in two sulphur-breasted toucans. *Proc Assoc Avian Vet* 1991;9–14.

Chapter 10

Necropsy

The information provided by a complete necropsy can include confirmation or disproval of a clinical diagnosis, identification of infectious agents, detection of flock or aviary problems, or identification of management problems. An important function of necropsy performance is continuing education. A complete necropsy allows a practitioner to compare clinical signs, physical examination findings, laboratory diagnostics, radiology, and endoscopy procedures with actual morphology. This information will allow a better understanding of the disease processes and enhance clinical diagnostic skills. Ancillary diagnostic testing (e.g., histopathology, bacterial cultures, virus isolation, and toxicology) is often required to make a definitive diagnosis.

To obtain the maximal useful information from a necropsy, an organized systematic protocol should be used every time. Use a checklist or necropsy report form to ensure that all tissues have been examined (Fig. 10–1).

EQUIPMENT

Designate instruments for necropsy use only. Clean and disinfect instruments after each use by steam, gas, or chemical disinfectants (e.g., glutaraldehyde or phenol). Rinse instruments disinfected with chemical disinfectants before use to avoid killing pathogens in tissues intended for culture.

Equipment needed to perform a necropsy includes forceps, scalpel, scissors, poultry shears, sterile slides, sterile culture swabs, culture and transport media, syringes, needles, sterile containers, tissue fixative, and marking pens to identify specimens and patient. Glass slides may be sterilized in an autoclavable container and autoclaving or sterilizing with gas. A flame source (e.g., Bunsen burner) and a spatula are needed for searing organ surfaces. Special transport media are required for *Chlamydia* and *Mycoplasma* cultures. A camera is useful for recording unusual abnormalities and reference photographs.

PREPARING THE DEAD BIRD

Immediate cooling is important to preserve tissue quality. Birds not necropsied immediately are soaked in cold soapy water. Soap will decrease the surface tension on the feathers and allow complete wetting of the carcass. This is important because dry feathers act as excellent insulators and slow cooling of the bird. Upon complete wetting, the bird is refrigerated until a necropsy is performed. Do not freeze the bird if histopathology samples will be submitted.

TISSUE SAMPLE COLLECTION AND HANDLING

Contact the diagnostic laboratory to which the samples will be submitted before performing the necropsy. Obtain specific directions for submission of specimens, including specimen collection, preparation, fixative, media, and shipment. Follow the directions.

Obtain fresh tissues and collect and submit a complete set of tissues (Table 10–1), not just tissues that appear abnormal. If monetary concerns prevent submission of a complete set of tissue samples, collect a complete set, fix the tissues for histopathology, and freeze samples that may be needed for virus isolation and toxicology. Send samples as needed to obtain a diagnosis.

Samples collected for histopathology are fixed in 10 times their volume of 10% neutral buffered formalin for 48 hours for fixation. After 48 hours, tissues are fixed and may be removed from the formalin and shipped with sufficient formalin to keep the tissues wet. Samples must be no thicker than 5 mm. Section congested tissue thinner. Small lungs may be put in formalin intact. Small and nestling birds may be submitted fixed whole. Open the body cavity, separate the organs, and place in adequate formalin. When submitting lesions, include a margin of normal tissue. Suspected gout lesions are fixed in absolute alcohol, because uric acid crystals may dissolve in formalin. Impression smears and cytology may also be used for identification of uric acid crystals.

Organ samples sent for bacterial culture must be kept refrigerated, including during shipment. The minimum tissue size is 2 cc. Place tissue samples in sterile containers and ship with a next-day courier service. Organs and tissue surfaces may also be cultured using a sterile swab placed in transport medium. Special transport media are required for *Chlamydia* and *Mycoplasma* cultures. If uncommon bacteria are suspected, contact the laboratory for instructions to optimize culture results.

Fresh tissues collected for virus isolation are placed in sealable plastic bags

---

TABLE 10–1 Tissues Routinely Collected for Histopathology at Necropsy

Air sac	Large intestine	Kidneys
Pancreas	Cloaca	Great vessels
Heart	Bursa of Fabricius	Thyroid glands
Spleen	Oviduct	Parathyroid glands
Liver	Ovary	Lung
Esophagus	Testes	Crop
Proventriculus	Adrenal glands	Trachea
Ventriculus	Muscle	Brain
Small intestine	Bone marrow	Thymus
Ceca		

Sample all other abnormal tissues, including bone, eye, peripheral nerves, tissues of the oropharynx and infraorbital sinus, and feather follicles (if feather abnormalities are noted).

Owner _____ Bird's name _____ Date _____

Species _____ Sex _____ Age _____ ID _____ Case # _____

External Exam	Thyroids	Ventriculus	Brain
Weight (wet/dry)	Parathyroids	Small intestine	Pituitary
Feathers	Gallbladder	Ceca	Miscellaneous
Skin	Proventriculus	Large intestine	Plexuses
Pectoral muscles	Ventriculus	Oviduct	Peripheral nerves
Mouth	Intestines	Cloaca	Bone strength
Beak	Pancreas	Bursa	Joints
Nares	Ceca	Gonads/adrenal/kidney	Bone marrow
Eyes	Spleen	Heart/great vessels	**Impression Smears**
Infraorbital sinuses	Collect heart blood	Thyroids/parathyroids	Air sacs
Ears	Kidneys	Lungs	Liver/spleen/heart
Cloaca	Adrenals	Oropharynx:	Other
Feet	Ovary	Tongue	**Culture Swabs**
Nails	Oviduct	Oral mucosa	Nasal aspirate
Skeletal palpation	Testes	Choana	Liver
Internal Exam	Lungs	Esophagus	Spleen
Pectoral muscles	Crop	Crop	Air sacs
Fat stores	**Dissection/Sample**	Larynx	Oviduct
Liver	Air sacs	Trachea	Trachea
Air sacs	Spleen	Syrinx	Intestinal
Pericardium	Liver	Thymus	Other
Heart	Proventriculus	Infraorbital sinuses	

NSF = No Significant Findings

Abnormalities: _____

_____

Diagnostics	Samples	Laboratory	Courier
Histopathology			
Cytology			
Bacteriology			
Virology			
Toxicology			
Other			

Owner to pick up body_____ Clinic disposal/date _____

Figure 10–1. Necropsy report form.

and frozen. Tissues collected for fungal culture may be refrigerated or frozen. If impression smears are to be sent to a laboratory for diagnostics, contact the laboratory for specific instructions on smear preparation and fixation. Samples not stained before submission must be protected from moisture and formalin fumes. Consult the laboratory for samples needed and handling of samples for toxicologic analysis. Liver, kidney, lung, brain, pancreas, adipose tissue, and gastrointestinal contents are generally collected when toxicoses are suspected. Place tissue samples in aluminum foil if pesticide or hydrocarbon toxicosis is suspected and in plastic bags if heavy metal toxicosis is suspected.

After the necropsy is completed and samples have been collected, freeze the leftover carcass until the case is completely evaluated. Samples may be discarded when the final report is received.

Provide a complete history, including signalment, history, and clinical, laboratory, and gross necropsy findings. This information improves histopathologic evaluation and interpretation of necropsy findings by the pathologist. Submit samples to a laboratory and pathologist experienced in the diagnosis of avian diseases.

SHIPPING CARCASSES

Refrigerate carcasses if histopathology is part of the examination; do not freeze. Send carcasses refrigerated if the carcass will reach the laboratory within 72 hours. Package with adequate coolant and insulation to ensure that it will remain cold until it arrives at the laboratory. Freeze carcasses and ship them frozen if more than 3 days will pass before arrival to the laboratory. Ship frozen carcasses packed in sufficient dry ice or freezer packs frozen in dry ice to remain frozen until reaching the laboratory. Ship carcasses overnight with a next-day courier service. Avoid Saturday deliveries because many laboratories do not process submissions on weekends.

PRECAUTIONS

Protect yourself and other hospital staff from zoonoses by using appropriate protection (e.g., surgical masks, gloves, eye protection). Wet the carcass with soapy water or disinfectant after the weight has been recorded to decrease aerosolization of potential pathogens.

THE NECROPSY RECORD

Record necropsy results on a written necropsy report form. The example provided may be used as a record as well as for a consistent protocol (see Fig. 10–1). Plain pages may be attached to describe multiple abnormalities. Write reports in present tense and describe lesions objectively.

NECROPSY PROCEDURE

Follow a written, systematic approach.

Weight

Weigh the bird and note if the weight is taken dry or wet.

External Structures

Examine the feathers, the pectoral musculature, skin, and all body orifices (mouth, nares, eyes, ears, and cloaca). If a nasal discharge is present, consider collecting a sample by sinus aspiration or nasal wash at this point. Assess the pericloacal area for feces or urate accumulation or lesions. Examine the beak, feet, and nails for abnormalities. Palpate the skeleton for current or previous fractures. Note leg band numbers, patagium (wing web) tattoos, or other identifying marks. Normal and abnormal external physical findings are discussed in Chapter 1.

If the bird is not already wet, saturate the feathers with soapy water or disinfectant to decrease aerosolization of pathogens and feather dander. Pluck feathers along the ventral body from the neck to the vent. Incise the skin of the medial thigh and cut the adductor muscles. The hips are disarticulated by forcing the stifle outward. The bird may then be pinned to a necropsy board in dorsal recumbency with the wings extended.

Subcutaneous and Pectoral Muscle Examination

Extend the skin incision from the inguinal area, past the lateral thorax, to the neck. Connect these two incisions caudally just cranial to the vent. Remove the skin from the abdominal and pectoral musculature to the mandible, with care to leave the thin abdominal musculature and crop intact.

Examine the subcutaneous tissue and pectoral musculature. Incise the pectoral musculature and observe for abnormalities. Observe for muscle wasting, hemorrhage, swelling, necrosis, pallor, or pale streaking. Muscle wasting may be caused by inadequate food intake or lack of absorption of nutrients. Hemorrhage or necrosis may be caused by injury, intramuscular or subcutaneous injections, septicemia, or some viral infections (e.g., polyomavirus). Pallor or pale streaking of the musculature may be caused by injury, inflammation, necrosis, anemia, neoplasia, or *Sarcocystis* infection. Collect samples of abnormal muscles for cytology and histopathology.

Opening the Coelomic Cavity

Open the body cavity by cutting with scissors through the abdominal muscles transversely caudal to the sternum. Then cut cranially through the pectoral

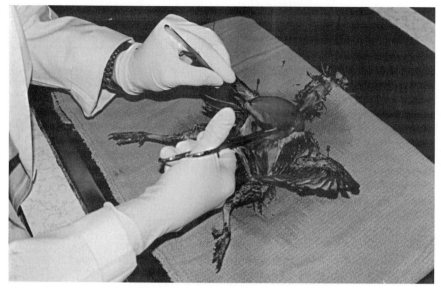

Figure 10–2. To open the body cavity, the skin is removed, the abdominal muscles are incised caudal to the sternum, and the muscles and ribs along the lateral thorax are cut.

muscles and ribs along the lateral thorax, extending through the coracoids and clavicles with scissors or poultry shears while lifting the sternum (Fig. 10–2). Note the size of the liver as the sternum is elevated. The normal liver does not extend beyond the edge of the sternum, except in some waterfowl.

Collect Microbiological Samples

Examine the exposed air sac membranes, pericardium, and liver. Normal air sac membranes are glistening and transparent. If lesions or exudates are present, the air sac membranes are cultured. Impression smears of the air sac membranes and surfaces of the liver and heart are taken if abnormalities are noted or chlamydiosis is suspected. Use a sterile slide. Culture samples may be taken, and cytology slides may be made with a swab. The sample is collected and rolled on a sterile slide, and the swab is placed in culture media.

If fluid is present in the body cavity, samples are collected for culture, cytologic evaluation, protein content evaluation, and cell count.

Examine the Viscera

Remove the sternum. Remove abdominal musculature cranial to the vent as needed to examine the viscera. Examine the air sac membranes, fat stores, heart, thyroid glands, parathyroid glands, liver, proventriculus, ventriculus, intestines, pancreas, spleen, kidneys, adrenal glands, gonads, lungs, and crop before removal of any organs.

Tissues are collected from abnormal air sac membranes. Air sac membrane samples collected for histopathology are placed on a piece of paper before fixation. Abnormalities that may be noted include fluid accumulation, exudates, opaque air sac membranes, granulomas, or mold growth. Fluid accumulation, exudates, or opaque air sac membranes may be the result of bacterial, chlamydial, viral, fungal, or parasitic infections. Granulomas may be caused by bacterial or fungal infection or foreign material. *Aspergillus* may appear as mold growth on the air sac membrane (a green or yellow area similar to bread mold).

In normal birds, a small amount of fat is usually present in the posthepatic septum (similar to the falciform ligament in mammals), in the mesentery, around the cloaca, at the heart base, and in the coronary groove. Excessive fat accumulation indicates obesity. Lack of fat indicates inadequate nutritional intake or absorption. Serous atrophy of fat appears as gelatinous fluid and indicates wasting.

The normal heart is somewhat triangular and the aorta curves to the right. The normal great vessels are smooth and white. Heart abnormalities include changes in the size, shape, color, appearance of petechiae, or the accumulation of fluid or white deposits. Pericarditis is commonly the result of bacterial, chlamydial, or viral infection or respiratory disease. Hydropericardium is commonly the result of viral infection, furazolidone toxicosis, or genetic defects. Myocarditis is commonly the result of bacterial, chlamydial, viral, or parasitic infection or vitamin E/selenium deficiencies. Cardiomegaly is commonly the result of bacterial or viral infection or hemochromatosis. Pale streaking may be the result of fibrosis, necrosis, inflammation, neoplasia, vitamin E/selenium deficiency, or parasitic infection (*Sarcocystis, Atoxoplasma*). White streaks on the pericardial sac and epicardium occasionally occur as a result of euthanasia by cardiac injection. Petechiae may be the result of bacterial septicemia, viral infection, or an agonal event. The accumulation of white gritty material may be uric acid crystal deposits (gout) or bacterial pericarditis. The normal pericardial sac contains minimal fluid. Collect fluid from the pericardial sac for culture, cytology, cell count, and protein determination if fluid is present. Note pericardial, heart, and great vessel abnormalities. Sear the right atrium with a hot spatula and collect heart blood for culture and blood smears with a sterile needle and syringe. Postmortem blood smears are useful for detection of blood parasites and bacteremia, and diagnostic cells may be observed in spite of cell lysis.

Examine the thyroid and parathyroid glands. The thyroid and parathyroid glands are immediately lateral to the carotid arteries at the thoracic inlet. Normal thyroid glands are oval and dark red. Enlarged thyroid glands are abnormal and may be the result of goiter, neoplasia, amyloidosis, or inflammation. A pair of parathyroid glands are associated with the caudal aspect of each thyroid gland. The normal parathyroid gland is yellow to off-white, very small, and may not be visible in small species. Enlarged parathyroid glands may be the result of calcium deficiency, vitamin D_3 deficiency, neoplasia, or possibly kidney disease (not proved to occur in birds). Calcium deficiency as a result of poor nutrition is a common cause of parathyroid enlargement. Note abnormalities of the thyroid and parathyroid glands.

Examine the liver. The normal liver is uniformly red-brown, bilobed, relatively large, and contacts the sides of the heart. In psittacines, the right lobe is generally larger than the left lobe. In raptors and gallinaceous birds, the lobes are similar in size. Gallinaceous birds, ducks, geese, toucans, and some passerine birds have gallbladders. Pigeons and psittacines do not have gallbladders. Abnormalities of the liver include hepatomegaly, decrease in size, granulomas, necrotic foci, discoloration, or mold growth. Hepatomegaly may be the result of chlamydial, bacterial, mycobacterial, viral, or parasitic infection; hepatic lipidosis; hemochromatosis; amyloidosis; gout; or neoplasia. A decrease in size may be the result of fibrosis (e.g., aflatoxicosis or resolved hepatic lipidosis). Multifocal white to yellow granulomatous or necrotic foci may be the result of bacterial, mycobacterial, chlamydial, viral, fungal, or parasitic infection or neoplasia. A pale to yellow enlarged liver is usually the result of hepatic lipidosis or a normal neonate-mobilizing egg yolk in the first 2 to 3 weeks of life. A dark brown to black enlarged liver is commonly the result of hemochromatosis or *Plasmodium* infection. *Aspergillus* may appear as mold growth on the surface of the liver (a green or yellow area similar to bread mold) or granuloma formation.

The liver, duodenum, and pancreas are elevated, and the proventriculus and ventriculus are examined (Fig. 10–3). These two organs make up the avian stomach. The shape of the proventriculus and ventriculus varies among species of birds. In granivorous, insectivorous, and herbivorous birds (e.g., psittacines, passerines, and pigeons), the normal proventriculus and ventriculus are easily distinguishable with a constriction between the two structures and muscular wall of the ventriculus. In carnivorous and piscivorous birds that eat soft foods (e.g., raptors and toucans), the ventriculus is thin walled and difficult to grossly differentiate from the proventriculus. Some birds have stomachs that grossly appear intermediate between the two. The normal proventriculus is located dorsal to the left liver lobe. If dilated, it may be visible without retracting the liver. Abnormalities of the proventriculus include dilatation, perforation,

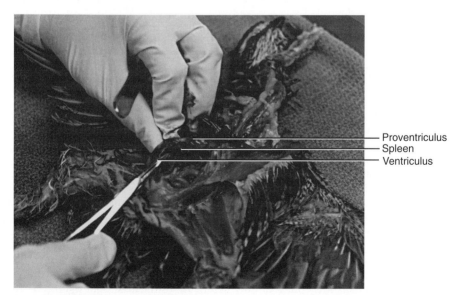

Proventriculus
Spleen
Ventriculus

Figure 10–3. Necropsy of a quail showing the ventriculus, proventriculus, and spleen.

congestion, or hemorrhage. Dilatation may be the result of impaction, proventricular dilatation syndrome, or bacterial infection.

The intestines, pancreas, and ceca are examined. In many birds the pancreas has three lobes: one in the duodenal loop, one lateral to the ascending duodenum, and one between the ventriculus and the spleen. There are variations among species of birds. Ceca may be large (toucans, gallinaceous birds, owls, and ostrich), small (passerines, diurnal raptors), or absent (psittacines and pigeons). Normal pancreatic tissue is light tan to pink. Abnormalities of the intestines include congestion, hemorrhage, thickened wall, distention with fluid, gas, foreign material (e.g., nesting substrate or grit), or nematodes. Congestion, hemorrhage, thickened wall, or distention with fluid may be the result of bacterial, viral, chlamydial, mycobacterial, or parasitic infection. Gas accumulation in the lumen of the intestine may be the result of vomiting, tube feeding, enteritis, or a postmortem change caused by gas production by enteric bacteria.

The ventriculus is elevated toward the bird's right side to expose the spleen. The shape of the normal spleen varies with the species. The normal spleen is dark purple/gray. The spleen of normal budgies is 1 mm, and up to 3 mm in English budgies. The normal cockatiel spleen is usually less than 4 mm. The normal Amazon parrot or African gray parrot spleen is usually less than 10 mm. Abnormalities include splenomegaly, discoloration, masses, or swellings. Splenomegaly may be the result of chlamydial, bacterial, viral, mycobacterial, or parasitic infection; lipidosis; hemochromatosis; amyloidosis; or neoplasia. Chlamydiosis is a common cause of splenomegaly in psittacines.

Retract the viscera to expose the kidneys, adrenal glands, and gonads. The kidneys lie in depressions of the synsacrum. Each kidney has three divisions; however, the boundaries between them are not always distinct. The normal kidney has a slightly granular surface and is brown to reddish brown. Abnormalities of the kidney include enlargement, discoloration, pallor, masses, or white foci. Renomegaly may be the result of bacterial, chlamydial, viral, or parasitic infection; dehydration; lipidosis; gout; amyloidosis; postrenal obstruction; congenital cysts; neoplasia; or lead or zinc toxicoses.

The adrenal glands are located at the cranial pole of the kidneys, dorsal to the gonads. The normal adrenal gland is yellow to pink and flattened round to triangular in shape. Abnormalities of the adrenal gland include enlargement, masses, or discoloration. Enlargement may be the result of chronic stress, chronic corticosteroid administration, adrenal neoplasia, or pituitary tumor.

In male birds, the testes are located at the cranial pole of the kidneys. They have a smooth surface, but vary in size, shape, and color. The testes of immature birds are small, bean shaped, and yellow to white. In some birds, they may be pigmented black or gray (e.g., some cockatoos, blue and gold Macaws, golden conures, mynahs, and toucans). During the breeding season, the testes of mature birds may enlarge from 10% to 500%. The large testes may be white, yellow, or gray, with a vascular surface. During the nonbreeding season, the testes atrophy and appear grossly similar to but slightly larger than the juvenile testes. Testicular abnormalities include swellings, tumors, atrophy (during the breeding season in adult males), and agenesis. Atrophy may be the result of inflammation, bacterial infection, septicemia, congenital, malnutrition, toxicosis, or lack of correct environmental stimuli. Enlargement or swelling may be the result of bacterial infection, inflammation, or neoplasia.

In most avian species the female has a single functional ovary. A smaller, second ovary is not uncommon. The ovary is located at the cranial pole of the left kidney. The oviduct courses over the ventral surface of the left kidney. The oviduct is very thin during reproductive inactivity, but becomes long, wide, and tortuous during active egg laying. In immature birds, the ovary is flattened and triangular and may be white, yellow, or pigmented black (e.g., some cockatoos, macaws, and conures), with a faintly granular surface. The immature ovary may resemble a piece of fat. The active ovary has follicles in varying stages of development, appearing as a cluster of variably sized grapes. The normal post-ovulatory follicle is devoid of blood clots. During the nonbreeding season, the ovary and oviduct regress, and many small follicles will be present on the ovary. Abnormalities of the ovary include inactive ovaries during breeding season; wrinkled, discolored, enlarged, firm, inspissated, pedunculated, or hemorrhagic ova; abnormal yolk that appears coagulated and flaking off into the abdominal cavity; congested or distorted follicles; swellings; or adhesions. Inactive ovaries during the breeding season may be the result of lack of correct environmental stimuli, immaturity, old age, severe stress, or aflatoxicosis. Large oviducts are examined for discolorations, swellings, hemorrhage, and the presence of eggs.

Examine the septal (ventromedial) surface of the lung. Normal lungs are pink. Abnormalities include discolorations, swellings, exudates, masses, and hemorrhage. Dark red and wet lungs may be the result of pulmonary edema and hemorrhage caused by bacterial infection, polytetrafluroethylene (Teflon) toxicosis, *Sarcocystis* infection, or inhalation of noxious gases or carbon monoxide. Multifocal white lesions may be caused by bacterial, fungal, or mycobacterial infection; neoplasia; or foreign material. *Aspergillus* may appear as mold growth on the surface of the lung (a green to yellow area similar to bread mold) or as granulomas. Postmortem extravasation of blood may enter the air sacs or lungs and may be confused with pulmonary hemorrhage.

The crop is examined. The normal crop wall is thin and uniform. When fully distended, the normal crop is almost transparent. Lesions include discolorations, thickening, swellings, foreign bodies, perforations, erosions, masses, and plaques.

The liver and spleen may be cultured at this time or after removing them from the body. The liver is routinely cultured, and the spleen is cultured if it is enlarged. The organ's surfaces are seared with a heated spatula, and the organ is incised through the capsule with the spatula in the seared region. Samples are collected from the exposed tissue. Remove and examine the spleen. Imprints may be made for cytologic evaluation. A portion of the spleen may be placed in a sterile container for culture. Splenic tissue should be collected and placed in formalin for histopathology.

Remove the proventriculus, ventriculus, liver, intestines, pancreas, cloaca, and vent as a single mass. The esophagus is transected just above the proventriculus. Lift and dissect these organs free from their attachments. Ligamentous attachments, air sac membranes, ureters, and oviducts (female birds) are severed with sharp dissection. A small amount of skin is excised with the vent.

The liver is removed from the mass of organs. Slices are made through the parenchyma of the organ every 0.5 cm to expose possible lesions. Lesions are noted and imprints are made for cytologic evaluation. A portion of the liver is placed in a sterile container or swabbed for culture, and tissue is collected and placed in formalin for histopathology. Samples may also be collected for toxologic analysis.

Open the proventriculus and ventriculus and examine the internal surface for erosions, ulcerations, discoloration, masses, or swellings. Collect samples of contents for toxologic evaluation if toxicosis is suspected. In granivorous, insectivorous, and herbivorous birds (e.g., psittacines, passerines, and pigeons), the ventriculus is thick walled and has a cuticle (koilin lining). The cuticle is often stained green if the bird has not been eating, but this is a normal finding in gallinaceous species and pigeons. Do not remove the cuticle. In carnivorous and piscivorous birds that eat soft foods (e.g., raptors and toucans), the ventriculus is thin walled and the koilin layer is thin and soft. Scrape the mucosal surface of the proventriculus and examine scraped material for parasite eggs (e.g., spirurids). Section the ventriculus, including cuticle and muscle wall, for histopathology. Examine the muscular wall of the ventriculus for pale striations in the muscle that may be associated with vitamin E deficiency.

If an intestinal culture is anticipated, aspirate the intestinal contents into a sterile needle and syringe before opening the intestines. In large birds, the intestines are opened and examined for erosions, ulcers, hemorrhage, parasites, masses, and thickening. Sections are taken for histopathology and microbiology. Handle sections for histopathology gently. Scrape the mucosal surfaces and examine the scraped material for parasites and eggs (e.g., coccidia, *Giardia, Cryptosporidium*). Impression smears are made when the intestinal mucosa is thickened and mycobacteriosis is suspected. Cytology of impression smears may reveal ghostlike nonstaining rods when stained with Wright's or Diff-Quick stains. A definitive diagnosis requires acid-fast staining and culture. Collect samples of contents for toxologic evaluation if toxicosis is suspected. In small birds, the intestines are fixed without opening; however, section at intervals to allow penetration of formalin.

Open and examine the ceca, if present, for hemorrhage, parasites, insipated exudates, discoloration, masses, or other lesions.

Open and examine the oviduct for thickening, masses, discolorations, or other lesions in adult female birds.

Examine the cloaca. In young birds, the bursa of Fabricius may be found on the dorsal wall of the cloaca. The bursa involutes with age and is difficult or impossible to identify grossly in adult birds. Open the cloaca and examine the mucosa for masses, erosions, hemorrhage, discoloration, or thickening. Section abnormalities, collect samples for microbiology, and fix samples for histopathology. Submit the bursa for histopathology in young birds.

The gonads, adrenal glands, and kidneys are removed from the body cavity as a single mass and submitted for histopathology without dissecting them apart. The fascia is grasped anterior to the gonads, adrenal glands, and kidneys, and attachments are dissected. The kidneys are removed from the renal fossa of the synsacrum (pelvis) with careful blunt dissection. The kidney parenchyma is examined for discoloration, pallor, masses, or white foci. White foci may be the result of gout. Collect tissue samples for toxologic evaluation if toxicosis is suspected. Samples are taken for culture if infection is suspected, and the tissues are fixed in formalin, remaining together.

The heart and associated great vessels are removed and examined. The four chambers of the heart are opened before fixing in formalin. In larger birds, the chambers of the heart and valves are examined. The right atrioventricular valve is a muscular, rather than membranous, flap. Open and examine the aorta and brachiocephalic trunks. Thickening, irregular shape, and yellow discolorations may be the result of arteriosclerosis. Collect samples of abnormal tissues. Longitudinal sections of the heart and great vessels are submitted for histopathology when the wall of the heart is thicker than 4 mm. The chambers of small hearts are opened, and the heart is fixed whole.

Thyroid and parathyroid glands are removed and placed in formalin.

The lungs are removed using blunt dissection and traction. Transect the parenchyma at 0.5 cm intervals to look for lesions in the parenchyma. Abnormalities include exudates, consolidation, hemorrhage, debris, and masses. Lesions associated with inhaled infections are most common in the dorsolateral areas of the lungs. Make impression smears of lesions for cytology. Collect samples for culture if bacterial infection is suspected. Collect samples for histopathology. Collect tissue samples for toxologic evaluation if toxicosis is suspected.

Open and examine the oropharynx, esophagus, and crop. Depending on the size of the bird, the commissure of the beak is cut on the right side using scissors or poultry shears. The cut is continued down the esophagus and the crop. Examine the tongue, oral mucosa, choana, larynx, esophagus, and crop for plaques, erosions, ulcers, masses, or discolorations. Abnormal tissues are collected for histopathology; impression smears may be made for cytologic evaluation. Collect samples of crop material if toxicosis is suspected.

The trachea is opened and examined. To open the avian trachea (with complete tracheal rings) for examination, an incision must be made on each side of the trachea. Examine the mucosa for hemorrhage, erosions, plaques, masses, or parasites. Tracheal swabs may be taken. If virus or *Mycoplasma* isolation is to be performed, a section of the trachea is removed aseptically. Closely examine the syrinx and main stem bronchi for keratin plaques and *Aspergillus* lesions. The thymus may be noted in young birds as pale tan to gray lobules of tissue adjacent to the trachea. Samples of thymic tissue are fixed for histopathology.

The nasal passages are examined by cutting through the skull at the base of the cere. Examine for exudates, masses, foreign bodies, swellings, and plaques. Collect samples of abnormal tissues for cytology, culture, and histopathology.

The bird is removed from the necropsy board. Pluck the feathers from the skull and reflect the skin from the calvarium. Sever the spinal cord at the atlanto-occipital joint. Cut away the calvarium with the tips of the scissors, starting at the foramen magnum, holding the scissors perpendicular to the surface of the calvarium (Fig. 10–4). Examine the brain for hemorrhage or congestion. Hemorrhage in the skull is a common finding and is often the result of postmortem extravasation of blood. Blood in or under the meninges warrants investigation.

Cut the dura mater midline and along the cranial cerebellum and reflect the dura. The brain is removed from the skull by careful dissection of the ventral surface of the brain with the head held upside down, letting gravity pull the brain away from the floor of the calvarium. The entire brain may be fixed for histopathology, or half of the brain may be fixed and the other half retained for cultures and virus isolation.

Examine the brachial plexuses, sacral plexuses, sciatic nerves, and intercostal nerves, especially in gallinaceous birds and birds with a history of neurologic

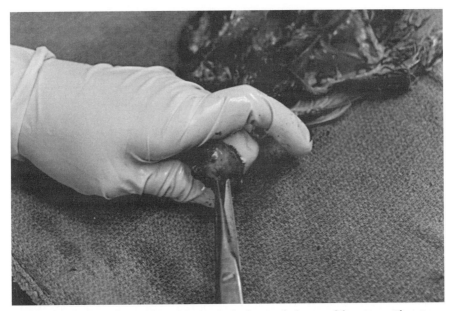

Figure 10–4. The calvarium is removed by cutting the bone with the tips of the scissors. The scissors are held perpendicular to the bone.

deficits. The brachial plexuses are located lateral to the thyroid glands. The sacral plexuses are imbedded in the middle division of the kidney. The sciatic nerve is medial to the medial thigh muscles.

Test the strength of a long bone by breaking one. Examine the coxofemoral, femorotibial, intertarsal, elbow, and carpal joints. Note the character of the synovial fluid and examine the articular cartilage. Crack the tibiotarsus and place it or a piece of the marrow in formalin for bone marrow evaluation, especially in birds with pale liver and kidneys, suggestive of anemia.

The spinal cord is difficult to extract without traumatizing the tissue. If a spinal cord lesion is suspected, the spinal column is removed intact, muscle and other soft tissue is removed, and the spinal column is fixed in formalin.

At the completion of the necropsy, go through the checklist to ensure that all tissues have been examined and samples collected. After all samples are collected, freeze the carcass and save it until histopathology and cultures are completed.

PEDIATRIC NECROPSY

Necropsies performed on pediatric birds are similar to those of adult birds. The same protocol is followed with the collection of the samples. Postmortem autolysis occurs rapidly in pediatric birds. Perform necropsies immediately upon death.

History of the bird and the aviary often provides assistance in making a diagnosis. Gross characteristic lesions may not be present in pediatric birds.

TABLE 10–2 Nursery History

Is the nursery located in a separate room or area of the aviary?
Are chicks from a single source or mixed with others from multiple sources?
Does cross contamination occur from quarantined, ill, and apparently healthy chicks?
Are visitors or customers allowed?
Are visitors or customers allowed to handle chicks?
Are chicks mixed from multiple parents from within the aviary?
Are small and large psittacine species allowed in the same nursery?
Review past medical history, including slow weight gains, slow crop emptying, and any other
   abnormalities. Review previous losses (species, age, when, where, cause).

Histologically, inflammatory responses may be minimal. Tables 10–2 and 10–3 contain important historical questions to be asked about the nursery and breeding facilities.

Pediatric birds have some anatomic differences. Compare the dead chick to a chick of the same age and species whenever possible to aid in identification of subtle external differences. Chicks younger than 24 hours normally appear misshapen. Examine external structures. Examine the body for developmental abnormalities. A large head in relation to body size is common in stunted or undersized birds. In newly hatched chicks, an egg tooth is present on the beak, and the hatching muscle along the back of the neck is very large and often edematous. This muscle may normally remain enlarged for up to 4 weeks. Beak abnormalities are common. Examine the oropharynx closely, looking for possible syringe punctures in hand-fed chicks. Eyes that are shut beyond the normal time of opening may be the result of a developmental anomaly, stunting, or artificial sealing with exudate or dried food. Ears are covered by a thin membrane at hatching in many species. Examine and palpate the crop for erythema, scabs, discoloration, foreign bodies, and consistency of crop contents.

Examine the skin and feathers for abnormalities. The normal skin in very young chicks is somewhat translucent. In older chicks, the skin is opaque, soft and pinkish-yellow. Some flaking of the skin is normal. Wrinkled or overly dry skin may indicate dehydration. Common causes of petechial hemorrhages in

---

TABLE 10–3 Breeding Facility History

Where are the adult breeders housed?
What are the sources of the birds?
What species of birds are housed within the aviary?
Are new arrivals quarantined?
Are ill birds isolated?
Does cross contamination occur from quarantined, ill, and established birds?
Are visitors allowed in the aviary?
Are visitors or customers allowed to handle chicks?
Investigate food storage location and conditions.
Review past medical history and previous losses (species, age, when, where, cause, any other
   abnormalities).
Review breeding and production records, including eggs produced, fertile eggs produced, dead in
   shell, percent successfully hatched, and percent successfully raised. Scrutinize first-time
   producers.

---

neonatal and pediatric birds include viral infections, bacterial septicemia, and bleeding problems (liver disease). Abnormal feather development may be the result of stunting or illness. Psittacine beak and feather disease, polyomavirus, and stunting are common causes of feather abnormalities in pediatric psittacines. Examine the umbilicus and the yolk sac in newly hatched chicks. The yolk sac is a diverticulum of the intestines and contains yolk that supplies nutrition and maternal antibodies to the neonate. The yolk sac is normally absorbed into the abdomen before completion of hatching. Subcutaneous soft tissue abnormalities such as swellings, lacerations, soft tissue calcification, or uric acid deposits may be noted with examination of the skin. Examine the body for musculoskeletal abnormalities (developmental abnormalities, fractures, etc.). The toes of a normal psittacine chick extend forward and are slightly curled until 10 to 20 days of age. Leg deviations are common. If constricted toes are noted, increase the humidity of the environment for the other birds in the brooder and nursery. Normal young birds do not have the large pectoral muscle mass of adult birds. Muscle mass and body stores are best assessed in young birds by the muscle and subcutaneous fat covering the elbows, toes, back, and hips. Examine the carcass for spinal and keel deviations. The abdomen of normal young birds is large and full. The liver, proventriculus, and ventriculus are large in comparison to body size and may be observed through the translucent abdominal skin.

Avoid rupturing the yolk sac when opening the body cavity. Incise the skin on the left lateral body from the mandible to the side of the vent. Carefully dissect the skin from the subcutaneous tissues to expose the crop, sternum, and pectoral and abdominal musculature. If the yolk sac is enlarged, cut the skin around the umbilicus. Remove the abdominal musculature and the sternum. Carefully move the yolk sac out of the way, and proceed with the necropsy protocol as in the adult bird.

Examination of the viscera is similar to the adult bird. Abnormalities to note include organs dark in color, petechial hemorrhage, and congestion of blood vessels. Congestion of the blood vessels of the upper portion of the proventriculus is normal in pediatric birds. Congested blood vessels are common in dehydrated chicks. The normal yolk sac is vascular and contains viscous yellow fluid. Yolk sacs are larger in precocial birds than altricial birds. Coagulation or discoloration may indicate bacterial infection. The yolk sac contents are normally absorbed within 10 days of hatching. The crop, proventriculus, and ventriculus are significantly larger in young birds. The normal liver is pale and slightly larger in size compared with body size in pediatric birds. The normal liver is yellow in birds mobilizing yolk material for the first 2 to 3 weeks of life. Hepatic hemorrhage may be the result of overzealous kicking to emerge from the egg in newly hatched chicks. Hepatic lipidosis is common. The duodenum contains food at all times in normal chicks. The spleen is pale and small in normal neonates. Examine the crop for erythema, discoloration, thickening, and ulcerations as a result of crop burns. Look for subcutaneous (paraesophageal) deposition of formula in the subcutaneous tissues of the neck. The thymus is enlarged in the cranial thorax.

Open the gastrointestinal tract after removal from the body cavity. Check proventricular and ventricular contents for foreign bodies and material. Ingestion of substrate is common and often results in impaction. The bursa of Fabricius is examined and collected for histopathology. Examine larger airways of the lung closely for presence of aspirated formula. Examine the contents of the crop for foreign bodies, ingested substrate, formula consistency, erythema, discoloration, thickening, masses, ulcerations, and perforations. Crop *Candida* infections are common and may be noted as white plaques in the crop. Confirm with cytology.

Viral or bacterial infections are suspected when multiple chicks die, especially clutchmates. Collect samples for virus isolation.

EGG NECROPSY

Be certain that the embryo is dead before performing the necropsy. Candle the egg and scrutinize the embryo for lack of development with continued incubation. Because of the rapid rate of autolysis in eggs, perform the necropsy as soon as possible after death. Obtain a complete history of the aviary, parents, incubation, and clutchmates before performing the necropsy. Note the external physical characteristics of the egg: weight, shape, size, cracks, irregular surfaces, and thinning of the shell. Note pip marks such as turning direction, location, and size. Chicks normally pip from the round end of the egg counterclockwise.

Perform the necropsy under sterile conditions until culture samples are obtained. Candle the egg to determine the best entry point for the necropsy. Open the egg over the air cell with sharp-blunt scissors, usually at the rounded end of the egg. Examine the shell membranes for abnormalities. Peel back the shell membranes with fine-tipped forceps and note the color, size, and location of the albumen, yolk, and allantois (Fig. 10–5). Note obvious microbial growth. Note circulatory tree presence and characteristics. Note abnormal odors. After the first third of incubation, the chorioallantoic membrane normally adheres to the inner shell membranes. Adhesions to the embryo are abnormal. Adhesions may occur if necropsies are not performed shortly after death. Avoid rupturing the yolk sac. Culture and examine the albumen and amnion. Use thumb forceps to enlarge the hole at the round end.

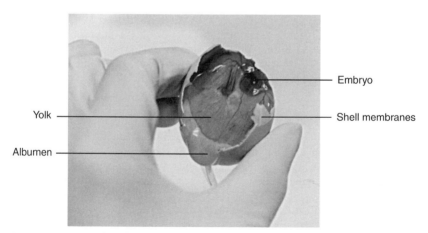

Figure 10–5. Necropsy of an egg demonstrating the shell membranes, albumen, yolk, and embryo.

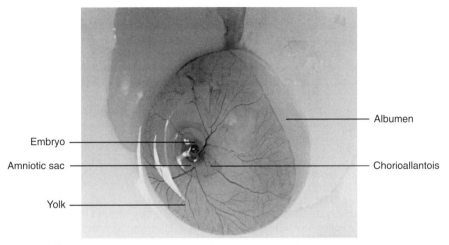

Figure 10–6. Structures of egg contents, including embryo, yolk, amniotic sac, chorioallantois, and albumen.

If a well-developed chick is present, note the position of the air cell in relation to the egg; orientation of the embryo within the egg; position of the head, beak, and neck in relation to the body; and position of the beak in relation to the air cell. The normal position at hatching is the head under the right wing with the tip of the beak directed toward the air cell. Psittacines may hold their head in the same plane as the wing. Note malpositions; consult Joyner (1994) for descriptions and classifications of malpositions. Positioning may affect hatching success. Perform a necropsy on the chick (see previous section).

If a small chick or no chick is present, pour the contents into a sterile container. Examine the contents, identify structures, and note abnormalities (Fig. 10–6).

References and Additional Readings

Abbott UK, Brice AT, Cutler BA, et al. Embryonic development of the cockatiel (*Nymphicus hollandicus*). *J Assoc Avian Vet* 1991;5(4):207–209.

Dorrestein GM. Diagnostic necropsy and pathology. In Altman RB, Clubb SL, Dorrestein GM, Quesenberry K (eds): *Avian Medicine and Surgery*. Philadelphia, WB Saunders, 1997, pp 158–169.

Freeman BM, Vince MA. *The Development of the Avian Embryo*. New York, John Wiley & Sons, 1974.

Graham DL. Necropsy procedures in birds. *Vet Clin North Am Small Anim Pract* 1984;14(2):173–177.

Graham DL. Check list for necropsy of the pet bird and preparation and submission of necropsy specimens: A mnemonic aid for the busy avian practitioner. *Proc Assoc Avian Vet* 1990;404–408.

Graham DL. A color atlas of avian chlamydiosis. *Semin Avian Exot Pet Med* 1993;2(4):184–189.

Graham DL. Necropsy procedures in birds. Schubot Exotic Bird Health Center, Texas A&M University.

Hamburger V, Hamilton HL. A series of normal stages in the development of the chick embryo. *J Morphol* 1951;88:49–89.

Joyner KL. Psittacine incubation and pediatrics. In Fowler ME (ed): *Zoo and Wild Animal Medicine, Current Therapy 3.* Philadelphia, WB Saunders, 1993, pp 247–260.

Joyner KL. Theriogenology. In Ritchie BW, Harrison GJ, Harrison LR (eds): *Avian Medicine: Principles and Application.* Lake Worth, FL, Wingers Publishing, 1994, pp 748–804.

Joyner KL, Abbott U. Egg necropsy techniques. *Proc Assoc Avian Vet* 1991;146–152.

Langenberg J. Pathological evaluation of the avian egg. *Proc Am Assoc Zoo Vet* 1989;78.

Latimer KS, Rakich PM. Necropsy examination. In Ritchie BW, Harrison GJ, Harrison LR (eds): *Avian Medicine: Principles and Application.* Lake Worth, FL, Wingers Publishing, 1994, pp 355–379.

Latimer KS, Rakich PM, Ritchie BW. Recognition and interpretation of selected gross necropsy lesions and anatomical variation. *J Assoc Avian Vet* 1992;6(1):31–33.

Lowenstine IJ. Necropsy procedures. In Harrison GJ, Harrison LR (eds): *Clinical Avian Medicine and Surgery.* Philadelphia, WB Saunders, 1986, pp 298–309.

McDonald SE. Anatomical and physiological characteristics of birds and how they differ from mammals. *1991 Manual of Basic Avian Medicine. Proc Assoc Avian Vet* 1991;1–18.

McKibben JD, Harrison GJ. Clinical anatomy with emphasis on the amazon parrot. In Harrison GJ, Harrison LR (eds): *Clinical Avian Medicine and Surgery.* Philadelphia, WB Saunders, 1986, pp 31–66.

McLelland J. *A Color Atlas of Avian Anatomy.* Philadelphia, WB Saunders, 1991.

Muser KK, Parrott T. Necropsy techniques on baby birds. *Proc Assoc Avian Vet* 1990;115–118.

Olsen GH, Nicolich JM, Hoffman DJ. A review of some causes of death of avian embryos. *Proc Assoc Avian Vet* 1990;106–111.

Phalen DN. Avian necropsy protocol. *Proceedings: Diagnostics and Therapeutics in Cage Birds and Avicultural Medicine.* Texas A&M University, 1995, pp 31–34.

Randall CJ. *Color Atlas of Diseases of the Domestic Fowl and Turkey.* Ames, Iowa, Iowa State University Press, 1985.

Romanoff AL. *The Avian Embryo.* New York, MacMillan Co, 1960.

Romanoff AL, Romanoff AJ. *Pathogenesis of the Avian Embryo.* New York, Wiley-Interscience, 1972.

Schmidt RE. Common gross lesions in non-psittacine birds. *J Assoc Avian Vet* 1992;6(4):223–226.

Chapter 11

Grooming and Medical Procedures

GROOMING

Providing grooming services for birds is an important part of avian practice. Basic grooming techniques include wing, nail, and beak trims. Correct performance of these techniques is important to the health of the bird. Each procedure is discussed, including indication, recommended equipment, and technique. It is important to take a history before grooming. Birds with malnutrition, such as birds on an all-seed diet, have increased risks of fractures and stress complications.

Beak Trim

Beak abnormalities resulting in overgrowth are most common in psittacine birds. The beak of normal birds usually does not overgrow. The tip of the beak may become sharp, necessitating trimming for the comfort of the owner. The tip of the beak may be ground off with a grinding tool with a cone-shaped stone (e.g., a Dremel tool). Take care to maintain the normal architecture of the beak.

Beak overgrowth may indicate illness or malocclusion. An ill bird may not use its beak for climbing, play, and eating in the same ways that a healthy bird will. This may result in general beak overgrowth. Liver disease or severe lesions associated with *Knemidokoptes* mites may also result in an overgrowth of the upper beak, especially in budgies. Malocclusions can result in overgrowth of the upper or lower beak or both, overgrowth of the side of the beak, crossed upper and lower beaks (scissors beak), and shortened upper beak (prognathism—tip of upper beak does not extend over the lower beak). When malocclusions are discovered and treated before hardening of the beak in young birds, abnormalities can often be corrected with physical therapy and manipulation of the beak (see Chapter 8). Severe abnormalities may require surgical correction. Once the bird becomes an adult, the beak is less amenable to permanent correction. Adult birds with malocclusions require repeated periodic beak trims during their entire lives. Extreme overgrowth can result in the bird being unable to eat.

When overgrowth occurs, trimming is used to re-establish the normal architecture of the beak. Knowledge of the normal shape of the beak for the species of bird is essential. The beak is carefully shaped with a grinding tool with a cone-shaped stone, such as a Dremel tool. Take care to prevent the bird from grasping the grinding stone with its foot or mouth. Control of the grinding tool can be increased by placing a finger on the beak or head, and the upper beak can be placed inside the lower beak to facilitate trimming the lower beak (Fig. 11–1). Flaking outer layers of the beak may be carefully ground off. Extreme beak trims may require anesthesia for trimming.

Birds that need their beak trimmed as a result of malocclusions may benefit from excessive trimming of the overgrown side of the beak. This can sometimes increase the time between trimmings.

If bleeding occurs as a result of grinding of the beak, a radiosurgical unit or ferric subsulfate may be used to control bleeding. Silver nitrate sticks are not recommended for use around the mouth because they can cause caustic burns. The grinding stone should be sterilized between birds, and dust created by grinding the beak can be a health hazard.

Nail Trim

The tip of the nails may become sharp, necessitating trimming for the comfort of the owner. The tip of the nails may be trimmed or ground without causing bleeding or pain. Small bird nails may be clipped with suture removal scissors or human nail clippers. Trimming of larger nails is best accomplished with a grinding tool with a cone-shaped stone (Dremel tool) (Fig. 11–2). Take care to prevent the bird from grasping the grinding tool stone with its foot or mouth. If bleeding occurs, cauterize the nail with silver nitrate or ferric subsulfate. The grinding stone should be sterilized between birds, and dust created by grinding the nails can be a health hazard.

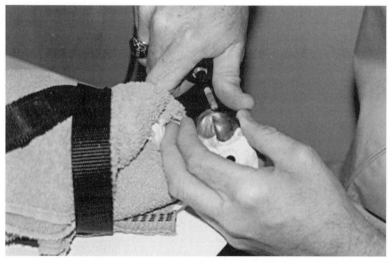

Figure 11–1. Restraint and beak trimming. The upper beak can be placed inside the lower beak to facilitate trimming of the lower beak.

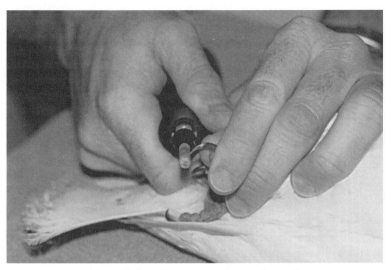

Figure 11–2. Nail trimming with a grinding tool.

Wing Trim

Trimming of some of the feathers on the wings is routinely performed in psittacine birds. Benefits include prevention of injury from flying, prevention of accidental escape, and aid in training and taming. When a wing trim is properly performed, the bird should not be able to fly or gain lift, but will gently glide to the ground over the distance of a few feet. Birds should not be taken outside with the assumption that a wing trim will keep them from flying. Owners should be warned that the bird may still be able to fly, especially in wind. Also, molting a few feathers can markedly improve a bird's ability to fly.

Improper clipping of wing feathers can result in irritation and cause some birds to preen excessively or begin to feather pick. Excessive trims may result in laceration of the skin and muscle of the keel, fractures of the wings or legs, or chipping off the tip of the beak in a fall.

Young birds should learn to fly and develop landing skills before their first trim. This allows them to develop balance, grace, and agility.

Each feather is clipped across the rachis proximal to the first vane (cut along the shaft of the feather proximal to the fluffy portion of the feather), below the level of the covert feathers (Fig. 11–3). Identify and visualize each feather before cutting. Avoid trimming blood feathers (growing feathers with a vascular shaft) because these will hemorrhage if cut. Cat claw clippers and White brand dog nail clippers are useful for clipping the feathers. Scissors may lacerate the skin if the bird flaps its wings or struggles. Most birds require approximately one-third to one-half of the primary feathers to be cut to prevent lift. Trim both wings symmetrically so the bird can maintain normal balance.

To perform a wing trim, the wing is extended while the bird is restrained. The wing is held gently and firmly, supporting the humerus to avoid fracturing the wing. Visualize the shaft of the feathers and cut the outer four feathers on

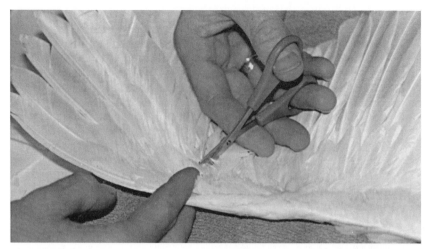

Figure 11–3. During wing trimming, the shaft of each feather is visualized and the rachis is cut proximal to the first vane.

both wings, beginning at the tip of the wing. Test the bird indoors to see if more feathers need to be removed. The bird can be held on a perch or arm and quickly dropped downward, causing the bird to flap its wings and jump off the perch. If the bird can gain lift, clip more primary feathers. Clip conservatively and remove additional feathers as needed to prevent the bird from gaining lift. Four to eight feathers usually require trimming on each wing to prevent lift. Heavy bodied birds, such as African gray parrots and Amazon parrots, usually require four or five feathers per wing removed. Powerful fliers, such as cockatiels and budgies, often need six to eight feathers trimmed per wing. Leave a feather on each side of a blood feather for support. The client may need to bring the bird back in a few weeks to finish the trim if multiple blood feathers are present. The bird may be able to fly until further trimming. Birds will require additional trimming 8 to 12 weeks after the start of a molt.

If a blood feather is accidentally cut, the bleeding feather is grasped with hemostats, and the feather is pulled straight out in the direction of growth while holding the wing and the bone firmly at the base of the feather. Hemorrhage is controlled with direct pressure. Do not place clotting powders in feather follicles.

Cosmetic wing trims differ in that the two primary feathers at the tip of the wing are left so that the wings look almost untrimmed when they are in a resting position. Leaving these feathers often does not keep strong fliers from flying, and these feathers are often damaged or caught in cage wires.

MEDICAL PROCEDURES

Common medical procedures are discussed in the following sections, including indications and techniques. Fluid therapy, oxygen therapy, and heat supplementation are discussed in Chapter 1. Air sac tube placement is discussed in Chapter 14.

Administration of Medications

Routes of administration of medications in birds include medicated water, medicated food, oral, injectable (intramuscular, intravenous, subcutaneous, intraosseous, intratracheal), topical, nebulization, and sinus and nasal flushes. Selection of route of administration is based on severity of infection, number of birds to be treated, the ability of the owner to administer the medication, and formulations available. Parenteral administration of medications is suggested for critically ill birds. Flocks of birds are often treated with medicated food or water, but therapeutic drug concentrations are seldom achieved in companion and aviary birds.

Medicated Water

Administration of medications through medicated water is not recommended. Psittacines often refuse to drink water with an abnormal taste, which may result in dehydration. Most infections in companion birds cannot be adequately treated with medicated water.

Medicated Food

It is difficult to achieve therapeutic concentration with medicated feeds. Sick birds eat less food. If the medication is placed in a food different from the usual diet of the bird, even palatable medicated food may be refused. Crushed tablets, oral suspensions, and powders can be mixed with moist foods; however, the energy content and palatability of the diet affect the amount consumed and therefore the dose of medication ingested. Chlortetracycline-medicated formulated commercial diets are available and can be used to treat chlamydiosis. Chlortetracycline impregnated millet seed is readily accepted by budgies and finches.

Oral Medication

Oral suspensions are difficult to administer to psittacines. It is difficult to get them to open their mouths, and some birds refuse to swallow medications. Medications can be mixed with a palatable liquid such as lactulose syrup or fruit juice to increase acceptance. Capsules that dissolve rapidly can be used in pigeons, waterfowl, and gallinaceous birds. Do not use oral medications in critically ill birds.

Intramuscular Injection

Intramuscular (IM) injection is usually the quickest and least stressful route of precise medication administration in companion birds. In most birds, IM injections are easier than oral administration. Owners can be taught to safely give injections. Some medications are irritating and may cause muscle necrosis. The volume of the injected medication must be considered. General guidelines for maximum injection volumes include: macaw and cockatoo, 1 ml; Amazon or

African gray parrot, 0.8 ml; cockatiel and small conure, 0.2 ml; and budgie, canary, and finch, 0.1 ml. Use multiple sites if larger volumes must be administered.

The pectoral muscles are the most common site for IM injections. Drugs injected in the leg muscles may be cleared by the renal portal system before reaching systemic circulation. Nestling birds and ratites have little pectoral muscle mass, and owners of racing pigeons, raptors, and some game birds may not allow pectoral IM injections.

Injections are given in the middle third of the pectoral muscle, 2 to 3 mm off the keel (carina of the sternum). The feathers are parted with an alcohol swab and the area is visualized. A 25- to 27-gauge × 3/8 in. needle and a tuberculin or insulin syringe is inserted at a 45-degree angle, and the medication is injected into the muscle (Fig. 11–4). Pressure is applied at the needle site to prevent leakage of medication through the puncture and to control any bleeding. Alternate sides with subsequent injections.

Intravenous Injection

Intravenous (IV) injections are used to achieve rapid therapeutic drug levels and should be reserved for emergencies and single dose drug administration. The most accessible veins for IV injections include the right jugular, basilic (wing), and medial metatarsal veins. The technique is similar to venipuncture to obtain blood samples (see Chapter 12). Anesthesia may simplify the procedure. Hematomas are common.

Subcutaneous Injection

Subcutaneous injections are useful when large volumes are injected. They are sometimes used for administration of irritating drugs. Subcutaneous injections

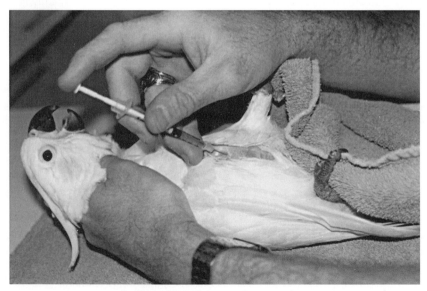

Figure 11–4. Intramuscular injection.

are often used by pigeon and game bird breeders. Subcutaneous injection of irritating drugs may cause skin necrosis and ulceration. Medication will often leak out of the skin at the injection site.

Intraosseous Injection

Intraosseous injections can be used for nonirritating medications. A catheter can be placed for repeated drug administration. Intraosseous injection technique is similar to intraosseous fluid therapy (see Chapter 1).

Intratracheal Injection

Intratracheal injection is used to inject amphotericin B to treat tracheal and lower respiratory tract *Aspergillus* infection. The mouth is held open with gauze loops or a speculum, and medication can be injected through the tracheal opening directly into the trachea with a small-diameter metal feeding needle. Injections can be made through the tracheal wall to dislodge proximal tracheal foreign bodies or to inject resuscitation drugs by isolating the trachea with the thumb and index finger. Insert the needle through the skin and into the tracheal lumen. An air sac breathing tube should be placed before attempting to remove tracheal foreign bodies.

Topical Medication

Use topical medications sparingly. Water-based medications are preferred. Oily medications may be preened over the body, resulting in loss of insulation properties of the feathers. Medications used topically must be nontoxic. Corticosteroids applied topically can be absorbed or ingested, resulting in immunosuppression.

Nebulization (Aerosol Therapy)

Nebulization of medications is indicated in sinus, tracheal, and lower respiratory tract infections. Ultrasonic nebulizers that produce particles smaller than 3 μm are recommended. A limited portion of the lower respiratory tract is likely to be penetrated by nebulization; however, clinical improvement often results. The benefits of nebulization also include humidification and hydration of the airways and respiratory epithelium.

The bird is placed in a container that will hold in the humidity that is produced by the nebulized particles. An alternative is to place the bird in a small cage or enclosure and place this in a plastic bag with the open end secured loosely. The container is placed in an incubator or warmed, if needed. The nebulizer flow hose is placed inside the container, and the air flow rate is adjusted to produce particles.

Some medications commonly nebulized are listed in Table 11–1. Initiate nebulization before culture and sensitivity results with a broad-spectrum antibiotic (e.g., cefotaxime or piperacillin). Alter selection of antibiotic based on sensitivity testing. Nebulize for 10 to 30 minutes, two to four times daily. Use in conjunction with systemic therapy.

TABLE 11–1. Some Medications Commonly Nebulized

Medication	Dosage	Administration Time and Frequency
Amikacin sulfate°	50 mg in 10 ml saline	15 min BID
Amphotericin B†	10 mg in 10 ml saline	15 min BID
Carbenicillin†	200 mg in 10 ml saline	15 min BID
Cefotaxime†	100 mg in 10 ml saline	10–30 min BID–QID
Erythromycin†	100 mg in 10 ml saline	15 min TID
Gentamicin°	50 mg in 10 ml saline	15 min TID
Piperacillin†	100 mg in 10 ml saline	10–30 min BID–QID
Tylosin	100 mg in 10 ml saline	10–60 min BID

°Discontinue use if polyuria develops.
†Injectable.

Nasal Flush

Nasal flushes are often important in the successful treatment of infraorbital sinus infections. Antibiotics can be added to the flushing solution for local therapy (e.g., 50 mg amikacin or gentamicin in 20 ml saline).

The bird is restrained and the head is held lower than the body. The syringe is pressed against the nostril, the fluid is flushed into the sinuses, and the fluid exits the opposite nostril and through the choana and mouth (Fig. 11–5). Use

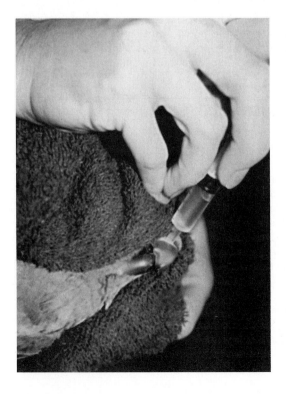

Figure 11–5. Nasal flush.

TABLE 11–2. Suggested Volumes for Nasal Flushes

Budgie, cockatiel, lovebird	1–3 ml
Amazon parrot, African gray parrot	4–10 ml
Macaw, cockatoo	10–15 ml

isotonic solutions and minimal pressure. Table 11–2 lists suggested amounts of fluid for nasal flushes.

Sinus Flush

A sinus flush is used to deliver medication directly into the infraorbital sinus for treatment of sinusitis. A sinus flush can also be used to dislodge exudate and foreign bodies from the sinuses or to obtain samples for cytology, culture, and sensitivity testing.

The bird is restrained with the head secure. The needle is inserted midway between the commissure of the beak and the medial canthus of the eye (Fig. 11–6). The needle is directed under the zygomatic arch at a 45-degree angle to the side of the head. The sinus is more easily entered if the mouth is held open. Once the sinus has been entered, sterile water and antibiotic solution may be injected. Take care to avoid penetration of the eye. Injectable antibiotics may be used for the treatment of sinusitis (e.g., 50 mg amikacin or gentamicin in 50 ml sterile saline). Inject only nonirritating solutions.

Blood Transfusion

Blood transfusions appear to be beneficial in birds with chronic anemia, for the purpose of stabilizing the bird while the cause of the anemia is being

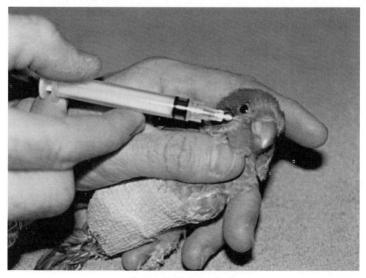

Figure 11–6. Sinus flush.

pursued. Birds with acute blood loss may better benefit from fluid replacement with lactated Ringer's solution. Birds with a packed cell volume less than 20% as a result of acute blood loss may benefit from a blood transfusion. Administration of iron dextran and B vitamins is also recommended for anemic birds and birds with acute blood loss.

Approximately 1% of the donor bird's weight can be safely collected in blood volume. For example, a 500-g pigeon can donate 5 ml of blood. The anticoagulant of choice is acid citrate dextrose (ACD) solution used at a rate of 0.15 ml of ACD per milliliter of blood. The calculated volume of ACD is drawn into an appropriate size syringe through a butterfly catheter. The ACD solution may be diluted with saline when very small volumes of ACD are to be used. The donor blood is slowly withdrawn, usually from the right jugular vein.

Transfusion of approximately 10% to 20% of the calculated blood volume is usually ideal for the blood recipient. Blood volume is approximately 10% of body weight. For example, a 450-g Amazon parrot should be given 4.5 to 9 ml of blood. A quick partial cross-match can be performed by mixing donor red blood cells with serum from the recipient. The absence of hemolysis or agglutination suggests compatibility. The blood may be administered intravenously or intraosseously.

Homologous (same species) blood transfusions are preferable; however, blood from pigeons, raptors, or chickens can be used for a single heterologous transfusion of blood to psittacines. Donor blood from a closely related species may remain in circulation longer in the recipient.

Cardiopulmonary Resuscitation

Prognosis associated with respiratory and cardiac arrest varies with the cause of the arrest. Isoflurane anesthetic overdose and acute illness (e.g., acute tracheal obstruction) often respond. Arrest as a result of chronic illness rarely responds to cardiopulmonary resuscitation (CPR).

If the bird arrests while on gas anesthesia, first stop anesthetic administration. Place an endotracheal tube and apply positive-pressure ventilation at the rate of once every 4 to 5 seconds. Once ventilation is started, the heartbeat and peripheral pulse are checked; ideally, electrical activity of the heart is observed with an electrocardiograph. If there is no heartbeat or peripheral pulse, begin firm and rapid compressions of the sternum, continue ventilation, and give epinephrine and atropine. Epinephrine and atropine can be given intravenously, followed by a bolus of saline or sterile water to encourage the drug transport to the heart. These drugs may also be administered by intratracheal, intraosseous, or intracardiac administration or sprayed into the thoracic cavity if the body wall is incised. Intratracheal administration is often the easiest route in arrested birds. The trachea is isolated with the fingers, and the needle is inserted into the tracheal lumen and drugs are injected.

Pulse oximeters can be used to monitor oxygen saturation, allowing evaluation of CPR effectiveness.

If acute tracheal obstruction is suspected, an air sac breathing tube is placed for positive-pressure ventilation.

Electrocardiography

Electrocardiography is useful for detection of cardiac enlargement, for the diagnosis and monitoring of treatment of cardiac arrhythmias, and for monitoring anesthesia. Cardiac pathology can be present without electrocardiographic abnormalities. The bird is placed in dorsal recumbency. The electrodes are attached to the prepatagium (wing web) of the right and left wings and the skin of the left medial thigh. The right leg is connected to the ground electrode. Electrode gel (preferable), alcohol, or saline is applied to the electrode sites. A paper speed of 50 mm/sec or 100 mm/sec is needed to record electrical activity because of the fast heart rates of birds.

A strip of lead II can be used to evaluate the rhythm. Evaluate the strip for a regular or irregular rhythm and normal or abnormal heart rate. Check for the presence of a P wave for each QRS complex, a QRS complex for each P wave, if P waves are related to the QRS complexes, if the P waves look alike, and if the QRS complexes look alike. The QRS complex is negative in normal birds. The T wave is always positive in lead II in normal birds. Normal electrocardiogram measurements in selected birds can be found in Table 11–3.

A tall P wave may be the result of right atrial hypertrophy. A wide P wave may be the result of left atrial hypertrophy. A tall, wide P wave is suggestive of both right and left atrial enlargement. Low voltage may be the result of pericardial effusion. Tall or wide QRS complexes may be the result of left ventricular hypertrophy. Prominent R waves may indicate right ventricular hypertrophy. The QRS complex may become positive in lead II and III with cardiomyopathy. Cardiomyopathy may also result in a shift in the mean electrical axis. A negative T wave may indicate myocardial hypoxia. A progressively increasing T wave may also indicate hypoxia and should be watched for during anesthesia monitoring. An increased T wave amplitude may be the result of hyperkalemia. Bradycardia may be the result of hypothermia, hypokalemia, hyperkalemia, thiamine deficiency, vitamin E deficiency, organophosphate toxicosis, polychlorinated biphenyl toxicosis, vagal stimulation, or some anesthetics (e.g., halothane, methoxyflurane,

TABLE 11–3. Reported Electrocardiogram Measurements in Selected Birds

Parameter	Budgie	Amazon Parrot	Racing Pigeon	African Gray Parrot
P-S (sec)	0.01–0.04	0.04–0.08	0.045–0.070	0.040–0.055
QRS (sec)	0.01–0.03	0.01–0.03	0.013–0.016	0.010–0.016
MEA	−83 to −108	−90 to −162	−18 to −99	−79 to −103
P (sec)	0.01–0.02	0.01–0.02	0.015–0.02	0.012–0.018
HR (bpm)	600–750	275–780	160–300	340–600
P (mV)	NA	NA	0.4–0.6	0.25–0.55
QS (mV)	NA	NA	1.5–2.8	0.9–2.2

From Rosenthal K, Miller M, Orosz S, et al. Cardiovascular system. In Altman RB, Clubb SL, Dorrestein GM, et al (eds): *Avian Medicine and Surgery.* Philadelphia, WB Saunders, 1997, p 496. (Data from Lumeij J, Ritchie B: Cardiology. In Ritchie B, Harrison G, Harrison L (eds): *Avian Medicine.* Lake Worth, FL, Wingers Publishing, pp 695–722; Miller M. Avian cardiology. *Proc Assoc Avian Vet* 1986, pp 87–102; Zenoble R. Electrocardiology in the parakeet and parrot. *Comp Cont Ed* 1981;3:711–714).

NA, not available; MEA, mean electrical axis; HR, heart rate.

xylazine, or acepromazine). For further information on interpretation of electro-cardiograms, see Lumeij and Ritchie (1994) or Rosenthal, Miller, Orosz, and Dorrestein (1997). Cardiac ultrasound is useful for visualization of suspected physical abnormalities.

Euthanasia

Humane euthanasia procedures in birds include intravenous administration of barbiturate (right jugular vein or cerebral sinus), gas anesthetic overdose, or gas anesthesia followed by exsanguination.

Microchipping

Microchips are tiny computer chips encapsulated in a biocompatible material. Each chip is programmed with a number that provides permanent identification. The microchips can be read by an appropriate scanner (Fig. 11–7). Not all scanners can read all available microchips. Microchips provide permanent and safe identification that cannot be altered.

Microchips are placed inside a hypodermic needle and injected into the muscle of the bird. In most birds, the chip is injected in the thickest portion of the pectoral (breast) muscle (Fig. 11–8). The bird is restrained, the feathers are parted, and the skin is swabbed with alcohol at the selected site. The needle is held at a 30-degree angle from the body of the bird with the bevel up. The needle is inserted until the bevel of the needle is covered by tissue. In smaller birds, the bevel is inserted until the bevel is mostly covered. The plunger of the syringe is slowly depressed, injecting the chip into the muscle. Pressure is applied at the injection site as the needle is withdrawn. Anesthesia is not required, but it is preferred by some avian veterinarians. In ratites, the chip is

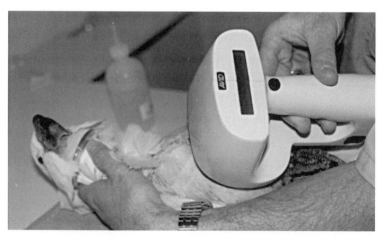

Figure 11–7. Reading of an AVID microchip after injection.

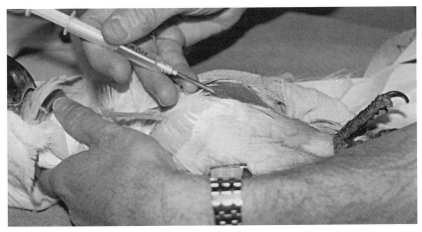

Figure 11–8. Injection of an AVID microchip. The chips are injected into the thickest portion of the pectoral muscle.

injected at hatching in the left side of the pipping muscle 2 to 3 cm below the ear. Microchips can be located with radiography, if needed.

Tube Feeding

Anorectic birds require nutritional support. Nutritional support is most commonly provided with tube feeding. Contraindications of tube feeding include crop stasis, ileus, gastrointestinal impaction, or other gastrointestinal abnormalities that do not allow the passage of ingesta or nutrient absorption.

Equipment required for tube feeding includes stainless steel feeding needles with rounded tips (10 to 18 gauge), rubber feeding cathethers, oral specula, syringes, and feeding formula. Equipment should be sterilized between uses to prevent spread of disease.

Perform all other procedures before tube feeding. Restraint after tube feeding may result in regurgitation and aspiration. Palpate the crop before each feeding. If food is present, do not tube feed (consult Chapter 4).

Commercial feeding formulas for birds are available (Table 11–4). Chick hand-feeding formula, human enteral nutritional formula, and homemade formulas may also be used for tube feeding. The commercial feeding formulas and formulas for hand feeding chicks are convenient and nutritionally balanced, and will pass through a feeding needle. Caloric density and nutritional content vary

---

TABLE 11–4. Some Commercial Feeding Formulas for Birds°

Emeraid I: Lafeber Co., Cornell, IL 61319 (815) 358-2301.
Emeraid II: Lafeber Co., Cornell, IL 61319 (815) 358-2301.
Formula AA: Roudybush Inc., Sacramento, CA 95821 (800) 326-1726.

°Hand-feeding formulas for chicks are found in Table 16–1.

among the human and homemade formulas, so they are less desirable. The feeding formulas for birds and chick hand-feeding formulas are mixed with warm water as directed. Feeding formulas are heated in hot water to a temperature between 101 and 104°F and fed immediately. Formulas are always fed warmed to prevent delayed crop emptying. To prevent crop burns, do not warm food in a microwave, and always stir the formula before measuring the temperature.

The bird is held in an upright position with the neck extended. If a rubber catheter is used for feeding, care must be taken to prevent the bird from biting the tube and swallowing the severed piece of tube. Speculums may be used or the beak may be manipulated to prevent the bird from biting the tube. The upper beak may be pushed to one side or inserted in the lower beak and held in position. The tube or feeding needle is gently passed into the left oral commissure, down the esophagus on the right side of the neck, and into the crop with the gruel-filled syringe attached (Fig. 11–9). If the beak is entered directly from the front, the bird will try to chew the tube or needle. Palpate the crop and verify that the tube or feeding needle is in the crop. The formula is infused into the crop, the tube or feeding needle is carefully withdrawn, and the bird is released. Maintain the neck in extension while the food is injected and until release of the bird to deter regurgitation. If food refluxes into the oral

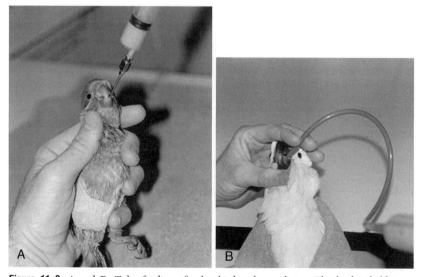

Figure 11–9. A and **B,** Tube feeding of a lovebird and a cockatoo. The bird is held in an upright position with the neck extended. The feeding needle is gently passed into the left oral commissure, down the esophagus on the right side of the neck, and into the crop with the gruel-filled syringe attached. Palpate the crop and verify that the tube or feeding needle is in the crop. The formula is infused into the crop, the feeding needle is carefully withdrawn, and the bird is released. If food refluxes into the oral cavity during the procedure, release the bird and allow the bird to clear the mouth of food on its own. When a tube is used, a speculum can be used or the tip of the upper beak can be placed into the lower beak to prevent biting of the tube.

TABLE 11–5. General Guidelines for Volumes and Frequency of Warmed Tube Feeding Formulas

Finch	0.1–0.5 ml 6×/day
Budgie	0.5–3 ml QID
Lovebird	1–3 ml QID
Cockatiel	1–8 ml QID
Small conure	3–12 ml QID
Large conure	7–24 ml TID–QID
Amazon parrot	5–35 ml TID
African gray parrot	5–35 ml TID
Cockatoo	10–40 ml BID–TID
Macaw	20–60 ml BID–TID

Neonates may require more frequent feedings.

cavity during the procedure, release the bird and allow the bird to clear the mouth of food on its own.

Frequency of feedings and amounts of formula to be fed vary with the age and size of bird. General guidelines for volumes and frequency of tube feedings are listed in Table 11–5. Neonates may require more frequent feedings.

Birds with crop, proventricular, or ventricular problems may require feeding through a proventricular tube or a duodenal catheter. Birds with gastrointestinal disease may require parenteral nutrition.

References and Additional Readings

Altman RB, Clubb SL, Dorrestein GM, et al (eds). *Avian Medicine and Surgery.* Philadelphia, WB Saunders, 1997.

Carpenter JW, Mashima TY, Rupiper DJ. *Exotic Animal Formulary.* Manhattan, KS, Greystone Publications, 1996.

Clipsham R. Surgical beak restoration and correction. *Proc Assoc Avian Vet* 1989;164–176.

Flammer K. Antimicrobial therapy. In Ritchie BW, Harrison GJ, Harrison LR (eds): *Avian Medicine: Principles and Application.* Lake Worth, FL, Wingers Publishing, 1994, pp 434–456.

Jenkins JR. Advanced procedures in avian medicine. *Proc Assoc Avian Vet Pract Labs* 1993;13–18.

Johnson-Delaney CA, Harrison LR (eds). *Exotic Companion Medicine Handbook.* Lake Worth, FL, Wingers Publishing, 1996.

Lumeij JT, Ritchie BW. Cardiology. In Ritchie BW, Harrison GJ, Harrison LR (eds): *Avian Medicine: Principles and Application.* Lake Worth, FL, Wingers Publishing, 1994, pp 695–722.

McCluggage DM. Basic avian medical techniques. *Proc Assoc Avian Vet Pract Labs* 1993;1–12.

Miller MS. Avian cardiology. *Proc ABVP, Avian Specialty Core Review Course* 1993;107–110.

Miller MS. Electrocardiography. In Harrison GJ, Harrison LR (eds): *Clinical Avian Medicine and Surgery.* Philadelphia, WB Saunders, 1986, pp 286–292.

Oglesbee BL, Atkinson R. Clinical avian techniques. *Proc Assoc Avian Vet Pract Labs* 1995.

Quesenberry KE, Hillyer EV. Supportive care and emergency therapy. In Ritchie BW,

Harrison GJ, Harrison LR (eds): *Avian Medicine: Principles and Application.* Lake Worth, FL, Wingers Publishing, 1994, pp 382–416.

Ritchie BW, Harrison GJ, Harrison LR (eds). *Avian Medicine: Principles and Application.* Lake Worth, FL, Wingers Publishing, 1994.

Rosenthal K, Miller M, Orosz S, Dorrestein GM. Cardiovascular system. In Altman RB, Clubb SL, Dorrestein GM, Quesenberry K. (eds): *Avian Medicine and Surgery.* Philadelphia, WB Saunders, 1997, pp 489–500.

Spink RR. Aerosol therapy. In Harrison GJ, Harrison LR (eds): *Clinical Avian Medicine and Surgery.* Philadelphia, WB Saunders, 1986, pp 376–379.

Wissman MA. Standardization of wing clipping for psittacines. *Newsletter Assoc Avian Vet* 1995;9(2):6–8.

Chapter 12

Clinical Pathology

HEMATOLOGY

Hematology is essential for the accurate diagnosis of illness in birds. In-house avian hematology can be performed with minimal investment to obtain a few materials in clinics where mammalian hematology is currently performed. Numerous laboratories are available for analysis of avian hematology samples; however, ill birds are often in critical condition, and the time required to obtain results often delays crucial therapy.

Blood collection and analysis is practical even in small birds. Up to 1% of the bird's body weight can safely be collected in blood unless the bird is anemic or hypovolemic. For example, a 500-g cockatoo can have a 5-ml sample of blood collected. Anemic and severely ill birds may require a reduced sample size.

Typically, when hematology is used to assist in making a diagnosis or to monitor response to treatment, a blood sample is drawn, blood smears are made immediately (preferably from blood without anticoagulant), and anticoagulated samples are refrigerated until a packed cell volume (PCV), total protein, and cell counts can be performed. A portion of the sample is immediately separated into cell and plasma components and refrigerated until biochemistries or other plasma diagnostic tests can be performed.

Sample Collection

Blood samples may be collected into a syringe, capillary tube, or microtainer collection system. Venipuncture can be performed with a 23- to 27-gauge needle. Use light suction when using a syringe because avian veins collapse easily. Ideally, blood collected for smears should be obtained without anticoagulant, because heparin can interfere with cell staining and EDTA can cause cell lysis in some birds. In practicality, lithium heparin may be used for obtaining blood, to make blood smears, and for performance of plasma biochemistries.

Sites for blood sample collection in birds include the jugular vein (right is larger), basilic (wing) vein, medial metatarsal vein, and nail clip. The preferred site for blood collection is the right jugular vein because the large size of the vein allows rapid collection of samples, and there is decreased incidence of hematoma formation. Excessive bleeding after blood collection with proper technique may indicate liver disease or other coagulopathy.

345

Jugular Venipuncture

For jugular sample collection, the bird may be restrained by an assistant. Small birds may be held with one hand and the blood collected with the other hand. The neck is extended to stabilize the vein. The feathers over the right jugular vein are parted with an alcohol swab, the vein is visualized, and the sample is collected (Fig. 12–1). The crop may need to be manipulated away from the venipuncture site. Typically, a needle and syringe are used to collect jugular samples (e.g., 25-gauge needle on a 3-ml syringe or 1-ml syringe). The vein may be entered in either direction. Pressure can be placed on the vein at the thoracic inlet to cause the vein to engorge with blood to allow sampling, but this is usually not needed. After sample collection, light pressure is applied to the venipuncture site to prevent hematoma formation. A large hematoma may form if the procedure is incorrectly performed. The left jugular vein is smaller, but it may be used for blood collection.

Basilic (Wing Vein) Venipuncture

Blood may be collected from the basilic vein in medium to large birds; however, prolonged pressure to the venipuncture site is required to prevent hematoma formation. For basilic venipuncture, the bird is restrained with the wing extended. The medial elbow (humeral radioulnar joint) is wiped with an alcohol swab to help visualization of the vein. The vein can be occluded to increase pressure in the vein. The sample can be collected dripping from the needle into a microcollection tube or into a syringe (Fig. 12–2). Apply pressure at the venipuncture site to aid in hematoma prevention. Hematoma formation is common even with proper technique.

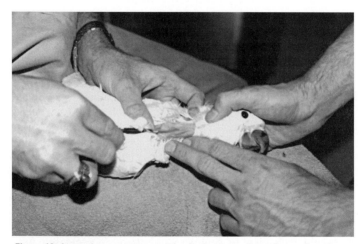

Figure 12–1. Jugular venipuncture. The feathers over the right jugular vein are parted with an alcohol swab, the vein is visualized, and the sample is collected. Apply light pressure when the needle is withdrawn.

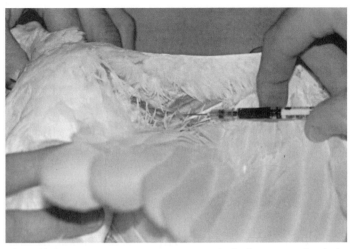

Figure 12–2. Basilic (wing vein) venipuncture. The bird is restrained with the wing extended. The medial elbow is wiped with an alcohol swab to help visualization of the vein. The sample is collected, and light pressure is applied at the venipuncture site to aid in hematoma prevention.

Medial Metatarsal Venipuncture

The medial metatarsal vein is located on the dorsomedial leg, just above or below the tarsal joint. To visualize the vein, apply digital pressure proximal to the collection site to occlude the vein. Venipuncture is accomplished with a needle (typically 25 gauge) and collected in a microcollection tube or syringe (Fig. 12–3). Apply pressure as the needle is withdrawn. Hematoma formation is usually inhibited by surrounding musculature.

Toenail Clip Collection

A toenail clip is the least desirable method of blood collection because of contamination with debris, increased incidence of clotting of the sample, and increased incidence of abnormal cell distributions. The nail should be clipped with sterile, sharp clippers and the blood collected without "milking" the blood. Hemostasis is accomplished with silver nitrate or ferrous subsulfate.

Blood Smear Preparation

Smears may be made using the standard two-slide wedge technique. Smears made with glass slides can result in an increase in ruptured cells, making results inaccurate. Glass coverslips may be used to make the blood smear to minimize rupturing of cells. A small drop of blood is placed in the center of one coverslip. A second coverslip is placed on the drop so that the edges do not match up. The two coverslips are pulled horizontally as the blood spreads (Fig. 12–4). If the blood pools at the edges, too large of a drop was placed on the coverslip. If

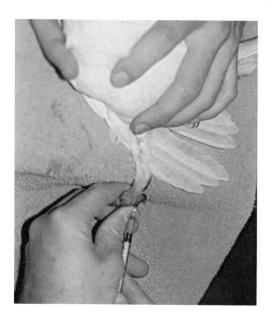

Figure 12–3. Dorsal metatarsal venipuncture. The dorsal metatarsal vein is located on the medial tibiotarsus, just above the tarsal joint. To visualize the vein, apply digital pressure proximally to the collection site to occlude the vein. Venipuncture is accomplished with a 25-gauge needle and collected in a microcollection tube or syringe. Apply pressure as the needle is withdrawn.

the blood does not spread, debris may be present on the coverslip or too small of a blood sample was used. Allow the slides to air dry before staining. Stains commonly used for examination of avian blood include quick stains (e.g., Diff-Quik, Hema-tek), Wright's, Wright's-Giemsa, and Giemsa (Table 12–1). Coverslips may be glued to slides after staining.

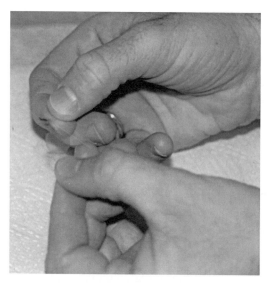

Figure 12–4. Making a coverslip smear. A small drop of blood is placed in the center of one coverslip. A second coverslip is placed on the drop so that the edges to not match up. The two coverslips are pulled horizontally as the drop spreads.

TABLE 12–1. Products Mentioned in the Text

Unopette: Becton-Dickinson and Co., Rutherford, NJ 07070.
Kodak DT60 Analyzer: Johnson-Johnson, Rochester, NY 14626; (800) 555-5234.
VetTest 8008: IDEXX, Westbrook, ME 04092; (800) 248-2483.
Reflotron: Boehringer-Mannheim, Indianapolis, IN 46250-0100; (800) 428-4674.
Mini-Tip Culturette: Becton-Dickenson and Co., Rutherford, NJ 07070.
Diff-Quik: American Scientific Products, Division of American Hospital Supply
  Corporation, McGraw Park, IL 60085.
Hema-tek: Ames Division, Miles Laboratories, Inc., Elkhart, IN 46515.
Gramcheck: Fisher Scientific, Houston, TX 77099; (800) 766-7000.
MicroScan Gram stain control slides: American Scientific Products, Lauderhill, FL 33313;
  (800) 922-5227.

Evaluating Blood Smears

Establish and consistently follow a routine to evaluate blood smears. Evaluate the quantity and morphology of erythrocytes, leukocytes, and thrombocytes. Evaluation of cell morphology is necessary in avian medicine because it may provide important information in the evaluation of the health of the bird. The relative leukocyte differential count is determined by counting 100 white blood cells (WBCs) and determining the percentage of each type of WBC. Do not include smudge cells when counting cells for differential counts, even if the cell can be identified. The percentage of each type of leukocyte is multiplied by the total WBC count to obtain the absolute count.

Cell Identification and Function

A general description of avian blood cells is listed in Table 12–2. Descriptions of staining characteristics are based on cells stained with Wright's stain. Rupturing of cells during preparation of the film result in smudge cells. These are most commonly erythrocytes. They appear as amorphous, pink to purple material on the slide. Preparation of smears using coverslips may reduce the number of smudges.

Erythrocytes

Erythrocytes are elliptical and contain a central oval nucleus (Fig. 12–5). The cytoplasm stains a uniform orange-pink. The nucleus of mature erythrocytes is condensed, stains dark purple, and contains uniformly clumped chromatin. In peripheral circulation, mature erythrocytes are uniform in color, size, and shape. The life span of avian erythrocytes is 28 to 45 days. Polychromatic erythrocytes are larger and contain cytoplasm that is more basophilic and nucleus that is less condensed than that of mature erythrocytes (see Fig. 12–5). Erythrocyte polychromasia indicates erythrocyte regeneration, and 1% to 5% of erythrocytes demonstrating polychromasia is considered normal. An increase in polychromasia is most commonly the result of anemia, but this may also occur as a result of myeloproliferative disorders, endotoxemia, or septicemia. When an anemia is

TABLE 12–2. Avian Blood Cells (Stained With Wright's Stain)

Erythrocyte
  Elliptical
  Cytoplasm: uniform orange-pink
  Nucleus: central oval dark purple with uniformly clumped chromatin
Thrombocyte
  Oval to round
  Cytoplasm: clear to pale blue reticulated or nonhomogeneous with fine red granules
  Nucleus: central and dark purple with dense clumped chromatin
Heterophil
  Round
  Cytoplasm: clear to faint pink cytoplasm filled with orange to red granules
  Nucleus: pale purple with two to three lobes and coarse, clumped chromatin
Eosinophil
  Round
  Cytoplasm: blue with red to orange granules
  Nucleus: light purple bilobed with clumped chromatin
Monocyte
  Round to irregularly shaped
  Cytoplasm: blue gray finely granular
  Nucleus: purple oval or bilobed eccentric nucleus with delicate chromatin
Lymphocyte
  Round
  Cytoplasm: homogeneous pale blue
  Nucleus: dark purple round to slightly dented centrally located and densely
    clumped or reticulated chromatin

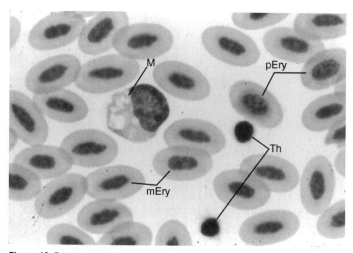

Figure 12–5. Mature erythrocytes *(mEry)*, polychromatic erythrocytes *(pEry)*, two thrombocytes *(Th)*, and a monocyte *(M)* from a barred owl. Wright's stain; original magnification, 100×. See Color Figure 12–5. (Photo courtesy of Terry W. Campbell, M.S., D.V.M., Ph.D.)

present, an incidence of 10% polychromasia indicates adequate response. Polychromasia may be graded as slight, 5 to 10 polychromatic cells per oil field; moderate, 10 to 20 polychromatic cells per oil field; or heavy, 40% to 50% of erythrocytes are at least slightly polychromatic. Anisocytosis indicates a variation in size and can be graded in a similar manner as polychromasia. Hypochromasia may be observed in blood smears of birds with heavy metal toxicosis (e.g., lead) or inflammation. Hypochromasia, marked poikilocytosis, and erythrocyte fragmentation are suggestive of severe iron deficiency.

Rubricytes (immature round erythrocytes) are seen with marked regenerative responses. Rubricytes are round to slightly oval cells with strongly basophilic, gray, or eosinophilic gray cytoplasm. The cell has a small nuclear-cytoplasmic ratio, the nucleus becomes increasingly pyknotic with maturity, and the nuclear chromatin stains coarse blue to black. Characteristics useful for differentiation from reactive lymphocytes are discussed in the section on lymphocyte cell identification.

Abnormal erythrocyte morphology may be the result of changes in maturation, disease, or improper slide preparation resulting in artifacts. Round erythrocytes with oval nuclei are occasionally observed in anemic birds. Binucleate erythrocytes have been associated with severe chronic inflammation and neoplasia. Basophilic stippling of the cytoplasm may be associated with a regenerative response or heavy metal toxicosis. Artifacts that may occur as a result of poor slide preparation or staining include smudge cells, perinuclear rings, and irregularly shaped erythrocytes.

Thrombocytes

Mature thrombocytes are small oval to round cells with clear to pale blue reticulated or nonhomogeneous cytoplasm and a central nucleus with dense clumped chromatin (see Fig. 12–5). Two to four eosinophilic polar granules may be present in the cytoplasm. Thrombocytes are often clumped together on the blood smear. Thrombocytes function in blood clotting and phagocytosis. Thrombocytes are differentiated from erythrocytes by their more round and dense and proportionally larger nucleus. Thrombocytes are differentiated from small mature lymphocytes based on cytoplasmic color and homogeneity and nuclear pyknosis. The cytoplasm of the thrombocyte is nonhomogeneous and colorless or pale blue and may contain small, round, red cytoplasmic granules. Small mature lymphocytes have a scant amount of blue homogeneous cytoplasm that contains azurophilic granules throughout the cytoplasm. Thrombocytes have a smaller nuclear-cytoplasmic ratio. Thrombocytes may be differentiated from nuclei of disrupted erythrocytes by the lack of a definite outline and absence of cytoplasm associated with the released nuclei of erythrocytes.

Reactive or immature thrombocytes are abnormal in peripheral blood. Reactive thrombocytes have diffusely eosinophilic cytoplasm and irregular cytoplasmic margins. Reactive thrombocytes are usually found in aggregates and tend to be more spindle-shaped than do nonreactive thrombocytes. Activation may also result in cytoplasmic vacuolation and alterations in outline. Reactive thrombocytes occur with chronic disease and contact with foreign surfaces.

Leukocytes

Leukocytes found in avian peripheral blood include granulocytes (heterophils, eosinophils, basophils) and mononuclear cells (lymphocytes, monocytes). There are some differences among species of birds, making exact descriptions difficult. However, some generalities apply to all birds.

HETEROPHILS. Mature heterophils are round with clear to faint pink cytoplasm filled with eosinophilic rod-, spindle-, or round-shaped granules and a pale basophilic nucleus that usually has two to three lobes and contains coarse, clumped chromatin (Fig. 12–6). The nucleus may or may not be visible through the cytoplasmic granules. The cytoplasmic granules often contain a central refractile body. These granules may degranulate in response to some staining techniques, resulting in cytoplasmic vacuoles.

For aid in differentiating heterophils from eosinophils, see the section on eosinophil cell identification.

Heterophils are the predominant granulocyte in birds. Heterophils appear to be the primary phagocytic leukocyte. They function in bacterial killing through chemotaxis, opsonization, ingestion, and lysis. Heterophils increase in the peripheral blood in response to inflammation, including bacterial, chlamydial, and fungal infections; tissue necrosis; metabolic disorders; stress; neoplasia; and paraneoplastic syndromes.

Toxic changes that occur in heterophils include cytoplasmic basophilia, vacuolation, nuclear degeneration, toxic granulation, and degranulation. The degree of toxicity usually increases with the severity of the illness. Toxicity is graded on a scale of +1 to +4 (Table 12–3). Toxic heterophils are usually associated with severe systemic illnesses, such as those with bacterial toxins, toxic products of metabolism, and products from tissue necrosis. Toxic heterophils are common with severe systemic bacterial, viral, and chlamydial infections and toxins.

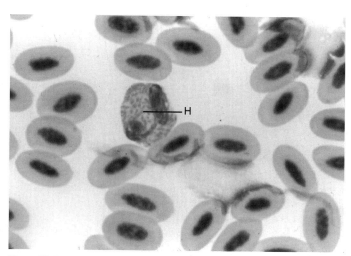

Figure 12–6. Heterophil (*H*) from a barred owl. Wright's stain; original magnification, 100×. See Color Figure 12–6. (Photo courtesy of Terry W. Campbell, M.S., D.V.M., Ph.D.)

TABLE 12–3. Heterophil Toxicity

+1	Slight cytoplasmic basophilia
+2	Darker cytoplasmic basophilia, vacuolization, and partial degranulation
+3	Dark cytoplasmic basophilia, moderate degranulation, abnormal granulation, and cytoplasmic vacuolation
+4	Deep cytoplasmic basophilia, moderate to marked degranulation, cytoplasmic vacuolation, and karyorrhexis or karyolysis

Heterophil artifacts that may occur on smears of peripheral blood include slight vacuolation, uneven distribution of cytoplasmic granules, irregular cell membranes, and pyknosis. These artifacts can be prevented by preparing blood smears within 1 hour after collection of blood.

IMMATURE HETEROPHILS. Band heterophils contain reduced nuclear lobulation and decreased numbers and rounding of cytoplasmic granules. Metamyelocytes are larger than band heterophils with round to slightly indented nuclei and reduced numbers of granules. Heterophil myelocytes are round cells with light blue cytoplasm that contains reduced numbers of typical heterophil granules. They contain magenta granules and rings and round to oval nuclei. The cell is larger, and the nucleus is less condensed than that of a metamyelocyte. Progranulocytes are large cells with light blue cytoplasm and eccentric nuclei with indistinct nuclear membranes. The nuclear chromatin is arranged in a delicate reticular pattern, and the cytoplasm contains orange spheres and dark magenta granules and rings.

Immature heterophils are rarely noted in blood smears from normal birds. Their presence usually indicates a severe inflammatory response, but can rarely be associated with a granulocytic leukemia.

EOSINOPHILS. Eosinophils are round cells that generally have round, brightly staining granules that lack a refractile body, contain pale blue cytoplasm, and contain a prominent staining, bilobed nucleus with clumped chromatin (Fig. 12–7). The granules are uniform and usually round but are occasionally rod-shaped. Granules vary in color between species of birds and type of stain. Granules may stain light blue, dark blue, or pink-orange, or they may be colorless. Eosinophil granules typically stain brighter or different from heterophil granules in the same blood smear and often appear brighter than heterophil granules. Eosinophil granules lack the central refractile body seen in heterophil granules.

Several characteristics can be used to differentiate eosinophils from heterophils. Eosinophils contain pale blue cytoplasm versus the colorless cytoplasm of normal heterophils. Eosinophil granules are usually brighter or duller than heterophil granules on the same blood smear. Eosinophil granules usually lack the central body that is often present in heterophils. The eosinophil nucleus appears darker blue and more distinct than the heterophil nucleus on the same blood smear. Eosinophils appear consistently similar to other eosinophils on the same blood smear and would rarely outnumber heterophils on a blood smear.

The functions of the avian eosinophil are unclear but may include modulation of type IV (delayed) hypersensitivity reactions and participation in inflammatory responses, phagocytosis, and bactericidal and parasiticidal activity.

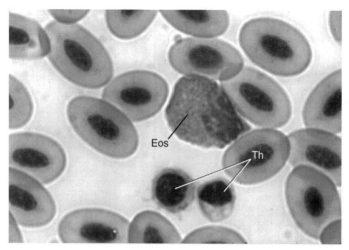

Figure 12–7. Eosinophil *(Eos)* and two thrombocytes *(Th)* from a red tail hawk. Wright's stain; original magnification, 1000 ×. See Color Figure 12–7. (Photo courtesy of Terry W. Campbell, M.S., D.V.M., Ph.D.)

BASOPHILS. Basophils are small- to medium-sized round cells with cytoplasm filled with intensely basophilic granules, with a round to oval light blue staining central nucleus that is often obscured by the cytoplasmic granules (Fig. 12–8). The granules frequently degranulate or coalesce with alcohol-based stains

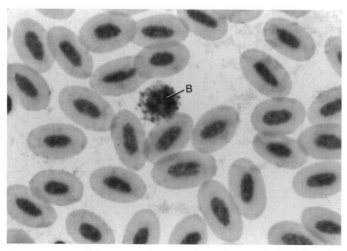

Figure 12–8. Basophil *(B)* from a barred owl. Wright's stain; original magnification, 100×. See Color Figure 12–8. (Photo courtesy of Terry W. Campbell, M.S., D.V.M., Ph.D.)

such as Wright's stain. Finches, canaries, and cockatiels have basophils that contain very small granules and can be easily overlooked.

The functions of avian basophils are not clearly understood. A basophilia may occur with tissue necrosis, chlamydiosis, respiratory disease, and hemolytic anemia.

MONOCYTES. Monocytes are large round to irregularly shaped cells, with blue-gray and finely granular cytoplasm and an oval to bilobed eccentric nucleus with delicate chromatin and few chromatin clumps (see Fig. 12–5). The cytoplasm is finely granular and may contain vacuoles and fine eosinophilic granules. There is often a pale perinuclear zone in the cytoplasm with a darker staining periphery. The presence of a large number of highly vacuolated monocytes is abnormal.

Monocytes are occasionally difficult to differentiate from large lymphocytes. Monocytes have abundant blue-gray cytoplasm that may contain vacuoles, and lymphocytes have a larger nuclear-cytoplasmic ratio and pale blue cytoplasm that appears homogenous and rarely contains vacuoles. The granules of monocytes are smaller than the occasional azurophilic lymphocytic granules. The monocyte nucleus is often flat on one side or bean-shaped, with finely granular to reticulated nuclear chromatin and a few dense clumps, whereas the lymphocytic nucleus is usually centrally located and round, with dense chromatin clumping.

Monocytosis can occur with bacterial, chlamydial, fungal, and mycobacterial infections; granulomatous diseases; chronic diseases; and in diseases with extensive tissue necrosis and debris.

LYMPHOCYTES. Normal mature lymphocytes are typically round, with homogenous and weakly basophilic cytoplasm, with a round to slightly dented and centrally located nucleus with densely clumped or reticulated nuclear chromatin (Fig. 12–9). Lymphocytes may be irregularly shaped as a result of molding around adjacent cells. Lymphocytes can be grouped according to size: small,

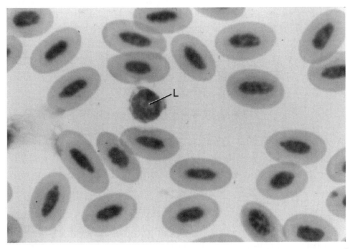

Figure 12–9. Lymphocyte *(L)* from a barred owl. Wright's stain; original magnification, 100×. See Color Figure 12–9. (Photo courtesy of Terry W. Campbell, M.S., D.V.M., Ph.D.)

medium, and large. Small lymphocytes are small round cells with a narrow band of cytoplasm. Medium and large lymphocytes have moderate amounts of cytoplasm that may contain a few eosinophilic granules. Lymphocytes often have cytoplasmic pseudopods (projections). Lymphocytes have a high nuclear-cytoplasmic ratio.

Lymphocytosis is normal in some species of birds (e.g., canaries, pigeons, doves, waterfowl, and some raptors and gallinaceous birds) or may occur as a result of chronic antigenic stimulation. Severe lymphocytosis suggests lymphoid leukemia.

Lymphocytes may become reactive as a result of antigenic stimulation. Reactive lymphocytes are characterized by an increased cell size, increased cytoplasmic basophilia, the presence of azurophilic (purple staining) cytoplasmic granules, and smooth nuclear chromatin. A clear perinuclear area is often present. Reactive lymphocytes are often associated with inflammatory diseases (e.g., chlamydiosis, mycobacteriosis, and aspergillosis).

Plasma cells are occasionally found in peripheral blood smears. They are characterized as large, round to oval lymphocytes with abundant, deeply basophilic cytoplasm, and an eccentric nucleus. A clear perinuclear area is often present.

Abnormal lymphocytes may occur in blood smears. Lymphocytes containing azurophilic granules (large purple), with cytoplasmic vacuolization, or with deep nuclear indentations or partial lobed nuclei are abnormal. Lymphocytes with scalloped cytoplasmic margins are occasionally observed in blood smears, but large numbers of vacuolated lymphocytes are considered abnormal. Immature lymphocytes in peripheral blood smears are abnormal.

For aid in differentiating large lymphocytes from monocytes, see the section on monocyte cell identification. For aid in differentiating small lymphocytes from thrombocytes, see the section on thrombocyte cell identification.

Reactive lymphocytes may appear similar to rubricytes. Reactive lymphocytes and some rubriblasts contain deeply basophilic cytoplasm, whereas other rubriblasts contain gray or eosinophilic gray cytoplasm. Reactive lymphocytes often have a distinct, clear perinuclear area. The nuclear chromatin of the rubricyte stains blue to black, compared with the purplish staining nucleus of the lymphocyte. Rubricytes have a small nuclear-cytoplasmic ratio; lymphocytes have a high nuclear-cytoplasmic ratio.

Cell Counting Techniques

The PCV and WBC counts are routinely performed on avian blood samples. Red blood cell (RBC) counts, hemoglobin determination, reticulocyte count, and thrombocyte count may be routinely performed or used when needed.

Erythrocyte Mass

The most common test used for the evaluation of RBC mass is the PCV. The total RBC count can be determined manually or with an automated cell counter. Manual RBC counts are performed using a hemocytometer and a diluent (e.g., Unopette or Natt and Herrick's solution) (see Table 12–1). If an automated counter is used for RBC count determination, the aperture of the counter must be adjusted for the size of the erythrocyte. Campbell (1995) describes the use of Natt and Herrick's solution to perform erythrocyte counts.

When the Unopette is used to determine RBC counts, the well-mixed blood is drawn into the Unopette pipette and discharged into the diluent, resulting in a 1:200 dilution. This solution is mixed by inverting several times and then discharged onto the hemacytometer counting chamber. The cells are allowed to settle for 5 minutes. The high-dry objective of the microscope is used to count the number of cells in the four corner and central squares of the center large square of the counting chamber. This number is multiplied by 10,000 to obtain the total erythrocyte count per microliter of blood.

Accurate hemoglobin determinations require lysis of the erythrocytes and separation of the nuclei by centrifugation. This allows calculation of RBC indexes.

Reticulocyte Count

The reticulocyte count is useful for the evaluation of the erythrocyte regenerative response. An equal amount of blood is mixed with 0.5% new methylene blue for 15 to 20 minutes. A smear is prepared and allowed to air dry. The ratio of reticulocytes to mature erythrocytes is calculated from the evaluation of 1000 erythrocytes. Reticulocytes are identified as erythrocytes that contain a distinct ring of aggregated reticulum surrounding the nucleus. Varying amounts of reticulum are normally present in mature erythrocytes. The normal reticulocyte count varies with the species of bird, but it is generally less than 10% of the total erythrocyte count in most normal adult psittacines and raptors, usually 2% to 3%. A general guide to interpretation of reticulocyte counts in anemic birds is that greater than 5% reticulocytes indicates a mild regenerative response and greater than 10% reticulocytes generally indicates a good regenerative response. Normal reticulocyte counts vary with the degree of anemia and probably vary with the species. An insufficient increase in reticulocytes for the severity and duration of the anemia indicates the presence of a nonregenerative anemia. Formal studies have not been published at this time regarding absolute normal, regenerative, and abnormal reticulocyte counts.

Leukocyte Counts

Three methods are available to evaluate the numbers of leukocytes in blood samples: automated counts, Unopette eosinophil system and hemacytometer counts, and WBC estimates. The presence of nucleated erythrocytes and thrombocytes complicates automated methods of counting leukocytes. Laser flow cytometry is available, allowing automated counting of WBCs. Campbell (1995) describes the use of Natt and Herrick's solution to perform leukocyte counts.

Leukocyte estimates are less accurate than counts. Estimates should be reserved for circumstances in which there is a suspicion of error in a value obtained from another method or when a count is unavailable (e.g., when only a drop of blood is available or when the count cannot be performed immediately). Estimates of WBCs are determined by counting the number of leukocytes at

40× (high dry) magnification in 10 monolayer fields. This number is multiplied by 2000 to give the estimated leukocytes per cubic millimeter.

The most common method of determining the WBC count in birds is an indirect method using the eosinophil Unopette 5877 system and a hemacytometer. Heterophils and eosinophils are stained with the diluent and can be counted. The total leukocyte count can be obtained by a formula using the leukocyte differential. Fill the Unopette pipette with blood (25 μl). Mix the blood with the diluent by inverting the Unopette several times for 30 seconds, fill both sides of the hemacytometer chamber, and let the loaded hemacytometer stand for 5 minutes. Do not allow the diluted blood to sit for an extended amount of time before performing the count because erythrocytes will stain with prolonged exposure to the stain and diluent will evaporate, altering the count. After the cells have settled, count the cells that appear red-orange and refractile in all 9 large squares on both sides of the hemacytometer, 18 squares total (Fig. 12–10). Perform the leukocyte differential count and calculate the total leukocyte count:

$$\text{Total WBC} = \frac{\text{no. of cells counted in 18 squares} \times 1.1 \times 16 \times 100}{\text{percentage of heterophils} + \text{eosinophils}}$$

Thrombocyte Estimates

Accurate thrombocyte counts are difficult to determine because thrombocytes tend to clump. An estimate can be obtained by determining the average number of thrombocytes in five oil immersion monolayer fields. An average of 2 to 3 per oil immersion field is normal if the PCV is normal. More accurate methods are available; consult Campbell (1995).

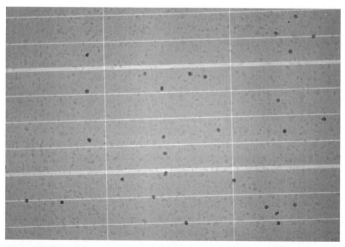

Figure 12–10. Indirect WBC count using Unopette. After the cells have settled, count the granulocytes on both sides of the hemacytometer that appear round, distinctly red-orange, and refractile. Eosinophil Unopette method; original magnification, 10×. See Color Figure 12–10. (Photo courtesy of Terry W. Campbell, M.S., D.V.M., Ph.D.)

Interpretation of Cell Counts

Normal values for various species are listed in Table 12–4.

Erythrocyte

ANEMIA. A decrease in the PCV, RBC count, or hemoglobin indicates anemia. Anemia may be the result of blood loss, increased erythrocyte destruction, or decreased erythrocyte production. Causes of blood loss anemia in birds include trauma, toxicosis resulting in coagulopathy (e.g., coumarin, aflatoxins), parasitism (ticks, *Dermanyssus* mites, coccidia), primary coagulopathy, and organic disease (e.g., gastrointestinal ulcers, organ rupture, ulcerated neoplasm). Causes of increased erythrocyte destruction include erythrocyte parasites (*Plasmodium, Aegyptianella, Haemoproteus, Leucocytozoon*), bacterial septicemia (salmonella, spirochetosis), toxicosis (mustards, petroleum products), and immune-mediated causes. Causes of decreased erythrocyte production include chronic disease (mycobacteriosis, chlamydiosis, aspergillosis, egg yolk peritonitis, hepatitis, nephritis, airsacculitis, neoplasia), hypothyroidism, toxicosis (lead, aflatoxins), nutritional deficiencies (starvation, iron, folic acid), and leukemia (lymphoid leukemia, erythroblastosis). Common causes of decreased erythrocyte production include trauma, chronic disease, septicemia, and parasitism. Blood loss anemias usually are seen with normal plasma protein levels, except in the early stages of acute hemorrhagic anemias when the total proteins may be decreased.

History and physical examination aid in the diagnosis of trauma, some parasites, and nutritional deficiencies. If other clinical signs or physical abnormalities are present, consult appropriate sections of the text for further diagnostic aid. A WBC count, leukocyte differential, and evaluation of blood smear for hemoparasites are the next step in the evaluation of the anemic bird and will often indicate a path to follow to pursue a diagnosis. If lead toxicosis is suspected, radiographs and blood lead levels may be performed. If a diagnosis is still not apparent, a reticulocyte count will allow classification of the anemia as regenerative or nonregenerative and help narrow differentials. Bone marrow aspirate and evaluation are also useful to determine the response to the anemia. Primary coagulopathies and immune-mediated anemias are rare in birds and are pursued as possible diagnoses when other causes are ruled out.

Treatment of anemia involves treatment of the underlying cause. Blood transfusions appear to be beneficial in birds with chronic anemia to stabilize the bird while a diagnosis of the etiology of the anemia is being pursued. Birds with an acute blood loss may better benefit from fluid replacement with lactated Ringer's solution. Birds with a PCV less than 20% as a result of acute blood loss may benefit from a homologous blood transfusion. Administration of iron dextran and B vitamins is also recommended for anemic birds and birds with acute blood loss.

INCREASED PCV OR ERYTHROCYTE COUNT. An increase in PCV or erythrocyte count can be the result of dehydration or absolute polycythemia. The plasma proteins will usually be elevated with dehydration. Polycythemia is the result of increased erythrocyte production and may occur with hemochromatosis, pulmonary disease, and heart disease.

TABLE 12–4. California Avian Laboratory Hematology/Chemistry Values*

	African Gray	Amazon	Budgie	Canary	Cockatiel	Cockatoo	Conure	Lovebird	Macaw
WBC × 1000	6–13	5–12.5	3–8	3–8	5–9	5–12	4–9	3–8	7–14
PCV (%)	42–52	41–53	45–57	45–59	43–57	42–54	42–54	43–55	43–54
Heterophil (%)	45–72	32–71	41–67	20–62	47–72	45–72	45–72	41–71	48–72
Lymphocyte (%)	20–50	20–65	22–58	40–70	27–58	20–50	22–49	28–52	18–52
Monocyte (%)	0–1	0–1	0–2	0–0.05	0–1	0–1	0–1	0–1	0–1
Basophil (%)	0–1	0–2	0–2	0–1	0–1	0–1	0–2	0–1	0–1
Eosinophil (%)	0–1	0–0.05	0–0.05	0–1	0–2	0–2	0–1	0–1	0–1
PP (g/dl)	3.2–4.5	3.2–4.5	3.0–4.4	3.2–4.6	2.9–4.2	3.1–4.4	3.2–4.4	3.1–4.4	2.7–4.7
AST (IU/L)	112–339	155–380	160–372	150–350	130–390	145–346	147–360	130–343	60–165
LDH (IU/L)	154–380	160–360	162–380	—	125–374	200–400	210–390	230–345	70–210
CK (IU/L)	120–410	120–410	120–360	—	167–420	150–400	150–397	160–320	90–360
Uric (mg/dl)	1.9–9.7	2.3–9.8	4–12.2	3–11	3.5–10.4	3.6–10.7	2.7–10.2	3.2–10.2	1.5–11
Calc (mg/dl)	8.3–11.7	8.5–13	8.5–11	—	8.3–10.9	8.4–11	8.4–11	8.6–11.5	8.3–11
Glucose (mg/dl)	280–354	250–370	210–450	—	230–440	210–410	230–400	210–390	210–360
Phos (mg/dl)	3.5–6.9	—	3.7–7.1	—	4.0–7.7	4.2–7.8	4.0–7.9	4.2–7.9	4.0–7.8
Alb (g/dl)	—	—	—	—	0.3–0.9	0.3–0.9	0.3–0.9	0.3–0.9	—
Glob (g/dl)	—	—	—	—	2.5–3.8	2.5–3.8	2.5–3.8	2.5–3.8	—
Chol (mg/dl)	—	150–220	120–220	—	90–195	90–200	83–190	125–195	—
Bile Ac (mg/L)	12–85	35–144	35–110	—	45–105	37–98	35–90	34–88	30–80

Courtesy of California Avian Laboratory, 6114 Greenback Lane, Citrus Heights, CA 95621. Telephone (916) 722-8428, FAX (916) 722-8490, World Wide Web: http://www.ns.net/avianlab.
WBC = white blood cell; PCV = packed cell volume; PP = plasma protein; AST = aspartate aminotransferase; LDH = lactate dehydrogenase; CK = creatine kinase; Calc = calcium; Phos = phosphorus; Alb = albumin; Glob = globulin; Chol = cholesterol; Bile Ac = bile acids. Dash (—) indicates that no values have been established.
*These values are provided as guidelines. Interpretation must be made in light of sample quality, clinical findings, and previous therapy. Juvenile birds tend to have somewhat lower PCVs and more variable WBCs.

Leukocytes

DECREASED LEUKOCYTE COUNT. Leukopenia is commonly the result of an overwhelming bacterial, fungal, chlamydial, or viral infection and septicemia. Other causes of leukopenia include toxicosis (plants, drugs, some chemicals), nutritional diseases, leukemia, anaphylaxis, radiation, and autoimmune disorders. Lymphopenia may be the result of stress, corticosteroid administration, or viremia.

INCREASED LEUKOCYTE COUNT. Classification of the types and numbers of the different WBCs resulting in a leukocytosis allow evaluation of the leukogram. Common causes of mature heterophilias include stress, mild bacterial infections, trauma, surgery, neoplasia, toxins, and metabolic diseases. A marked leukocytosis and heterophilia (often in excess of 40,000/mm^3) is common with chlamydiosis, mycobacteriosis, aspergillosis, and egg yolk peritonitis. Many juvenile psittacines normally have a mature heterophilia. A reversal of the lymphocyte-to-heterophil ratio may be the only sign of an inflammatory response in birds that typically have a greater percentage of lymphocytes than heterophils (e.g., pigeons, doves, canaries, waterfowl, and some raptors and gallinaceous birds).

Regenerative left shifts (the presence of immature heterophils in circulation combined with leukocytosis) may occur with severe or chronic bacterial, fungal, and chlamydial infections; erythroid regeneration after severe blood loss; and occasionally toxins and neoplasia. Degenerative left shifts (immature heterophils in circulation combined with leukopenia) may occur as a result of septicemia, toxicosis, and many viral infections.

Lymphocytosis may occur with chronic antigenic stimulation or lymphocytic leukemia. Reactive lymphocytes indicate antigenic stimulation and are common with chronic infections and viral diseases.

Eosinophilias have been reported to be associated with allergic reactions and parasitic infections.

Basophilias may occur with tissue necrosis, chlamydiosis, respiratory disease, and hemolytic anemia.

Monocytosis can occur with bacterial, chlamydial, fungal, and mycobacterial infections, granulomatous diseases, chronic diseases, and in diseases with extensive tissue necrosis and debris. Monocytosis may occur in some species of birds with zinc deficiency.

Thrombocytes

Thrombocytopenias are usually the result of peripheral demand. Other causes include depression of thrombocytopoiesis, septicemia, and disseminated intravascular coagulopathy. Thrombocytosis may result after a marked erythrocyte response to anemia.

Identification of Common Blood Parasites

Hemoparasites are most common in imported and wild birds and those that are housed outdoors. Common blood parasites of birds include *Haemoproteus,*

Plasmodium, Leucocytozoon, and microfilaria. Less common blood parasites include *Atoxoplasma, Aegyptianella, Borrelia,* and *Trypanosoma.* The most common parasites are discussed in this section; consult Campbell (1995) for descriptions of *Aegyptianella, Borrelia,* and *Trypanosoma.* Descriptions of disease syndromes and treatment of various blood parasites are discussed in Chapter 9.

Hemoproteus

Hemoproteus gametocytes appear as pigmented intracytoplasmic inclusions in erythrocytes (Fig. 12–11). The mature gametocyte occupies over half the erythrocyte cytoplasm and causes little displacement of the erythrocyte nucleus. The pigment may appear yellow to brown or black and is refractile. Macrogametocytes stain blue, and microgametocytes stain pale blue and pink with Romanowsky stains (e.g., Wright's and quick stains), and both contain pigment granules.

Plasmodium

Plasmodium gametocytes, trophozoites, and schizonts may be observed in erythrocytes, thrombocytes, and leukocytes (Fig. 12–12). Gametocytes appear as yellow to brown or black intracytoplasmic refractile inclusions. The gametocyte of some species of *Plasmodium* usually displaces the host cell nucleus; other species do not tend to displace the cell nucleus. The gametocyte usually occupies less than half the cytoplasm of the host cell cytoplasm. Trophozoites appear as small, round to oval intracytoplasmic inclusions with a large vacuole. Schizonts appear as intracytoplasmic basophilic (dark purple staining) round to oval inclusions in erythrocytes. A buffy coat smear may be used to concentrate the parasite to aid detection because numbers may be low in acute infections.

Plasmodium can be differentiated from *Haemoproteus* by the presence of

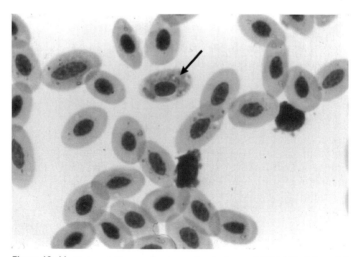

Figure 12–11. *Haemoproteus* mature gametocyte *(arrow).* Wright's stain; original magnification, 100×. See Color Figure 12–11. (Photo courtesy of Terry W. Campbell, M.S., D.V.M., Ph.D.)

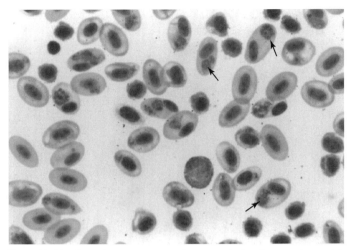

Figure 12–12. *Plasmodium* gametocytes (some marked with *arrows*). Wright's stain; original magnification, 100×. See Color Figure 12–12. (Photo courtesy of Terry W. Campbell, M.S., D.V.M., Ph.D.)

schizonts in peripheral blood, the occurrence of forms in blood cells other than erythrocytes, and the fact that gametocytes of *Plasmodium* are more likely to displace the host cell nucleus than those of *Haemoproteus.*

Leucocytozoon

Leucocytozoon appears as round to elongated intracytoplasmic inclusions usually in erythrocytes (Fig. 12–13). The presence of the parasite in the host cell causes the host cell to appear distended and elongated with two nuclei, that of the host cell pushed to the margin of the cell and the pale pink nucleus of the parasite. Only the gametocyte stage occurs in the peripheral blood, and the gametocyte does not contain refractile pigment. Parasitized cells may have tapered ends or long tails.

Atoxoplasma

Atoxoplasma appears as pale staining round to oval intracytoplasmic inclusions in lymphocytes and monocytes. The parasite causes indentation of the host cell nucleus, resulting in a crescent-shaped host cell nucleus. Sporozoites do not contain pigment.

PLASMA BIOCHEMISTRIES

Plasma is commonly used for avian clinical biochemistries. Blood must stand for a period of time to allow coagulation, which can result in changes in the sample to obtain serum. Cells and plasma should be separated immediately. Lithium heparin is the anticoagulant of choice for most avian blood samples.

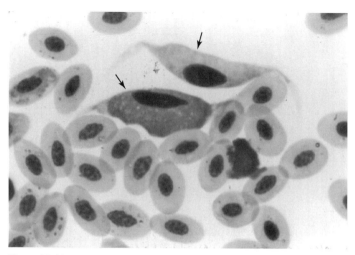

Figure 12–13. *Leucocytozoon (arrows).* Wright's stain; original magnification, 100×. See Color Figure 12–13. (Photo courtesy of Terry W. Campbell, M.S., D.V.M., Ph.D.)

Dry chemistry systems that require very small sample size are especially well suited for avian medicine, some of which include Kodak DT60 Analyzer, VetTest 8008, and Reflotron (see Table 12–1).

Blood sample collection is discussed in the previous section on hematology. Table 12–4 lists normal values for some species of birds. Commonly used and most useful plasma biochemistry tests are discussed in this section.

Amylase

Primary sources of amylase include the pancreas, liver, and small intestine. Amylase activity in birds is not well understood. Increases can occur with acute pancreatitis, typically greater than three times the upper limit of normal reference ranges. Enteritis may result in elevations less than twice the upper limit of the normal reference range. Proventricular dilatation syndrome may result in normal or slight elevation of amylase levels.

Aspartate Aminotransferase

Sources of aspartate aminotransferase (AST) include liver, skeletal muscle, heart, brain, and kidney cells. Elevated levels usually indicate liver or muscle damage. Marked increases in AST levels (>4 times the upper limit of normal) are usually the result of liver necrosis. Mild to moderate increases (2 to 4 times the upper limit of normal) are usually associated with skeletal muscle injury. Skeletal muscle causes of AST elevation may be differentiated from liver origin by measuring creatine kinase (CK) levels, which will increase with skeletal muscle damage. Slight increases in AST may be associated with glucocorticosteroid excess in some birds. Other causes of elevation of AST include vitamin E, selenium, or methionine deficiencies and pesticide and carbon tetrachloride toxicoses.

The magnitude of the elevation of AST roughly correlates to the number of hepatocytes damaged. Marked AST increases suggest severe diffuse liver damage; however, liver damage and inadequate liver function may be present with normal levels of AST.

The plasma half-life of AST in pigeons is 7 to 9 hours.

Bile Acids

Elevated levels of bile acids indicate impaired liver function. Absolute normal ranges are not available at this time and probably vary with the species of bird. Samples obtained after fasting, postprandial, or after random food consumption may affect values somewhat. In general, bile acid levels are a sensitive indicator of liver function, but exact values for interpretation of results are unavailable at this time. In general, mild elevations should be managed with diet and monitored. Persistent and moderate elevations indicate a need for liver biopsy. Marked elevations (500 to 700 mg/L) indicate that disease has progressed past the usefulness of liver biopsy.

Calcium and Phosphorus

Decreased calcium concentration may occur as a result of inadequate calcium in the diet and excessive egg laying; however, calcium is usually mobilized from bone to maintain calcium blood concentration within normal limits. Other causes of hypocalcemia include nutritional hyperparathyroidism, secondary renal hyperparathyroidism, hypovitaminosis D_3, hypoalbuminemia, hypoparathyroidism, and hypercalcitonism. Glucocorticoid therapy can decrease calcium concentration.

Elevated calcium concentrations may occur with vitamin D toxicosis (dietary or other sources), osteolytic bone tumors, dehydration, primary hyperparathyroidism, pseudohyperparathyroidism, and some plant toxicoses. Normal ovulating hens may have elevated calcium levels. Calcium levels should be interpreted along with albumin concentration. Hypoalbuminemia will result in decreased measured calcium concentration, without reducing biologically active calcium. Dehydration resulting in hyperproteinemia may cause an increase in measured calcium levels.

Decreased phosphorus levels may occur with hypovitaminosis D_3, starvation, malabsorption resulting from phosphate binding agents in the diet, long-term glucocorticosteroid therapy, early primary hyperparathyroidism and pseudohyperparathyroidism, and diabetes mellitus complicated by ketoacidosis. Calcium levels will be decreased with hypovitaminosis D_3 but normal with malabsorption caused by phosphate binding agents.

Increased phosphorus levels may occur with vitamin D toxicosis, nutritional secondary hyperthyroidism, renal disease, excessive dietary phosphorus intake, osteolytic bone lesions, severe tissue trauma, and hypoparathyroidism. False elevations occur with hemolysis.

Cholesterol and Triglycerides

Decreased cholesterol levels may occur with bacterial septicemia, liver disease, intestinal disease, aflatoxicosis, and reduced fat in the diet.

Increased cholesterol can be associated with starvation, high levels of dietary fat, hypothyroidism, liver disease, bile duct obstruction, and xanthomatosis. Increased cholesterol levels have been reported in conjunction with atherosclerosis.

Increased triglycerides may occur with starvation, egg-related peritonitis, hepatic lipidosis, hyperadrenocorticism, and exercise.

Creatine Kinase

Increased CK levels occur primarily as a result of muscle cell damage. Levels of CK can be used to differentiate elevations in AST as a result of muscle or liver damage. Elevation of both CK and AST levels may be the result of muscle cell damage only or both muscle and liver damage. Elevations of CK may be associated with muscle injury, intramuscular injections, exercise, convulsions, vitamin E and selenium deficiencies, neuropathies, lead toxicosis, and chlamydiosis.

The half-life of CK in pigeons is 3 to 4 hours.

Electrolytes

Decreased sodium levels may be associated with increased sodium loss (e.g., renal disease, severe diarrhea) or overhydration (e.g., psychogenic polydipsia, intravenous fluid therapy with low sodium or sodium free fluids). Lipemia may result in reported decreased sodium levels.

Elevated sodium levels are usually the result of dehydration caused by inadequate water intake or excessive water loss (e.g., gastrointestinal or renal loss). Hypernatremia may be the result of increased sodium intake (e.g., peanuts, crackers, ornamental dough ingestion).

Decreased potassium levels may be associated with decreased potassium intake, chronic diarrhea, diuretic therapy, or alkalemia. Prolonged storage of unseparated blood may result in pseudohypokalemia.

Elevated potassium levels may be associated with increased intake, renal failure, severe tissue damage, acidemia, adrenal disease, hemolytic anemia, or dehydration. Hemolysis, delayed separation of cells from plasma, and the use of potassium heparin may result in pseudohyperkalemia.

Decreased chloride levels may be associated with vomiting and metabolic acidosis.

Increased chloride levels may be associated with dehydration and renal tubular necrosis.

Glucose

Decreased levels of glucose may be associated with starvation, malnutrition, liver disease, septicemia, neoplasia, aspergillosis, or endocrinopathies. Some birds can tolerate prolonged fasting without resulting in hypoglycemia (e.g., pigeons). Other birds, such as raptor neonates, become hypoglycemic after a few days of fasting. Vitamin A deficiency, high-protein diets, and urea-containing diets may result in hypoglycemia.

Increased glucose levels may be associated with stress, diabetes mellitus, or glucocorticosteroid administration. Transient glucose elevations may occur with egg-related peritonitis. Definitive diagnosis of diabetes mellitus requires finding persistently elevated blood glucose levels (>800 mg/dl).

Lipase

Increased lipase levels may occur with acute pancreatitis. No reference values are currently available; therefore, a blood sample from a clinically normal bird of the same species should be used for comparison.

Total Protein/Albumin

Decreased levels of total protein may occur with chronic renal and hepatic disease, malnutrition, malabsorption (e.g., enteritis, tumors, parasitism), chronic blood loss, and neoplasia.

Increased levels of total protein may occur with dehydration or hyperglobulinemia (e.g., chronic infectious diseases that stimulate production of globulins).

Decreased levels of albumin may be associated with chronic liver disease, chronic inflammation, loss through renal disease, protein malnutrition, loss through gastrointestinal disease, parasitism, or sequestration (increased hydrostatic pressure or reduced oncotic pressure).

Increased levels of albumin may occur with dehydration.

Hyperproteinemia with a normal albumin-to-globulin (A:G) ratio indicates dehydration. Hypoproteinemia with a normal A:G ration can occur with overhydration, acute blood loss, external plasma loss, and internal plasma loss. An increased A:G ration indicates decreased globulins. A decreased A:G ratio can be the result of hypoalbuminemia or hyperglobulinemia. Causes of hypoalbuminemia are listed in the previous paragraph. Hyperglobulinemia may be the result of increases in α-, β-, or γ-globulins. Interpretation of plasma protein levels is aided by protein electrophoresis (EPH) (see section on protein electrophoresis).

Uric Acid

Increased levels of uric acid may occur with starvation, gout, massive tissue necrosis, renal disease, or prerenal causes (e.g., dehydration). Elevations may be the result of primary renal disease or renal disease secondary to aminoglycoside toxicosis, vitamin D toxicosis, vitamin A deficiency–induced damage, and some bacterial and viral infections. Loss of two thirds of the functional mass of the kidney is required for uric acid increases to occur as a result of renal disease. Renal disease may be present with normal levels of plasma uric acid. Contamination of the sample with urates during sample collection with a toenail clip may result in false elevations.

PROTEIN ELECTROPHORESIS

Interpretation of plasma protein levels is aided by EPH. Hyperglobulinemia may be the result of increases in α-, β-, or γ-globulins. An increase in α- and β-globulins may occur with acute inflammation, systemic mycoses, acute nephritis, and active hepatitis. An increase in γ-globulins may be polyclonal, which may occur with chronic inflammation, immune-mediated disease, or suppurative disease, or monoclonal, which may occur with plasma cell dyscrasia. A lack or loss of γ-globulins may indicate an immunodeficient state.

Protein electrophoresis is useful as a diagnostic tool, to monitor disease progression, and to monitor response to treatment. Electrophoresis may be used to diagnose systemic mycotic diseases (e.g., aspergillosis), chlamydiosis, mycobacteriosis, chronic active hepatitis, egg-related peritonitis, and acute nephritis.

MICROBIOLOGY

Avian microbiology is an essential aid in the diagnosis of disease. Having properly trained staff members with experience in avian microbiology is necessary for in-house culture and sensitivity testing. Samples should be sent to a laboratory with experience in avian microbiology unless properly trained staff members and adequate equipment are available. Consult Joyner (1989) and microbiology texts for information on in-house bacterial and fungal identification, culture, and sensitivity testing. Gram's stains are discussed in the section on cytology.

Sample Collection

Samples collected for culture and sensitivity testing can be obtained with sterile swabs in larger birds, but specialized small swabs (Mini-Tip Culturette) are available for collection of samples from smaller birds (see Table 12–1). Samples should be set up immediately or placed in transport medium, refrigerated, and transported to an outside laboratory. The sample should be kept cool during transport. Common sites cultured in live birds include cloaca, choana, crop, eye, trachea, ear, joints, air sacs, and skin. Sinus aspirates, feces, oviduct, and uterus are sometimes cultured.

Cloacal cultures are indicated when signs of gastrointestinal or reproductive disease are present, during routine health checks and postpurchase examinations, and whenever infection is suspected. Cloacal samples are collected with the appropriately sized swab moistened with transport medium or sterile saline. The bird is restrained, and the feathers are parted away from the vent to prevent contamination of the swab. The swab is gently inserted into the cloaca with a twisting motion (Fig. 12–14). In larger birds, the opening of the oviduct or

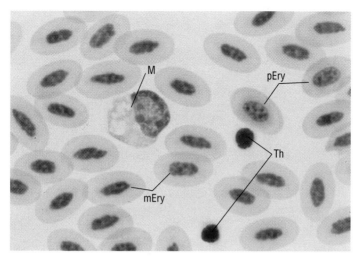

Color Figure 12–5. Mature erythrocytes *(mEry)*, polychromatic erythrocytes *(pEry)*, two thrombocytes *(Th)*, and a monocyte (M) from a barred owl. Wright's stain; original magnification, 100×. (Photo courtesy of Terry W. Campbell, M.S., D.V.M., Ph.D.)

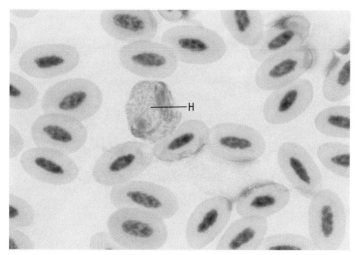

Color Figure 12–6. Heterophil *(H)* from a barred owl. Wright's stain; original magnification, 100×. (Photo courtesy of Terry W. Campbell, M.S., D.V.M., Ph.D.)

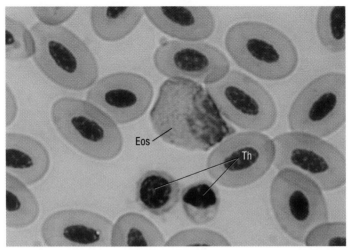

Color Figure 12–7. Eosinophil *(Eos)* and two thrombocytes *(Th)* from a red tail hawk. Wright's stain; original magnification, 1000×. (Photo courtesy of Terry W. Campbell, M.S., D.V.M., Ph.D.)

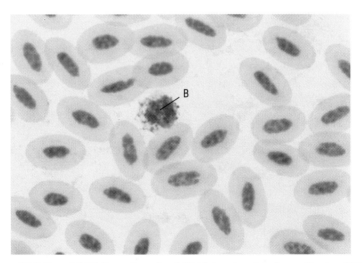

Color Figure 12–8. Basophil *(B)* from a barred owl. Wright's stain; original magnification, 100×. (Photo courtesy of Terry W. Campbell, M.S., D.V.M., Ph.D.)

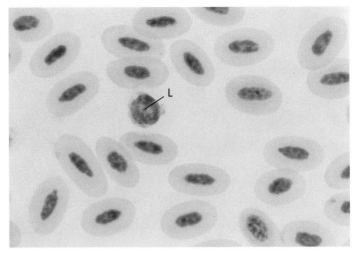

Color Figure 12–9. Lymphocyte *(L)* from a barred owl. Wright's stain; original magnification, 100×. (Photo courtesy of Terry W. Campbell, M.S., D.V.M., Ph.D.)

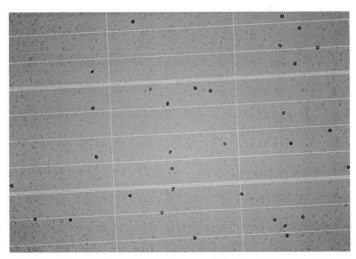

Color Figure 12–10. Indirect WBC count using Unopette. After the cells have settled, count the granulocytes on both sides of the hemacytometer that appear round, distinctly red-orange, and refractile. Eosinophil Unopette method; original magnification, 10×. (Photo courtesy of Terry W. Campbell, M.S., D.V.M., Ph.D.)

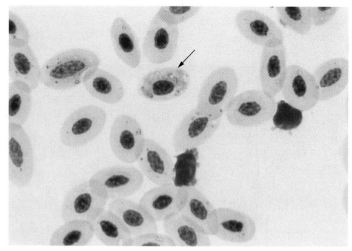

Color Figure 12–11. *Haemoproteus* mature gametocyte *(arrow)*. Wright's stain; original magnification, 100×. (Photo courtesy of Terry W. Campbell, M.S., D.V.M., Ph.D.)

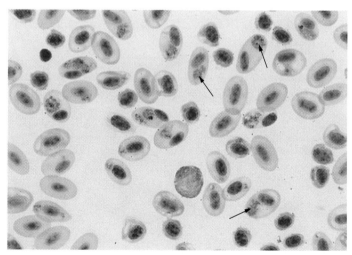

Color Figure 12–12. *Plasmodium* gametocytes (some marked with *arrows*). Wright's stain; original magnification, 100×. (Photo courtesy of Terry W. Campbell, M.S., D.V.M., Ph.D.)

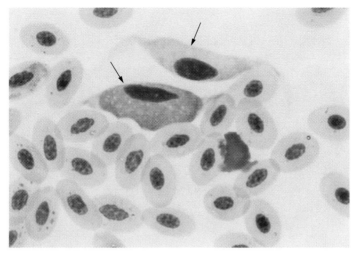

Color Figure 12–13. *Leukocytozoon (arrows)*. Wright's stain; original magnification, 100×. (Photo courtesy of Terry W. Campbell, M.S., D.V.M., Ph.D.)

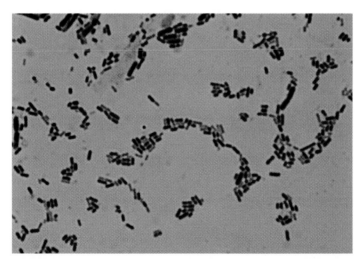

Color Figure 12–16. Gram's stain. Gram-positive organisms stain deep violet and gram-negative organisms stain red. This photograph shows approximately 50% gram-positive organisms and 50% gram-negative organisms. Original magnification, 1000×. (Photo courtesy of Terry W. Campbell, M.S., D.V.M., Ph.D.)

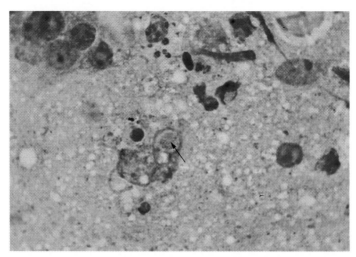

Color Figure 12–17. Macchiavello's stain: numerous *Chlamydia* inclusions. Chlamydia elementary bodies stain red and the larger initial bodies stain blue. (Photo courtesy of Terry W. Campbell, M.S., D.V.M., Ph.D.)

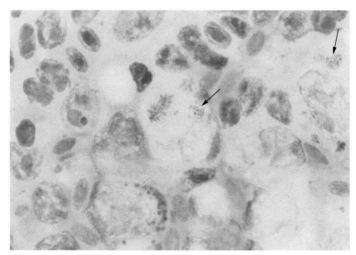

Color Figure 12–19. Chlamydial inclusions *(arrows)* in a liver impression smear. Wright's stain; original magnification, 100×. (Photo courtesy of Terry W. Campbell, M.S., D.V.M., Ph.D.)

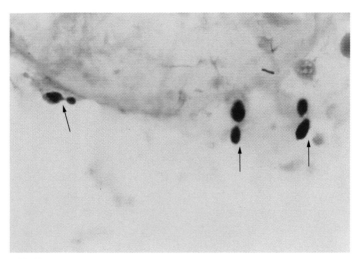

Color Figure 12–20. Budding yeast *(Candida)* from the crop of a cockatoo chick. Wright's stain; original magnification, 100×. (Photo courtesy of Terry W. Campbell, M.S., D.V.M., Ph.D.)

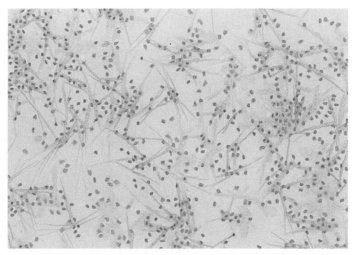

Color Figure 12–22. Uric acid crystals from the joint of a bird with articular gout. Wright's stain; original magnification, 20×. (Photo courtesy of Terry W. Campbell, M.S., D.V.M., Ph.D.)

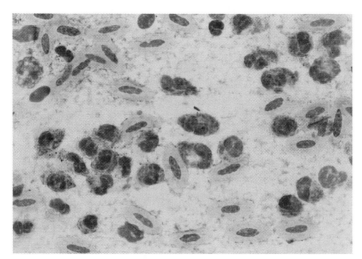

Color Figure 12–23. Smear from a sinus aspirate demonstrating heterophilic inflammation. Wright's stain; original magnification, 100×. (Photo courtesy of Terry W. Campbell, M.S., D.V.M., Ph.D.)

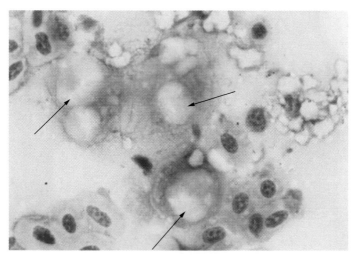

Color Figure 12–24. Poxvirus inclusions *(arrows)* from a flamingo chick. Wright's stain; original magnification, 100×. (Photo courtesy of Terry W. Campbell, M.S., D.V.M., Ph.D.)

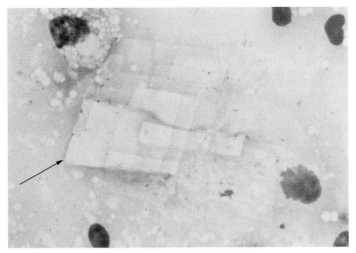

Color Figure 12–25. Cholesterol crystals from a xanthoma on a macaw. Wright's stain; original magnification, 100×. (Photo courtesy of Terry W. Campbell, M.S., D.V.M., Ph.D.)

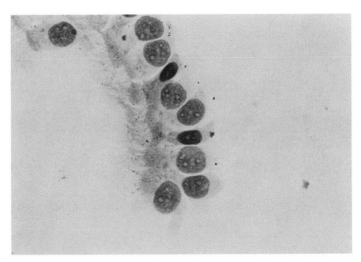

Color Figure 12–27. Respiratory epithelial cells. Wright's stain; original magnification, 100×. (Photo courtesy of Terry W. Campbell, M.S., D.V.M., Ph.D.)

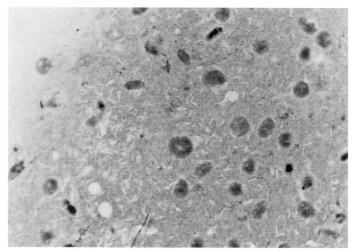

Color Figure 12–28. *Mycobacterium* appears as numerous nonstaining rods in the background on an impression smear from the liver of an Amazon parrot with mycobacteriosis. Wright's stain; original magnification, 100×. (Photo courtesy of Terry W. Campbell, M.S., D.V.M., Ph.D.)

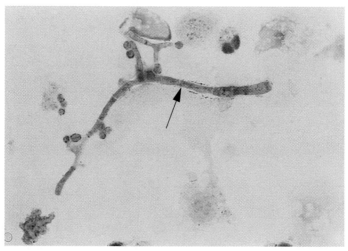

Color Figure 12–29. *Aspergillus* hyphae *(arrow)* in a tracheal wash from an African gray parrot. Wright's stain; original magnification, 100×. (Photo courtesy of Terry W. Campbell, M.S., D.V.M., Ph.D.)

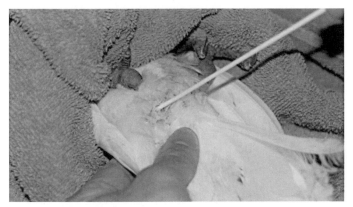

Figure 12-14. Cloacal sample collection.

ureters can be isolated and specifically cultured with the use of a speculum or endoscope.

Cultures of the choana are indicated when signs of respiratory disease or choanal pathology are present, during routine health checks and postpurchase examinations, and whenever infection is suspected. The swab is moistened with transport medium or sterile saline, and the bird is restrained. A mouth speculum or gauze is used to hold the mouth open. The swab is inserted in the anterior choana (Fig. 12-15). Contamination by oral and environmental bacteria occurs and must be considered when interpreting choanal culture results (see the section on interpretation of bacterial and fungal cultures). When infection of the sinus is suspected, superior samples can be obtained with a sinus aspirate that prevents contamination of the sample with oral bacteria.

To perform a sinus aspirate, the bird is restrained with the head secure. A 22-

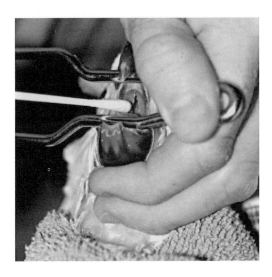

Figure 12-15. Choanal sample collection.

to 27-gauge needle on a 3- or 5-ml syringe is used to collect the sample. The needle is inserted midway between the commissure of the beak and the medial canthus of the eye (see Fig. 11–6). The needle is directed under the zygomatic arch at a 45-degree angle to the side of the head. The sinus is more easily entered if the mouth is held open with a speculum. Take care to avoid penetration of the eye.

Crop cultures may be indicated when signs of gastrointestinal disease are present, especially delayed crop emptying or crop stasis; however, bacterial ingluvitis (crop infection) is rarely the primary cause of the illness. Samples for culture of the crop are obtained as described for crop cytology (see the section on cytology).

Cultures of the conjunctiva or ear are indicated when discharge, swelling, erythema, an ulcer, or a lesion is present or infection is suspected. For collection of a conjunctival sample, a moistened swab is inserted into the fornix of the eye and moved from side to side, carefully avoiding injury to the cornea. Lesions of the ear are directly swabbed for culture.

Tracheal cultures are indicated when signs of respiratory infection are present. Samples for tracheal culture may be obtained in awake or anesthetized birds. The bird is restrained, a speculum or gauze is used to hold the mouth open, and the sample can be collected with a Mini-Tip Culturette from the trachea. In anesthetized birds, samples may be obtained through the endotracheal tube if the diameter of the tube is large enough to allow passage of the culturette through the lumen of the endotracheal tube. Samples can also be obtained with tracheal washings (see the section on cytology).

Culture of joints is indicated when bacterial or fungal infection is suspected based on cytology. The bird is anesthetized unless severely depressed. The skin over the joint is surgically prepped, and a needle and syringe are used to obtain a sample of fluid. The sample is expressed onto a swab, placed in transport media, and shipped to the laboratory.

Air sac cultures are indicated in birds with respiratory signs or evidence of infection based on radiographic or endoscopic appearances. The bird is anesthetized and placed in lateral recumbency. The area caudal to the last rib is surgically prepped. A nick is made in the skin just caudal to the last rib ventral to the flexor cruris medialis muscle, and the muscles are bluntly separated with hemostats. An endoscope or sterile otoscope cone is passed into the caudal thoracic air sac. The air sac membrane and lesions are swabbed with a Mini-Tip Culturette, or a sterile soft catheter may be passed and the air sac membrane irrigated with a small amount of sterile saline. The fluid is then removed with the catheter and cultured.

Culture of the skin is indicated when signs of infection are present. A moistened swab is rolled over the lesion. Feather follicles and pulp from a growing feather can also be cultured.

Interpretation of Bacterial and Fungal Culture Results

Interpretation of culture results are based on the presence or absence of clinical signs, the type of bacteria or fungi isolated, and the number of bacteria isolated. Whether clinical signs are present is a critical factor in determining if the bird should be treated. When unusual bacteria are isolated in ill birds, treatment with an appropriate antibiotic will probably be beneficial.

The type of bacteria or fungus isolated must be compared with likely normal flora for that site. Normal flora must be differentiated from pathologic organisms. Normal flora can vary with the species, aviary, and between the same species of birds within the same aviary. Populations of bacteria change as a result of many factors, including the type of food fed, level of bacteria in the food, bacteria in the environment, diseases, the use of antibiotics, and stress. Interpretation of culture results is complicated by the fact that the normal flora for the bird may include organisms that are pathogenic for other birds. Cockatoos have more gram-negative bacteria than most other psittacines, and gram-negative bacteria are isolated more frequently from raptors.

Routine aerobic fecal cultures from healthy passerines usually grow no bacteria. Common normal flora of toucans include *Escherichia coli, Staphylococcus,* and *Streptococcus. Klebsiella* was isolated from half of the clinically normal toucans in one study.

In general, the normal flora of the psittacine intestinal tract and choana contains predominantly gram-positive bacteria, including *Streptococcus, Staphylococcus, Lactobacillus, Cornyebacterium,* and *Bacillus.* Varying concentrations of gram-negative bacteria can also be found in healthy psittacines, including *E. coli, Enterobacter, Klebsiella, Citrobacter, Pasteurella,* and *Moraxella.* Other gram-negative bacteria such as *Pseudomonas* are rarely found in healthy birds. Conjunctival and ear cultures of healthy birds usually grow nothing or gram-positive organisms. Gram-negative bacteria are occasionally isolated from normal eyes and ears.

In general, isolation of *Proteus, Salmonella, Pseudomonas, Klebsiella, Listeria, Erysipelothrix,* hemolytic *Staphylococcus aureus, Cryptococcus neoformans,* or *Aspergillus fumigatus* is clinically significant in ill birds.

The number of bacteria isolated is important when interpreting culture results. Isolation of large numbers of a single organism from a bird without growth of any normal flora can indicate abnormal bacterial colonization.

Treatment

Many bacterial and fungal infections are the direct result or partially the result of malnutrition and poor management techniques. The diet should be scrutinized and corrected in all birds with bacterial or fungal infections. Management techniques that may contribute to microbial infections include contaminated or spoiled food, contaminated water, contact with other birds or their droppings, rodent droppings, and contaminated nest material. Humans are also a source of spread of disease.

Treatment of infections should be based on sensitivity testing. Post-treatment cultures should be performed to determine effectiveness of therapy. If antibiotics are used in young birds or for long periods of time (e.g., treatment of chlamydiosis), monitor for *Candida* overgrowth or prophylactically treat with an antifungal agent (e.g., nystatin, ketoconazole).

Mycoplasma and Chlamydial Cultures

Isolation of *Mycoplasma* or *Chlamydia* requires special transport media. Contact the laboratory for instructions and to obtain transport media.

CYTOLOGY

Cytology is a simple, rapid, and inexpensive diagnostic technique. Discharges, masses, and swellings should be evaluated cytologically. Cytology is also useful in postmortem examinations.

Equipment

Equipment needed to perform cytologic examinations includes a microscope with good resolution and oil immersion capabilities, microscope slides, cover slips, stains, needles, syringes, sterile swabs, sterile saline, and sterile feeding needles or red rubber catheters. Sterile glass slides are convenient because a single sample can be collected and used for both cytology and culture. Slides can be placed in a container (e.g., plastic slide container) and autoclaved or gas sterilized. Samples collected with a sterile swab can be rolled onto a sterile slide, and the swab can be placed in transport media or set up for culture.

Stains and General Staining Techniques

Stains routinely used in avian medicine include Gram's stain, Wright's stain, and quick stains such as Diff Quick or Hema-tek (see Table 12–1). Other useful stains include Macchiavello's, Gimenez, Giemsa, and acid-fast stains.

Gram's Stain

Gram's stain is used to determine if bacteria or fungi are present and for the classification of bacteria present (gram-negative or gram-positive). Samples are collected and rolled onto a slide. The slide is air dried. The staining procedure for Gram's stain is listed in Table 12–5. A Bunsen burner or lighter may be used

---

TABLE 12–5. Staining Procedure for Gram's Stain

1. Heat fix the air-dried smear by passing the slide (smear side up) through a low flame five or six times. Allow to cool.
2. Flood the smear with crystal violet for 1 minute, then gently rinse with water for 1 to 5 seconds. Drain excess water from the slide.
3. Flood the smear with Gram's iodine solution and let stand for 1 minute. Gently rinse with water.
4. Flush the smear with decolorizer until the runoff is relatively clear. Rinse with water.
5. Flood the smear with safranin O, and let stand for 1 to 2 minutes. Rinse the slide with water and let dry.

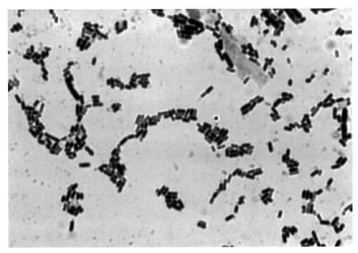

Figure 12–16. Gram's stain. Gram-positive organisms stain deep violet and gram-negative organisms stain red. This photograph shows approximately 50% gram-positive organisms and 50% gram-negative organisms. Original magnification, 1000×. See Color Figure 12–16. (Photo courtesy of Terry W. Campbell, M.S., D.V.M., Ph.D.)

for a flame source. The slide should be warm to the touch but not hot when touched immediately after heating. The length of time the slide requires for decolorization is dependent on the thickness of the slide. Overdecolorization is common and results in gram-positive organisms appearing red.

Gram-positive organisms and yeast stain deep violet, and gram-negative organisms stain red (Fig. 12–16). Gram-negative bacteria are predominantly rod or coccobacillic shaped and are usually much smaller than gram-positive rods in birds. Spirochetes are gram-negative spiral bacteria. Commercially prepared slides of gram-positive and gram-negative organisms can be used for ensuring accuracy of results on collected samples (e.g., Gramcheck, MicroScan; see Table 12–1).

Organisms are classified by morphologic type (shape of organism and gram-negative or gram-positive) and relative percentages of each type under oil immersion. Table 12–6 lists a method of quantitation of bacteria noted on smears. For a sample Gram's stain report form, see Table 12–7. The thickness of the smear will affect results. Superior staining and consistent quantitation require thin uniform smears.

TABLE 12–6. Method of Quantitation of Bacteria on Gram's Stains

0 = no organisms present
1 = 1 organism per oil immersion field
2 = 2 to 5 organisms per oil immersion field
3 = 6 to 20 organisms per oil immersion field
4 = greater than 20 organisms per oil immersion field

TABLE 12–7. Sample Gram's Stain Report Form

Morphology	Quantity (0 to 4+)	Percentage
Gram + cocci		
Gram + rods		
Gram − rods		
Gram − coccobacilli		
Yeast		
Hyphae		
WBCs		
RBCs		

Wright's, Wright-Giemsa, Diff-Quik, and Hema-tek

Wright's, Wright-Giemsa, Diff-Quik, and Hema-tek stains are used for routine cytology, as well as for staining of peripheral blood smears. The staining procedure for Diff-Quik and Hema-tek stains is listed in Table 12–8. For staining procedures for the other stains, consult manufacturers directions or Campbell (1995).

Wright's stain results in dark violet staining of nuclei. Wright-Giemsa, Diff-Quik, and Hema-Tek stains result in reddish purple staining of nuclei. For further description of staining results, see hematology section.

Macchiavello's Stain

Macchiavello's stain is used to identify *Chlamydia* and *Mycoplasma* inclusions. *Chlamydia* elementary bodies stain red, and the larger initial bodies stain blue (Fig. 12–17). *Mycoplasma* inclusions resemble *Chlamydia* inclusions. Heterophil granules, eosinophil granules, and other nonchlamydial particles may stain red, making interpretation difficult.

Gimenez Stain

Gimenez stain is used to identify *Chlamydia* inclusions. Chlamydial inclusions stain red and are circular. The cellular background stains blue-green.

Giemsa Stain

Giemsa stain is used to aid in detection of some blood parasites, chlamydial elementary and initial bodies, and *Mycoplasma* inclusions. Chlamydial elemen-

TABLE 12–8. Staining Procedure for Diff-Quik and Hema-tek Stains

1. Dip the air-dried smear in fixative for five 1-second dips. Drain excess.
2. Dip the smear into Solution I (red) for five 1-second dips. Drain excess.
3. Dip the smear into Solution II (purple) for five 1-second dips. Drain excess.
4. Rinse the slide with distilled or deionized water. Allow to air dry.

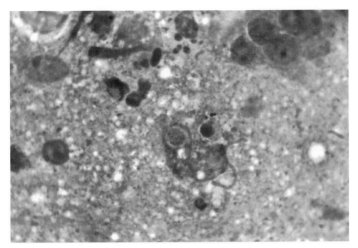

Figure 12–17. Macchiavello's stain: *Chlamydia* inclusions. *Chlamydia* elementary bodies stain red, and the larger initial bodies stain blue. See Color Figure 12–17. (Photo courtesy of Terry W. Campbell, M.S., D.V.M., Ph.D.)

tary bodies stain purple and initial bodies stain blue. Mycoplasmal inclusions stain pink or purple.

Acid-Fast Stain

Acid-fast stain is used to demonstrate mycobacterial organisms that cause mycobacteriosis. *Mycobacterium* stain red, and other bacteria and cells stain blue. Feces or liver biopsies are the samples often used for acid-fast staining in live birds.

Cytologic Responses

Smears are stained with Wright's, Wright-Giemsa, Diff-Quik, or Hema-tek stain and allowed to dry. Scan the slide on low power for large diagnostic structures such as fungal hyphae and small fragments of tissue and to determine variation in distribution and content of the smear. After scanning on low power, begin evaluation of cells. Locate areas of the smear that are thin and have intact, well-stained individual cells. Scan the slide on high power, looking for diagnostic structures such as bacteria, fungi, and tissue fragments. Determine cell populations of various cell types and record in percentages. Determine if the cell population is primarily inflammatory or noninflammatory. Inflammatory cells are categorized according to inflammatory cell types. If the cell population is primarily tissue cells, determine the cell types present and evaluate cells for malignant characteristics.

Classification of cytologic response is based on the majority of the cell types, the morphology of the cells, and the character of the noncellular background.

Cellular responses include inflammation, tissue hyperplasia or benign neoplasia, and malignant neoplasia.

Inflammation

Inflammatory cells include heterophils, lymphocytes, macrophages, eosinophils, and plasma cells.

Heterophilic inflammation is characterized by a 70% heterophil population or greater. Heterophilic inflammation indicates an acute inflammatory response. Degenerate heterophils suggest sepsis (i.e., bacterial infection), but can occur with severe inflammation. Nondegenerate heterophils suggest bacterial infection or severe irritation, but microbial toxins are not present. Degenerative changes include increased cytoplasmic basophilia, vacuolization, degranulation, karyolysis, and karyorrhexis. Karyolysis appears as swollen nuclei with a wider, more irregular shaped, lighter staining nucleus. Karyorrhexis appears as fragmentation of the nucleus. Degenerative changes must be differentiated from trauma to fragile cells during making of the smear or partial lysis caused by storage of the sample. Nondegenerate heterophils resemble normal cells in a blood smear. Nuclear pyknosis may be present. Pyknosis appears as small dense nuclei that stain deeply basophilic.

Mixed-cell inflammation is characterized by the presence of heterophils (>50%), mixed with variable numbers of lymphocytes, macrophages, and plasma cells. Heterophils are usually nondegenerate. Mixed-cell inflammation indicates active inflammation and is common with foreign bodies, fungal infections, chlamydiosis, and ulcerated neoplasms.

Macrophagic inflammation is characterized by a population of primarily macrophages (>50%), with variable numbers of lymphocytes, plasma cells, and heterophils. Macrophagic inflammation may occur with chronic or acute stages of disease and is common with foreign bodies, xanthomatosis, and mycobacterial, chlamydial, and fungal infections. Examine the smear for the presence of fungal elements, chlamydial inclusions in macrophages, and multinucleate giant cells with large ghostlike bacterial rods that may occur with mycobacteriosis.

Eosinophilic inflammation, which is rare in birds, is characterized by the presence of primarily eosinophils.

Tissue Hyperplasia or Benign Neoplasia

Tissue hyperplasia cannot be differentiated from benign neoplasia with cytology. Cells from these lesions may have increased cytoplasmic basophilia and pale vesicular nuclei. An increase in normal mitotic figures may occur. Their uniform nuclear to cytoplasmic ratio and appearance are used to differentiate these cells from malignant neoplastic cells. Common causes of tissue hyperplasia in birds include chronic inflammation, vitamin A deficiency, and iodine deficiency (causing thyroid hyperplasia in budgies). Lipomas are common benign neoplasms in budgies.

Malignant Neoplasia

A definitive diagnosis of malignant neoplasia most often requires histopathology. A suspicion of malignancy can be obtained with cytology. Suspicious lesions should be biopsied and samples submitted for histopathology because many inflammatory lesions show some cellular changes. The consequences of a diagnosis of malignant neoplasia can be severe.

Nuclear changes suggestive of malignancy include increased nuclear size, increased nuclear-cytoplasmic ratio, nuclear anisocytosis (variable size), nuclear pleomorphism (variable shape), coarse hyperchromatic nuclear chromatin, large nucleoli (greater than one-third the diameter of the nucleus), multiple nucleoli (more than five), irregular nuclear margins, abnormal or increased mitotic figures, and abnormal lobation. Multinucleated giant cells with nuclei that are enlarged, irregularly arranged, and pleomorphic are also suggestive of neoplasia. Cytoplasmic changes suggestive of malignancy include increased basophilia, abnormal vacuolation, abnormal inclusions, small cytoplasmic volume, variations in staining quality, and variable cytoplasmic margins.

Malignant neoplastic cells may be classified as carcinomas, sarcomas, discrete cell neoplasms, or poorly differentiated neoplasms. Carcinomas are characterized by exfoliation in cellular aggregates. Adenocarcinomas often have cytoplasmic secretory vacuoles (e.g., ovarian adenocarcinoma). Sarcomas tend to exfoliate poorly and as individual cells. They tend to have indistinct cytoplasmic margins, possess one or more nuclei, have prominent nucleoli, and are often elongated or spindle shaped (e.g., fibrosarcoma). Discrete cell neoplasms tend to be round or oval cells that exfoliate as individual cells (e.g., lymphosarcoma).

Sample Collection and Interpretation

Abdominocentesis/Abdominal Effusions

Abdominocentesis is performed to collect abnormal abdominal fluid accumulation for evaluation and to relieve clinical signs of dyspnea. The area caudal to the sternum is surgically prepped. A 21- to 25-gauge needle on a syringe is inserted at the midline immediately caudal to the sternum directed to the right side of the abdomen to avoid the ventriculus (Fig. 12–18). Only enough fluid is withdrawn to evaluate and relieve dyspnea.

Little or no fluid can be collected from the abdomen of normal birds. Normal fluid contains few cells such as an occasional mesothelial cell and macrophage. Normal mesothelial cells are flat, polygonal cells with homogeneous, weakly basophilic cytoplasm and a centrally placed round or oval nucleus. They may occur singly or in clusters or sheets. Reactive mesothelial cells are round or oval, may contain cytoplasmic vacuoles, and have scalloped margins or villuslike eosinophilic cytoplasmic margins. They are larger and more basophilic than nonreactive mesothelial cells. The nuclei often contain coarsely granular chromatin and prominent nucleoli, and they may be multinucleate and show mitotic activity. Reactive mesothelial cells occur with irritation or after having been present in abdominal fluid for an extended period of time. Reactive mesothelial cells may occur singly or in clusters. These cells should not be mistaken for malignant neoplasia. Macrophages are large variably shaped cells with abundant granulated cytoplasm. They may contain phagocytic vacuoles or foreign material. Macrophages can reproduce in fluids; therefore, mitotic figures may be observed.

Abdominal fluids can be classified as transudates, modified transudates, exu-

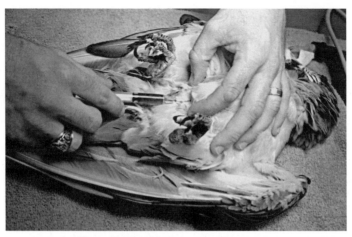

Figure 12–18. Abdominocentesis in a macaw.

dates, hemorrhage, or malignant effusions. Transudates are transparent, clear to pale yellow, odorless, and are characterized by low cell count (<1000 cells/μl), specific gravity of 1.020 or less, and total protein less than 3.0 g/dl. Transudates are rare in birds but may occur as a result of hepatic cirrhosis, cardiac insufficiency, or hypoproteinemia. Transudates are common in mynahs with hemochromatosis.

Modified transudates are characterized by increased cellularity (1000 to 5000 cells/μl). Cells usually consist primarily of macrophages and lymphocytes, with occasional mesothelial cells and rare heterophils. Mesothelial cells are usually reactive. Modified transudates occur as a result of changes in hydrostatic pressure or irritation from transudates present for extended periods of time. Modified transudates may occur as a result of hepatic cirrhosis, hemochromatosis, cardiac insufficiency, or hypoproteinemia.

Exudates vary in color and turbidity. They often have a foul odor and are viscous. Exudates are characterized by increased cellularity (>5000 cells/μl), a specific gravity greater than 1.020, and total protein greater than 3.0 g/dl. Acute exudative effusions of less than a few hours contain primarily heterophils. Within a few hours, cells typically are of a mixed-cell inflammatory response. Septic exudates may contain intracellular bacteria or degenerate heterophils. Chronic exudates often contain lymphocytes and plasma cells. Plasma cells are oval cells with abundant, deeply basophilic cytoplasm, eccentric nucleus, and perinuclear clear space. Exudates occur as a result of inflammatory or infectious processes. Common causes of abdominal exudates include septic peritonitis, egg-related peritonitis, and abdominal malignancies.

Hemorrhagic effusions are characterized by the presence of fluid containing leukocytes and erythrocytes in the same proportions as in peripheral blood. Thrombocytes may be present if there is active hemorrhage or if peripheral blood contamination of the sample has occurred. Erythrophagocytosis by macrophages or heterophils may occur. Iron pigment may be noted in macrophages or heterophils and stains gray to blue-black.

Malignant effusions may contain exfoliated malignant cells and may be exudative or hemorrhagic.

Contamination of the abdomen with urates occasionally occurs. Samples from the abdomen have a milky appearance and contain abundant urate crystals and few cells. Urate crystals are spherical, have a spoke-wheel appearance, and are birefringent under polarized light (see Joint Aspirate). Chronic urate peritonitis contains inflammatory cells.

Air Sac Swab/Air Sac Washing

Indications for air sac sampling and cytology include lower respiratory clinical signs, radiographic evidence of air sac involvement, or observation of abnormalities during laparoscopy or laparotomy. Bacterial, fungal, and chlamydial infections may be diagnosed through the use of air sac cytology when airsacculitis is present.

Equipment needed to perform endoscopic sampling of the air sac include sterile swabs and an endoscope or otoscope with an operating head and sterile cones. A left or right lateral approach is used, depending on radiographic evidence of the affected site. The bird is anesthetized and placed in lateral recumbency. The area over and caudal to the last rib is surgically prepped. A nick is made in the skin just caudal to the last rib or between the last two ribs, and the muscles are bluntly separated with hemostats. An endoscope or sterile otoscope cone is passed into the caudal thoracic air sac space. The air sac membrane and lesions are swabbed with a Mini-Tip Culturette, or a sterile soft catheter may be passed and the air sac membrane irrigated with a small amount of sterile saline. The fluid is then removed with the catheter. Grasping or biopsy forceps can be used to collect caseous debris with an endoscope. The swab is rolled onto a slide and air dried. Cells can be concentrated with slow speed centrifugation. The supernatant is poured off, and the cells are suspended by tapping the tube. A small amount is placed on a slide, and a smear is made using another slide and push technique. The smear is then allowed to air dry.

The smear is stained with Wright's, Modified Wright's, Diff-Quik, or Hematek stain. Normal air sac cytology contains occasional noncornified squamous epithelial cells with a clear background. Inflammatory cells, bacterial phagocytosis by leukocytes, and heavy staining background material indicate septic airsacculitis.

The presence of fungal elements, multinucleated giant cells, and mixed cell or macrophagic inflammation indicates fungal infection. The most common fungal air sac infection in birds is *Aspergillus*. *Aspergillus* may be identified as branching septate hyphae. Hyphae may stain poorly or basophilic with Wright's or quick stain. New methylene blue stain may be used to visualize hyphae better. Basophilic staining conidiophores or spores may be seen when stained with Wright's or quick stains. *Candida* air sac lesions are uncommon, but can be identified by the presence of many oval budding yeasts. Yeast cells stain basophilic with Wright's or quick stains. The presence of hyphae in *Candida* infections indicates tissue invasion and is associated with a poor prognosis.

Mixed-cell or macrophagic inflammation and chlamydial inclusions indicate chlamydiosis. Chlamydial inclusions appear as small blue or purple spheres in the cytoplasm of macrophages or epithelial cells when stained with Wright's or

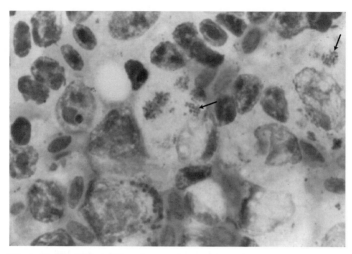

Figure 12–19. Chlamydial inclusions *(arrows)* in a liver impression smear. Wright's stain; original magnification, 100×. See Color Figure 12–19. (Photo courtesy of Terry W. Campbell, M.S., D.V.M., Ph.D.)

quick stains (Fig. 12–19). Confirm chlamydial inclusions with special stains (e.g., Macchiavello's, Gimenez, or Giemsa).

Bone Marrow Aspirate

Bone marrow cytology is useful for the evaluation of hematopoiesis. Equipment needed to collect a sample for bone marrow aspiration cytology includes syringe, scalpel blade, and bone marrow aspiration needles or spinal needles with stylets. For proper evaluation of the bone marrow, bone marrow cytology must be compared with a peripheral blood sample collected the same day. Samples may be collected from the tibiotarsus or sternum. Collection from the proximal tibiotarsus is discussed in the following paragraph; consult Campbell (1995) for sample collection procedures from the sternum and discussion of interpretation of bone marrow aspirates.

The bird is anesthetized. The proximal cranial tibiotarsus is surgically prepped. The site is the same as in intraosseous catheter placement and a similar technique (see Fig. 1–13). The tibiotarsus is grasped, a small stab incision is made in the skin at the collection site, and the needle is inserted into the marrow cavity with gentle pressure and twisting motion of the needle. The stylet is removed, and the sample is aspirated with a syringe. The needle is removed from the syringe, and air is drawn into the syringe. The needle is placed back on the syringe with air, and the sample is expelled onto a slide. A smear is then made using another slide pulled horizontally.

Choanal Swab

Choanal swabs are commonly collected for evaluation of the upper respiratory tract. Samples are stained with Gram's stain and evaluated for the presence of abnormal populations of bacteria and yeast. The mouth is held open with a speculum or gauze strips. A swab moistened with transport media or sterile saline is introduced into the rostral choana. The swab is rolled onto a slide. The slide is air dried, fixed, and stained with Gram's stain. Choanal Gram's stains from most normal birds contain mixed populations of gram-positive bacteria and occasional yeast, with or without occasional gram-negative bacteria. *Alysiella filiformis* is a coccobacillus, often associated with squamous epithelial cells in pairs or chains, that is part of the normal flora. Large numbers of gram-negative bacterial rods, gram-negative spirochetes, abundant yeast organisms, budding yeast, and protozoa are abnormal. See the sections on Gram's stain and interpretation of bacterial and fungal culture results for aid in interpretation of results. Choanal swabs can be evaluated cytologically when stained with Wright's, modified Wright's, Diff-Quik, or Hema-tek stain; see oral lesion smears.

Cloacal Swab/Fecal Swab

Cloacal and fecal Gram's stains are useful for evaluation of the gastrointestinal, urinary, or reproductive tracts, but they may also contain bacteria affecting the respiratory tract. Samples are stained with Gram's stain and evaluated for the presence of abnormal populations of bacteria or yeast. To obtain a cloacal sample, a swab is moistened with transport medium or sterile saline and gently inserted into the cloaca with a twisting motion. Fecal samples are collected onto a swab from a fresh dropping. The sample is rolled onto a slide to make a thin uniform smear. The slide is air dried, fixed, and stained with Gram's stain. Cloacal Gram's stains from most normal birds contain mixed populations of gram-positive bacteria and occasional yeast, with or without occasional gram-negative bacteria. Large numbers of gram-negative bacterial rods, abundant yeast organisms, budding yeast, protozoa, and parasite eggs are abnormal. See the sections on Gram's stain and interpretation of bacterial and fungal culture results for additional aid in interpretation of results.

Cloacal smears can be made and evaluated cytologically when stained with Wright's, Modified Wright's, Diff-Quik, or Hema-tek stain. Normal cloacal cytology contains occasional noncornified squamous or columnar epithelial cells with centrally or eccentrically placed nuclei. Inflammatory cells are indicative of inflammation of the cloaca, lower intestinal tract, reproductive tract, or urinary tract. Leukocytic bacterial phagocytosis indicates bacterial infection. The presence of basal epithelial cells and erythrocytes indicates traumatic collection or the presence of ulcerative lesions. Basal cells are round with large, round nuclei and a high nuclear-cytoplasmic ratio. They may occur in sheets or as individual cells.

Conjunctiva and Corneal Smear/Scraping

Corneal or conjunctival cytology is indicated in birds with conjunctivitis or keratoconjunctivitis. Technique of sample collection and interpretation of results are discussed in Chapter 5.

Crop Wash/Aspirate

Indications for crop aspirates include vomiting, regurgitation, delayed crop emptying, crop stasis, or other crop disorders. Crop washes may be used to obtain samples from crops when crop aspirates yield little fluid for evaluation. Equipment needed to perform crop aspirates and washes include stainless steel feeding needles with rounded tips (10 to 18 gauge) or red rubber catheters, oral specula, syringes, and sterile saline. The bird is restrained. If a rubber catheter is used, care must be taken to prevent the bird from biting the tube and swallowing the severed piece of tube. A speculum may be used or the beak may be manipulated to prevent the bird from biting the tube. The upper beak may be pushed to one side, or the upper beak may be inserted in the lower beak and held in position. The tube or feeding needle is gently passed into the left oral commissure, down the esophagus on the right side of the neck, and into the crop (see Fig. 11–9). If the beak is entered directly from the front, the bird will try to chew the tube or needle. Crop contents are aspirated into a syringe. Sterile saline can be infused and aspirated if the crop is empty or if the contents are too viscous for aspiration.

Crop aspirates and washings can be evaluated cytologically or with Gram's stain to evaluate bacterial and fungal populations. Wright's, Modified Wright's, Diff-Quik, or Hema-Tek stains are used for cell evaluation, and a wet mount can be used to look for protozoa.

Samples are stained with Gram's stain and evaluated for the presence of abnormal populations of bacteria and yeast. The sample is collected, and a swab is used to make a thin, uniform smear. The smear is air dried, fixed, and stained with Gram's stain. Crop Gram's stains from most normal birds contain mixed populations of gram-positive bacteria and occasional yeast, with or without occasional gram-negative bacteria. *Alysiella filiformis* is a coccobacillus, often associated with squamous epithelial cells in pairs or chains, that is part of the normal flora. Large numbers of gram-negative bacterial rods, a homogeneous population of bacteria, abundant yeast organisms, budding yeast (Fig. 12–20), and protozoa are abnormal. Some commercial formulated diets contain large

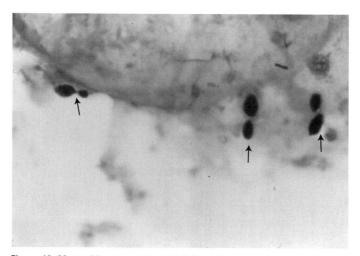

Figure 12–20. Budding yeast *(Candida)* from the crop of a cockatoo chick. Wright's stain; original magnification, 100×. See Color Figure 12–20. (Photo courtesy of Terry W. Campbell, M.S., D.V.M., Ph.D.)

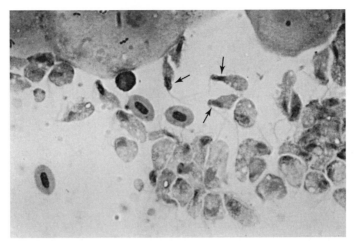

Figure 12–21. *Trichomonas* (some marked with *arrows*). Wright's stain; original magnification, 100×. (Photo courtesy of Terry W. Campbell, M.S., D.V.M., Ph.D.)

numbers of nonpathogenic nonbudding yeast. A sample of the food can be evaluated for the presence of yeast. See the sections on Gram's stain and interpretation of bacterial and fungal culture results for additional aid in interpretation of results.

Smears are stained with Wright's, Modified Wright's, Diff-Quik, or Hema-tek stains for cell evaluation. Cytologic evaluations from normal birds commonly demonstrate squamous epithelial cells, bacteria, and debris with or without occasional yeast. Inflammatory cells, bacterial phagocytosis by leukocytes, a homogeneous population of bacteria, basal cells, and protozoa are abnormal. Inflammatory cells indicate inflammation. Bacterial phagocytosis indicates primary or secondary bacterial infection. The presence of basal cells in samples indicates ulceration of the epithelium.

A wet mount is performed to look for protozoa. A fresh sample of crop contents is mixed with sterile saline and placed on a slide with a cover slip. *Trichomonas* appears as a motile, piriform protozoa with anterior flagella and an undulating membrane (Fig. 12–21).

Feather Pulp

Indications for feather pulp cytologic evaluation include feather picking, feather abnormalities, and follicular abnormalities. A smear can be made by squashing the proximal end of an affected developing feather between two slides. Abnormalities include bacteria, fungal elements, inflammatory cells, and inclusion bodies. Psittacine beak and feather disease can result in basophilic intranuclear and intracytoplasmic inclusion bodies. Intranuclear inclusion bodies may occur in epithelial cells, and intracytoplasmic inclusion bodies may occur in macrophages. Large basophilic or amphophilic intranuclear inclusion bodies can occur with polyomavirus infection. To definitively diagnose these two viral infections, DNA probe testing is recommended when inclusions are demonstrated.

Joint Aspirate

Indications for joint aspiration include joint swelling and fluid distention. The site is surgically prepped. Fluid is aspirated with a small-gauge needle and syringe. The sample is placed on a slide or cover slip and a smear is made. Normal joint fluid contains mucin and few cells. Cells can be macrophages, leukocytes, and synovial-lining cells. Mucin results in a granular background appearance. Increased numbers of leukocytes are abnormal. An increase in leukocytes may occur with septic arthritis, traumatic arthritis, or gout. Heterophils and bacteria or bacterial phagocytosis indicate septic arthritis. Erythrocytes may be present as a result of joint trauma, traumatic joint tap, or peripheral blood contamination of the sample. The presence of thrombocytes indicates peripheral blood contamination or continued hemorrhage. The presence of monosodium urate crystals is diagnostic of articular gout. When articular gout is present, aspirated fluid is cream to yellow colored. Urate crystals are needle shaped and birefringent under polarized light (Fig. 12–22).

Oral Lesion Smears

Abnormalities in the oropharynx can be aspirated, scraped, or excised to obtain a sample for cytologic examination. Cytologic evaluation from normal birds commonly demonstrate squamous epithelial cells, bacteria, and debris with or without occasional yeast. Inflammatory cells, bacterial phagocytosis by leukocytes, increased numbers of yeast, large aggregates of highly cornified squamous epithelial cells, and protozoa are abnormal. Inflammatory cells indicate

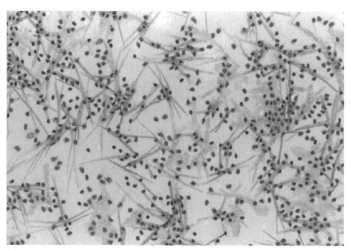

Figure 12–22. Uric acid crystals from the joint of a bird with articular gout. Wright's stain; original magnification, 20×. See Color Figure 12–22. (Photo courtesy of Terry W. Campbell, M.S., D.V.M., Ph.D.)

inflammation or infection. Bacterial phagocytosis indicates primary or secondary bacterial infection. Squamous cell hyperplasia or metaplasia as a result of vitamin A deficiency may result in aggregates or sheets of highly cornified squamous epithelial cells that stain basophilic. Secondary bacterial infection can occur as a result of vitamin A deficiency.

Sinus Aspirate/Flush

Indications for sinus aspirates include nasal discharge, swelling over the infraorbital sinus or around the eye, or other evidence of sinus abnormality. The bird is restrained with the head secure. A needle on a syringe is inserted midway between the commissure of the beak and the medial canthus of the eye (see Fig. 11–6). The needle is directed under the zygomatic arch at a 45-degree angle to the side of the head. The sinus is more easily entered if the mouth is held open. Avoid penetration of the eye. Once the sinus is entered, a sample is aspirated. Flushing of the sinus with a small amount of sterile saline may be necessary to obtain a sample in some birds. Bilateral aspiration may be necessary in birds with sinuses that do not communicate, such as passerines (e.g., canaries, finches, mynahs).

Cytologic evaluations of a normal sinus usually demonstrates few cells and no intracellular bacteria. A few extracellular bacteria and an occasional squamous epithelial cell with associated bacteria may be present in a cytologic sample from a normal infraorbital sinus. An increase in inflammatory cells indicates sinusitis (Fig. 12–23). The number and type of inflammatory cells present depends on the etiology. Bacterial phagocytosis in leukocytes indicates primary or secondary bacterial sinusitis. Secondary bacterial sinusitis may occur as a result of vitamin A deficiency, neoplasia, allergy, fungal infection, or a foreign body. Bacterial cocci in chains suggests *Streptococcus* sinusitis. Fungal elements may be identified.

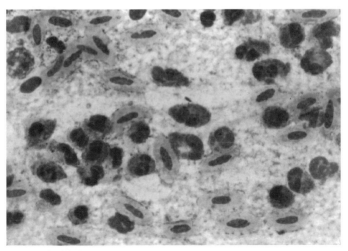

Figure 12–23. Smear from a sinus aspirate demonstrating heterophilic inflammation. Wright's stain; original magnification, 100×. See Color Figure 12–23. (Photo courtesy of Terry W. Campbell, M.S., D.V.M., Ph.D.)

Aspergillus is characterized by septate branching hyphae. Hyphae may stain poorly or basophilic with Wright's or quick stains. New methylene blue stain may be used to better visualize hyphae. Basophilic staining fungal spores or conidiophores may be seen. *Candida* is identified by the presence of many oval budding yeasts. *Cryptococcus neoformans* is an oval to round yeast with a mucopolysaccharide capsule. Yeast cells stain basophilic with Wright's or quick stains. The *Cryptococcus* capsule portion of the yeast does not stain with Wright's or quick stains but forms a clear halo around the yeast.

Intracytoplasmic inclusions in macrophages or epithelial cells may be observed with *Chlamydia* or *Mycoplasma* infection. *Chlamydia* inclusions appear as small blue or purple spherules when stained with Wright's or quick stains. *Mycoplasma* inclusions are basophilic coccoid intracytoplasmic inclusions when stained with Wright's or quick stains. Gimenez or Macchiavello's stain aid in cytologic identification of *Chlamydia* inclusions.

Large macrophages or giant cells containing phagocytized foreign material may be seen with nasal, sinus, or choanal foreign bodies. Because foreign bodies may be secondarily infected, aspirates may contain inflammatory cells and bacteria.

Aspirates may contain inflammatory cells without an etiologic agent being apparent. Culture or other diagnostic tests are used to make a diagnosis.

Skin Aspirate/Impression Smear

Indications for skin aspirates include cutaneous or subcutaneous swellings, masses, ulceration, or other suspected abnormality. Samples can be collected by aspiration or imprinting of exposed or excised lesions. Ulcerated lesions may be scraped to obtain a sample. Bacterial phagocytosis by leukocytes indicates bacterial infection and typically results in large numbers of inflammatory cells (heterophilic inflammation). Fungal elements indicate mycotic infection, which is typically associated with macrophagic inflammation. Multinucleated giant cells may be noted in fungal infections. Multinucleated giant cells and macrophages containing phagocytized debris with a mixed-cell or macrophagic inflammatory response are consistent with a foreign body or mycobacteriosis. Nonstaining bacterial rods may be observed in the background with mycobacteriosis (see tracheal wash/aspirate). Swollen squamous epithelial cells with large eosinophilic intracytoplasmic inclusion bodies are consistent with poxvirus (Fig. 12–24). Inflammatory cells may be present if secondary bacterial or fungal infection has occurred. The presence of numerous highly vacuolated macrophages, multinucleated giant cells, and cholesterol crystals is consistent with cutaneous xanthomatosis. Cholesterol crystals are angular, translucent, and variable in shape (Fig. 12–25), and may dissolve with alcohol fixatives of some stains such as Wright's and Diff-Quik. Mixed-cell inflammation, debris, feather fragments, and occasional multinucleated giant cells are consistent with feather cysts. Erythrocytes or erythrophagocytosis may occur. The presence of primarily lymphocytes is consistent with lymphoid neoplasia. Erythrophagocytosis is suggestive of a hematoma. Cells containing melanin granules on a background of rod-shaped black melanin pigment granules may occur with normal pigmentation of skin, chronic skin irritation, or melanoma formation. Smears of lipomas appear greasy before staining. Fat droplets may dissolve in alcohol-based stains such as Wright's or

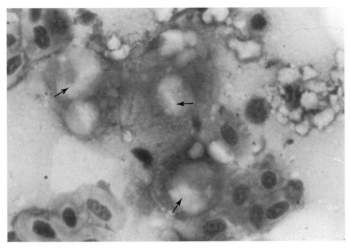

Figure 12–24. Poxvirus inclusions *(arrows)* from a flamingo chick. Wright's stain; original magnification, 100×. See Color Figure 12–24. (Photo courtesy of Terry W. Campbell, M.S., D.V.M., Ph.D.)

quick stains. Suspected lipomas may be stained with Sudan IV or new methylene blue stain to observe characteristic fat cells and lipid material.

Skin Scraping

Indications for skin scrapings include proliferative lesions with the characteristic honeycomb appearance of *Knemidokoptes* mites or flaking on the head and

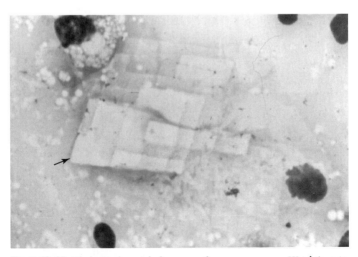

Figure 12–25. Cholesterol crystals from a xanthoma on a macaw. Wright's stain; original magnification, 100×. See Color Figure 12–25. (Photo courtesy of Terry W. Campbell, M.S., D.V.M., Ph.D.)

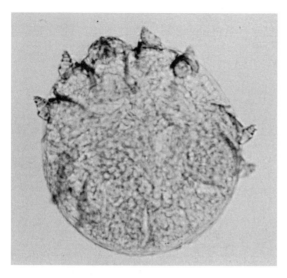

Figure 12–26. *Knemidokoptes* mite from a parakeet. (Photo courtesy of the Clinical Parasitology Laboratory, College of Veterinary Medicine, University of Tennessee, Knoxville, TN 37901.)

neck. The skin is scraped with a scalpel blade, and samples are placed in a drop of oil on a slide. *Knemidokoptes* mites are easily demonstrated (Fig. 12–26).

Tracheal Wash/Aspirate

Tracheal aspirates and washes are indicated when clinical signs of tracheal or syringeal disease are present (e.g., change in voice, coughing), when radiographic evidence of tracheal or pulmonary disease is present, or when other evidence of tracheobronchial disease is present. The bird is anesthetized, and an appropriately sized sterile rubber catheter is passed directly through the glottis or through the endotracheal tube into the distal trachea as far as possible. Sterile saline is infused into the trachea and quickly aspirated. A dose of 1.0 to 2.0 ml/kg body weight can be safely infused in most birds. An air sac breathing tube may be placed, and anesthesia can be maintained through this tube. Some birds will tolerate tracheal washes without anesthesia. A speculum is used to prevent biting of the tube and to allow visualization of the glottis. Samples can also be obtained with sterile cotton swabs passed down the trachea in larger birds or with an endoscope.

Cytologic samples from normal birds contain few cells and little background debris. Respiratory epithelial cells and goblet cells with occasional macrophages, lymphocytes, heterophils, eosinophils, and squamous epithelial cells are normal. Cornified squamous epithelial cells are contaminants from the oropharynx and may have bacteria attached. Respiratory epithelial cells are ciliated and columnar but may vary in size and shape. They occur singly or in clusters and may be identified by their eosinophilic cilia and oval nuclei (Fig. 12–27). Goblet cells exfoliate singly or in clusters. They have abundant cytoplasm with vacuoles and eosinophilic granulation. Noncornified squamous epithelial cells may be observed, originating from the syrinx.

Abnormal tracheal washes may result from bacterial, viral, or fungal infections.

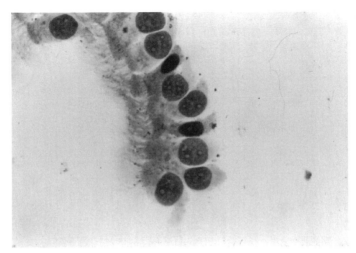

Figure 12–27. Respiratory epithelial cells. Wright's stain; original magnification, 100×. See Color Figure 12–27. (Photo courtesy of Terry W. Campbell, M.S., D.V.M., Ph.D.)

Parasite eggs (tracheal and air sac mites, gapeworms) and neoplastic cells also may be found in washes from affected birds. Tracheal washes with abundant heterophils and macrophages indicate tracheobronchitis or lower respiratory infection. An increase in the number of goblet cells and amount of mucin often occurs with tracheobronchitis, causing the background of mucin to stain purple with Wright's and quick stains. Degenerate respiratory epithelial cells with loss of cilia, cytoplasmic vacuolation, and karyolysis indicate severe tracheobronchitis.

The presence of intracellular bacteria in leukocytes indicates bacterial tracheobronchitis or pneumonia. Mononuclear leukocytes with fragmented respiratory epithelial cells in which a ciliated fragment and a nucleated fragment form are indicative of a viral infection. Abundant plasma cells and macrophages may be seen with chronic infections, although increased numbers of macrophages occur with some acute diseases such as chlamydiosis and avian mycobacteriosis. Increased numbers of macrophages and multinucleate giant cells with nonstaining bacterial rods in the background may be seen with mycobacteriosis (Fig. 12–28). Acid-fast staining can be used to identify acid-fast positive *Mycobacterium.*

Multinucleate giant cells and macrophages may also be seen with upper respiratory tract foreign bodies. These cells often contain phagocytized foreign material.

Fungal elements may be present in tracheal samples. Aspergillosis is the most common fungal infection of the avian respiratory tract, and the organism can be identified by the septate branching hyphae (Fig. 12–29). Hyphae may stain poorly or basophilic with Wright's or quick stains. New methylene blue stain may be used to visualize hyphae better. Basophilic staining conidiophores or spores may be seen when stained with Wright's or quick stains. *Mucor* hyphae are nonseptate. *Candida* is identified by the presence of many oval budding yeasts (see Fig. 12–20). Candidiasis infrequently extends into the larynx with a severe oropharyngeal infection or may occur as a systemic infection. *Cryptococ-*

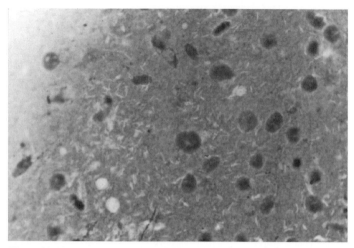

Figure 12–28. *Mycobacterium* appears as numerous nonstaining rods in the background on an impression smear from the liver of an Amazon parrot with mycobacteriosis. Wright's stain; original magnification, 100×. See Color Figure 12–28. (Photo courtesy of Terry W. Campbell, M.S., D.V.M., Ph.D.)

cus neoformans is an oval to round yeast with a mucopolysaccharide capsule. Yeast cells stain basophilic with Wright's or quick stains. The *Cryptococcus* capsule portion of the yeast does not stain with Wright's or quick stain, forming a clear halo around the yeast.

Basophilic intracytoplasmic inclusions from *Chlamydia* infection may be seen in macrophages or epithelial cells stained with Wright's or quick stains. They

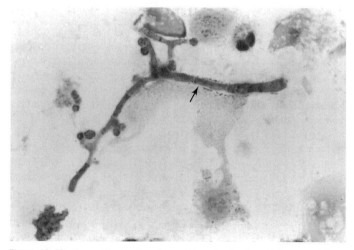

Figure 12–29. *Aspergillus* hyphae *(arrow)* in a tracheal wash from an African gray parrot. Wright's stain; original magnification, 100×. See Color Figure 12–29. (Photo courtesy of Terry W. Campbell, M.S., D.V.M., Ph.D.)

may occur in packets. Gimenez or Macchiavello's stain aids in cytologic identification of inclusions.

An increase in eosinophils and goblet cells indicates an allergic response or parasitic infection.

Malignant cells are occasionally found in cytologic samples when neoplasia involves the trachea or syrinx.

Proventricular Wash

Proventricular wash is used to obtain samples from the proventriculus. A tube may be passed blindly to the level of the proventriculus or an endoscope may be used to place a tube within the lumen of proventriculus via an ingluvotomy (see Chapter 14). A small amount of saline is infused and then aspirated. This sample is useful for cytology and culture. This procedure is most commonly used to demonstrate megabacteria in suspected cases where tests on samples from the crop or oropharynx are inconclusive.

VIRUS TESTS

Many methods are available to detect viral infections in birds. The sample needed varies with the type of virus and stage of infection. Samples from live birds may include feces, swabs, skin biopsies, feather samples, organ biopsies, plasma, serum, or blood. Samples to detect viral infection at necropsy include serum, whole blood, formalin-fixed tissues, fresh-frozen tissues, and swabs of organs. Consult the laboratory that will perform a specific viral diagnostic test for the correct method of collection and transporting the sample.

Direct techniques used for detection of a virus include isolation of the virus from a tissues or samples, demonstration of viral particles by electron microscopy, demonstration of viral antigen with viral-specific antibodies, and demonstration of viral nucleic acid with viral-specific nucleic acid probes. Indirect virus detection may be demonstrated with detection of antibodies to a particular virus. Demonstration of an increase in antibody titer in paired serum samples is necessary to differentiate an active infection from a previous infection.

URINALYSIS

Indications for urinalysis include polyuria, hematuria, abnormal kidney appearance on radiographics, and suspected renal disease. A common cause of polyuria is stress. Evaluation of stress-induced polyuria is unnecessary. Samples can be collected by placing a water-resistant material below the cage or by placing the bird in a cage with a nonporous surface (e.g., aquarium, steel cage). The liquid portion of the dropping is aspirated, avoiding gross feces and urates.

Urine characteristics that are evaluated include color, turbidity, specific gravity, chemical analysis, and microscopic evaluation of the sediment. Table 12–9 lists normal findings in avian urine. In most birds, normal urine is clear. Ratites and waterfowl may normally pass opaque, cloudy, or slightly flocculent urine. Yellow or green urine may indicate liver disease. Brown or red urine can be the result of lead toxicosis. Normal specific gravity is 1.005 to 1.020.

TABLE 12–9. Normal Urinalysis Findings

Color	Clear
Specific gravity	1.005–1.020
pH	6.0–8.0
Protein	Negative–trace
Glucose	Negative–trace
Ketones	Absent
Bilirubin	Absent
Urobilinogen	0.0–0.1
Blood	Negative–trace
Sediment	
Epithelial cells	Absent
Casts	Absent
RBCs	0–3 per high power field
WBCs	0–3 per high power field
Bacteria	Negative unless fecal contamination

Chemical analysis can be accomplished using multitest dipsticks. The pH of normal bird urine is 6.0 to 8.0. Carnivorous birds (e.g., raptors) have acidic urine, and granivorous birds (e.g., psittacines, passerines) tend to have more alkaline urine. Trace amounts of protein can be normal in bird urine. Causes of mild to moderate proteinuria include hematuria, hemoglobinuria, hyperproteinemia, and renal disease (increased glomerular permeability). False-positive protein results can occur if the urine is alkaline (most psittacines) or if the strip is soaked in urine. Trace amounts of glucose can be normal in bird urine. Increased glucose levels in the urine can occur with diabetes mellitus, egg-related peritonitis, and Fanconi's syndrome. A diagnosis of diabetes mellitus requires demonstration of elevated plasma glucose levels. Ketones are absent from normal avian urine. Catabolic processes may result in ketonuria, including diabetes mellitus and severe hepatitis. Bilirubin is normally absent from avian urine. Normal urobilinogen levels are 0.0-0.1 Ehrlich unit. Elevations may occur with intravascular hemolysis or severe liver disease. False elevations can occur as a result of some drugs (e.g., vitamin B_{12}, sulphonamides). Negative or trace amount of blood can be normal in avian urine. Sources of blood can include the cloaca or urinary, digestive, or reproductive tracts.

Examine sediment from urine relatively free of feces and urates. Normal avian urinary sediment contains no epithelial cells or casts. Renal disease may result in cast formation. Granular, cellular, and hyaline casts may be observed in avian urine. Normal urine contains 0 to 3 RBCs per high power field and 0 to 3 WBCs per high power field. Sources of elevated blood cell numbers in the urine include the cloaca or urinary, digestive, or reproductive tracts. Normal avian urine does not contain bacteria, but contamination from feces often occurs. Gram's stains or cultures of the urine and feces can be compared to determine the source of bacteria found in urine.

ANALYSIS FOR PARASITES

Methods for parasite detection include fecal flotation, fecal sedimentation, and direct smears of feces, crop contents, oropharyngeal mucous, or skin scrapings.

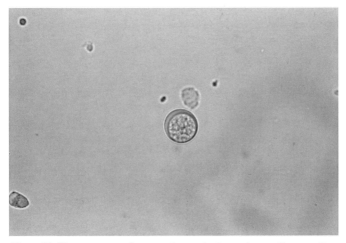

Figure 12–30. *Isospora* sp. from a Bali mynah. Original magnification, 40×. (Photo courtesy of the Clinical Parasitology Laboratory, College of Veterinary Medicine, University of Tennessee, Knoxville, TN 37901.)

Flotation of feces with supersaturated salt solutions will concentrate the eggs of some parasites, including coccidia (Figs. 12–30 and 12–31), trematodes (flukes) (Fig. 12–32), ascarids (Fig. 12–33), *Capillaria* (Fig. 12–34), spirurids *(Dispharynx, Spiroptera)* (Fig. 12–35), *Syngamus* (Fig. 12–36), and cestodes (tapeworms) (Fig. 12–37). Fecal flotations are usually negative for cestode eggs because eggs are contained in proglottids. Direct smear of fresh feces mixed with saline may allow detection of *Giardia* (Fig. 12–38). Direct smears of crop contents may

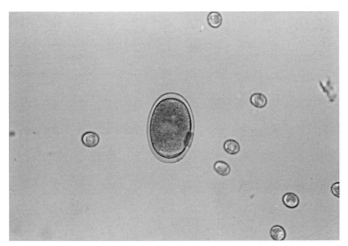

Figure 12–31. *Eimeria* sp. and *Heterakis* egg (larger single egg). Original magnification, 20×. (Photo courtesy of the Clinical Parasitology Laboratory, College of Veterinary Medicine, University of Tennessee, Knoxville, TN 37901.)

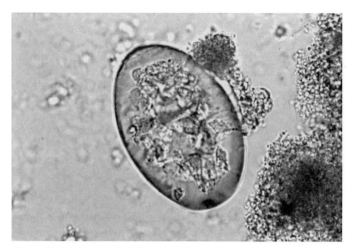

Figure 12–32. Trematode (fluke) egg. (Photo courtesy of the Clinical Parasitology Laboratory, College of Veterinary Medicine, University of Tennessee, Knoxville, TN 37901.)

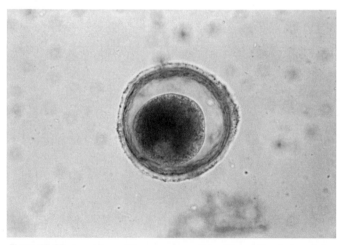

Figure 12–33. Ascarid egg. (Photo courtesy of the Clinical Parasitology Laboratory, College of Veterinary Medicine, University of Tennessee, Knoxville, TN 37901.)

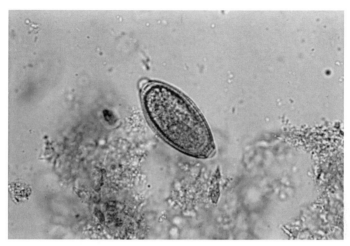

Figure 12–34. *Capillaria* egg. Original magnification, 40×. (Photo courtesy of the Clinical Parasitology Laboratory, College of Veterinary Medicine, University of Tennessee, Knoxville, TN 37901.)

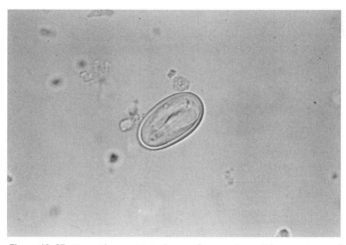

Figure 12–35. Spirurid egg. Original magnification, 40×. (Photo courtesy of the Clinical Parasitology Laboratory, College of Veterinary Medicine, University of Tennessee, Knoxville, TN 37901.)

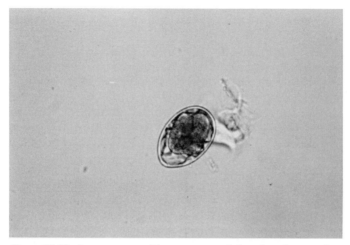

Figure 12–36. *Syngamus* egg. (Photo courtesy of the Clinical Parasitology Laboratory, College of Veterinary Medicine, University of Tennessee, Knoxville, TN 37901.)

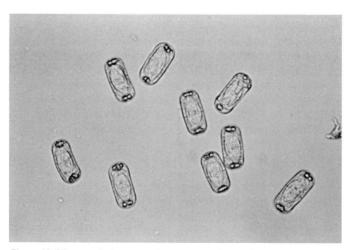

Figure 12–37. Cestode (tapeworm) eggs. Original magnification, 20×. (Photo courtesy of the Clinical Parasitology Laboratory, College of Veterinary Medicine, University of Tennessee, Knoxville, TN 37901.)

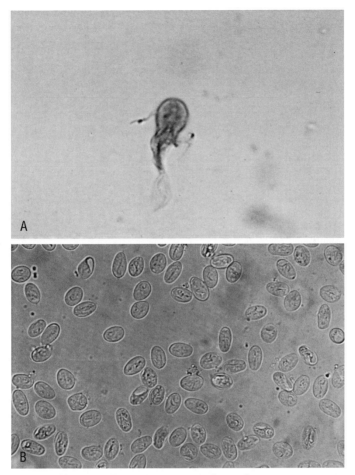

Figure 12–38. A, *Giardia* trophozoite. Original magnification, 40×. **B,** *Giardia* cysts. (Photos courtesy of the Clinical Parasitology Laboratory, College of Veterinary Medicine, University of Tennessee, Knoxville, TN 37901.)

allow detection of *Trichomonas* (see Fig. 12–21). Direct smear of oropharyngeal mucus may allow detection of *Trichomonas, Syngamus,* and tracheal mites. *Knemidokoptes* and other external mites are detected by scraping affected areas (see Fig. 12–26). The exfoliated material is mixed with a small amount of oil and examined for parasites.

Hemoparasites are discussed in the section on hematology. Treatments for parasites are discussed in Chapters 9 and 17.

AVIAN LABORATORIES

Submit samples to a laboratory experienced in the diagnosis of avian diseases. Use of an avian experienced laboratory will result in detection of diseases

TABLE 12–10. Diagnostic Laboratories With Avian Experience

Laboratory	Tests Performed
Animal Health Diagnostic Laboratory Michigan State University PO Box 30076 Lansing, MI 48909 (517) 353-1683	Biochemistries, *Chlamydia*, cytology, hematology, histopathology, microbiology, necropsy, nutritional analysis, parasitology, toxicology, virology
Antech Diagnostics 10 Executive Blvd. Farmingdale, NY 11735 (800) 872-1001	Biochemistries, *Chlamydia*, cytology, EPH, hematology, histopathology, microbiology, parasitology, virology
Antech Diagnostics 17672-A Cowan Ave. Irvine, CA 92714 (800) 745-4725	Biochemistries, *Chlamydia*, cytology, EPH, hematology, histopathology, microbiology, parasitology, virology
Avian and Exotic Animal Clin/Path Labs 3701 Inglewood Ave., Suite 106 Redondo Beach, CA 90278 (800) 350-1122	Biochemistries, *Chlamydia*, cytology, hematology, histopathology, microbiology, parasitology, toxicology, virus tests
Avian Genetic Sexing Lab 6551 Stage Oaks Dr., Suite 3A Bartlett, Tenn 38134	Genetic sexing
Avian Research Associates 100 TechneCenter Dr., Suite 101 Milford, OH 45150 (513) 248-4700	DNA testing (polyomavirus, psittacine beak and feather disease, *Chlamydia*, sexing)
Avian Wildlife Lab University of Miami Division of Comparative Pathology 1550 NW 10th Ave. Room 105 Miami, FL 33136 (800) 232-1056 (305) 547-6594	Biochemistries, *Chlamydia*, cytology, EPH, hematology, histopathology, parasitology, necropsy, virology
California Avian Laboratory 6114 Greenback Lane Citrus Heights, CA 95621 (800) 783-2473 (916) 722-8428 FAX (916) 722-8490 www.ns.net/avianlab	Biochemistries, *Chlamydia*, cytology, hematology, histopathology, microbiology, necropsy, parasitology, radiology, sexing, virus tests
Consolidated Veterinary Diagnostics 2825 Kovar Dr West Sacramento, CA 95605 (800) 444-4210	Biochemistries, *Chlamydia*, cytology, DNA sexing, EPH, hematology, histopathology, microbiology, necropsy, parasitology, toxicology, virology
Indiana Veterinary Diagnostic Lab 11837 Technology Dr. Fishers, IN 46038 (800) 955-6353 FAX (317) 579-6355	Biochemistries, *Chlamydia*, cytology, EPH, hematology, histopathology, microbiology, parasitology, toxicology, virology

TABLE 12–10. Diagnostic Laboratories With Avian Experience *(Continued)*

Laboratory	Tests Performed
Marshfield Laboratories Vet Division 1000 North Oak Ave. Marshfield, WI 54449-5795 (800) 222-5835	Biochemistries, cytology, electrophoresis, hematology, histopathology, microbiology, necropsy, parasitology, toxicology (lead)
Schubot Exotic Bird Health Center College of Veterinary Medicine Texas A&M University College Station, TX 77843-4467 (409) 845-4177	Cytology, histopathology, necropsy (including microbiology and virology on specimens submitted for necropsy)
Texas Veterinary Medical Diagnostic Laboratory PO Drawer 3040 College Station, TX 77841 (409) 845-3414	Biochemistries, *Chlamydia*, cytology, hematology, histopathology, microbiology, necropsy, parasitology, toxicology, virology
University of Minnesota Raptor Center 1920 Fitch Ave. St. Paul, MN 55708 (612) 624-4745	*Aspergillus*
Veterinary Diagnostic Laboratory Oregon State University PO Box 429 Corvallis, OR 97339-0429 (503) 737-3261	Biochemistries, *Chlamydia*, cytology, hematology, histopathology, microbiology, necropsy, parasitology, virus testing
Zoogen 1105 Kennedy Place, Suite 4 Davis, CA 95616 (800) 995-BIRD (916) 756-8089 FAX (916) 756-5143	DNA sexing

unfamiliar to many mammal laboratories. A list of some diagnostic laboratories with avian experience is found in Table 12–10. Many laboratories will provide guidance for sample collection and result interpretation.

References and Additional Reading

Aranaz A, Leibana E, Mateos A, Dominguez L. Laboratory diagnosis of avian mycobacteriosis. *Semin Avian Exot Pet Med* 1997;6(1):9–17.

Brown PA, Redig PT. Incorporating laboratory tests into diagnostic strategies. *Proc Assoc Avian Vet* 1993;41–45.

Campbell TW. Cytology in avian diagnostics. In Kirk RW (ed): *Current Veterinary Therapy IX, Small Animal Practice*. Philadelphia, WB Saunders, 1986, pp 725–731.

Campbell TW. Avian hematology and cytology. *Proc Assoc Avian Vet* 1991;357–361.

Campbell TW. Avian cytodiagnosis. *Proc ABVP Avian Specialty Core Review Course* 1993;149–157.

Campbell TW. Avian hematology and blood chemistries. *Proc ABVP Avian Specialty Core Review Course* 1993;139–148.

Campbell TW. Cytology. In Ritchie BW, Harrison GJ, Harrison LR (eds): *Avian Medicine: Principles and Application.* Lake Worth, FL, Wingers Publishing, 1994, pp 199–222.

Campbell TW. Hematology. In Ritchie BW, Harrison GJ, Harrison LR (eds): *Avian Medicine: Principles and Application.* Lake Worth, FL, Wingers Publishing, 1994, pp 176–198.

Campbell TW. *Avian Hematology and Cytology,* ed 2. Ames, IA, Iowa State University Press, 1995.

Carpenter JW, Kolmstetter CM, Bossart G, et al. Use of serum bile acids to evaluate hepatobiliary function in a cockatiel *(Nymphicus hollandicus). Proc Assoc Avian Vet* 1996;73–75.

Clipsham R. Avian pathogenic flagellated enteric protozoa. *Semin Avian Exot Pet Med* 1995;4(3):122–125.

Clipsham RC. Restraint, sample collection and surgical preparation in the avian patient. *Proc Assoc Avian Vet* 1991;331–340.

Clubb SL, Schubot RM, Joyner K, et al. Hematologic and serum biochemical reference intervals in juvenile eclectus parrots *(Eclectus roratus). J Assoc Avian Vet* 1990;4(4):218–225.

Clubb SL, Schubot RM, Wolf S. Hematologic and serum biochemical reference values for juvenile macaws, cockatoos, and eclectus parrots. In Schubot RM, Clubb SL, Clubb KJ (eds): *Psittacine Aviculture: Perspectives, Techniques and Research.* Loxahatchee, FL, Avicultural Breeding and Research Center, 1992.

Clyde VL, Patton S. Diagnosis, treatment, and control of common parasites in companion and aviary birds. *Semin Avian Exot Pet Med* 1996;5(2):75–84.

Cornelissen JM, et al. Cloacal microflora of healthy hornbills, toucans and aracaris. *Proc First Conf Europ Assoc Avian Vet* 1991;453–460.

Cray C, Bossart G, Harris D. Plasma protein electrophoresis: Principles and diagnosis of infectious disease. *Proc Assoc Avian Vet* 1995;55–59.

Cray C, Bossart G, Harris D. Plasma protein electrophoresis: An update. *Proc Assoc Avian Vet* 1996;97–100.

Degernes LA. A clinical approach to ascites in pet birds. *Proc Assoc Avian Vet* 1991;131–136.

Dein JF. *Laboratory Manual of Avian Hematology.* Orlando, FL, Association of Avian Veterinarians, 1984.

Dorrestein GM, Zwart P, Hage MH. Cytology in avian medicine. *Proc Assoc Avian Vet* 1989:274–283.

Flammer K. Serum bile acids in psittacine birds. *Proc Assoc Avian Vet* 1994;9–12.

Fudge AM. Avian hematology, identification, and interpretation. *Proc Assoc Avian Vet* 1989;284–292.

Fudge AM. How to get the most from your avian diagnostic laboratory. *J Assoc Avian Vet* 1990;4(4):208–211.

Fudge AM. Blood testing artifacts: Interpretation and prevention. *Semin Avian Exot Pet Med* 1994;3(1):2–4.

Gerlach H. Bacterial diseases. In Harrison GJ, Harrison LR (eds): *Clinical Avian Medicine and Surgery.* Philadelphia, WB Saunders, 1986, pp 434–456.

Gonzalez A, Bladow R, Cray C. Comparison of techniques for bile acid determination. *Proc Assoc Avian Vet* 1996;65–71.

Graham DL. Acute pancreatic necrosis in quaker parrots *(Myiopsitta monachus). Proc Assoc Avian Vet* 1994;87–88.

Greiner EC, Ritchie BW. Parasites. In Ritchie BW, Harrison GJ, Harrison LR (eds): *Avian Medicine: Principles and Application.* Lake Worth, FL, Wingers Publishing, 1994, pp 1005–1029.

Harrison GJ, Harrison LR (eds): *Clinical Avian Medicine and Surgery.* Philadelphia, WB Saunders, 1986.

Harrison GJ, Harrison LR. Reference values of clinical chemistry tests. In Harrison GJ, Harrison LR (eds): *Clinical Avian Medicine and Surgery.* Philadelphia, WB Saunders, 1986, pp 658–661.

Hawkey CM, Dennett TB. *Comparative Veterinary Hematology.* Ames, IA, Iowa State University Press, 1989.

Hochleithner M. Reference values for selected psittacine species using a dry chemistry system. *J Assoc Avian Vet* 1989;3(4):207–209.

Hochleithner M. Biochemistries. In Ritchie BW, Harrison GJ, Harrison LR (eds): *Avian Medicine: Principles and Application.* Lake Worth, FL, Wingers Publishing, 1994, pp 223–245.

Hoefer HL. The use of bile acids in the diagnosis of hepatobiliary disease in the parrot. *Proc Assoc Avian Vet* 1991;118–119.

Hoefer HL. Bile acid testing in psittacine birds. *Semin Avian Exot Pet Med* 1994;3(1):33–36.

Jenkins JR. Avian metabolic chemistries. *Semin Avian Exot Ped Med* 1994;3(1):25–32.

Joseph V. Laboratory diagnostics: An update of specimen collection and processing. *Proc Assoc Avian Vet* 1990;501–505.

Joyner KL. Microbiologic techniques for the avian practitioner. In Kirk RW, Bonagura JD (eds): *Current Veterinary Therapy X, Small Animal Practice.* Philadelphia, WB Saunders, 1989, pp 780–786.

Joyner KL. Practical approaches to diagnostics in avian medicine. *Proc Assoc Avian Vet* 1990;394–403.

Joyner KL. The use of Gram stain results in avian medicine. *Proc Assoc Avian Vet* 1991;78–97.

Klappenbach KM. Cerebral spinal fluid analysis in psittacines. *Proc Assoc Avian Vet* 1995;39–41.

Kossoff S, Bladow R, Luya M, Cray C. Standardization of avian diagnostics in hematology and chemistry. *Proc Assoc Avian Vet* 1996;57–63.

Lane R. Use of Gram's stain for bacterial screening. *J Assoc Avian Vet* 1990;4(4):214–217.

Lane R. Basic techniques in pet avian clinical pathology. *Vet Clin North Am* 1991;21(6):1157–1179.

Lane R. Gram's stains: Theory and practice. *Proc Assoc Avian Vet* 1991;316–320.

Lane RA. Sampling procedures: Do's and don'ts. *Proc Assoc Avian Vet* 1992;463–467.

Lane RA. Clinical techniques and diagnostics: The quality of results are directly proportional to the quality of the samples sent. *Proc Assoc Avian Vet* 1993;318–322.

Lane RA, Rosskopf WJ, Allen KL. Avian pediatric hematology: Preliminary studies of the transition from the neonatal hemogram to the adult hemogram in selected psittacine species—African greys, amazons and macaws. *Proc Assoc Avian Vet* 1988;231–238.

Lind PJ, Wolff PL, Petrini KR, et al. Morphology of the eosinophil in raptors. *Assoc Avian Vet* 1990;4(1)33–38.

Lumeij JT. Avian plasma chemistry in health and disease. *Proc Assoc Avian Vet* 1993;20–26.

Lumeij JT. Avian clinical enzymology. *Semin Avian Exot Pet Med* 1994;3(1):14–24.

Lumeij JT, Maclean B. Total protein determination in pigeon plasma and serum: Comparison of refractometric methods with the Biuret method. *J Avian Med Surg* 1996;10(3):150–152.

McCluggage D. Parasitology in caged birds. *Proc Assoc Avian Vet* 1988;98.

McCluggage DM. Basic avian medicine. *Proc Assoc Avian Vet* 1990;344–354.

Merritt E, Fritz CL, Ramsay EC. Hematologic and serum biochemical values in captive american flamingos *(Phoenicopterus ruber ruber). J Avian Med Surg* 1996;10(3):163–167.

Mitzner BT. In-house laboratory testing for the avian practice. *J Assoc Avian Vet* 1992;6(2):88–90.

Page CD, Haddad K. Coccidial infection in birds. *Semin Exot Pet Med* 1995;4(3):138–144.

Pokras MA, Zupke K. Normal exfoliative cytology of the avian cloaca. *J Assoc Avian Vet* 1991;5(2):77–82.

Powers LV. Current techniques in assessing avian coagulation. *Proc Assoc Avian Vet* 1996;109–111.

Quesenberry K. Plasma electrophoresis in psittacine birds. *Proc Assoc Avian Vet* 1991;112–117.

Rae M. Hemoprotozoa of caged and aviary birds. *Semin Avian Exot Pet Med* 1995;4(3):131–137.

Reidarson TH, McBain J. Serum protein electrophoresis and *Aspergillus* antibody titers as an aid to diagnosis of aspergillosis in penguins. *Proc Assoc Avian Vet* 1995;61–64.

Romangnano A, Sudo S, Barnes HD. Thrombocytopenia in psittacines. *Proc Assoc Avian Vet* 1994;77–81.

Rosskopf WJ, Shindo MK. The laboratory workup: Tips on convincing the client of its necessity and value. *Proc Assoc Avian Vet* 1992;468–470.

Rosskopf WJ, Woerpel RW. Pet avian hematology trends. *Proc Assoc Avian Vet* 1991;98–111.

Smith SA. Parasites of birds of prey: Their diagnosis and treatment. *Semin Avian Exot Pet Med* 1996;5(2):97–105.

Speer BL, Kass PH. The influence of travel on hematologic parameters in hyacinth macaws. *Proc Assoc Avian Vet* 1995;43–53.

Stadler CK, Carpenter JW. Parasites of backyard game birds. *Semin Avian Exot Pet Med* 1996;5(2):85–96.

VanDerHeyden N. Identification, pathogenicity and treatment of avian hematozoa. *Proc Assoc Avian Vet* 1985;163–174.

VanDerHeyden N. The hematology of nestling raptors and psittacines. *Proc Assoc Avian Vet* 1986;347–354.

VanDerHeyden N. Evaluation and interpretation of the avian hemogram. *Semin Avian Exot Pet Med* 1994;3(1):5–13.

Woerpel WW, Rosskopf WJ. Clinical experience with avian laboratory diagnostics. *Vet Clin North Am* 1984;14:254–255, 260.

Chapter 13

Imaging

Imaging techniques available include radiology, ultrasound, fluoroscopy, computed tomography (CT), and magnetic resonance imaging (MRI). Radiology is a useful and frequently used diagnostic tool in avian medicine. Ultrasound is commonly used when organomegaly is suspected or an effusion is present. Computed tomography, MRI, and fluoroscopy may be limited to referral centers, but they are useful in some cases.

TECHNIQUE

High-quality radiographs with a high degree of detail are needed to accurately interpret avian radiographic films. Short exposure times are required because of the high respiratory rates of most avian species. Short exposure times can be achieved by using a machine with high milliampere capability. The mA required varies with the type of screen. Low kilovolts (45 to 55) are recommended to provide high contrast. High-detail screen and film combinations are suggested. Screens with greater intensifying capacity are advocated to minimize exposure times (e.g., rare-earth screens). Single emulsion film combined with high-detail, rare-earth screens are recommended.

Birds are usually not measured to determine the exposure. Exposure charts must be determined based on x-ray machine capabilities and film and screen used.

POSITIONING

Whole body radiographs are commonly taken in birds. Specific areas such as the head or feet may be the center of focus for study. A minimum of two views taken at 90-degree angles is necessary for accurate radiograph interpretation. For positioning of ventrodorsal (VD) views of the body, the wings are extended laterally, the legs are extended caudally, and the carina of the sternum (keel) is perpendicular to the table. When positioned correctly, the keel is superimposed on the spine. Lateral views of the body are taken with the wings extended over the back, the legs pulled caudally, and the keel parallel to the table. The wing and leg closer to the table can be placed slightly cranial to the up limb to allow evaluation of each limb and for consistency in radiographic evaluations. When

403

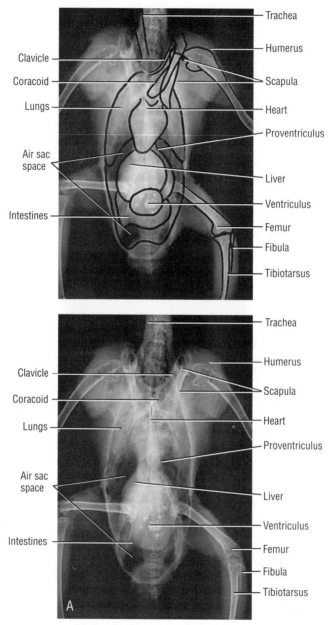

Figure 13–1. A and **B,** Radiographs of a normal Moluccan cockatoo. (Photos courtesy of Stephen Fronefield, D.V.M.)

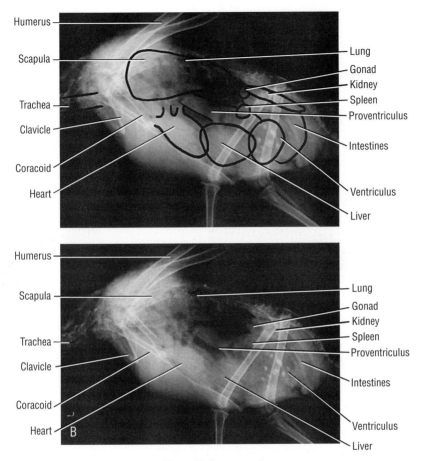

Humerus
Scapula
Trachea
Clavicle
Coracoid
Heart

Lung
Gonad
Kidney
Spleen
Proventriculus
Intestines
Ventriculus
Liver

Humerus
Scapula
Trachea
Clavicle
Coracoid
Heart

B

Lung
Gonad
Kidney
Spleen
Proventriculus
Intestines
Ventriculus
Liver

Figure 13–1 *Continued*

positioned correctly, the acetabuli are superimposed. Radiographs of the head usually require anesthesia and additional views (lateral, VD, dorsoventral [DV], rostral, and obliques). Figure 13–1 shows radiographs of a normal cockatoo.

A horizontal radiograph may be taken on a standing bird that is in critical condition when routine radiography is deemed too risky. Celomic fluid, air sac and lung lesions, and heavy metal densities in the gastrointestinal tract may be noted. Other structures are difficult to evaluate in this position. Scans for heavy metal densities in the ventriculus may be taken with the bird standing on the cassette when restraint is risky (Fig. 13–2).

Birds may be held in position with tape or a mechanical restraint device. Birds may be taped to a thin acrylic sheet or a piece of clear developed x-ray film. Part the wing feathers before taping. Fold the ends of the tape so it can be quickly removed. When securing a bird in a mechanical restraint device, restrain the head first, the wings next, and the legs last. Several commercial restraint

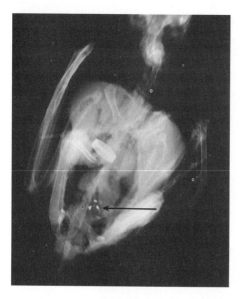

Figure 13–2. Heavy metal densities (three) in the ventriculus in a bare-eyed cockatoo standing on the cassette. (Photo courtesy of Stephen Fronefield, D.V.M.)

devices are available.* If birds are manually restrained, the restrainer should not be exposed to the primary beam, even when covered with protective clothing.

Anesthesia is often used to prevent injury to the bird and to decrease personnel exposure to radiation. Birds should be evaluated before administration of anesthesia (see Chapter 14).

INTERPRETATION

Develop a routine for examining radiographs and consistently follow the routine. Two approaches are commonly used: concentric circles and organ systems. Routine use of both approaches is recommended. With the concentric circles system, the film is examined using concentric circles until the middle of the film is reached. With the systems approach, the film is examined by organ systems (e.g., respiratory—sinuses, trachea, air sacs, lungs, pneumatized bones). Study the entire radiograph, not just the lesion.

RESPIRATORY SYSTEM

Normal sinuses are clear and symmetrical. Soft tissue opacity within the sinus without bone destruction may occur with vitamin A deficiency or bacterial infection. Soft tissue density with osteolysis is commonly the result of aspergillo-

---

*Henry Schein Inc., Port Washington, NY 11050 (800) 443-2756; Veterinary Specialty Products Inc., Boca Raton, FL 33481 (800) 362-8138.

sis or mycobacteriosis, but it may be the result of other bacterial infection (abscess, osteomyelitis), neoplasia, or foreign body.

The normal trachea courses down the right side of the neck and is free of soft tissue or fluid densities. Tracheal rings may ossify in older birds. The trachea of mynahs and toucans deviates ventrally at the thoracic inlet. Narrowing of the lumen may occur with extrinsic or intrinsic masses or strictures. Intraluminal masses may be the result of aspergillosis, foreign bodies, bacteria, vitamin A deficiency, parasites, or neoplasia.

The normal syrinx is difficult to visualize and can best be evaluated on lateral radiographs. It is located between the second and third thoracic vertebrae in most birds. An increased radiodensity indicates pathology; however, care must be taken in interpreting this sign because of superimposition of the coracoid, cranial cardiac vessels, and pectoral muscles. Increased radiodensity is commonly the result of granuloma formation (e.g., aspergillosis, vitamin A deficiency) or foreign body (e.g., aspirated food or granuloma).

Radiographs of normal lung have a prominent reticular or honeycombed pattern appearance. Terminology used in mammalian radiography, such as alveolar and interstitial patterns, does not apply to avian radiology because of differences in anatomy. Atelectasis does not occur. The cranial portions of the lungs are often opacified by the pectoral muscles. A blotchy appearance may be the result of infiltration around parabronchi. Obliteration of the reticular pattern may be the result of pulmonary consolidation from exudates, edema, blood, abscesses, or granulomas (Fig. 13–3). Focal increased radiodensities are commonly the result of aspergillosis or abscesses. Diffuse homogeneous increased radiodensities are often the result of bacterial pneumonia. An increase in the reticular pattern may be the result of pneumonia.

Normal air sac spaces should have slightly more density than does the background. Generalized nonhomogeneous opaqueness of the abdominal or thoracic air sac spaces indicates airsacculitis and is often the result of chlamydiosis or aspergillosis (Figs. 13–4 and 13–5). Generalized homogeneous opaqueness of the caudal thoracic and abdominal air sac spaces is commonly the result of ascites or peritonitis (Figs. 13–6 and 13–7). Focal densities of the abdominal or thoracic air sacs are commonly the result of aspergillosis (see Fig. 13–3) or mycobacteriosis, but they may be the result of yolks or eggs free in the abdomen or a mass (tumor). Normal air sac membranes or walls cannot be visualized radiographically. Thickened air sac membranes of the caudal thoracic and abdominal air sacs indicate chronic airsacculitis and are commonly the result of aspergillosis or chlamydiosis, but other etiologies include bacterial, parasitic, or other fungal infection (Fig. 13–8). Overinflation of the abdominal air sacs indicates obstruction of air flow through the upper respiratory tract. End-on vessels anterior to the heart should not be confused with lung or air sac densities.

Normal pneumatized bones should show a radiolucent region. Densities within the pneumatic area are often *Aspergillus* or mycobacterial granulomas.

GASTROINTESTINAL SYSTEM

Plain radiography may reveal abnormal densities, organomegaly, or changes in locations of organs. Single or double contrast studies are often helpful to further

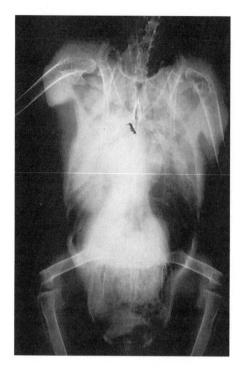

Figure 13–3. Pulmonary consolidation of the right lung and right thoracic and abdominal air sacs. (Photo courtesy of Connie Orcutt, D.V.M., A.B.V.P.-Avian.)

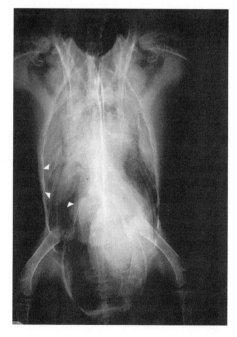

Figure 13–4. Airsacculitis *(arrowheads)* in an African gray parrot. (Photo courtesy of Connie Orcutt, D.V.M., A.B.V.P.-Avian.)

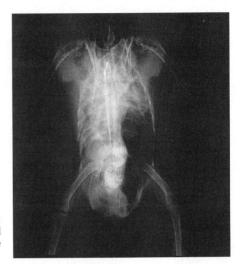

Figure 13–5. Severe airsacculitis in an African gray parrot involving the right thoracic and abdominal air sacs. (Photo courtesy of Connie Orcutt, D.V.M., A.B.V.P.-Avian.)

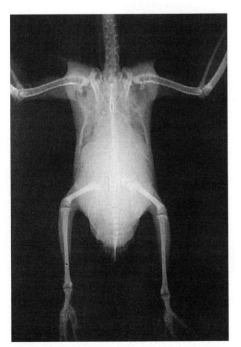

Figure 13–6. Ascites in a cockatiel. A renal adenocarcinoma was identified on necropsy. Polyostotic hyperostosis is also present. (Photo courtesy of Connie Orcutt, D.V.M., A.B.V.P.-Avian.)

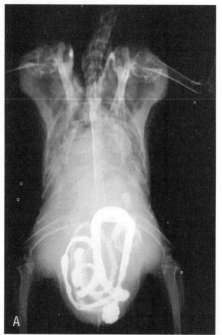

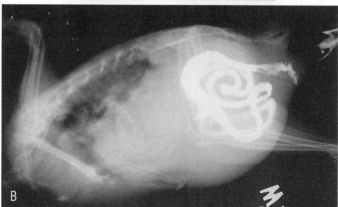

Figure 13–7. A and **B,** Cardiomegaly and ascites in an Indian Hill mynah (gastrointestinal barium series). (Photo courtesy of Connie Orcutt, D.V.M., A.B.V.P.-Avian.)

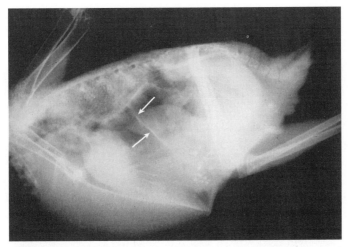

Figure 13–8. Thickened contiguous membrane of the caudal thoracic and abdominal air sac *(arrows)*. This is commonly the result of aspergillosis or chlamydiosis, but other etiologies include bacterial, parasitic, or other fungal infection. (Photos courtesy of Connie Orcutt, D.V.M., A.B.V.P.-Avian.)

identify the source of a mass, dislocations, or wall thickness. Contrast studies are discussed in the section on Special Procedures.

The crop is located at the thoracic inlet, but it is usually not visible radiographically unless it contains food or other material. Food in the crop usually appears as a soft tissue density. Focal crop densities may be the result of granulomas, foreign bodies, or ingluvioliths (crop stones). Gas in the crop may be the result of gas anesthesia, dyspnea, tube feeding, or a penetrating wound or crop burn infected with a gas-producing organism. Crop distention may be the result of infection, impaction, or obstruction (crop, proventricular, ventricular, intestinal). Pigeons normally have large crops.

The cervical esophagus is usually not visible radiographically. The thoracic esophagus can be visualized dorsal to the heart on lateral views.

The size and shape of the proventriculus varies among species and age of the bird. The proventriculus is more readily observed on lateral views and typically appears as an elliptical or funnel-shaped density dorsal to the liver and cranial to the ventriculus. The proventriculus may be indistinguishable from the left lateral liver on VD views on plain films (Fig. 13–9). Contrast radiography can be used to distinguish the proventriculus from the liver when an enlargement is noted in this area (Fig. 13–10). The proventriculus in hand-fed young psittacines is large and can be normally enlarged until 1 year of age. Air in the proventriculus (Fig. 13–11) can be the result of dyspnea, tube feeding, gas anesthesia, or proventricular dilatation syndrome (PDS). Distention of the proventriculus can be the result of PDS, impaction, ileus, foreign body, neoplasia, infection, or intestinal obstruction (see Fig. 13–10). Radiographic signs of proventricular dilatation syndrome include distended proventriculus, air in the proventriculus, and dilated isthmus (loss of narrowing at the ventriculus or proventriculus junction). The ventriculus and intestines may also be distended. An enlarged

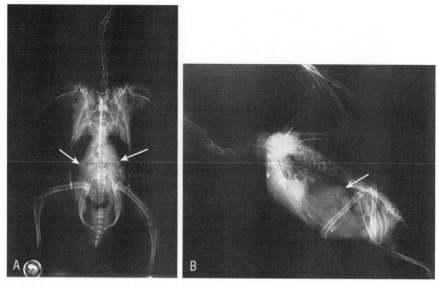

Figure 13–9. A and **B,** Enlarged proventricular/hepatic silhouette *(arrows)* in a Moluccan cockatoo. (Photos courtesy of Stephen Fronefield, D.V.M.)

proventriculus may distend caudal to the ventriculus. Radiographic signs are not pathognomonic for PDS; definitive diagnosis requires biopsy. Proventricular dilatation syndrome can be present without radiographic signs. Dilatation of the proventriculus may occur without PDS infection (e.g., lead toxicosis). Dorsal displacement of the proventriculus may occur with hepatomegaly. Cranial dis-

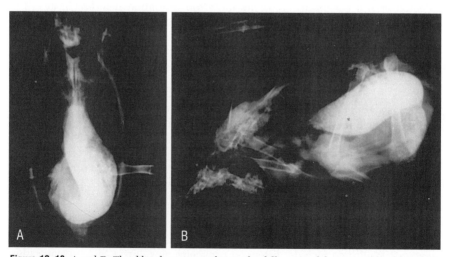

Figure 13–10. A and **B,** The dilated proventriculus can be differentiated from an enlarged liver with a gastrointestinal barium series. This macaw with a distended proventriculus was diagnosed with PDS on necropsy. (Photos courtesy of Connie Orcutt, D.V.M., A.B.V.P.-Avian.)

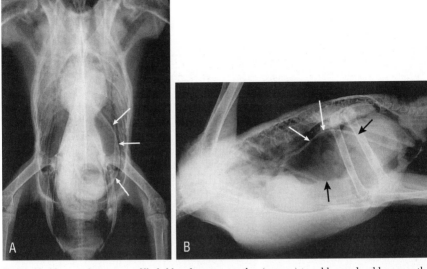

Figure 13–11. **A** and **B,** An air-filled dilated proventriculus *(arrows)* in a blue and gold macaw that was diagnosed with PDS on necropsy. (Photos courtesy of Connie Orcutt, D.V.M., A.B.V.P.-Avian.)

placement of the proventriculus may occur with enlargement of the ventriculus, intestines, or oviduct or with other abdominal masses.

The ventriculus may be visualized as a large oval density in the left caudal abdomen on VD views. The ventriculus is normally at the level of the acetabula and slightly to the left of midline on VD views. On lateral views it is normally located caudal and ventral to the proventriculus. It often contains grit, allowing identification of its location. Ingested heavy metal particles are often retained in the ventriculus, providing prolonged exposure to toxins. Heavy metal (e.g., lead, zinc) densities are usually easily differentiated from grit and stones that are often found in normal birds (Figs. 13–12 and 13–13). If heavy metal densities are noted radiographically, a blood sample should be collected and submitted for lead and zinc levels (see Chapter 9). Chelation therapy should be administered while waiting for these results if clinical signs are present. Dilatation of the ventriculus can occur with impaction, PDS, or intestinal obstruction. Displacement of the ventriculus may indicate organomegaly elsewhere in the abdomen or an egg. Dorsocranial or caudal displacement of the ventriculus may result from hepatomegaly. Ventrocranial or caudal displacement of the ventriculus may result from splenomegaly or enlargement of the kidneys or gonads. Ventrocaudal displacement indicates dilatation of the proventriculus. Ventrocranial displacement indicates dilatation of the intestines or an egg in the oviduct.

Normal intestines usually appear as a mass of mixed density dorsal to the ventriculus on lateral views and between the ventriculus and right abdominal air sac on VD views. Normal intestines do not contain air. Gas in the intestines can occur as a result of bacterial enteritis (most commonly), dyspnea, tube feeding, gas anesthesia, PDS, ileus, or a heavy infestation of intestinal worms. Fluid distention of the intestines is normal in mynahs and toucans, but it is pathologic

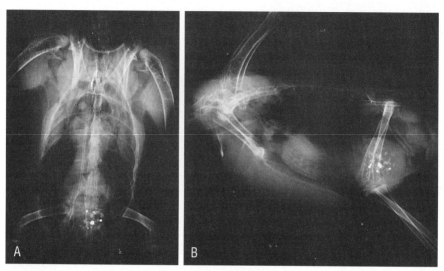

Figure 13–12. **A** and **B,** Heavy metal densities in the ventriculus of a vasa parrot. The heavy metal densities are the five radiopaque particles. Grit is also present in the ventriculus. (Photos courtesy of Taffi Tippit, D.V.M.)

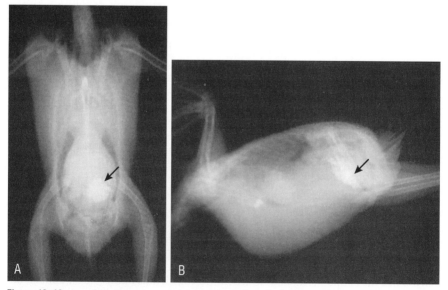

Figure 13–13. **A** and **B,** Excessive grit in the ventriculus of a budgie. (Photos courtesy of Connie Orcutt, D.V.M., A.B.V.P.-Avian.)

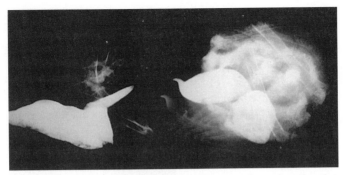

Figure 13–14. Increased intestinal wall thickness is demonstrated with a gastrointestinal barium contrast study in this Amazon parrot that was diagnosed by biopsy as having mycobacteriosis. (Photo courtesy of Connie Orcutt, D.V.M., A.B.V.P.-Avian.)

in most other birds and may occur with ileus or an obstruction. Ileus may occur as a result of viral or bacterial infections, heavy metal toxicosis (lead, zinc), septicemia, hypoxemia, peritonitis, or anesthesia. Thickening of the wall of the intestines is commonly the result of *Mycobacteria* infection (Fig. 13–14). Ventral displacement of the intestines may be the result of kidney, ovarian, testicular, or splenic masses, and the intestines may also be displaced cranially or caudally. Peritonitis may result in adhesions and intestinal displacement.

The normal cloaca may or may not be visible. If visible it appears as an oval density in the caudal coelom. Distention of the cloaca may occur as a result of papillomas, cloacaliths, neoplasia, idiopathic atonic dilatation, or an egg. A double contrast study of the cloaca can be used to better visualize the cloaca.

LIVER

The liver shadow joins the heart shadow cranially and ventriculus shadow caudally on lateral views. On VD views, the cranial liver is contrasted with the air sacs and the caudal liver shadow blends with the ventriculus and intestines. The cranial margin of the liver contacts the caudal heart. The superimposed shadow produces an hourglass-shaped shadow referred to as the cardiohepatic silhouette. The proventriculus may be indistinguishable from the left lateral liver on VD views on plain films. Contrast radiography can be used to distinguish the proventriculus from the liver when an enlargement is noted in this area. When properly positioned, the normal psittacine liver should not extend beyond a line connecting the lateral coracoid and acetabulum on VD views (Fig. 13–15). On lateral views, the dorsal border of the normal liver should not extend above the level of the base of the heart and does not extend beyond the sternum. Radiographic signs of hepatomegaly on the VD view include loss of the hourglass silhouette, extension of the liver beyond the coracoid/acetabulum line, cranial displacement of the heart, and compression of the abdominal air sacs (Figs. 13–16 and 13–17). On the lateral view, radiographic signs of hepatomegaly include extension of the liver beyond the sternum or dorsal to the level of the

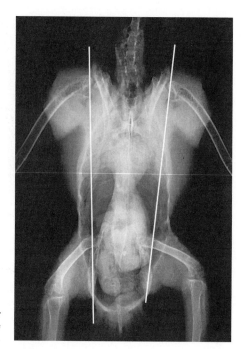

Figure 13–15. The normal psittacine liver should not extend beyond a line connecting the lateral coracoid and acetabulum on VD views.

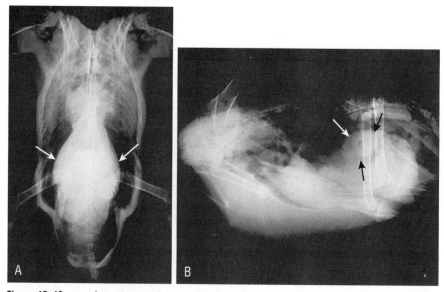

Figure 13–16. **A** and **B,** Hepatosplenomegaly in a macaw with chlamydiosis. The margins of the liver are marked with *white arrows* and the spleen is marked with *black arrows*. (Photos courtesy of Connie Orcutt, D.V.M., A.B.V.P.-Avian.)

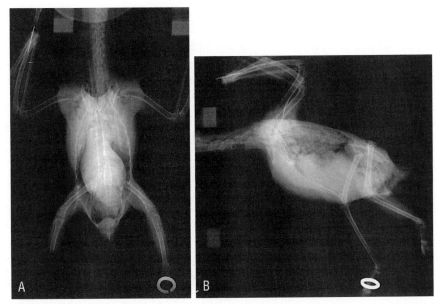

Figure 13–17. A and **B,** Hepatomegaly in an African gray parrot as a result of *Sarcocystis* infection. (Photos courtesy of Stephen Fronefield, D.V.M.)

base of the heart, cranial displacement of the heart, dorsal displacement of the proventriculus, caudodorsal displacement of the ventriculus, compression of the abdominal air sacs, and rounding of the liver lobes. Hepatomegaly may be the result of infectious disease (chlamydial, viral, bacterial, mycobacterial, fungal, parasitic), metabolic disease (hepatic lipidosis, hemochromatosis, amyloidosis, gout), neoplastic disease (primary, metastatic), toxicosis, or cardiac disease. Hepatomegaly with decreased hepatic radiopacity is suggestive of hepatic lipidosis. A decrease in liver size is commonly the result of fibrosis. Irregular borders of the liver are abnormal and are usually the result of granuloma formation, hepatic lipidosis, or neoplasia. Neonates have relatively large livers. Raptors often have comparatively small hepatic silhouettes. Pigeons normally have wide hepatic silhouettes.

SPLEEN

The spleen is located dorsal to the junction of the proventriculus and ventriculus on lateral views. On VD views, the spleen is typically oval or round and on the right side between the proventriculus and ventriculus. Splenomegaly should be suspected when the spleen appears larger than normal (see Fig. 13–16). Some normal sizes include budgie, 1 mm; Amazon and African gray parrots, 6 mm; and umbrella cockatoos, 8 mm. Splenomegaly may be the result of infectious (chlamydial, bacterial, mycobacterial, viral), metabolic (lipidosis, hemochromatosis), or neoplastic diseases.

URINARY SYSTEM

The kidneys lie ventral to the ileum and synsacrum. On lateral views, the cranial divisions extend into the radiolucent air sacs. The kidneys are superimposed with the gastrointestinal tract on VD views. There is an air space of the abdominal air sac between the kidneys and synsacrum in normal birds. Loss of the air space can be the result of renomegaly, dorsal displacement of abdominal organs, or the presence of abdominal fluid or fat. Renomegaly may be noted radiographically by an enlarged kidney shadow or loss of the dorsal air space (Fig. 13–18). Care must be taken to differentiate kidneys from gonads, which are anterioventral to the cranial division of the kidneys. Renomegaly may be the result of infection (bacterial, chlamydial), metabolic disease (vitamin A deficiency, gout, lipidosis), dehydration, postrenal obstruction, or neoplasia. Irregular borders are commonly the result of neoplasia or abscesses. An increase in density of the kidneys can occur as a result of dehydration, gout, or calcification (Fig. 13–19).

REPRODUCTIVE SYSTEM

The radiographic appearance of the reproductive organs varies with the sex and reproductive state of the bird. During the nonbreeding season, the gonads will be small. Testicles may or may not be visible ventral and cranial to the cranial division of the kidneys. The ovary and oviduct are typically not visible during the nonbreeding season. During breeding season, gonads increase in size. Testicles can normally become massive and should not be mistaken for abnormal. The ovary and oviduct enlarge and fill the dorsal coelom from the lungs to the caudal body wall. Individual follicles may be distinguishable. An enlarged ovary and oviduct may fill the coelom so that abdominal structures may not be

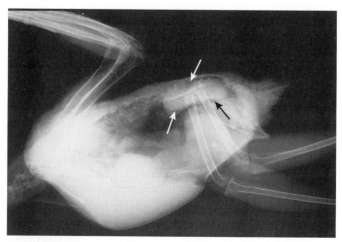

Figure 13–18. Renomegaly *(arrows)* in a Goffin's cockatoo. (Photo courtesy of Connie Orcutt, D.V.M., A.B.V.P.-Avian.)

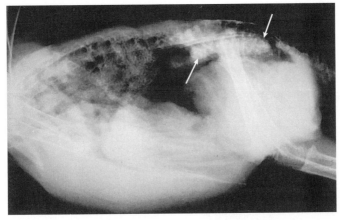

Figure 13–19. Increased opacity of the kidneys *(arrows)* in an African gray parrot. (Photo courtesy of Connie Orcutt, D.V.M., A.B.V.P.-Avian.)

identifiable (Fig. 13–20). Calcified eggs may be identified in the oviduct or free in the abdomen (Figs. 13–20 and 13–21). Soft-shelled eggs are difficult to distinguish from other soft tissue densities (see Fig. 13–20). Increased medullary density (polyostotic hyperostosis) may occur in the long bones with reproductive activity in female birds (Fig. 13–22). Ultrasound is useful to further evaluate reproductive abnormalities.

CARDIOVASCULAR SYSTEM

The heart forms the cranial portion of the cardiohepatic hourglass-shaped silhouette on VD views and contacts the sternum on lateral views. The heart is best evaluated in conjunction with ultrasound examination. An electrocardiogram is required to observe electrical abnormalities. Heart disease may be noted radiographically as an enlarged cardiac silhouette, a change in shape of the cardiac silhouette, change in the cardiohepatic hourglass-shaped silhouette, enlarged systemic or pulmonary vessels, or enlargement of the shadow of the left atrium (Figs. 13–7 and 13–23). Cardiomegaly may be the result of infectious diseases (viral, bacterial), hemochromatosis, valvular degeneration, chronic anemia, or heart defects. Microcardia occurs as a result of hypovolemia (acute volume loss or endotoxemia). Vascular calcification may occur in older psittacines.

MUSCULOSKELETAL SYSTEM

Examine the skeleton for fractures, thinning of the cortices, endosteal filling, osteolytic lesions, and sclerosis. Acute fractures appear radiographically as distinct sharp edges of bone fragments and soft tissue swelling at the fracture site (Fig. 13–24, A–C). Chronic fractures show endosteal filling and indistinct fracture fragments. Healing occurs primarily by endosteal callus with minimal perios-

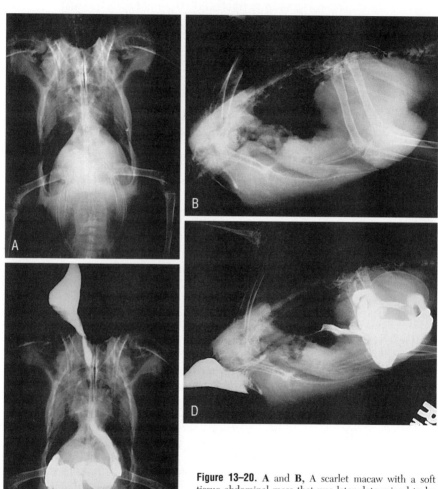

Figure 13–20. **A** and **B,** A scarlet macaw with a soft tissue abdominal mass that was later determined to be an egg before calcification. **C** and **D,** A gastrointestinal barium series demonstrating the now partially calcified egg. (Photos courtesy of Connie Orcutt, D.V.M., A.B.V.P.-Avian.)

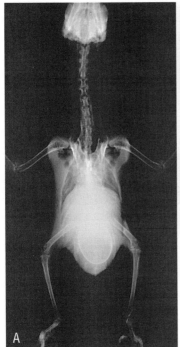

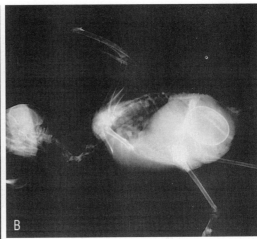

Figure 13–21. A and **B,** Egg binding in an Amazon parrot. (Photos courtesy of Connie Orcutt, D.V.M., A.B.V.P.-Avian.)

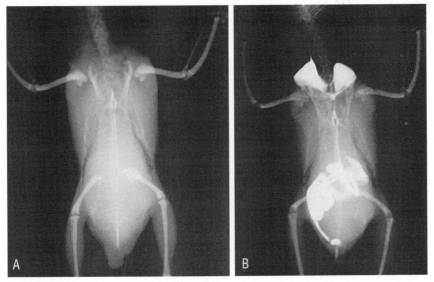

Figure 13–22. A and **B,** Polyostotic hyperostosis and soft tissue abdominal mass in a budgie. (Photo courtesy of Connie Orcutt, D.V.M., A.B.V.P.-Avian.)

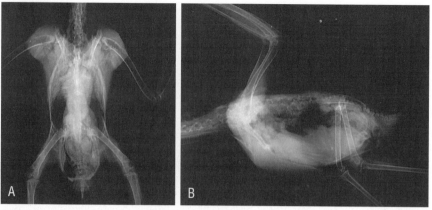

Figure 13–23. **A** and **B,** Cardiomegaly in a cockatoo. (Photos courtesy of Stephen Fronefield, D.V.M.)

teal response. Healing is indicated radiographically by development of an endosteal callus and elimination of the radiolucent fracture line (Fig. 13–24, D). The most common site of spinal fractures is the neck and just cranial to the synsacrum (pelvis). Fractures are discussed more extensively in Chapter 7.

Decreased skeletal density, bending of the long bones, or pathological fractures indicate metabolic bone disease (Fig. 13–25). Normal avian long bones typically have thin cortices, faint trabecular patterns, and relatively less calcium than mammals, so care should be taken when evaluating the skeletal opacity.

Focal increased medullary densities within pneumatic areas of bones are often *Aspergillus* or mycobacterial granulomas. A periosteal response is common.

Focal osteolytic disease may be the result of mycobacteriosis, bacterial osteomyelitis, or neoplasia. Mycobacteriosis typically causes multiple punctate areas of osteolysis surrounded by a thin rim of sclerotic bone. A single area of punctate radiolucency of bone may occur with mycobacteriosis. Chronic osteomyelitis may result in sclerotic lesions with thickened cortex that will persist and not return to normal after infection is resolved. Primary tumors of bone are rare and tend to cause bone destruction with little or no periosteal response. Severe osteolysis of the joint indicates septic arthritis. A narrowed joint cavity, subchondral sclerosis, periosteal reactions, and soft tissue swelling indicate primary arthritis. Severe osteolysis, soft tissue swelling, and a sharp zone of demarcation between affected and normal bone commonly indicate neoplasia. Biopsy is required to distinguish neoplasia from infectious processes.

Increased medullary density of the long bones occurs as a result of high estrogen levels (polyostotic hyperostosis) (see Fig. 13–22). The densities can be diffuse or mottled. Polyostotic hyperostosis can be normal in laying hens or occur as a result of ovarian cysts, ovarian tumors, oviductal tumors, sertoli cell tumors, and abdominal hernias.

FAT

Abdominal fat appears as a nonhomogeneous celomic density and can result in loss of serosal detail. Pigeons normally have increased abdominal fat.

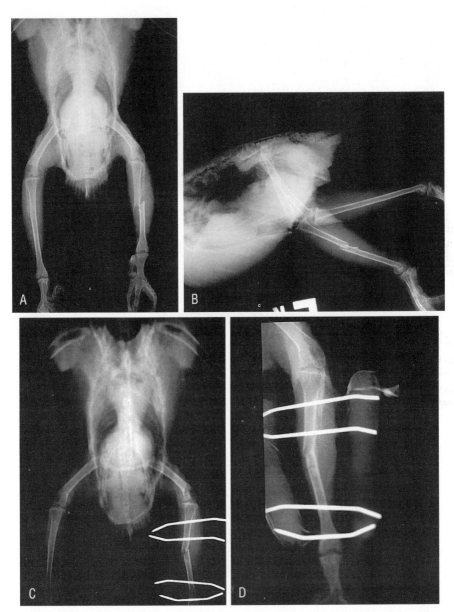

Figure 13–24. A and **B,** An acute tibiotarsal fracture in a cockatoo demonstrating distinct sharp edges of bone fragments and soft tissue swelling. **C,** Postsurgical radiograph. **D,** Healed fracture, 6 weeks after surgical repair. (Photo courtesy of Connie Orcutt, D.V.M., A.B.V.P.-Avian.)

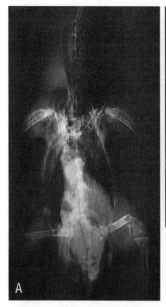

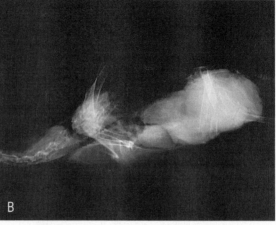

Figure 13–25. **A** and **B,** Metabolic bone disease, with decreased skeletal density and fractures of both femurs in a Moluccan cockatoo. (Photos courtesy of Taffi Tippit, D.V.M.)

SPECIAL PROCEDURES

Barium Series

Single- or double-contrast studies of the gastrointestinal tract may be performed. Contrast studies are performed for the examination of an organ's size, shape, or position; to delineate an organ from other organs; to examine the thickness and condition of the wall of hollow organs; and to evaluate the function of an organ. Single-contrast studies are most commonly used. Double-contrast studies better demonstrate the thickness and condition of the walls of the gastrointestinal tract.

Anesthesia is not recommended because it can result in aspiration of barium that may leak from the crop into the oropharynx and may decrease gastrointestinal motility.

Plain radiographs should always be taken before contrast administration to note abnormalities and to visualize heavy metal particles in the gastrointestinal tract that may be obscured by contrast agents. Dehydrated birds are rehydrated before contrast radiography. The bird is fasted for 2 to 4 hours before barium administration. If present, excessive fluid in the crop should be aspirated before contrast administration. For single-contrast studies, a 25% to 45% barium sulfate solution is administered directly into the crop or esophagus at a rate of 20 ml/kg of bodyweight, similar to tube feeding (see Chapter 11). Pressure applied to the proximal esophagus and slow withdrawal of the tube discourages barium reflux into the oropharynx. The contrast fluid is warmed before administration to young birds. Regurgitation and aspiration of barium sulfate may result in dyspnea if large amounts are aspirated. Small amounts usually do not result in clinical problems. Barium sulfate should not be administered when perforation of the gastrointestinal tract is suspected.

For double-contrast studies, 10 to 20 ml/kg of air is infused into the crop and is followed by a 25% barium sulfate solution at a rate of 10 ml/kg of bodyweight while digital pressure is applied to the proximal esophagus. The crop is gently massaged to milk the barium/air mixture into the more distal gastrointestinal tract while continued pressure is applied to the proximal esophagus.

Radiographs are usually taken immediately after contrast administration and at 30 minutes, 1, 2, 4, 8, and 24 hours after contrast administration. Times are adjusted based on findings and type of bird. In general, the crop should be empty by 4 hours in psittacines. Some normal transit times are listed in Table 13–1.

Normal transit times vary with the size and species of the bird. Decreased transit times may occur with gastroenteritis or stress, small birds, or in birds on a soft diet, or that are cachectic. Prolonged transit times may occur with anesthesia and in obese birds, large birds on a seed diet, hand-fed birds, and birds with large amounts of food in the proventriculus. Pathologic causes of prolonged transit times include obstruction (foreign body, extraluminal or intraluminal masses, strictures, massive worm infestation), ileus (viral or bacterial infections, lead or zinc toxicosis, septicemia, hypoxemia, peritonitis, neoplasia, anesthesia), and dilatation (PDS, *Candida* infection). Intraluminal masses (granulomas, intussusception, papilloma, abscess, granuloma, tumor) will cause filling defects. Thickening of the wall of the digestive tract may occur with chronic infectious processes (bacterial, mycobacterial, fungal, parasitic), neoplasia, or vitamin A deficiency (see Fig. 13–14). Mycobacteriosis is a common cause of thickening of the intestinal walls. Proventricular dilatation can easily be differentiated from hepatomegaly with contrast radiography (see Fig. 13–10). Abdominal hernias are readily identified with gastrointestinal barium studies (Fig. 13–26).

Radiographic abnormalities should be present on more than one film (i.e., be repeatable) before making a diagnosis.

TABLE 13–1 Some Normal Barium Sulfate Transit Times*

	Stomach	Small Intestines	Large Intestines	Cloaca
African gray parrot	10–30	30–60	60–120	120–130
Budgerigar	5–30	30–60	60–120	120–240
Racing pigeon	5–10	10–30	30–120	120–240
Indian Hill mynah	5	10–15	15–30	30–90
Hawk	5–15	15–30	30–90	90–360
Amazon parrot	10–60	60–120	120–150	150–240
Canary	5	10–15	15–30	30–90
Pheasant	10–45	45–120	120–150	150–240

Courtesy of McMillan MC. Imaging techniques. In Ritchie BW, Harrison GJ, Harrison LR (eds): *Avian Medicine: Principles and Application.* Lake Worth, FL, Wingers Publishing, 1994, p 258. Used by permission.
*Time in minutes for barium sulfate administered by crop gavage to reach and fill various portions of the gastrointestinal tract.

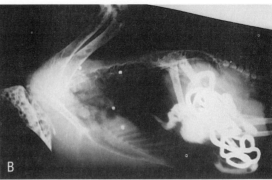

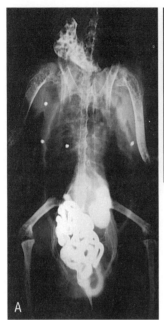

Figure 13–26. A and B, Gastrointestinal barium study demonstrating an abdominal hernia in a scarlet macaw. (Photos courtesy of Stephen Fronefield, D.V.M.)

Other Contrast Studies

Double-contrast studies of the cloaca can be performed to outline the cloacal mucosa. A 25% barium sulfate solution is administered retrograde into the cloaca at a rate of 10 ml/kg of bodyweight, and this is immediately followed by 10 to 20 ml/kg of air while digital pressure is applied to the vent. Filling defects may be the result of papillomas, ulcerations, tumors, cloacaliths, or air.

Contrast urography, rhinosinography, and angiocardiography have been used in avian medicine. Intravenous excretory urography is useful to delineate the size and shape of the kidneys if they cannot be adequately visualized with routine radiography. Positive contrast rhinosinography is useful for evaluation of the nasal cavity and infraorbital sinuses. Angiocardiography is useful for evaluation of the heart for enlargement, shunts, and valvular disease. Consult McMillan (1994) for further information.

Ultrasonography

Ultrasonography is usually performed without anesthesia. The feathers are parted and a water-soluble acoustic gel is used. Ascites allows better visualization of many organs. Peritonitis results in a heterogeneic hyperechoic appearance in the coelomic cavity. Effusions as a result of other causes is often anechoic or hypoechoic.

The liver is examined from a ventromedial approach (transducer placed just caudal to the sternum) with the beam angled cranially. The normal liver is homogeneous, delicately granular, and of average echogenicity, containing anechoic channels of blood vessels. Hepatomegaly may be present if the liver extends beyond the caudal edge of the sternum. Increased echogenicity and hepatomegaly may indicate hepatic lipidosis or hepatic lymphoma. Focal hyperechoic masses may occur with granulomas, abscesses, or neoplasia. Hypoechoic masses may occur with abscesses, granulomas, necrosis, hematomas, or subcapsular bleeding.

The heart can usually be visualized from the ventromedial or lateral approach. The chambers, valves, and great vessels can be visualized, and the motility of the heart and valves can be evaluated. Hypertrophy, pericardial effusion, and other abnormalities can be noted. Pericardial effusion can be recognized as an anechoic band separating the pericardium and the epicardium.

The normal spleen is difficult to visualize with ultrasound. When enlarged, the spleen can be easily demonstrated from the ventromedial approach. Homogeneous enlargement may occur with infection or trauma. Hypoechoic areas may occur with hemorrhage. Focal or diffuse nonhomogeneous masses may occur with splenic tumors.

The normal kidney is difficult to visualize with ultrasound. Massive lesions may be demonstrated using the ventromedial approach. Tumors are typically round nonhomogeneous masses, and cysts appear as rounded anechoic structures.

The inactive reproductive tract cannot be visualized sonographically. Eggs appear as two layers of differing echogenicity with the ventromedial or lateral approach. Eggs lacking a shell appear as oval or round areas with differing echogenicity.

Visualization of the gastrointestinal tract can be enhanced by administering water. The proventriculus may be visualized with the ventromedial or lateral approach. The ventriculus may be identified from the ventromedial or lateral approach and may contain hyperechoic grit particles. The proventriculus, intestinal loops, and cloaca may be identified by their echogenic walls, hypoechoic contents, and typical shape. Dilatation of the proventriculus may occur with PDS, impaction, ileus, foreign bodies, or intestinal obstruction. Thickening of the intestinal walls may occur with enteritis, mycobacteriosis, or neoplasia. The ventromedial approach is used to visualize the cloaca. Ultrasound examinations of the cloaca are facilitated by retrograde administration of fluid. Cloacaliths, papillomas, and other tumors may be noted. Consult Krautwald-Junghanns and Enders (1994) for further information on diagnostic ultrasound.

Computed Tomography and Magnetic Resonance Imaging

Currently, CT and MRI are seldom used and are limited to referral, research, or university facilities. Computed tomography is sometimes useful for the diagnosis of central nervous system and respiratory diseases. Magnetic resonance imaging may prove to be useful for imaging many parts of the body.

References and Additional Readings

Blue-McLendon A, Homco LD. Ultrasound determination of yolk sac size in ostrich chicks. *Proc Assoc Avian Vet* 1995;311–312.

Enders F, Krautwald-Junghanns M, Duhr D. Sonographic evaluation of liver diseases in birds. *Proc 1993 European Con Avian Med Surg* 1993;155–163.

Greenacre CB, Watson E, Ritchie BW. Choanal atresia in an African grey parrot *(Psittacus erithacus erithacus)* and an umbrella cockatoo *(Cacatua alba)*. *J Assoc Avian Vet* 1993;7(1):19–22.

Jenkins JR. Use of computed tomography (CT) in pet bird practice. *Proc Assoc Avian Vet* 1991;276–279.

Kostka V, Krautwald ME, Tellheim B. Radiology of the avian skull: Techniques, radiographic anatomy and pathology. *Proc Assoc Avian Vet* 1989;333–336.

Kostka V, Krautwald ME, Tellhelm B, et al. A contribution to radiologic examination of bone alterations in psittacines, birds of prey and pigeons. *Proc Assoc Avian Vet* 1988;37–59.

Krautwald ME, Enders F. Ultrasonography in birds. *Semin Avian Exot Pet Med* 1994;3(3):140–146.

Krautwald-Junghanns ME. Radiology of the respiratory tract and the use of computed tomography in psittacines. *Proc Assoc Avian Vet* 1992;366–373.

Krautwald-Junghanns ME, Enders F. Ultrasonography. In Altman RB, Clubb SL, Dorrestein GM, Quesenberry K (eds): *Avian Medicine and Surgery*. Philadelphia, WB Saunders, 1997, pp 200–209.

Krautwald-Junghanns ME, Riedel U, Neumann W. Diagnostic use of ultrasonography in birds. *Proc Assoc Avian Vet* 1991;269–275.

Krautwald-Junghanns ME, Schulz M, Hagner D, et al. Transcoelomic two-dimensional echocardiography in the avian patient. *J Avian Med Surg* 1995;9(1):19–31.

Krautwald-Junghanns ME, Schumacher F, Tellhelm B. Evaluation of the lower respiratory tract in psittacines using radiology and computed tomography. *Vet Radiol Ultrasound* 1993;34(6):382–390.

Krautwald-Junghanns ME, Tellhelm B. Advances in radiography of birds. *Semin Avian Exot Pet Med* 1994;(3):115–125.

Love N, Flammer K, Spaulding K. The normal computed tomographic (CT) anatomy of the African grey parrot *(Psittacus erithacus)*: A pilot study. *Proc Am Coll Vet Radiol* 1993.

McMillan MC. Radiographic diagnosis of avian abdominal disorders. *Compend Cont Educ Pract Vet* 1986;8(9):616–632.

McMillan MC. Avian radiographic diagnosis. *Proc Assoc Avian Vet* 1988;301–308.

McMillan MC. Imaging of avian urogenital disorders. *AAV Today* 1988;2(2):74–82.

McMillan MC. Imaging techniques. In Ritchie BW, Harrison GJ, Harrison LR (eds): *Avian Medicine: Principles and Application*. Lake Worth, FL, Wingers Publishing, 1994, pp 247–326.

McMillan MC, Petrak ML. Retrospective study of aspergillosis in pet birds. *J Assoc Avian Vet* 1989;3(4):211–215.

Morgan RV, Donnell RL, Daniel GB. Magnetic resonance imaging of the normal eye and orbit of a screech owl *(Otus asio)*. *Vet Radiol Ultrasound* 1994;35(5):362–367.

Murphy JP, Koblik P, Stein G, et al. Psittacine skull radiography. *Proc Assoc Avian Vet* 1986;81–85.

Pokras MA, Blackmer R. Understanding the syringeal bulla. *AAV Today* 1988;2(3):134–135.

Riedel U. Ultrasonography in birds. *Proc First Conf Europ Assoc Avian Vet* 1991;190–198.

Romagnano A, Shiroma JT, Heard DJ, et al. Magnetic resonance imaging of the avian brain and abdominal cavity. *Proc Assoc Avian Vet* 1995;307–308.

Rosenthal K, Stefanacci J, Quesenberry K, et al. Computerized tomography in 10 cases of avian intracranial disease. *Proc Assoc Avian Vet* 1995;305.

Rosenthal K, Stefanacci J, Quesenberry K, et al. Ultrasonographic findings in 30 cases of avian celomic disease. *Proc Assoc Avian Vet* 1995;303.

Rubel GA, Isenbugel E, Wolvekamp P (eds). *Atlas of Diagnostic Radiology of Exotic Pets*. Philadelphia, WB Saunders, 1992.

Silverman S. The principles of avian radiographic interpretation. *Proc Assoc Avian Vet* 1985;147–152.

Silverman S. Advanced avian radiographic interpretation. *Proc Assoc Avian Vet* 1987;539–544.

Silverman S. Advanced avian radiographic interpretation. *Proc Assoc Avian Vet* 1989;303–306 and 1990;339–342.

Silverman S. Advances in avian and reptilian imaging. In Kirk RW, Bonagura JD (eds): *Current Veterinary Therapy X, Small Animal Practice*. Philadelphia, WB Saunders, 1989, pp 786–789.

Silverman S. Basic avian radiology. *Proc Assoc Avian Vet* 1989;298–302, and 1990;334–338.

Silverman S. Selected tips on radiography in birds. *J Assoc Avian Vet* 1990;4(4):202–204.

Smith BJ, Smith SA. Radiology. In Altman RB, Clubb SL, Dorrestein GM, Quesenberry K (eds): *Avian Medicine and Surgery*. Philadelphia, WB Saunders, 1997, pp 170–199.

Smith SA, Smith BJ. *Atlas of Avian Radiographic Anatomy*. Philadelphia, WB Saunders, 1992.

Storm J, Greenwood AG. Fluoroscopic investigation of the avian gastrointestinal tract. *Proc Europ Conf Avian Med Surg* 1993;170–177.

Tully TN, Hillman D, Williams J. Anatomic examination of an emu *(Dromauis novaehollandiae)* using diagnostic imaging: Techniques and anatomic cross sections. *Proc Assoc Avian Vet* 1995;313–315.

Turrel JM, McMillan MC, Paul-Murphy J. Diagnosis and treatment of tumors of companion birds II. *AAV Today* 1987;1(4):159–165.

Wack RF, Kramer L, Anderson. Cardiomegaly and endocardial fibrosis in a secretary bird *(Sagittarius serpentarius)*. *J Assoc Avian Vet* 1994;8(2):76–80.

Walsh MT. Radiology. In Harrison GJ, Harrison LR (eds): *Clinical Avian Medicine and Surgery*. Philadelphia, WB Saunders, 1986, pp 201–233.

Chapter 14

Surgery

Anesthesia, endoscopy, and surgery are common procedures used in the practice of avian medicine. With the correct use of proper equipment and safe anesthetic agents, anesthesia is a safe procedure in birds. A thorough knowledge of monitoring, induction, maintenance, support, and recovery from anesthetic is required. Excellent endoscopic equipment is available to make endoscopy safe and useful. Current surgical techniques and surgical and monitoring equipment make avian surgery safe and effective. Adequate surgical and endoscopic skills should be gained through continuing education classes and practice on cadavers before operating on client animals.

ANESTHESIA

Before anesthesia, all birds should be evaluated as thoroughly as their condition will allow. Before elective surgical procedures and those surgical procedures where time permits (all but absolute emergency procedures), a complete history, physical examination, and laboratory work-up should be performed. A complete history and physical examination will allow identification of possible problems. Preanesthetic work-ups will identify many birds at risk of dying as a result of the stress of anesthesia, surgery, or postsurgical complications. Birds should be stabilized before anesthesia unless the anesthetic procedure is important in stabilizing the birds (e.g., air sac breathing tube placement for tracheal obstruction). A minimum data base should include a complete history, physical examination, hematocrit, plasma protein, uric acid level, aspartate aminotransferase (AST), glucose, and white blood cell count (WBC). When history, physical examination, or laboratory data indicate possible abnormalities, further pertinent testing such as additional plasma biochemistries, radiographs, electrocardiogram, and cultures are recommended. Respiratory recovery time can be used to evaluate respiratory stability. The respiratory rate should return to normal within 3 to 5 minutes after capture and restraint for at least 2 minutes.

Noted laboratory abnormalities should be evaluated and possible etiologies considered and weighed against possible complications from anesthesia and surgery. Elective procedures may have to be delayed and therapy administered before surgical intervention. Dehydration should be corrected before anesthesia. Fluid therapy should be administered to patients with a hematocrit above 60%. Anesthesia should be delayed in birds with a hematocrit less than 20%, or whole blood should be administered. Birds with plasma protein levels below 2 mg/dl

431

are poor surgical candidates. Elective surgery should be postponed and therapy pursued to treat the underlying cause. Intraoperative 5% dextrose should be administered intravenously (IV) in birds with a glucose below 200 mg/dl.

Fasting is recommended before anesthesia to allow the upper gastrointestinal tract to empty. Psittacines should be fasted for a minimum of 3 hours (usually 5 to 8 hours) and raptors for 24 to 36 hours. Prolonged fasting is not recommended in psittacines. If the bird cannot be fasted before anesthesia, the crop can be emptied with a tube or the bird can be induced in an upright position with digital pressure over the proximal esophagus, intubated with a properly sized endotracheal tube, and the crop emptied. The crop can be emptied by holding a gauze pad over the choana, turning the bird upside down, and manually expressing the crop contents. Placing gauze in the upper esophagus during anesthesia will further inhibit aspiration of crop contents. The head and neck should be elevated for the duration of the anesthesia.

Preanesthetics are generally not used in birds. Atropine can cause increased heart rates, decreased gastrointestinal motility, and thickening of respiratory secretions. These secretions can occlude endotracheal tubes.

Support

Rapid loss of heat can occur with anesthesia and may result in arrhythmias, increased recovery time, and death. Body heat loss should be minimized during surgery with the use of supplemental heat (e.g., circulating warm water blankets, warm water bottles, heat lamps, heated lavage solutions, heated IV fluids). Minimize the amount of alcohol used for the surgical prep. The normal body temperature is 105 to 107° F. A tympanic scanner or cloacal probe can be used to monitor temperature.

Fluid therapy during anesthesia will speed postanesthetic recovery time and is useful to replace fluids lost during surgery. Lactated Ringer's solution is most commonly used. Fluids should be warm when infused and may be administered IV or intraosseously (IO). Infusion pumps or periodic small boluses are recommended for IV and IO routes. The maximum administration rate tolerated by healthy birds is 90 ml/kg/hr IV or IO.

Intermittent positive-pressure ventilation (IPPV) is recommended at 20 to 40 per minute at 10 to 24 cm H_2O. This is especially important in birds placed in dorsal recumbency, where even healthy birds may be poorly oxygenated.

Monitoring

The most important aid in anesthetic monitoring is a trained technician. Clear drapes allow visual monitoring (Table 14–1). Care should be taken to ensure that the bird's ability to move the sternum is not restricted.

The depth of anesthesia can be evaluated by heart rate, respiratory rate, respiratory effort, toe pinch reflex, palpebral and corneal reflexes, cloacal tone, and wing tone. A light plane of anesthesia is characterized by positive palpebral and toe pinch reflexes and wing tone. At a surgical plane of anesthesia, respirations should be slow, even, and deep, the heart rate should be slow and even,

TABLE 14–1. Products Mentioned in the Text

Clear drapes: Incise, Johnson and Johnson, Arlington, TX 76004; Veterinary Specialty Products, Boca Raton, FL 33481, (800) 362-8138; Steri-drapes, 3M Animal Care Products, St. Paul, MN 55144, (612) 733-0072.

Respiratory monitors: Medical Engineering, Jackson, MI (517) 783-5851.

Small reservoir bags (50 ml, 100 ml, 250 ml): Exotic Animal Medical Products, Watkinsville, GA 30677.

Endoscopes: Karl Storz Veterinary Endoscopy, Goleta, CA 93117, (800) 955-7832, Fax (805) 968-1553.

Focuscope: MDS Inc, Brandon, FL 33509, (813) 653-1180.

Self-adherent bandaging material: Vetwrap Bandaging Tape, 3M Animal Care Products, St. Paul, MN 55144, (612) 733-0072.

Hemostatic clips: Solvay Animal Health Inc, Mendota Heights, MN 55120, (800) 247-1139.

Surgical spears: Weck-Cell Surgical Spears, Solvay Animal Health Inc, Mendota Heights, MN 55120, (800) 247-1139.

Gelatin sponges: Gelfoam, Upjohn Co, Kalamazoo, MI 49001, (616) 323-4000.

Restraint boards: Henry Schein, Port Washington, NY 11050, (800) 443-2756; Veterinary Specialty Products, Boca Raton, FL 33481, (800) 362-8138; Silverdust Bird Positioner, El Granada, CA 94122.

Radiosurgical equipment: Ellman Surgitron, Ellman International Inc, Hewlett, NY 11557, (516) 569-1482.

Tegaderm bandage: 3M Animal Care Products, St. Paul, MN 55144, (612) 733-0072.

Hydroactive dressing: DuoDerm Ulcer Pack; Bristol-Myers Squibb, New Brunswick, NJ.

---

the corneal reflex should be present, a slight withdrawal reflex may be present, and pain reflexes and response to positional changes should be absent. The corneal reflex is slow and the pupils are mydriatic, with a delayed but present pupillary light response in a surgical plane of anesthesia. Deep anesthesia is characterized by the loss of the corneal reflex, decreased heart rate, and decreased respiratory rate and volume and requires an immediate decrease in anesthetic flow rate.

The normal respiratory and heart rate should be determined for the specific surgical patient before induction of anesthesia. The respiratory rate should be slow, deep, and regular under anesthesia. An increase in rate may indicate light anesthesia, obstruction of the endotracheal tube, or build-up of CO_2. Respiratory monitors are available for use in birds (see Table 14–1). Monitoring cardiac electrical activity with an electrocardiogram (ECG) is recommended. As anesthesia deepens, T waves become smaller and R waves increase in magnitude. Pulse oximeters are useful for monitoring oxygen saturation and provide an early indication of a problem. Oxygen saturation levels should ideally remain above 90%. Levels below 80% are life threatening. Self-ventilating birds typically maintain an oxygen saturation between 80% to 85%. The use of IPPV is important in maintaining a desirable oxygen saturation.

Anesthetic Agents

Inhalation and injectable anesthetics are available for avian anesthesia. Isoflurane is the anesthetic of choice in birds. Inhalation anesthetics are generally safer than injectable anesthetics in birds. They can be titrated to effect, allow rapid changes in anesthetic level, and have consistent therapeutic indices. Inhalation anesthetics provide smoother and generally more rapid recoveries.

Inhalation Anesthetics

Induction should be accomplished with a face mask. The patient is manually restrained, and the nostrils and mouth or head are placed in the face mask (Fig. 14–1). Some macaws, owls, and gallinaceous birds are sensitive to gas anesthetics and may become apneic.

Commercial dog and cat face masks may be used; however, these are easily torn with the bird's beak and fit poorly. Disposable face masks can be made from clear plastic drinking cups or from the top part of soda bottles. Latex gloves or plastic can be stretched over the large open end, and a T cut made to allow introduction of the head or just the beak and nares. Alternately, paper towels or a cloth towel can be used to fill the space between the head and cup. If face masks are reused, they should be sterilized between each patient.

Intubation is relatively simple. The glottis is located immediately caudal to the tongue (Fig. 14–2). The glottis can be elevated to ease intubation with digital pressure between the mandibles. The tube is gently inserted into the trachea and taped to the beak to secure. Cuffless endotracheal tubes should be used in birds due to their complete tracheal rings. Birds cockatiel size and larger can be intubated with a standard endotracheal tube or modified tube. Tubes should be of appropriate length (the distance from the tip of the beak to the thoracic inlet). Endotracheal tubes for smaller birds can be made from red rubber catheter feeding tubes. The end is cut to the correct length at an angle and then blunted by heating. Intubation is recommended if the procedure requires anesthesia for longer than 10 minutes. Birds in critical condition should be intubated so that breathing can be assisted as needed.

A nonrebreathing system should be used in birds less than 7 to 8 kg. A Bain's or Ayre's T is appropriate. In most pet birds, small reservoir bags allow better monitoring of respiration. Small reservoir bags are available or can be made

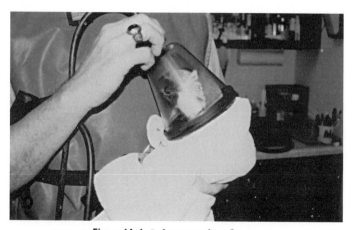

Figure 14–1. Induction with isoflurane.

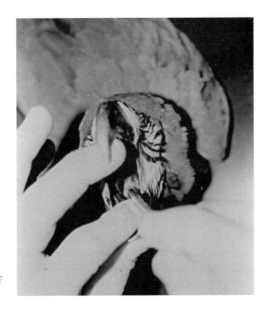

Figure 14–2. Endotracheal intubation of a macaw.

from small plastic bags (see Table 14–1). The maintenance oxygen flow rate minimum should be 0.5 to 1 L/min. In large birds, the oxygen flow rate is based on body weight size, at 0.5 to 1 L/kg/min with a minimum rate listed previously. The flow rate for induction of most pet birds is 1 L/min, depending on the size of the bird.

Isoflurane is the anesthetic recommended for birds. It allows rapid alterations in anesthetic levels, has a large margin between respiratory and cardiac arrest, allows rapid inductions, and provides rapid and smooth recoveries without postrecovery depression. Many birds will eat and drink immediately after recovering from isoflurane anesthesia. Isoflurane is also the safest anesthetic when organ pathology is present. Birds may be induced at 4% to 5%. Induction typically takes 1 to 3 minutes. Alternately, birds can be induced at 2.5% to 3%, taking 1 to 5 minutes. Most birds can be maintained at about 2%. Some macaws, owls, and gallinaceous birds may be maintained at much lower levels (as low as 0.25%). Recovery typically takes 2 to 8 minutes. The bird is usually held until it can stand alone. Most birds quickly return to normal behaviors.

Halothane allows for rapid induction and recovery. However, apnea and cardiac arrest often occur at the same time with halothane. Also, halothane sensitizes the heart to catecholamines, increasing the risk of arrhythmias and cardiac arrest. Birds may be induced at 2% to 3% and are typically maintained at 0.5% to 1.5%. Induction typically takes 2 to 5 minutes. Recovery usually takes 3 to 8 minutes, but may take up to 20 minutes with longer anesthetic times. Birds are usually held until recovery is complete. Postrecovery depression may last several hours.

Methoxyflurane anesthesia requires relatively long induction and results in prolonged recovery times. Responses to changes in vaporizer settings are prolonged. Birds are induced at 3% to 4%, and maintained at 1% to 2%. Induction takes 5 to 15 minutes and recovery usually takes 10 to 30 minutes. Because recovery is prolonged, birds are not held for recovery. The bird is wrapped loosely in a towel, the oropharynx is dried with swabs, and the bird is placed in a quiet and warm (80–90°F) environment to recover. The bird should be checked and turned frequently, removing any oropharyngeal secretions. Postrecovery depression may last several hours.

Injectable Anesthetics

The level of anesthesia and oxygenation of the bird are more difficult to control with injectable anesthetics. Recoveries are often rough and prolonged, and birds may remain depressed for many hours after recovery. Injectable anesthetics should not be used in ill birds. Short procedures in healthy birds are the only acceptable uses of injectable anesthetics. Isoflurane is the best anesthetic for use in all birds. Supplemental oxygen via a face mask is recommended.

Combinations of ketamine with diazepam or xylazine may be used in healthy birds for short procedures. Accurate body weight is essential when determining the dose of injectable anesthetic. Ketamine combinations can be administered IV or intramuscularly (IM). Ketamine (100 mg/ml) and diazepam (5 mg/ml) are mixed in the same syringe in equal volumes and administered at a dose of 0.2 to 0.6 ml/kg IM or 0.1 to 0.2 ml/kg IV. Ketamine (100 mg/ml) and xylazine (20 mg/ml) are mixed in the same syringe in equal volumes and administered at a dose of 0.2 to 0.5 ml/kg IM or 0.1 to 0.3 ml/kg IV. Birds weighing less than 250 g generally require a higher dose than birds weighing more than 250 g. Intramuscular induction is facilitated by placing the bird in a quiet, dark environment for 3 to 5 minutes immediately after injection. For IV administration, half of the calculated dose should be administered, then titrated to effect. Start at the lower end of the dosage range when dosing injectable anesthetics. These injectable combinations have narrow therapeutic indices. Response varies with the species and with individual birds. Difficulties have been reported with the use of ketamine/xylazine combination anesthesia in waterfowl and some owls and hawks.

These two combinations generally provide 10 to 45 minutes of anesthesia. If longer anesthesia is needed, small additional doses can be administered or the patient may be changed to gas anesthesia. Xylazine should not be used in debilitated birds. Recovery from IV administration of these combinations generally takes 15 to 45 minutes. Recovery from IM administration may take hours. Recoveries can be violent. For recovery, the bird is wrapped loosely in a towel, the oropharynx is dried with swabs, and the bird is placed in a quiet and warm (80–90° F) environment to recover. The bird should be checked and turned frequently, removing any oropharyngeal secretions. Postrecovery depression may last several hours.

Air Sac Breathing Tube Anesthesia

Inhalation anesthetics can be administered through an air sac breathing tube. Common indications for air sac anesthesia include surgery of the trachea, syrinx, or head and for relief of tracheal obstruction. Birds typically do not respire during the anesthetic period. For method of placement of air sac breathing tubes, see the section on air sac breathing tube placement.

Emergencies

Prognosis associated with respiratory and cardiac arrest varies with the cause of the arrest. Isoflurane anesthetic overdose and acute illness (e.g., acute tracheal obstruction) often respond. Arrest as a result of chronic illness rarely responds to cardiopulmonary resuscitation (CPR). Respiratory arrest during inhalation anesthesia requires immediate attention. Stop anesthetic administration. Place an endotracheal tube if the bird is not intubated, place the bird in sternal recumbency, and apply positive-pressure ventilation at the rate of once every 4 to 5 seconds. Once ventilation has been instigated, the heart beat and peripheral pulse are checked; and ideally the electrical activity of the heart is observed with an ECG. If there is no heart beat, place the bird in dorsal recumbancy and begin firm and rapid compressions of the sternum, continue ventilation, and give epinephrine and atropine. Epinephrine and atropine can be given IV, followed by a bolus of saline or sterile water to encourage drug transport to the heart. These drugs may also be administered by intratracheal, IO, or intracardiac administration, or sprayed into the thoracic cavity if the body cavity is open. Intratracheal administration is often the easiest route in arrested birds. The trachea is isolated with the fingers, and the needle is inserted into the tracheal lumen and drugs are injected.

If acute tracheal obstruction is suspected, an air sac breathing tube is placed for positive-pressure ventilation.

If excessive hemorrhage occurs during an anesthetic procedure, increase fluid therapy (warm fluids), control bleeding, and give IV or IO blood transfusions (see Chapter 11).

ENDOSCOPY

Endoscopy in birds is facilitated by the unique design of their respiratory system; the presence of air sacs and lack of a diaphragm. The best endoscope for general avian practice is a 2.7-mm rigid endoscope 170 to 190 mm in length. This diameter scope is useful in birds weighing 55 to 4000 g. A 1.9-mm diameter endoscope is the smallest available endoscope with high-quality optics and is useful in small birds (less than 100 g) and in small spaces (e.g., sinuses, choana, trachea, oviduct), but it is fragile and has limited light transmission, limiting its usefulness in larger body cavities. A beveled distal lens element allows easier and less traumatic passage through air sacs and the abdominal wall. It also allows better visualization of concurrently used instruments (e.g., biopsy forceps). Visualization of small structures is enhanced with the magnification features of endoscopes. An excellent system as described above with an instrument channel is available through Karl Storz Veterinary Endoscopy (Fig. 14–3) (see Table 14–1). Endoscopes used for human endoscopy, otoscopes, and tubular endoscopes (Focuscope) have also been used in avian medicine. Size, light quality, clarity of image, and decreased magnification make these instruments less useful

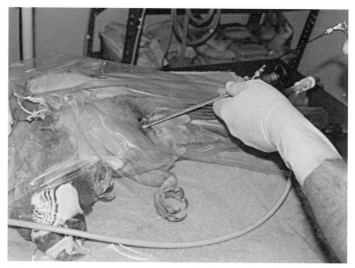

Figure 14–3. Collection of a biopsy sample using a Karl Storz Veterinary Endoscopy endoscope. (Karl Storz Veterinary Endoscopy, 175 Cremona Dr, Goleta, CA 93117; 800 955-7832.)

than the system described above, which was designed for use in birds. Otoscopes were commonly used in the past. The low level of light available with use of an otoscope allows very limited visualization of structures. Tubular endoscopes allow transmission of more light than otoscopes, but still considerably less than the new endoscopes. Critically examine the quality and completeness of any equipment before purchase.

It is important to obtain quality instruments and adequate surgical skills before performing endoscopy on client birds. Experience can be gained through hands-on laboratories offered at various seminars (e.g., Association of Avian Veterinarians, North American Veterinary Conference) and/or practice with pigeons, dead birds, or birds to be euthanized (with owner consent). Consistent positioning allows rapid orientation.

Proper instrument care will prolong the life and maintain the quality of the optics of an endoscope. Rigid endoscopes must be handled carefully during transport, use, and cleaning. Always handle the scope with the eyepiece. Avoid torsion stress on the long axis of the endoscope. Follow manufacturers' recommendations for cleaning and storage. In general, rigid endoscopes should be stored in a sleeve and padded storage container. They may be rinsed with distilled water to clean. A nonabrasive cleanser can be used to remove debris and fat, if needed. The instrument channel should be flushed to remove debris. Lens paper is used to clean lens surfaces. An alcohol flush can be used to dry the scope before storage.

The endoscope should be sterilized before each use. Follow manufacturers' recommendations for sterilization. Ethylene oxide or a specific 2% gluteralde-hyde solution is recommended. For most practices, a manufacturer-recommended gluteraldehyde solution is most practical. The endoscope is soaked for a minimum of 15 to 20 minutes. Stacking instruments is not recommended because the solution must contact all surfaces. Soaking times greater than 2 hours are not recommended. The scope must be rinsed with sterile water before use. Instruments can be placed in a sterile container of sterile water for rinsing. The instrument is wiped dry before use.

Anesthesia with isoflurane is recommended for all procedures. Ketamine combined with diazepam or xylazine has been used successfully for anesthesia in healthy birds. A complete history and physical examination are necessary before anesthesia and endoscopy (see section on anesthesia). Preanesthetic laboratory tests will identify many birds at risk of dying as a result of the stress of anesthesia or organ failure. Psittacines should be fasted for a minimum of 3 hours, raptors for 24 to 36 hours. Heat support should be provided during endoscopic procedures. Elective endoscopy of hand-fed neonates is not recommended because the proventriculus is large and is predisposed to trauma because of its enlarged size.

Common uses of endoscopy include gender identification in monomorphic birds, visualization of organs and tissues, collection of samples (exudates, biopsies), foreign body removal, granuloma removal, and to monitor response to treatment. Sites accessible with an endoscope in many birds and commonly examined include the celom (gonads, air sac, liver, lung, spleen, kidney, ventriculus), oral cavity, trachea, choana, crop, proventriculus, ventriculus, cloaca, external ear canal, and nares.

Laparoscopy

Many approaches have been described for laparoscopy in birds. The left lateral approach allows visualization of many celomic structures, including gonads, air sacs, liver, lungs, spleen, pericardium, kidneys, proventriculus, and ventriculus. The bird is anesthetized and restrained in right lateral recumbancy. The wings are extended dorsally and taped to a restraint board or table. The left leg is extended cranially, and self-adhering tape (e.g., Vetwrap; see Table 14–1) is wrapped around the tarsometatarsus and then bound to the neck (Fig. 14–4). The entry site is just caudal to the last rib and just ventral to the flexor cruris medialis muscle (Fig. 14–5). Clear drapes are recommended. A small skin incision is made and the muscle is bluntly dissected with mosquito forceps (Fig. 14–6). The forceps are gently pushed through the body wall in a craniomedial direction. The scope can then be inserted through this opening in a craniodorsal direction into the caudal thoracic air sac space (Fig. 14–7). From this view looking cranially, the confluent walls of the caudal thoracic and abdominal air sacs can be visualized. The proventriculus and dorsal liver can be observed ventrally, and the heart, lung, and the opening of the lung into the caudal thoracic air sac (ostium) are visible craniodorsally (Fig. 14–8). The confluent walls of the caudal thoracic and abdominal air sacs usually must be penetrated to view the gonads, kidney, and intestines. The air sac wall can be penetrated with steady pressure on an avascular area in the central portion of the air sac wall. Once this membrane has been penetrated, the gonad, adrenal gland, kidney, ureter, and oviduct or vas deferens can be visualized caudodorsally (Fig. 14–9).

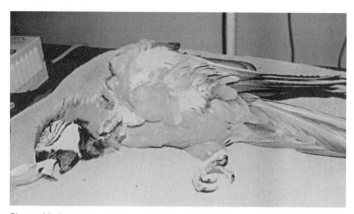

Figure 14–4. Positioning for a left lateral endoscopic approach in a macaw. The left leg is extended cranially, and self-adhering tape (e.g., Vetwrap) is wrapped around the tarsometatarsus and then bound to the neck.

Organs and air sacs should be evaluated for location, color, size, and shape. Note lesions and abnormalities. Normal air sac membranes are transparent with minimal vascularity. Abnormalities that may be noted include thickening or opaque air sac membranes, fluid accumulation or exudates, granulomas, or mold growth. Fluid accumulation, exudates, or opaque air sac membranes may be the result of bacterial, chlamydial, viral, fungal, or parasitic infection. Granulomas may be caused by bacterial or fungal infection or foreign material. *Aspergillus* may appear as mold growth on the air sac membranes (a green or yellow area similar to bread mold). Samples of exudate may be collected, or granulomas or air sac membrane may be biopsied and used for cytologic preparations, microbi-

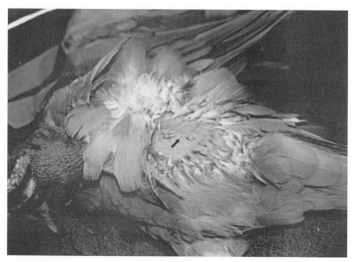

Figure 14–5. The entry site for a left lateral endoscopic examination is just caudal to the last rib and just ventral to the flexor cruris medialis *(arrow)*.

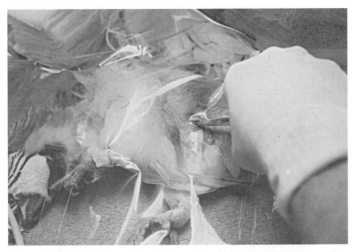

Figure 14–6. Dissection of the body wall with mosquito forceps to allow insertion of the endoscope lens into the celom (left lateral approach).

ology, and/or histopathology. The normal proventriculus is pale and vascular. Proventricular abnormalities include congestion, hemorrhage, and perforation. Dilatation is difficult to accurately evaluate endoscopically. The normal liver is uniformly red-brown and contacts the heart. Abnormalities of the liver include hepatomegaly, decrease in size, granulomas, necrotic foci, discoloration, or mold growth. Hepatomegaly may be the result of chlamydial, bacterial, mycobacterial, viral, or parasitic infection; hepatic lipidosis; hemochromatosis; amyloidosis; gout; or neoplasia. A decrease in size may be the result of fibrosis (e.g., aflatoxicosis,

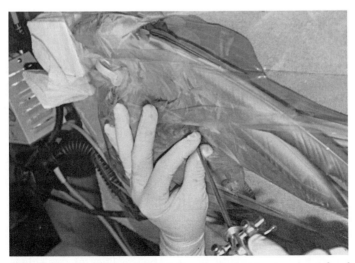

Figure 14–7. The scope is inserted through the incision in a craniodorsal direction into the caudal thoracic air sac space.

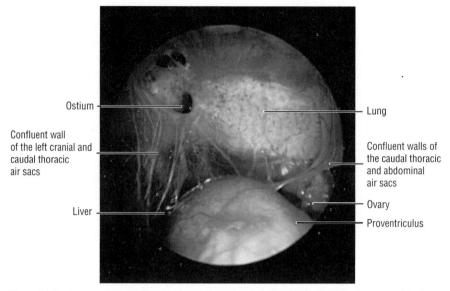

Figure 14–8. A view of a left lateral endoscopic approach looking cranially. The lung is visible from 11 to 2 o'clock. An ostium associated with the lung is visible at 11 o'clock. The confluent walls of the left cranial thoracic and caudal thoracic air sacs are visible from 7 to 11 o'clock. The proventriculus and the edge of the left lobe of the liver are visible at the bottom from 4 to 7 o'clock. The confluent wall of the caudal thoracic and abdominal air sacs is visible at the right border from 4 to 1 o'clock. This confluent wall has been perforated. The ovary can be seen at 3 o'clock. (Photo courtesy of Michael Taylor, D.V.M.)

resolved hepatic lipidosis). Multifocal white to yellow granulomatous or necrotic foci may be the result of bacterial, mycobacterial, chlamydial, viral, fungal, or parasitic infection or neoplasia. A pale to yellow enlarged liver is usually the result of hepatic lipidosis or a normal neonate mobilizing egg yolk in the first 2 to 3 weeks of life. A dark brown to black enlarged liver is commonly the result of hemochromatosis or *Plasmodium* infection. *Aspergillus* may appear as mold growth on the surface of the liver or granuloma formation. The accumulation of white gritty material on the pericardium may be uric acid crystal deposits (gout) or bacterial pericarditis. Normal lungs are pink and ostei are clear of exudates. Abnormalities include discoloration, swellings, exudates, masses, and hemorrhage. Dark red and wet lungs may be the result of pulmonary edema and hemorrhage caused by bacterial infection, polytetrafluoroethylene (Teflon) toxicosis, *Sarcocystis* infection, or inhalation of noxious gases or carbon monoxide. Multifocal white lesions may be caused by bacterial, fungal, or mycobacterial infection; neoplasia; or foreign material (e.g., inhalation pneumonia). *Aspergillus* may appear as mold growth on the surface of the lung or as granulomas.

In the caudodorsal celom, the kidney, adrenal gland, gonads, and associated structures are visible once the confluent membranes of the abdominal and caudal thoracic air sac have been penetrated. A normal kidney has a slightly granular surface and is brown to reddish brown. Abnormalities of the kidney include discoloration, pallor, enlargement, masses, or white foci. Renomegaly may be

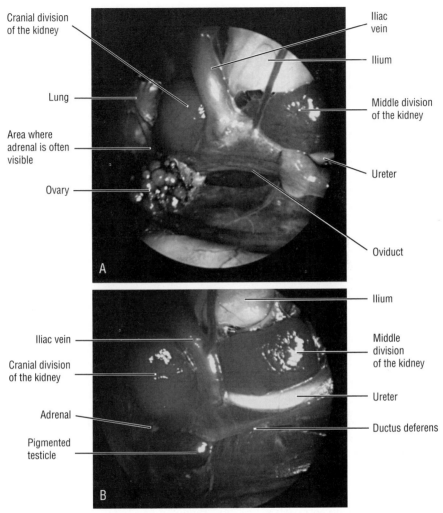

Cranial division of the kidney

Iliac vein

Ilium

Lung

Middle division of the kidney

Area where adrenal is often visible

Ovary

Ureter

Oviduct

A

Ilium

Iliac vein

Middle division of the kidney

Cranial division of the kidney

Ureter

Adrenal

Ductus deferens

Pigmented testicle

B

Figure 14–9. A, A caudodorsal view of the left lateral endoscopic approach in a female cockatoo. The black ovary contains numerous small follicles. The cranial and middle divisions of the kidney, oviduct, ureter, and iliac vein are also visible. **B,** A caudal view of the left lateral endoscopic approach in a male cockatoo. The testis, adrenal gland, kidney, ureter, and ductus deferens can be visualized. (Photos courtesy of Michael Taylor, D.V.M.)

the result of bacterial, chlamydial, viral, or parasitic infection; dehydration; lipidosis; gout; amyloidosis; postrenal obstruction; congenital cysts; neoplasia; or lead or zinc toxicosis. The adrenal gland is located at the cranial pole of the kidney and lateral to the gonad. A normal adrenal gland is yellow to pink and flattened round to triangular in shape. Abnormalities of the adrenal gland include enlargement, masses, or discoloration. Enlargement may be the result of chronic stress, chronic corticosteroid administration, adrenal neoplasia, or pituitary tumor.

In male birds, the testes are located at the cranial pole of the kidneys. They have a smooth surface, but vary in size, shape, and color. In general, testes are bean shaped, with distinct rounded cranial and caudal poles. The right testicle can often be visualized through the dorsal mesentery from the left lateral approach. The testes of immature birds are small, bean shaped, and yellow to white. In some birds they may be pigmented black or gray (e.g., some cockatoos, blue and gold macaws, golden conures, mynahs, and toucans). During the breeding season, the testes of mature birds may enlarge from 10% to 500%. The large testes may be white, yellow, or gray, with a vascular surface. During the nonbreeding season, the testes atrophy and appear similar to but slightly larger than juvenile testes. Testicular abnormalities include swellings, tumors, atrophy (during the breeding season in adult males), and agenesis. Atrophy may be the result of inflammation, bacterial infection, septicemia, toxicosis, malnutrition, congenital abnormality, or lack of correct environmental stimuli. Enlargement or swelling may be the result of bacterial infection, inflammation, or neoplasia.

In most avian species, the female has a single functional ovary. It is located at the cranial pole of the left kidney. In immature birds, the ovary is flattened and triangular and may be white, yellow, or pigmented black (e.g., some cockatoos, macaws, and conures) with a granular surface. The immature ovary may resemble a piece of fat. The active ovary has follicles in varying stages of development, appearing as a cluster of variably sized grapes. The oviduct courses over the ventral surface of the left kidney. The oviduct is very thin during reproductive inactivity, but becomes long, wide, and tortuous during active egg laying. During the nonbreeding season, the ovary and oviduct regress, and many small follicles will be present on the ovary. Abnormalities of the ovary include inactive ovaries during breeding season; wrinkled, discolored, enlarged, insupated, pedunculated, or hemorrhagic ova; abnormal yolk that appears coagulated and flaking off into the body cavity; congested or distorted follicles; swellings; or adhesions. Inactive ovaries during the breeding season may be the result of lack of correct environmental stimuli, immaturity, old age, severe stress, or aflatoxicosis.

The right kidney, lung, liver lobe, testis, and thoracic and abdominal air sacs may be visualized with a right lateral approach. This approach is similar to the left lateral approach discussed above only performed on the right side with the bird in left lateral recumbancy.

A ventral midline approach is best for examining and biopsying the liver. The bird is placed in dorsal recumbancy. Feathers are plucked just caudal to the sternum. The area is surgically prepped and an incision is made on the midline just caudal to the sternum. The linea alba is incised and the caudal border of the membrane of the ventral hepatic peritoneal cavity is bluntly penetrated. A large fat pad may be present in this area in some birds. Both liver lobes may be examined.

A postischial approach can be used to visualize the kidneys, gonads, adrenal gland, spleen, intestines, ventriculus, and proventriculus. Entry is dorsal to the pubic bone, caudal to the ischium, and dorsolateral to the vent. The endoscope first enters the intestinal peritoneal cavity. The confluent membrane of the intestinal peritoneal cavity and abdominal air sac membrane must be penetrated to enter the abdominal air sac space.

A prepubic approach is commonly used to visualize and biopsy the caudal pole of the kidney. The incision is made ventral to the acetabulum, midway between the last rib and the pubis, at the ventral border of the flexor cruris medialis muscle.

Trachea

In patients larger than a cockatiel, a 2.7-mm endoscope can be used to examine the tracheal lumen. In small birds, a 1.9-mm endoscope is recommended. The bird is anesthetized and placed in sternal recumbency, with the neck extended. An abdominal air sac breathing tube can be placed for respiration and anesthesia before tracheal endoscopy; however, this is usually not necessary for a quick examination of the tracheal lumen.

The scope is passed through the glottis and the tracheal lumen is examined for abnormalities (hemorrhage, erosions, plaques, masses, parasites, foreign bodies). The syrinx may be examined at the tracheal bifurcation when an appropriately sized endoscope is used. The syrinx is a common site of bacterial and fungal infection and inhaled foreign bodies. Grasping forceps or biopsy cups may be used to grasp foreign bodies or to remove granulomas and biopsy growths. The tip of the endoscope may be wiped with a culture swab immediately after the procedure to obtain a sample for bacterial or viral cultures.

Esophagus, Crop, Proventriculus, and Ventriculus

The esophagus can be examined by passing the endoscope past the glottis in an anesthetized patient. The degree of longitudinal folding varies among species of birds. Abnormalities include hemorrhage, erythema, ulceration, erosions, and plaques.

The crop can be examined in birds with crops (psittacines, pigeons, doves, gallinaceous birds, and some passerines) by passing the endoscope through the cervical portion of the esophagus. The bird should be fasted for several hours before the procedure to increase visualization when possible. Insufflation of the crop with air will increase visualization. The instrument channel or a flexible feeding tube attached to a syringe is passed into the crop, and the air is injected while pressure is maintained on the proximal esophagus. The normal mucosa is pale, smooth, and even colored and may contain clear mucus or food. The mucosa is examined for hemorrhage, erosions, ulceration, plaques, and masses, and the lumen is examined for foreign bodies. Grasping forceps or basket can be used to remove foreign bodies and masses can be biopsied with biopsy cups.

An ingluvotomy (crop incision) is used to examine the proventriculus. The bird is anesthetized, intubated, and placed in dorsal recumbency. An incision is made in the skin and crop. The telescope is introduced into the thoracic esophagus, located on the caudodorsal midline of the crop and is gently passed into the proventriculus. A saline-filled syringe connected to a no. 3 to 5 French rubber catheter can be inserted into the instrument channel or along the side of the telescope and used for flushing debris from the field of vision. Grasping forceps or basket can be used to grasp and remove foreign bodies. The crop is closed with a two-layer closure (see section on surgery).

The bird should be fasted for 5 to 6 hours before the endoscopy when possible. When fasting is not possible, food can be flushed from the ventriculus with sterile saline into the crop and then aspirated. This is facilitated by lowering the head below proventriculus level. Gauze sponges should be placed in the cervical esophagus, and an endotracheal tube should be placed to help prevent aspiration of flushed contents.

The ventriculus may be entered by gently inserting the telescope through the proventricular ventricular junction. Air or saline may be used to improve visualization. Grasping forceps or basket can be used to remove foreign bodies.

Oviduct and Cloaca

The three chambers of the cloaca can be examined with the aid of an endoscope. The urodeum can be flushed with saline and then insufflated with air to improve visualization. Pressure must be applied around the vent to retain air in the cloaca. The distal oviduct can be examined in reproductively active birds. Visualization of oviductal disease and collection of samples for culture are possible.

Endoscopic Biopsy Techniques

All visible structures should be evaluated before collection of biopsy samples. Commonly biopsied organs include air sac, liver, kidney, testis, lung, ventriculus, and spleen. Collect biopsy samples from borders of lesions. Samples collected for culture or immunologic tests should be handled according to instructions from the laboratory to which the sample will be sent. Prepare impression smears before fixing biopsied tissues. The small samples obtained through endoscopic biopsy techniques are best fixed and stored in small glass vials, such as small stoppered blood collection containers without anticoagulant.

Air Sac and Lung

Indications for air sac or lung biopsy include persistent, nonresponsive respiratory disease based on abnormal physical examination findings and radiographic abnormalities or visualization of lesions on an endoscopic examination. Pieces of air sac can be removed for culture, cytology, and histopathology evaluation. Cup biopsy forceps are used to grasp a small piece of the air sac membrane from the border of a puncture site. Lesions may be collected with biopsy forceps. Exudates may be collected with forceps for culture and cytology. An air sac wash can be performed by infusing a small amount of saline over the air sac membrane and aspirating this fluid with an infusion needle or catheter. The caudal surface of the lungs can be biopsied from a left or right lateral approach. The costal surface of the lung may be sampled through an intercostal approach. Size 5 Fr. elliptical forceps are recommended for lung sample collection in small birds and 7 Fr. in larger birds. The degree of hemorrhage as a result of sample collection is related to the size of the biopsy forceps used and the depth of penetration into the parenchyma of the lung; however, the diagnostic quality of the sample can be affected by inadequate sample size.

Liver

Indications for liver biopsy includes evidence of liver disease based on the history, physical examination findings, persistent elevation of bile acids (2 weeks), radiographic abnormalities, and visualization of abnormalities noted on endoscopic examination. Vitamin K administration prior to liver biopsy may aid in prevention of excessive hemorrhage. The liver can be biopsied through a ventral midline approach or a right or left lateral approach. A ventral midline approach is best when the liver is the only organ of interest because both liver lobes may be examined and sampled through a single incision. The liver frequently appears grossly normal, even when significant histologic lesions are present. Size 5 or 7 Fr. biopsy forceps are used to collect samples. Care should be taken to not open the forceps too wide when collecting the sample; this can result in crushing artifacts. Collect samples from the borders of lesions. The borders of the liver are most easily sampled with generalized disease.

Kidney

Indications for renal biopsy include kidney disease based on history, physical examination findings, renal plasma biochemistries, and abnormal radiographic findings; abnormalities noted during endoscopic examination; increasing uric acid levels; or unexplained persistent polyuria. A left or right lateral approach is used to gain access to the cranial and middle lobes of the kidney. The confluent wall of the caudal thoracic and abdominal air sac is penetrated to access the kidney. The caudal lobe of the kidney is best accessed through a prepubic approach. Biopsy samples can be collected with a size 3, 5, or 7 Fr. forceps. Round cup forceps are recommended.

Testes

Indications for testicular biopsy include suspected dysfunctional testes. A lateral, postischial, or prepubic approach can be used. Size 5 or 7 Fr. round forceps are recommended for sample collection.

Ventriculus

Ventricular biopsies are performed when proventricular dilatation syndrome (PDS) is suspected. Samples of the serosa and muscularis can be endoscopically collected because the thick ventricular muscularis prevents perforation into the lumen. Sites heal well. A lateral approach is recommended. At least two samples are collected along the greater curvature of the ventriculus along the caudoventral surface near a branching blood vessel. Size 7 or 9 Fr. biopsy forceps are recommended for sample collection.

Spleen

Indications for splenic biopsy include persistent systemic disease without an etiologic diagnosis, unexplained persistent splenomegaly, granulomatous inflammation of the spleen, or visualization of lesions on endoscopic examination. A left lateral or postischial approach may be used to biopsy the spleen. The spleen is located near the junction of the proventriculus and ventriculus. Size 5 Fr. elliptical biopsy forceps are recommended to harvest tissue.

SURGERY

Techniques and equipment have been developed that make performance of surgical procedures on birds safe, effective, and often lifesaving. The relatively small size of avian patients requires careful attention to hemostasis and loss of body heat. The presurgical evaluation, use of proper surgical equipment, proper patient preparation, proper surgical technique, and excellent postoperative care help ensure a favorable outcome.

Presurgical Evaluation

Before elective surgical procedures and those surgical procedures where time permits (all but absolute emergency procedures), a complete history, physical examination, and laboratory work-up should be performed. This will identify many birds at risk of dying as a result of the stress of anesthesia, surgery, or postsurgical complications. Birds should be stabilized before surgery unless the surgical procedure is important in stabilizing the bird (e.g., air sac breathing tube placement for tracheal obstruction). A minimum data base should include a complete history, physical examination, hematocrit, plasma protein, uric acid, AST, glucose, and WBC count. When history, physical examination, or laboratory data indicate possible abnormalities, further testing such as additional plasma biochemistries, radiographs, ECG, and cultures are recommended. Respiratory recovery time can be used to evaluate respiratory stability. The respiratory rate should return to normal within 3 to 5 minutes after capture and restraint for at least 2 minutes. A clotting disorder should be suspected if bleeding occurs when mature feathers are pulled during the surgical preparation.

Noted laboratory abnormalities should be evaluated and possible etiologies considered and weighed against possible complications from surgery. Elective procedures may have to be delayed and therapy administered before surgical intervention. Dehydration should be corrected before surgery. Fluid therapy should be administered to patients with a hematocrit above 60%. Surgery should be delayed in birds with a hematocrit less than 20%, or whole blood should be administered. Birds with plasma protein levels below 2 mg/dl are poor surgical candidates. Elective surgery should be postponed and therapy pursued to treat underlying cause. Intraoperative 5% dextrose should be administered IV in birds with a glucose less than 200 mg/dl.

Surgical Equipment

Supplies and equipment suited for avian medicine are recommended. Clear plastic drapes are available and allow better monitoring of the patient (see Table 14–1). A large cloth or paper drape with a large fenestration that allows viewing of the body should be placed over the clear drape to provide a large sterile field. Do not allow drapes to impede respiration.

Instruments should be of appropriate size for the patient. Ophthalmic instruments are often useful. Toothed forceps are seldom appropriate for handling the delicate tissues of birds. Microsurgical instruments can be used. The tips of microsurgical instruments are miniaturized; their handles are rounded, and they do not have clasps for comfortable and smoother use. Hemostatic clips are useful in controlling hemorrhage. Sterile cotton-tipped applicators, surgical spears, and small gauze sponges are useful to absorb fluids. Absorbable gelatin sponges are valuable for hemorrhage control (see Table 14–1).

Magnification instruments are recommended for avian surgery. Binocular magnification loupes or operating microscopes are commonly used. Individual vessels are more easily identified. Support wrists to decrease hand tremors.

Restraint boards facilitate positioning and transport for postoperative radiography (see Table 14–1).

Radiosurgical equipment such as the Ellman Surgitron is recommended for avian surgical procedures (Fig. 14–10). Radiosurgical units aid in the control of hemorrhage. Radiosurgical units cannot be used close to someone with an unshielded pacemaker or in the presence of explosive gases or flammable

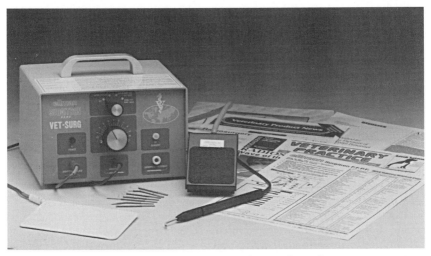

Figure 14–10. An Ellman Surgitron is an excellent radiosurgical unit for use in avian surgery. (Photo courtesy of Ellman International, 1135 Railroad Ave., Hewlett, NY 11557; 516 560-1482.)

fluids (e.g., alcohol). Improper grounding can result in burns or shock. Follow manufacturers' directions and precautions. Cadavers should be used to acquire adequate skills before use on patients.

Wire and fine-tip electrodes are used for removal of delicate tissues and skin incisions. Loop electrodes are used for removing heavier tissues. The current should be activated before contacting tissue when making an incision with a wire electrode. The electrode handle should be held like a writing pen. The handpiece should be held so the electrode is at a right angle to the tissue being incised. The electrode should glide effortlessly through the tissue—pressure does not need to be applied to incise. Use sufficient current, because insufficient current will result in drag. When properly performed, only a slight color change will occur in the tissue. Electrodes should be kept clean to decrease tissue drag. Power settings vary with type of tissue, electrode size, tissue moisture, and the electrosurgical unit used. The Harrison modified ophthalmic bipolar electrode (Ellman) is excellent for creating a skin incision and provides hemostasis for the majority of blood vessels in the skin.

The electrode should be activated after contacting the tissue when used for coagulation. Coagulation should result in a white spot in the tissue. Ball electrodes are used only for coagulation. Bipolar forceps may also be used for coagulation. Larger vessels must be ligated with suture material or hemostatic clips.

Suture Selection

Size 3-0 to 6-0 sutures are commonly used in avian surgery. Catgut and polyglactin 910 cause marked inflammatory responses in birds. Catgut should not be used in avian surgery. Polydioxanone, nylon, and steel cause minimal tissue reaction. Polydioxanone, polyglactin, and catgut are absorbable suture materials, and nylon and steel are nonabsorbable. Monofilament nylon is recommended for contaminated or infected wounds. Multifilament sutures are contraindicated in contaminated or infected wounds. Use of the fewest and finest sutures possible and minimizing surgically induced tissue trauma are important factors in decreasing the risk of wound infection. Birds generally do not traumatize suture lines, allowing the use of continuous suture patterns in the skin. Tie adequate secure knots. Medical-grade tissue adhesives are also useful.

Patient Prep

Fasting is recommended for elective procedures. A fast of 5 to 8 hours is usually sufficient to allow the upper gastrointestinal tract to empty. In birds that cannot be fasted before surgery, the crop should be emptied, the bird induced in an upright position, intubated with a properly sized endotracheal tube, and the head elevated during surgery. Placing gauze in the upper esophagus will further inhibit aspiration of crop contents.

If antibiotics are indicated, perioperative antibiotic therapy should be administered 1 to 2 hours before surgery and maintained for 8 to 16 hours after the surgical procedure.

To prepare the skin for surgery, the feathers should be plucked 2 to 3 cm from the surgical site. Feathers are gently plucked to avoid tearing and bruising the skin. Small feathers may be plucked three or four at a time. Contour and covert feathers should be plucked individually in the direction of their growth. Primary feathers (long wing and tail feathers) are attached to the periostium. These large feathers must be pulled one at a time in the direction of growth while securing the skin, muscle, and bone at the base of the feather. Avoid removal of large feathers. Masking tape, self-adhering tape, water-soluble gel, and/or stockinette can be used to retract feathers. Feathers can be cut if the skin is damaged or torn, to prevent further injury. A clotting disorder should be suspected if bleeding occurs when mature feathers are pulled during the surgical preparation. Excessive feather removal will result in a decrease in insulation and an increase in metabolic demand postsurgically.

Chlorhexidine or povidone iodine can be used for skin preparation. The use of excessive amounts of water, alcohol, or scrub solution may result in hypothermia. Alcohol predisposes to hypothermia and may be hazardous when used with radiosurgery.

Body heat loss should be minimized during surgery with the use of supplemental heat (e.g., circulating warm water blankets, warm water bottles, heat lamps) and by using heated lavage and IV or IO fluids.

If excessive hemorrhage is expected during surgery, intravenous fluids can be administered before or during surgery.

Postoperative Care

Recovering birds should be monitored. Patients should be left intubated as long as their level of anesthesia allows. Recovering birds should be kept in a warm environment at about 85°F (e.g., incubator, intensive care unit). Intravenous or intraosseous fluids should be administered to birds with excessive blood loss. Blood transfusions should be considered in birds with a packed cell volume (PCV) less than 20%. If antibiotics are indicated, therapy should be administered 1 to 2 hours before surgery and maintained for 8 to 12 hours postoperatively. Pain relief should be considered postoperatively. Butorphanol and buprenorphine hydrochloride have been used for pain control in avian patients. Food and water should be placed where they are easily accessible once the bird is alert. Tube feeding or proventricular or duodenal feeding tubes may be indicated in anorectic birds.

Surgical Techniques

Standard aseptic surgical technique is essential in avian surgery. Care should be taken during the surgical procedure that the weight of drapes and placement of the surgeon's hands and instruments do not compromise respiration. A review of many of the surgical techniques commonly performed in avian practice are discussed in the following section; additional information may be found in the references. Referral of surgical cases are recommended until adequate skills have been acquired through continuing education or work on cadavers.

SURGERY OF THE SKIN
Skin Incision

Skin incisions should be made between feather tracts, avoiding feather folli-cles. Skin incisions are best made using the Harrison modified ophthalmic bipolar electrode. Gently grasp the skin with atraumatic forceps, lightly close the tips of the bipolar forceps on the fold of skin, activate the electrode, and withdraw the bipolar forceps. This will create a small incision in the skin. The skin incision is extended by inserting one of the poles of the bipolar forceps subcutaneously, lightly opposing the tips of the forceps, activating the current, and withdrawing the forceps. Close the tips, activate, and withdraw the tips repeatedly until the incision is of adequate length. This technique can be used to create skin incisions and provide hemostasis for the majority of blood vessels.

Skin Wound Repair

Cat and dog bites and scratches should be treated with antibiotics. Secondary bacterial septicemia is common. Puncture wounds should be left open to drain. Small wounds need not be sutured. Large lacerations treated within a few hours are flushed with chlorhexidine solution and sutured closed. Older wounds should be cleaned, debrided, and bandaged twice daily and closed when infection is under control.

Self-mutilation wounds on the trunk are debrided, skin edges trimmed, rolled slightly inverted, sutured, and covered with tissue glue. Wounds on the feet and legs are cleaned and then covered with Tegaderm bandages or hydroactive dressing covered by self-adherent tape (see Table 14–1). Tegaderm bandage is cut into strips and applied in two or three layers. It is left on for 1 to 7 days depending on the condition of the wound. Wounds too extensive to close are left to granulate. Skin grafts can be used. Full-thickness skin grafts revascularize rapidly and can be collected from the flank folds on the inner thighs.

Trauma-induced lacerations of the wing web are sutured. If the associated tendons are transected, the function of the wing web is often affected and return of flight capabilities may not be possible. Lacerations on the legs often require plastic surgical techniques to close. Techniques such as Z-plasty and Y-plasty can be used to close large wounds on the legs and chest. Lacerations on the wings and back often lack adequate skin to allow surgical repair and may be covered with tissue glue and allowed to granulate. Laceration of the ventral surface of the tail caudal to the vent and granulomas of the carina of the sternum (keel) may occur when birds fall with excessive wing trims or have plucked primary flight feathers. Deep debridement and removal of the extensive fat and connec-tive tissue in the caudal tail area will allow wound closure. Two or more horizontal mattress sutures are placed to approximate the edges of the wound, and then the defect is closed with a continuous suture pattern. Granulomas of the carina are debrided of granulation and scar tissue. Digital pressure is used to control the extensive hemorrhage that commonly occurs with debridement in this area. The skin is then dissected free overlying the pectoral muscles and closed.

Skin and Feather Biopsies

Skin biopsies may aid in the diagnosis of the etiology of feather and skin disorders. Skin biopsies are indicated in birds that pluck or chew feathers and in those with chronic dermatoses. Radiosurgery or scissors can be used to collect samples. If radiosurgery is used, minimal power should be used to limit destruction of collected tissue. Biopsies of skin lesions should contain an area that includes normal and abnormal tissue. Feather biopsies should include an actively growing feather, feather follicle, and surrounding skin. The follicle is elevated with hemostats and the skin is cut under the level of the follicle with scissors below the end of the follicle.

Feather Cyst Removal

Feather cysts are hereditary (canaries) or trauma induced. Blade excision appear superior to radiosurgical removal to prevent damage to surrounding follicles. Entire feather tracts may be involved in canaries and can be removed using a fusiform incision. These incisions generally are easily closed and usually do not result in abnormal appearances. Removal of primary feathers requires removal of the entire follicle, including attachments to bone. Take care to preserve adjacent follicles and their blood supply. A tourniquet may be used on the wing to aid in control of hemorrhage.

Constricted Toe Syndrome

Circumferential constrictions may be caused by fibers, scabs, or necrotic tissue and may result in avascular necrosis of the digit distal to the constriction. The affected area is examined with magnification to identify and aid in removal of any fibers, if present. A 25-gauge needle with a bent tip can be used to remove the fibers. The wound should be covered by a hydroactive dressing to prevent desiccation and formation of a constricting scab. In neonates, an increase in humidity, hot moist compresses, and massage of the affected toe may reestablish circulation. If a circular indention is identified, this indented tissue is excised with the aid of magnification. A circumferential skin anastomosis is performed. Two to three subcutaneous sutures are used to hold the skin in apposition, and then the incision is closed with simple interrupted shallow skin sutures. Release incisions are then made on the medial and lateral aspects of the digit longitudinally across the anastomosis. The wound is covered with a hydroactive dressing to keep tissues moist and prevent formation of a constricting scab.

SURGERY OF THE RESPIRATORY TRACT

Infraorbital Sinusitis

Abscessation of the infraorbital sinus is a common sequella to untreated sinusitis. Surgical exploration and curettage are recommended. A horizontal incision is made over the suborbital arch with radiosurgery. Purulent material is removed by curettage and flushing with sterile saline. The exudate should be cultured, and appropriate antibiotics should be initiated. Gelatin sponges and digital pressure are used to control hemorrhage.

Air Sac Breathing Tube Placement

The left lateral approach is commonly used. The bird is anesthetized and restrained in right lateral recumbancy. The procedure can be performed without anesthesia in birds in critical condition; however, oxygen administration during induction of anesthesia often improves oxygenation and results in increased response and struggling, making anesthesia preferable. The wings are extended dorsally and taped to a restraint board or table. The left leg is extended cranially. The skin is incised just caudal to the last rib and just ventral to the flexor cruruis medialis muscle (as in a left lateral endoscopic approach). The muscle is bluntly dissected with mosquito forceps. The forceps are gently pushed through the body wall in a craniomedial direction and are held open to allow passage of a sterile tube. The tube is inserted through this opening in a craniomedial direction into the caudal thoracic air sac space. Feeding tubes, plastic intravenous catheters, or small endotracheal tubes can be used for breathing tubes. A tape butterfly is placed on the tube to allow suturing of the tube to the skin with small nonabsorbable suture material. The tube is removed when no longer needed and the defect is surgically closed.

SURGERY OF THE GASTROINTESTINAL TRACT

Celiotomy

Birds should be positioned with the head elevated to prevent the flow of fluids into the lungs. Moistened cotton or gauze sponges can be placed in the caudal oropharynx to prevent crop and proventricular reflux from entering the trachea and aspiration. Fluid should be removed from the body cavity before opening the air sacs in birds with ascites. Stirrups can be placed around the tarsometatarsus of the legs for positioning. Incision of air sac membranes will result in release of anesthetic gases and may cause difficulty in maintaining adequate anesthetic levels. The incision can be covered with saline moistened gauze sponges for several breaths while increasing the level of anesthesia to increase depth of anesthesia. An air sac breathing tube can be placed in the contralateral side for anesthesia maintenance.

The celiotomy approaches commonly used include left lateral, ventral midline, and transverse. These are modified or combined for increased exposure.

A left lateral celiotomy provides exposure to the proventriculus, ventriculus, female reproductive tract, and left kidney. The bird is placed in right lateral recumbancy. The wings are extended dorsally and taped. The right leg is pulled ventrally, and the left leg is rotated at the hip and pulled as far caudally and dorsally as is possible. The skin is incised from the cranial extent of the pubis craniodorsally to just dorsal to the uncinate process of the fifth or sixth rib (Fig.

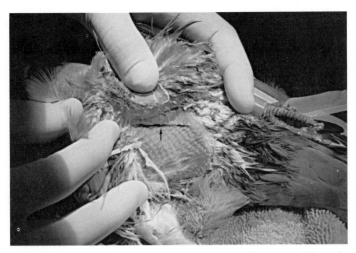

Figure 14–11. A left lateral celiotomy approach. The skin is incised from the cranial extent of the pubis craniodorsally to just dorsal to the uncinate process of the fifth or sixth rib (*arrow*).

14–11). Care must be taken to incise only the skin. The left leg can then be repositioned further dorsal and caudal to allow access to the left lateral body wall. Identify and coagulate or ligate the superficial medial femoral artery and vein that passes over the lumbar fossa toward the ventral midline. The vessels are identified and can be coagulated by grasping the vessels with bipolar forceps and activating the current in two places along the vessels. The intercostal blood vessels associated with the last two or three ribs should be coagulated in a similar manner. The vessels run along the cranial border of the ribs and should be coagulated where they will be transected just dorsal to the junction between the sternal and vertebral ribs (where they make a sharp bend). The vessels are coagulated, the ribs transected, and the abdominal wall is incised using bipolar forceps. In larger birds, the vessels may require clamping to achieve hemostasis and the caudal two or three ribs may need to be removed to gain adequate exposure. Care must be taken to incise only the musculature and ribs. In some birds, the lungs extend to the seventh rib, and care must be taken to avoid laceration of the lung. Small retractors are used to maintain exposure. The air sac membranes are incised as needed to obtain exposure. The intestines can be gently retracted with saline moistened cotton tipped applicators. To close, the body wall and skin are closed separately with 4-0 to 6-0 absorbable suture material in a continuous or interrupted pattern. Release of the left leg will allow apposition of the muscles. Closure of large incisions may be facilitated by passing sutures around the pubis. If ribs have been removed, tension sutures may be placed from the body wall musculature around the last intact rib.

A ventral midline celiotomy is used primarily for procedures requiring exposure of both sides of the celomic cavity (e.g., surgery of the small intestine, liver biopsies, peritonitis, abdominal masses, egg binding, repair of cloacal prolapse). The bird is placed in dorsal recumbancy. The wings are extended and taped into position. The legs are pulled caudally and taped into position using tape stirrups.

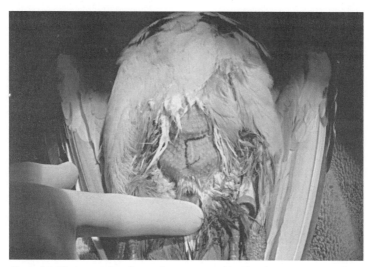

Figure 14–12. A ventral midline celiotomy approach. The skin incision is made on the midline several millimeters caudal to the apex of the sternum and cranial to the vent. Flaps may be created cranially and/or caudally by incising a few millimeters from the sternum and/or pubic bone.

The skin incision is made on the midline several millimeters caudal to the apex of the sternum and cranial to the vent (Fig. 14–12). The linea alba appears as a thin layer of fibrous tissue. The linea alba is incised by picking up the linea with nontraumatic forceps and making an incision with bipolar forceps between the pubic bones. Care must be taken to incise only the linea alba, because the duodenum lies directly inside the body wall. The incision can be extended for greater exposure by incising the body wall approximately 2 mm from the sternal border, creating a flap. The body wall can be incised cranial to the pubis to create a caudal flap. The body wall and skin are closed separately with 4-0 to 6-0 absorbable suture material in a continuous or interrupted pattern.

A transverse celiotomy provides exposure to a large area of the celom. The bird is placed in dorsal recumbancy. The wings are extended and taped into position. The legs are pulled caudally and taped into position using tape stirrups. A transverse skin incision is made midway between the sternum and the vent. The body wall is lifted and incised taking care to avoid lacerating the underlying intestines. The duodenum and ventriculus can be retracted using a saline-moistened cotton-tipped applicator to expose the kidneys, cloaca, and female reproductive tract. The body wall and skin are closed separately with 4-0 to 6-0 absorbable suture material in a continuous or interrupted pattern.

Crop Surgery

Common crop surgeries include ingluvotomy (crop incision), crop biopsy, and crop burn repair. Indications for ingluvotomy include crop foreign body, food retention, or to gain access to the caudal esophagus to allow endoscopy of the proventriculus and ventriculus. To perform an ingluvotomy, the bird is intubated and placed in dorsal recumbancy with the head elevated and the esophagus occluded with moist cotton or gauze to prevent aspiration of refluxed crop material. The wings are extended and taped into position. The legs are pulled caudally and taped into position using tape stirrups. The site is surgically prepped. Clear drapes are recommended. The skin is incised over the cranial edge of the left lateral sac of the crop. The crop is incised with a blade in an avascular area approximately half the desired length because the crop easily stretches. Use of radiosurgery for the crop incision results in needless trauma, but radiosurgery is used to coagulate vessels as needed. The crop incision is closed using an inverting pattern with an absorbable suture material on an atraumatic needle. A two-layer closure may be necessary to prevent leakage. The crop can be inflated with air or saline to check for leakage before closure of the skin. The skin is closed with 4-0 to 6-0 absorbable suture material in a continuous pattern.

A crop biopsy is used to provide a tissue sample for histopathology of abnormal lesions or for diagnosis of PDS. Crop biopsy is a lower-risk procedure than proventricular and ventricular biopsies. In birds with clinical signs of PDS that involve the crop (e.g., vomiting, delayed crop emptying) histopathology of a sample of crop tissue frequently identifies PDS-affected birds. A negative result does not rule out PDS. The technique for crop biopsy is similar to an ingluvotomy. The skin is bluntly dissected from the crop to expose a portion of the crop. The section of crop to be harvested should include a blood vessel to increase chances of obtaining nerve tissue. The crop is incised approximately 2 cm and another incision is made parallel to and 1 cm from the first. This section is removed and submitted for histopathology. The crop is closed using the technique for ingluvotomy.

Crop burns are a common problem in hand-fed neonates. Identification of crop burns is discussed in Chapter 4. Treatment includes feeding reduced volumes of food more frequently, placing the bird on antibiotics and antifungals (e.g., enrofloxacin and ketoconazole), and monitoring the bird until the wound contracts and a fistula appears (7 to 14 days postinjury). Food and water may leak from the fistula. When the wound contracts, the scab is removed and the necrotic portion of the skin and crop are surgically excised. All necrotic tissue is removed. The area is flushed to remove all debris. The skin and crop are meticulously dissected apart. The crop and skin are closed as described for an ingluvotomy. A simple continuous appositional pattern over sewn with an inverting pattern can be used when reduced crop size is a concern. Surgery before wound contraction is often unsuccessful because devitalized and healthy tissue cannot be differentiated. Surgical adhesives can be used to close the wound if food begins to leak before wound contracture. Severe burns may require feeding via a proventricular feeding tube before surgery.

Proventricular (Pharyngostomy) Feeding Tube Placement

A proventricular feeding tube can be used to supply nutrition when the mouth, esophagus, or crop must be bypassed. The skin is surgically prepped at the caudal extent of the right mandible. A moistened cotton tipped applicator is inserted through the mouth into the esophagus. A small incision is made through the skin, and a stab incision is made into the esophagus. A feeding tube is passed through the incision and advanced through the crop and lower esophageal sphincter. The tube is sutured in place and a bandage is used to hold the tube on the dorsal cervical area. Feed the amount the proventriculus will accommodate every 2 hours (approximately 20 ml in macaws). When the tube is removed, the esophagus and skin defects are allowed to heal by second intention.

Proventriculotomy

Proventriculotomy is most commonly indicated for the removal of foreign bodies and toxic material. A left lateral approach is used. The abdominal musculature is incised and retracted, exposing the ventriculus and proventriculus. Air sac membranes and suspensory ligaments are bluntly dissected to allow the proventriculus to be retracted caudally. Two stay sutures can be placed in the white tendonous portion of the ventriculus to aid in exteriorization of the ventriculus and manipulation of the proventriculus. Stay sutures should not be placed in the proventriculus. The liver can be gently retracted with saline-moistened cotton-tipped applicators. The proventriculus and ventriculus should be isolated with moist gauze sponges to prevent contamination of the body cavity with gastric contents. An incision is made in an avascular area of the isthmus of the proventriculus with a blade, scissors, or bipolar forceps. The isthmus is the constriction between the proventriculus and ventriculus. Suction and flushing are used to evacuate gastric contents. The incision is extended cranially as needed. The incision can be extended caudally if a ventriculotomy is required. Curettes or small spoons may be used to remove objects. The proventriculus is closed with a simple continuous appositional pattern oversewn with a continuous or interrupted inverting pattern with a fine absorbable suture material using a small atraumatic needle. The incision should be closed beyond the limits of the incision to achieve a seal. Meticulous closure is important to prevent leakage. An orogastric tube can be placed and the proventriculus and the stomach inflated with air or sterile saline to check for leakage. Food and water are offered upon recovery from anesthesia. A duodenal feeding tube can be placed to allow alimentation if the proventricular wall appears thin and friable.

Ventriculotomy

Ventriculotomy is commonly used to retrieve foreign bodies. The approach for proventriculotomy is used for exposure. The ventriculus can be entered as described with the proventriculotomy, or an incision can be made transversely across the muscle fibers in the lighter colored elliptical area of the ventriculus. The ventriculus is closed using 3-0 to 5-0 absorbable suture material on a swaged on atraumatic needle in a simple interrupted pattern. Place sutures close together to help prevent leakage of gastric contents.

Intestinal Surgery

Intestinal surgery is not commonly performed on birds. Closure of an accidental enterotomy site, an intestinal anastamosis, and placement of duodenal feeding tubes are occasionally performed on avian patients. Closure of an enterotomy site may be required as a result of an accidental enterotomy during a celiotomy. A poor prognosis is associated with enterotomies. A ventral midline, ventral midline with a flap, or transverse celiotomy may be used, depending on the location of the lesion. Microsurgical techniques and equipment are recommended. The intestines are closed using 6-0 to 10-0 monofilament absorbable suture material on a swaged on atraumatic needle in a simple interrupted appositional pattern.

An intestinal anastamosis may be performed to remove constrictions or necrotic bowel. See VanDerHeyden (1993) for techniques to perform intestinal anastamoses.

Intestinal feeding tubes may be used to provide nutritional supplementation in birds in which a portion of the gastrointestinal tract must be bypassed. A ventral midline celiotomy is used to place a through the needle catheter (such as a jugular catheter) in the descending duodenum. The needle is first passed through the left abdominal wall and then into the descending duodenum. The duodenal loop can be identified by the presence of the pancreas between the descending and ascending segments. The catheter is advanced into the ascending duodenum and the needle is withdrawn from the intestine and body wall. The duodenum is sutured to the body wall with an absorbable suture material at the site of catheter placement. The catheter is sutured to the outside body wall by passing the suture ends around the catheter three or four times. The needle is protected within the snapguard, and the catheter is flushed and then routed behind the leg and wing and attached at the base of the neck with sutures. Commercially available liquid diets can be slowly injected into the intestine through the catheter. The catheter should be flushed and capped after each feeding. Four to six feedings per day are typically required.

Cloacal

Common cloacal surgeries include cloacapexy and treatment of cloacal papillomas. Cloacal papillomas are discussed in Chapter 9.

Cloacal prolapse may occur as a result of enteritis or may be idiopathic. Minor prolapses of the cloaca are reduced and held in place with stay sutures while the underlying cause is treated. Two mattress sutures or two transverse sutures of nonabsorbable suture material are placed perpendicular to the vent. Care must be taken to allow the normal passage of droppings. Severe prolapses or recurring prolapses may require cloacapexy. A ventral midline celiotomy is performed. The urodeum can be more easily identified if moistened, cotton-tipped applicators or a gloved finger of an assistant is placed in the cloaca. The fat is excised from the ventral aspect of the cloaca. Size 3-0 polyglactin 910 is recommended to anchor the cloaca to the ribs. Sutures are passed around the last rib and then full thickness through the cloaca and tied with enough tension to invert the vent slightly. Two sutures are placed on each side. It is important to penetrate the cloacal lumen and to take large bites of urodeum tissue in the sutures. The cloacal wall is incorporated into the closure of the body wall to allow the formation of adhesions. The suture is passed through one side of the body wall, then through the full thickness of the cloaca, and then through the other side of the body wall. The skin is closed over the body wall in a separate layer in a routine manner.

Liver Biopsy

A ventral midline celiotomy is performed to gain access to the liver. The tissue sample can be harvested with a wire loop radiosurgical tip or with suture material. For radiosurgical collection, the unit is changed from bipolar to mono-polar and the current is activated before contact with liver tissue. The current is activated and the loop is passed through the tissue, excising a section of liver tissue and coagulating blood vessels. If suture material is used to collect the tissue sample, a loop of suture material is placed around a point of the liver. The suture is tightened, cutting through the liver parenchyma. The sample is transected distal to the suture. If any residual hemorrhage occurs, gelatin sponges may be applied to help control bleeding.

FEMALE REPRODUCTIVE TRACT

Common female reproductive tract surgeries include salpingohysterectomy, ovocentesis, and correction of egg binding. Ovocentesis and egg binding are discussed in Chapter 15. Salpingohysterectomy is performed to treat egg binding when medical therapy and ovocentesis fail, to remove an infected or ruptured oviduct, to treat a prolapsed oviduct, and to treat recurring egg-related peritonitis. It is commonly used in cockatiels to stop chronic egg laying and prevent complications associated with chronic egg laying when husbandry and medical therapies have failed and the risk of complications from the chronic egg laying outweigh the surgical risks. The oviduct and uterus are removed, but the ovary is left intact because of the difficulty in removal and because uterine control of ovarian development apparently occurs in most pet birds. A left lateral celiotomy is performed. The proventriculus and ventriculus are retracted to expose the reproductive tract along the dorsal aspect of the body cavity. The avascular ventral suspensory ligament is identified and dissected to allow the oviduct and uterus to be stretched out. The ventral suspensory ligament causes the oviduct and uterus to convolute into numerous folds. The blood vessel coursing from the ovary to the infundibulum is identified and coagulated or clipped with two small hemostatic clips at the ovary. If this vessel is accidentally torn, a gelatin sponge can be applied to stop the hemorrhage. The vessels in the dorsal suspensory ligament can then be visualized and coagulated with bipolar forceps or clips applied to larger vessels. The infundibulum is bluntly dissected from the ovary, and the dorsal suspensory ligament is dissected to the level of the junction of the uterus with the vagina near the cloaca. The uterus is ligated at its junction with the vagina with one or two hemostatic clips or a ligature. If vaginal tissue has been damaged, clips may be applied at the cloaca, with care not to entrap the ureter. The body cavity is inspected for hemorrhage before routine closure of the body wall and skin.

MISCELLANEOUS PROCEDURES

Abdominal Hernia

Abdominal hernias occur most commonly in middle-aged or older female birds. Budgies, cockatiels, and sulphur-crested cockatoos appear most commonly affected. Hormone imbalance, chronic egg laying, and altered calcium metabolism have been suggested as possible causes. Nutritional deficiencies should be corrected, and concurrent diseases (e.g., hepatic lipidosis, obesity) should be treated before surgical correction whenever possible. Most abdominal hernias are of little clinical significance; however, many will enlarge and are generally easier to repair when they are small. Closure of the body wall may result in respiratory compromise as a result of the replaced abdominal viscera compression on the abdominal and thoracic air sacs. To minimize recurrence, a salpingo-hysterectomy is recommended at the time of surgery. A mesh implant may be used to reinforce the abdominal wall.

Fracture Repair

Fracture repair is discussed in Chapter 7.

References and Additional Readings

Altman RB. Electrosurgery. *Proc Assoc Avian Vet* 1990;360–364.

Altman RB. Avian neonatal and pediatric surgery. *Semin Avian Exot Pet Med* 1992;1(1):34–39.

Altman RB. A method for reducing exposure of operating room personnel to anesthetic gas. *J Assoc Avian Vet* 1992;6(2):99–101.

Altman RB. Beak repair, acrylics. In Altman RB, Clubb SL, Dorrestein GM, Quesenberry K (eds): *Avian Medicine and Surgery*. Philadelphia, WB Saunders, 1997, pp 787–799.

Altman RB. General surgical considerations. In Altman RB, Clubb SL, Dorrestein GM, Quesenberry K (eds): *Avian Medicine and Surgery*. Philadelphia, WB Saunders, 1997, pp 691–703.

Altman RB. Radiosurgery (electrosurgery). In Altman RB, Clubb SL, Dorrestein GM, Quesenberry K (eds): *Avian Medicine and Surgery*. Philadelphia, WB Saunders, 1997, pp 767–772.

Altman RB. Soft tissue surgical procedures. In Altman RB, Clubb SL, Dorrestein GM, Quesenberry K (eds): *Avian Medicine and Surgery*. Philadelphia, WB Saunders, 1997, pp 704–732.

Bauck L. Analgesics in avian medicine. *Proc Assoc Avian Vet* 1990;239–244.

Bennett RA. A review of avian soft tissue surgery. *Proc Assoc Avian Vet* 1993;65–71.

Bennett RA. Instrumentation, preparation, and suture materials for avian surgery. *Semin Avian Exot Pet Med* 1993;2(2):62–68.

Bennett RA. Surgical considerations. In Ritchie BW, Harrison GJ, Harrison LR (eds): *Avian Medicine: Principles and Application*. Lake Worth, FL, Wingers, 1994, pp 1081–1095.

Bennett RA. Avian soft tissue surgery wet lab. *Proc Assoc Avian Vet Lab Manual* 1995;43–47.

Bennett RA. Review of orthopedic surgery. *Proc Assoc Avian Vet* 1995;291–296.

Bennett RA, Harrison GJ. Soft tissue surgery. In Ritchie BW, Harrison GJ, Harrison LR (eds): *Avian Medicine: Principles and Application.* Lake Worth, FL, Wingers, 1994, pp 1121–1124.

Bennett RA, Kuzma AB. Fracture management in birds. *J Zoo Wildl Med* 1991;23(1):5–38.

Bennett RA, Yeager M, Trapp A, et al. Tissue reaction to five suture materials in pigeons *(Columba livia). Proc Assoc Avian Vet* 1992;212–218.

Brown RE, Klemm RD. Surgical anatomy of the propatagium. *Proc Assoc Avian Vet* 1990;176–181.

Castro L, Speer BL. Anesthesia for the avian technician. *Proc Assoc Avian Vet* 1991;311–313.

Clipsham R. Surgical beak restoration and correction. *Proc Assoc Avian Vet* 1989:164–176.

Clipsham R. Surgical correction of beaks. *Proc Assoc Avian Vet* 1990:788–789.

Clipsham R. Beak repair, rhamphorthotics. In Altman RB, Clubb SL, Dorrestein GM, Quesenberry K (eds): *Avian Medicine and Surgery.* Philadelphia, WB Saunders, 1997, pp 773–786.

Cooper JE. Avian endoscopy. In Brearley MJ, Cooper JE, Sullivan M (eds): *Colour Atlas of Small Animal Endoscopy.* St. Louis, Mosby–Year Book, 1991, pp 97–109.

Cooper JE. Endoscopy in avian medicine. In Raw ME, Parkinson TJ (eds): *The Veterinary Annual,* vol 32. London, Blackwell, 1992, pp 129–137.

Cooper JE. Biopsy techniques. *Semin Avian Exot Pet Med* 1994;3(3):161–165.

Cooper JE, Schildger BJ. Endoscopy in exotic species In Brearley MJ, Cooper JE, Sullivan M (eds): *Colour Atlas of Small Animal Endoscopy.* St. Louis, Mosby, 1991, pp 111–122.

Degernes LA, Redig PT. Soft tissue wound management in avian patients. *Proc Assoc Avian Vet* 1990;182–190.

Doolen M. Crop biopsy: A low risk diagnosis for neuropathic gastric dilatation. *Proc Assoc Avian Vet* 1994;193–196.

Doyle JE. Introduction to microsurgery. In Harrison GJ, Harrison LR (eds): *Clinical Avian Medicine and Surgery.* Philadelphia, WB Saunders, 1986, pp 568–576.

Dustin LR. Surgery of the avian respiratory system. *Semin Avian Exot Pet Med* 1993;2(2):83–90.

Flammer K. Update on avian anesthesia. In Kirk RW, Bonagura JD (eds): *Current Veterinary Therapy X, Small Animal Practice.* Philadelphia, WB Saunders, 1989, pp 776–780.

Greenacre CB, Watson E, Ritchie BW. Choanal atresia in a African grey parrot *(Psittacus erithacus erithacus)* and an umbrella cockatoo *(Cacatua alba). J Assoc Avian Vet* 1993;7(1):19–22.

Hannon DE, McGehee NW, Weber TD. Use of a single pedicle advancement flap for wound repair in a great horned owl *(Bubo virginianus). Proc Assoc Avian Vet* 1995;285–289.

Harris JM. Teflon dermal stent for the correction of subcutaneous emphysema. *Proc Assoc Avian Vet* 1991;20–21.

Harrison GJ. Anesthesiology. In Harrison GJ, Harrison LR (eds): *Clinical Avian Medicine and Surgery.* Philadelphia, WB Saunders, 1986, pp 549–559.

Harrison GJ. Evaluation and support of the surgical patient. In Harrison GJ, Harrison LR (eds): *Clinical Avian Medicine and Surgery.* Philadelphia, WB Saunders, 1986, pp 543–548.

Harrison GJ. Selected surgical procedures. In Harrison GJ, Harrison LR (eds): *Clinical Avian Medicine and Surgery.* Philadelphia, WB Saunders, 1986, pp 577–586.

Harrison GJ. Surgical instrumentation and special techniques. In Harrison GJ, Harrison

LR (eds): *Clinical Avian Medicine and Surgery.* Philadelphia, WB Saunders, 1986, pp 560–567.

Harrison GJ. Surgical repair of crop injuries. *AAV Today* 1987;1(2):63.

Harrison GJ. Anesthesia and common surgical procedures. *Proc Assoc Avian Vet* 1990; 460–488.

Heard DJ. Anesthesia and analgesia. In Altman RB, Clubb SL, Dorrestein GM, Quesenberry K (eds): *Avian Medicine and Surgery.* Philadelphia, WB Saunders, 1997, pp 807–827.

Hochleithner M. Cystadenoma in an African grey parrot *(Psittacus erithacus).* *J Assoc Avian Vet* 1990;4(3):163–165.

Hochleithner M. Endoscopy. In Altman RB, Clubb SL, Dorrestein GM, Quesenberry K (eds): *Avian Medicine and Surgery.* Philadelphia, WB Saunders, 1997, pp 800–806.

Howard PE, et al. Surgical removal of a tracheal foreign body from a whooping crane *(Grus americana).* *J Zoo Wildl Med* 1991;22(3):359–363.

Hunter DB, Taylor M. Lung biopsy as a diagnostic technique in avian medicine. *Proc Assoc Avian Vet* 1992;207–211.

Jenkins JR. Avian soft tissue surgery: Part I and part II. *Proc Am Coll Vet Surg* 1992;631–636.

Jenkins JR. Postoperative care of the avian patient. *Semin Avian Exot Pet Med* 1993;2(2):97–102.

Jones BD. Laparoscopy. *Vet Clin North Am Small Animal Pract* 1990;20:1243–1263.

Kenny D, Cambre RC. Indications and technique for the surgical removal of the avian yolk sac. *J Zoo Wildl Med* 1992;23(1):55–61.

King AS, McLelland J. *Birds: Their Structure and Function.* Philadelphia, Bailliere Tindall, 1984.

King WW, Tully TN. Management of a large cutaneous defect in a moluccan cockatoo. *Proc Assoc Avian Vet* 1993;142–145.

Kollias GV, Harrison GJ. Biopsy techniques. In Harrison GJ, Harrison LR (eds): *Clinical Avian Medicine and Surgery.* Philadelphia, WB Saunders, 1986, pp 245–249.

LaBonde J. The medical and surgical management of domestic waterfowl collections. *Proc Assoc Avian Vet* 1992;223–233.

LaBonde J, Michel C. Anesthesia monitoring and intraoperative support of the avian patient. *Proc Assoc Avian Vet* 1995;271–274.

Lloyd M. Heavy metal ingestion: Medical management and gastroscopic foreign body removal. *J Assoc Avian Vet* 1992;6(1):25–29.

MacCoy DM. General principles of avian surgery. *Compend Contin Ed* 1991;13:989–993.

MacWhirter P. A review of 60 cases of abdominal hernias in birds. *Proc Assoc Avian Vet* 1994;27–37.

Martin HD, Ritchie BW. Orthopedic surgical techniques. In Ritchie BW, Harrison GJ, Harrison LR (eds): *Avian Medicine: Principles and Application.* Lake Worth, FL, Wingers, 1994, pp 1137–1169.

McCluggage D. Hysterectomy: A review of select cases. *Proc Assoc Avian Vet* 1992;201–206.

McCluggage D. Proventriculotomy: A study of select cases. *Proc Assoc Avian Vet* 1992;195–200.

McCluggage DM. Surgery of the integument: Selected topics. *Semin Avian Exot Pet Med* 1993;2(2):76–82.

Mulloy P. The avian surgical patient. *Proc Assoc Avian Vet* 1996;327–330.

Murray MJ, Taylor M. Retrieval of proventricular and ventricular foreign bodies with rigid endoscopic equipment. *Proc Assoc Avian Vet* 1995;281–284.

Orosz SE, Ensley PK, Haynes DJ. *Avian Surgical Anatomy: Thoracic and Pelvic Limbs.* Philadelphia, WB Saunders, 1992.

Phalen DN, Mitchell ME, Cavazos-Martinez ML. Evaluation of three heat sources for their ability to maintain core body temperature in the anesthetized patient. *J Avian Med Surg* 1996;10(3):174–178.

Rich GA. Surgery of the head. *Semin Avian Exot Pet Med* 1993;2(2):69–75.

Ritchie BW, Doyle JE, Harrison GJ. Micro Techniques for the Surgical Management of Avian Disease. Lake Worth, FL, Research Institute for Avian Medicine, Nutrition and Reproduction, 1990, pp 13–18.

Rode J, Bartholow S, Ludders J. Ventilation through an air sac cannula. *J Assoc Avian Vet* 1990;4:98–101.

Rosskopf WJ, Woerpel RW. Cloacal conditions in pet birds with a cloaca-pexy update. *Proc Assoc Avian Vet* 1989;156–163.

Rosskopf WJ, Woerpel RW. Abdominal air sac breathing tube placement in psittacine birds and raptors: Its use as an emergency airway in cases of tracheal obstruction. *Proc Assoc Avian Vet* 1990;215–217.

Rosskopf WJ, Woerpel RW. Avian obstetrical medicine. *Proc Assoc Avian Vet* 1993;323–336.

Rosskopf WJ, Woerpel RW. Avian obstetrical medicine. In Birchard SJ, Sherding RG (eds): *Saunders Manual of Small Animal Practice.* Philadelphia, WB Saunders, 1994, pp 1302–1311.

Rosskopf WJ, Woerpel RW, Blake SR. Sinus trephination of the supra-orbital sinuses in psittacine birds: An aid in the treatment of chronic sinus infections. *Proc Assoc Avian Vet* 1986;295–301.

Rosskopf WJ, Woerpel RW, Shindo MK, et al. Surgery of the avian respiratory system. *Proc Assoc Avian Vet* 1993;199–206.

Sinn L. Anesthesiology. In Ritchie BW, Harrison GJ, Harrison LR (eds): *Avian Medicine: Principles and Application.* Lake Worth, Wingers, 1994, pp 1066–1080.

Satterfield WC. Avian endoscopy. *Vet Clin North Am Small Anim Pract* 1990;20:1356–1363.

Suedmeyer WK, Bermudez. A new approach to renal biopsy in birds. *J Avian Med Surg* 1996;10(3):179–186.

Taylor M. A morphologic approach to the endoscopic determination of sex in juvenile macaws. *J Assoc Avian Vet* 1989;3(4):199–201.

Taylor M. Endoscopy. *Proc Assoc Avian Vet* 1990;319–324.

Taylor M. A new endoscopic system for the collection of diagnostic specimens in the bird. *Proc Assoc Avian Vet* 1993;83–86.

Taylor M. Endoscopic examination and biopsy techniques. In Ritchie BW, Harrison GJ, Harrison LR (eds): *Avian Medicine: Principles and Application.* Lake Worth, FL, Wingers, 1994, pp 327–354.

Taylor M. Endoscopic techniques. *Semin Avian Exot Pet Med* 1994;3(3):126–132.

Taylor M. Biopsy techniques in avian medicine. *Proc Assoc Avian Vet* 1995;275–280.

Thorstad CL. Anesthesia and monitoring of the surgical patient. *Proc Assoc Avian Vet* 1992;471–475.

VanDerHeyden N. Jejunostomy and jejunocloacal anastomosis in macaws. *Proc Assoc Avian Vet* 1993;72–77.

Van Sant F. Surgery of the avian gastrointestinal tract. *Semin Avian Exot Pet Med* 1993;2(2):91–96.

Wheler C. Avian anesthetics, analgesics, and tranquilizers. *Semin Avian Exot Pet Med* 1993;2(1):7–12.

Chapter 15

Aviculture and Obstetrics

Reproductive disorders are common in birds. Diagnosis of the etiology of reproductive disorders requires an understanding of avian theriogenology. Theriogenology in birds includes aviculture practices, reproduction, obstetrics, egg production, and incubation.

Husbandry, nutrition, the environment, and reproductive organ health play major roles in reproductive success and failure. Aviary management critically affects production and must be evaluated in addition to the health of reproductive organs. Clinical and subclinical disease identification, education, and management flaws are areas in which veterinarians can play an important role in aviary production.

Determination of gender is important for production in birds and is hindered by the fact that many species of birds are monomorphic (males and females appear similar). Pairing of same sex birds is a common cause of lack of reproductive success in psittacines.

Some species of birds are monogamous (bond into pairs), whereas others are polygamous. In general, psittacines, passerines, toucans, swans, geese, and some gallinaceous birds are monogamous. Some gallinaceous birds are polygamous. Ducks pair for a season, but they may pair with different partners the next season.

The veterinarian can provide individual bird medical expertise, avicultural management knowledge, nutritional recommendations, and record-keeping systems and their review for aviculturists. An aviary file should be maintained with individual bird medical information; this is essential for avicultural medical management. The veterinarian should provide a reminder system for physical examinations, laboratory sampling, vaccinations, and breeder performance reviews. Make use of specialists to aid in increasing production, including species specialists, nutritionists, toxicologists, reproductive physiologists, virologists, immunologists, environmental and mechanical engineers, and others knowledgeable in associated areas.

AVIARY MANAGEMENT

Flock health is oriented to the group of birds rather than the individual bird. Diseases of individual birds must be identified and used to determine management changes necessary for future disease prevention. Most diseases, infectious and noninfectious, are the result of management problems. Because multiple

465

birds may be involved, fast and accurate diagnosis of diseases is essential. Search for management practices that allowed the development of the illness or the introduction of the disease. Stop the losses as soon and effectively as possible, but recommend management changes to prevent further losses and introduction of other diseases. Persistent or frequent drug therapy warrants evaluation for an underlying management problem.

Limiting species variety aids in disease control. Requirements, disease susceptibilities, management requirements, and nutritional needs vary with the species of bird. Concentration on a few species often allows better concentration on the needs of those species and increases production. Table 15–1 lists average breeding characteristics of some common psittacine species.

Evaluate birds according to the goals of the aviary. Birds not meeting these goals are evaluated medically (management or husbandry changes, behavior analysis, and infertility examination), relocated, or culled. Make recommendations of management changes based on the goals of the aviary, weighing the cost against the benefits.

Common problem areas in aviary management include lack of record keeping, malnutrition, poor sanitation and disinfection protocols, inappropriate flock therapy, lack of a quarantine area, unrealistic overhead, lack of understanding of the needs of each species being bred (behavioral and psychological demands), improper housing of specific species relative to their needs, lack of a culling protocol, and lack of accurate sex determination. As mentioned above, most flock diseases are a symptom of management problems. Common infectious diseases of economic impact in avicultural settings include polyomavirus, psittacine beak and feather disease (PBFD), proventricular dilatation syndrome (PDS), chlamydiosis, Pacheco's disease, and parasitism (tapeworms, roundworms, giardia, lice, mites, etc.). Common noninfectious diseases include infertility and suboptimal production.

Purchasing Birds for the Aviary

Aviculturists should never purchase birds without first examining them. Some things the buyer should look for include overall appearance, stance, body mass, vision evaluation, leg and wing abnormalities, early lesions of PBFD in commonly affected species, and choanal and cloacal papillomas in macaws, mini-macaws, and Amazon parrots.

A written contract should be part of the sales agreement. All stipulations and agreements should be listed, including price, number of birds, species, identification, return/replacement policy and terms (or sold "as is"), and financial and medical responsibility for diagnosis of preexisting disease or postpurchase development of disease within a stated period of time.

All purchased birds should enter the aviary through the quarantine area of the facility.

Aviary Construction

Outdoor aviaries are limited to areas of constant year-round mild climate. Enclosed aviaries must provide both insulation and ventilation. Appropriate

TABLE 15–1 Average Breeding Characteristics of Some Common Psittacine Species

Species	Breeding Season	Eggs per Clutch/Offspring	Incubation Period (days)	Fledging Age (days)*	Weaning Age Parent-Raised (days)†	Weaning Age Hand-Reared (days)‡	Breeding Age§
Budgerigar	All year	4-9/4-8	16	22-26	30-40	30	6 mo.
Cockatiel	All year	3-7/4-5	18	32-38	47-52	42-49	6 mo.
Australian parakeet	Spring	3-5/3-5	18-19	30-45	50-65	NA	1-3 yr.
Princess parakeet	Spring/late spring/summer	3-5/3-5	18	32-38	50-55	NA	1 yr.
Ring-neck parakeet	Early summer	3-5/4	23-24	40-45	55-65	NA	3 yr.
Lovebirds	All year	2-6/3-5	18	30-35	45-55	40-45	6 mo.
Lories/lorikeets	Early spring/spring	2-4/2	21	42-50	62-70	50-60	2 yr.
Conures	Spring/late spring/summer	2-8/2-6	21-23	35-40	45-70	60	2-3 yr.
Amazon parrots	Spring/late spring/summer	2-4/2	23-24	45-60	90-120	75-90	4-6 yr.
Small-sized macaws	Spring/late spring/summer	2-4/2	23-24	45-60	90-120	75-90	4-6 yr.
Large-sized macaws	Early spring/spring/late spring/summer	2-4/2-3	26-28	70-80	120-150	95-120	5-7 yr.
African gray	Spring/late spring/summer	2-4/2-4	24-26	50-65	100-120	75-90	4-6 yr.
Medium-sized cockatoos	Early spring/spring/late spring/summer	2-4/2	23-25	45-60	90-120	75-100	3-4 yr.
Galah cockatoo	Early spring/spring/late spring/summer	2-4/2-3	24	45-55	90-120	80-90	1 yr.
Large-sized cockatoos	Early spring/spring/late spring/summer	2-4/2	24-26	60-80	120-150	95-120	5-6 yr.
Eclectus parrot	All year	1-2/1-2	26	72-80	120-150	100-110	4 yr.

Courtesy of Flammer K. Average breeding characteristics of some common psittacine species. In Harrison GJ, Harrison LR (eds): *Clinical Avian Medicine and Surgery.* Philadelphia, WB Saunders, 1986, p 663. Used by permission.

Note: These data are provided as an approximate guide only. Some species may vary from these values, depending on individual characteristics and environmental conditions. In general, larger birds have older fledging, weaning, and breeding ages, and longer egg incubation periods.

*Time when the young leave the nest.

†Time when the young no longer require parental care in captivity.

‡NA—not applicable; rarely hand-reared.

§Age of sexual maturity—corresponds to the best age to encourage breeding except for budgerigars, cockatiels, and lovebirds. These birds mature earlier, but should not be set up for breeding until 9 months of age (budgerigars), or 12 months (cockatiels and lovebirds).

enclosure and cage construction can decrease spread of disease between birds within the collection, between wild and aviary birds, and between birds and other disease vectors (opossums, raccoons, roaches, mosquitos, etc.). Roof heights should be designed so that perches are at head height. The floor should be constructed with drainage and sanitation in mind (cement is recommended). Floors should be sloped so wash water flows easily toward drains (½ inch per foot or more). Drains should be located at close intervals so that infectious wastes are restricted to the areas producing them.

Bowls should be placed away from perches in recessed feeding chambers or hung above perch level to decrease fecal contamination. Hood devices or side ports will also reduce contamination with feces. Food and water bowls should be placed several feet apart to discourage dunking of food (especially in cages for macaws, Amazon parrots, and conures). Water sources should be cultured. Tap water should run for 1 to 2 minutes before filling bowls to flush out bacteria, and faucet screens should be disinfected routinely. Well water should be cultured before initial use.

Soft food items should be prepared daily. Fruits, vegetables, soft mixes, soak and scratch grains, primate biscuits, and sprouted seeds should be offered as soon after dawn as possible. Birds generally eat soon after daylight, and they fill babies early morning and late afternoon. Portions should be small so that soft foods are totally consumed. Scoops and ladles, not hands, should be used to fill bowls. Mobile carts with food and water on top and used dishes below work well.

Vector control is essential for disease control. Vectors of concern include insects, rodents, opossums, raccoons, wild birds, food carts, shoes, hands, and other contaminated items. Foot baths containing glutaraldehyde solutions are well suited for foot baths, which should be placed at all entrances.

The Closed Aviary Concept

A closed aviary restricts introduction of infectious disease agents and controls traffic flow within the aviary. To control disease introduction and spread, the aviary needs designated areas and controlled flow of human, animal, and supplies traffic. Prevention of disease is less costly than treatment and losses from disease.

Ideally, the aviary should have well-defined areas within it, including breeding aviary, nursery, isolation, quarantine, and food storage.

Any bird leaving the premises must be considered a new bird to the aviary if it returns.

Breeding Aviary

The breeding aviary is where the adult breeding birds are housed. Products of the breeding aviary include baby birds, eggs, feathers, and adult birds removed from the aviary.

Birds may enter the breeding aviary from quarantine (after proper protocol is followed), the nursery, or isolation (after required treatment and affirmation of health). All birds entering the breeding aviary should already be adjusted to a proper diet, have gender determined by a reliable method, and be determined to be healthy (through quarantine or from the aviary nursery). All birds entering the breeding aviary should be placed in a flight that has been designed according to the needs known for the species. The veterinarian should initiate a permanent breeder record at this time and keep individual productivity records for each separately housed pair of birds. Important information that should be recorded for each pair includes identification of the clutch and egg numbers, dates laid (if known), eggs broken or lost, eggs infertile (clear), eggs fertile, dead-in-shell embryos, date of hatch, any medical diagnoses of chicks, causes of death, date weaned, age at weaning, date sold, buyer information, and sale price (Fig. 15–1).

Birds may leave the breeding aviary to enter the nursery (baby birds and eggs), be isolated (because of illness), or be sold or die.

Any bird showing signs of illness is immediately transferred to the isolation area. Prompt diagnosis of the etiology of the illness is important so the threat to the breeding flock may be evaluated.

Year_____ Breeder Pair _____ Flight # _____

Bird ID   Male _____ Species _____

         Female _____ Species _____

# eggs in clutch				
Date laid				
Eggs broken				
# Infertile				
# Fertile				
Dead in shell				
Hatch date				
Date weaned				
Age weaned				
Date sold				
Buyer				
Cause of death				
Medical diagnoses				

Figure 15–1. Productivity record. (Courtesy of Speer BL. Avicultural medical management. *Proc Parrot Mgmt Semin* 1991; 125–152. Used by permission.)

Plan annual vaccinations, physical examinations, and beak and nail grooming for the nonbreeding season. Postbreeding evaluations, infertility examinations, papilloma checks, and PBFD checks are common annual breeding stock procedures. Do not use chloramphenicol, penicillin, tetracycline, oxytetracycline, or sulfa drugs in breeding female birds near or during the breeding season because these drugs may cause deformities in embryos.

Encourage breeders to limit species to related groups or a few different groups. Discourage raising of cockatiels, budgies, conures, and lovebirds on the same premises as larger psittacines, because the smaller birds are often carriers of infectious diseases and are often not deemed valuable enough to maintain free of infectious diseases.

Cages should be constructed with the vertical wire axis to the inside of the cage and wire floor at least 1 inch by 3 inches to decrease trapping of food and feces. Vegetable oil spray may be applied to the floor and sides of the cages to make cleaning easier. Cages should be at least 4 feet above the ground, with the ceiling at least 8 feet above the ground. This allows the perch to be placed at 6 feet or higher, giving the birds a feeling of security. A solid roof over cages and small screening around cages can be used to prevent entry of rodents, which can carry disease (e.g., *Sarcocystis*). Cages may be placed on legs or hung.

Nest boxes may be made from wood or metal. Entry doors and interiors may be lined with sheet metal to prevent rapid box destruction (especially important with macaws, cockatoos, and conures). Metal is a poor insulator and should be lined with wood and shaded. The size and shape of the box varies with the species. The box should be placed at a sufficient height so that the bird considers the box to be out of the reach of predators. A ladder may be required for box inspection ports. All boxes should have wire mesh ladders extending to the lower level of the box. Perches should never extend inside the box, and they should run parallel, not perpendicular, to the box faces. Nesting material should consist of clean wood chips or shavings (white pine or fir). Avoid cedar, peat moss, potting soil, and mulch. Nesting material should be removed and replaced each season so that bacteria and fungi do not accumulate.

Cage and nest box construction need to supply isolation and security for breeding pairs. Stress and energy spent defending territory inhibit production. Different species have different needs. Cockatoos should not be housed with raucous species (e.g., macaws or Amazon parrots). Eclectus and African gray parrots should not be housed with loud species. Eclectus and *Pionus* species can be housed with African gray parrots or some cockatoos on a selective basis. Amazon parrots, macaws, and other screamers may be housed together. Pigeons are common carriers of *Chlamydia;* therefore, care must be taken when breeding psittacines and pigeons. Cockatoos (especially all sulphur-crested varieties), African gray parrots, and macaws should be visually shielded from each other. One side of the cage and 50% to 60% of the opposite side and rear sections should be covered to provide the pairs with a psychologically defensible nesting area. Antagonistic and nervous species (e.g., rosellas and great-billed parrots) should be isolated, or less aggressive species should be interspersed between them. An L-shaped flight is ideal for nervous or highly territorial species (e.g., macaws or African gray parrots). The back of the flight should have a side compartment with the nest box attached to the front wall, allowing the mate guarding the nest a nonthreatening view. Male Australian parakeets housed side-by-side may neglect the females during breeding season because they are defending their territory.

A closed-circuit video camera is an excellent tool to help observe courtship or lack of courtship behaviors. These behaviors are often inhibited by the presence of people, and birds will more readily display courtship behaviors when people are out of view.

Nursery

The nursery is where chicks are hand fed and raised. The nursery may also house the hatchery and juvenile holding rooms. The offspring are the primary product and goal of the breeding aviary and are of great value.

Only birds produced from the breeding aviary and kept at the facility may enter the nursery. Birds from other sources are housed in a separate nursery or quarantine area. Birds may leave the nursery as product sold, enter the breeding aviary as a producer, enter isolation in the nursery (in cases of noninfectious disease), enter isolation in another area of the facility (in cases of infectious disease), or die.

An individual record is started upon entry into the nursery that includes identification, species, parents, date of hatch, date entering nursery, date and age hand feeding was initiated, formula used, weight, time, volume fed, and comments (see Fig. 16–1 for a sample pediatric record). All birds entering the nursery require identification. Microchip implants provide permanent identification. Closed banding may be used. Very young birds may be temporarily identified with removable plastic leg bands, with color coding by nontoxic, water-soluble colored marking pens along the back, or in labeled individual containers.

Perform a routine health examination and medical workup on each chick entering the nursery, including a complete physical examination, review of parent performance, hatching and nursery performance, fecal and crop cytology and/or Gram's stains, and oral/crop/cloacal bacterial cultures. If any abnormalities are found, more extensive diagnostics may be performed, including a complete blood count (CBC), biochemistries, fungal cultures, and cytology; investigation of the history of the chick, parents, aviary, and hatch group; and the management of the nursery. The growth of the chick should be monitored and evaluated through comparison with established normal growth parameters from the aviary or other sources (Flammer, 1986b; Hanson, 1987; Joyner, 1993; Abramson, Speer, and Thomsen, 1995; Schubot, Clubb, and Clubb, 1992).

Perform another full examination and testing as birds leave the nursery. This examination decreases the chances of selling an ill bird and also provides information about the success of the management procedures of the nursery.

Heat and cold stress are the most common sources of disease origin in psittacine nurseries. A high-quality thermometer and hygrometer are essential. Relative humidity should be maintained at 55% to 75%, which can be accomplished with water pans. Formula should be fed at 104° to 105° F, measured with a thermometer. The entire room may be heated and humidified to act as a giant brooder, or chicks may be housed in individual brooders, separately or by clutch. Chicks are kept in small plastic containers inside the brooder with cloth diapers or disposable paper towels for bedding to provide support and traction (Fig. 15–2). Bedding should be replaced when soiled. Older chicks may be

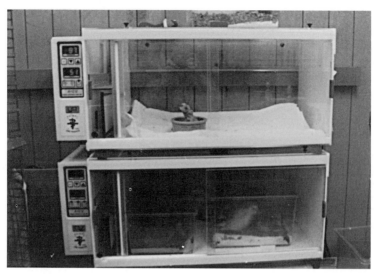

Figure 15–2. Chicks are kept in small plastic containers inside the brooder with cloth diapers or disposable paper towels for bedding to provide support and traction. (Photo courtesy of Jean Jordan, Adventures in Birds. Used by permission.)

housed in cages with plastic-coated raised wire floors (Fig. 15–3). The mesh must be small enough to prevent the leg from extending through the bottom of the cage. Because particulate bedding may be ingested and is constantly contaminated with droppings, it should not be used. Further information on pediatrics is provided in Chapter 18.

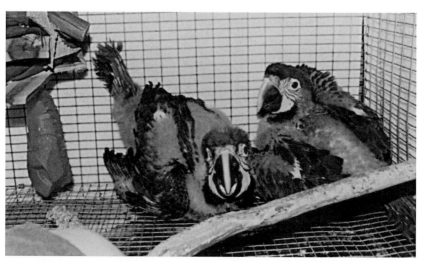

Figure 15–3. Older chicks may be housed in cages with plastic-coated, raised wire floors. (Photo courtesy of Jean Jordan, Adventures in Birds. Used by permission.)

It is important to help the aviculturist develop a nursery protocol and insist that it is followed. Food and water are available within the nursery so that outside contact does not occur. Ideally, nursery personnel are restricted to the nursery, without contact with the rest of the aviary. Street shoes should be left outside.

Areas of food preparation and water sources should be monitored with periodic cultures. Tap water should run freely for 1 to 2 minutes before use if a sterile water source is not used.

Dirty working surface areas, mixing cups, blender O rings, and feeding syringes are common sources of pathogens in the nursery. Disinfect equipment with glutaraldehyde, chlorine washes, or steam sterilization. Chlorhexidine or quaternary ammoniums are poor disinfectants against many viruses, *Pseudomonas*, and some other pathogenic organisms.

Hatchery

Hatching rooms may be a separate part of the nursery, but no contact should occur between them.

Gross fecal contamination of eggs can be removed with fine sandpaper. If eggs are disinfected with a dip or spray, the solution must be warm. Correct incubation is crucial for normal development. During artificial incubation, temperature and humidity must be appropriate for the species. Inappropriately high temperatures may result in an early weak hatch, dehydrated chicks, and facial malformations. Inappropriately low temperatures can result in late, weak, wet hatches; failure to absorb the yolk; and neuromuscular disorders. Humidity allows for optimal water loss through the eggshell pores, which is generally about 16%. Excessively high humidity during incubation may result in late hatching of wet, weak chicks; poor positioning; and failure of the umbilicus to close. Excessively low humidity may result in early hatching of dry, weak chicks. The egg must be rotated at intervals appropriate for the species to prevent the embryo from sticking to the egg membranes and to allow proper development of the shell membrane vasculature. Inadequate rotation can result in poorly positioned chicks or difficult hatches (see Abramson, Speer, and Thomsen, 1995; Clubb, Clubb, and Schubot, 1992; Dhillon, 1991; Jordan, 1990; Joyner, 1993; Stewart, 1991 for further discussion of incubation procedures). Egg necropsy procedures are discussed in Chapter 10.

Isolation

Isolation is the area where clinically ill or diseased birds from the collection are housed. The treatment area is included in the isolation area, as is the hospital if one exists. Isolation must be separate from the quarantine area. Birds leave isolation and go back to the breeding aviary or nursery (when deemed healthy following a set protocol), are sold, or die.

Only birds from the breeding aviary and nursery are allowed into isolation. Birds that become ill in quarantine are housed and treated in the quarantine area.

Quarantine

Quarantine is where all new arrivals to the aviary are housed until they are deemed admissible into the breeding aviary. New breeding stock always enters the collection through the quarantine area. All new flock additions, returning birds, members of the original collection as it is being assembled, and birds used to replace culls enter through the quarantine area. This area is the primary defense against introduction of infectious disease agents.

The quarantine area should be physically isolated from all other areas, with limited access, and be serviced with separate personnel or at the end of the shift. Birds are held in quarantine for varying periods of time, depending on the protocol of the aviary (typically 45 to 60 days, minimum 6 weeks). Eighteen months is used for very valuable collections. All diagnostic tests are done while the bird is in quarantine, and no bird is released from quarantine until all results are known. Many of the most significant infectious diseases of economic importance are viral, and detection is not always possible at the time the bird first enters the quarantine area. A prolonged observation period is of great value. Stress plays a vital role in the onset of pathogen shedding and sepsis. A prolonged acclimation period should be encouraged, especially in larger, sensitive, and highly intelligent species such as cockatoos and macaws. Repeated testing is of great potential value for those species with well-documented carrier states, such as cockatiels and budgies (*Chlamydia, Giardia,* and *Mycoplasma*), conures (Pacheco's disease), cockatoos (PBFD), and macaws (PDS).

Birds leave the quarantine area when they move to the breeding aviary (only after the set protocol has been followed), are returned to the seller, or die. Birds in quarantine should not be sold.

Birds that become ill in the quarantine are isolated in an area of the quarantine area, not transferred to the aviary isolation area.

All birds in quarantine should have a quarantine record that includes the source of the bird, conditions of the sale, medical and breeder past history, date entering quarantine, sex and method of determination, comments pertinent to the individual bird (e.g., examinations, medical tests, treatments, observation), and date released from quarantine. All birds in quarantine should be permanently identified (e.g., microchip implants, leg bands, tattoos).

Each bird in quarantine should be visually inspected at rest in the holding cage daily. Food intake, character of droppings, stance, and behavior should be observed; any abnormalities should be noted in the quarantine record. During the quarantine period, necessary diet changes can be made and the sex of the bird can be determined. Routine immunizations used in the aviary should be administered (poxvirus, Pacheco's, etc.).

The health status of the bird should be determined through a set protocol that should be followed on every bird. Diagnostic tests to be performed on each bird to determine the health status are established by the aviculturist and the veterinarian. Cost must be balanced with the goals and desires of the aviculturist. Knowledge of common diseases affecting the species involved and of infectious diseases posing the greatest potential threat is used by the veterinarian in making management recommendations. Discuss the pros and cons of prophylactic treatment for chlamydiosis. Necropsy of all birds that die in quarantine is highly recommended.

Food Storage

Food storage is the area within the facility where food supplies are stored. No birds should be housed in this area. The food preparation area may be located in the food storage area.

Food should be stored in metal containers with tight-fitting lids to protect against contamination by pests.

METHODS OF GENDER DETERMINATION (SEXING)

Determination of sex is important in bird reproduction. Many species of birds are monomorphic (males and females appear similar), whereas others are dimorphic. Differences between the sexes in dimorphic birds may include feather color, iris color, and bill color and size. Immature birds typically appear similar to adult female birds. Table 15–2 lists characteristics of some dimorphic psittacine species. In monomorphic birds, subtle differences in weight, body size, head size, and bill size may vary between the sexes and may allow gender determination. With most monomorphic species, definitive gender determination requires laparoscopic examination, chromosomal evaluation, or DNA testing. Gender determination by behavior or width of the pelvic bones is unreliable.

Advantages of gender determination by laparoscopy include visualization of reproductive organs and other celomic structures. Disadvantages include increased risk of complications caused by anesthesia and surgical technique, occasional inability to determine the gender because of uncontrollable circumstances, and the invasive nature of the procedure. Gender determination in mature birds is relatively conclusive. Gonadal differences between the sexes in mature birds are prominent. Laparoscopic gender determination is possible in young birds; however, experience and knowledge of juvenile gonadal anatomy is required for accuracy. Laparoscopy on preweaned birds carries increased risks because of the increased proventricular and intestinal contents. Adipose tissue in obese birds may make laparoscopic gender determination difficult or impossible. The technique for laparoscopic gender determination is described in Chapter 14.

Chromosomal analysis is used to determine the gender of monomorphic birds without invasive procedures. Feather pulp of growing feathers is used as the source of chromosomes. Multiple growing feathers are shipped overnight in a preservative to the laboratory (Table 15–3). Chromosomal abnormalities are sometimes noted. Disadvantages include the difficulty of obtaining an adequate number of growing feathers, requirement of overnight mailing, and the time required to process the sample.

DNA testing uses a small amount of blood for gender determination. Blood is placed in a preservative and may be stored or shipped immediately to the laboratory (see Table 15–3). Advantages include ease and safety of sample collection, accuracy at any age, long shelf life of samples, rapid laboratory processing time, and the noninvasive nature of the procedure. The sample may also be used for DNA fingerprinting and identification.

Gross morphological differences allow vent sexing in some birds. Ducks, geese, pigeons, and monomorphic gallinaceous birds may be sexed by examination of the cloaca. In ducks and geese, the cloaca is everted by placing pressure on both

TABLE 15–2 Sexual Dimorphic Characteristics of Some Psittacine Species

Parrots of Australian and Pacific Distribution

Loridae—Most species are monomorphic. The head is usually larger in male birds.

    Monomorphic genera

        Pseudeos—**dusky lory**

        Chalcopsitta—**black lory, duivenbode's lory**

        Eos—**red lories**

        Lorius—**chattering lories**

        Vini—**blue lories**

        Most *Trichoglossus* spp.–**rainbow lories**

    Dimorphic genera (species)

        Charmosyna—**Stella lory** *(Charmosyna papou)*—The female has a yellow patch on the rump and lower back that is absent in the male. Apparent in red and black color morphs.

        —**red-flanked lory** *(Charmosyna placentis)*—The male has bright red patches on the flank that are absent in the female. The male has bright blue cheek patches, whereas the female has yellow-streaked cheek patches. Other less common members of the genus are also dimorphic.

        Trichoglossus (T. flavoviridis meyeri)—**Meyer's lorikeet**—The male has a larger and brighter yellow ear patch than the female.

Cacatuidae—Psittaci-formes

    Cacatuinae

        Monomorphic genera

            Probosciger—**palm cockatoo**—Male is usually larger and has a larger beak. Size also varies geographically and with subspecies.

        Dimorphic genera

            Calyptorhynchus—**black cockatoos**—Dimorphism is striking in some species and barely noticeable in others. In the Banksian cockatoo *(C. magnificus)*, the male plumage is black except for bands of red in the tail, whereas the female is dotted and barred with orange yellow.

            Callocephalon—**gang gang cockatoo**—The male is slate gray with a red head and crest. The female has a gray head and crest and plumage that is barred with yellow orange.

            Cacatua and *Eolophus*—**white and pink cockatoos**—Adult birds, except for the bare-eyed cockatoo *(C. sanguinea)*, can usually be sexed by eye color. The female has a red iris, whereas the iris of the male is dark brown to black. A bright light may be needed to determine eye color in some species such as the Moluccan cockatoo *(C. moluccensis)*. The female of most species is smaller than the male. Red-eyed males and dark-eyed females have been reported and are more common in captive-reared birds. The iris is brown in immature birds of both sexes.

    Nymphicinae

        Nymphicus—**cockatiel**—Sex is easily determined in the wild type (gray), because the male has a large yellow facial patch and crest that is gray in the female. The primary flight feathers and tail feathers of the female are diagonally barred with white. Immature birds resemble females. Cinnamon, lutino, and fallow cockatiels can be sexed by the faint diagonal barring of the primary flight feathers in the females, and in cinnamons, a faint yellow mask in the male. Pied cockatiels can be sexed as grays unless heavily pied, and these areas are white. Pearl cockatiel males lose their pearling when mature. White-faced cockatiels are sexed as grays.

Psittacidae

    Psittacinae

        Monomorphic genera

            Cyanoramphus—**kakarikis**

        Dimorphic genera

            Melopsittacus—**budgerigar**—In the normal green variety, the cere of the adult male is blue, whereas the cere of the adult female is pinkish brown. This is not dependable in color mutations such as lutino, blue, or white birds.

TABLE 15–2 Sexual Dimorphic Characteristics of Some Psittacine Species *(Continued)*

Parrots of Australian and Pacific Distribution *(Continued)*

Psittacidae *(Continued)*

Platycercus—**rosellas**—The male of most rosella species is slightly brighter than the female or immature. Female and young of several species have a row of white spots on the ventral surface of seven or eight primary and secondary flight feathers. These are lost by the males at the time they reach sexual maturity. Wing spots are retained in adult female yellow rosellas *(P. flaveolus)*, golden-mantled rosellas *(P. eximius)*, mealy rosellas *(P. adscitus)*, and Stanley's rosellas *(P. icterotis)*. Male Stanley's rosellas have red heads and bright yellow cheek patches, whereas females have green heads and dull cheek patches.

Psephotus—**red-rumped parakeet** *(P. haematonotus)*—Most species in the genus exhibit sexual dimorphism. The male red-rumped parakeet has a red patch on the rump, whereas the female is drab. Other species are uncommon in aviculture.

Neophema—**grass parakeets**—Sexual dimorphism varies from a slight variation in the Bourke's parakeet *(N. bourkii)* (the male has more blue and pink on the breast) to extreme sexual dimorphism in the scarlet-chested parakeet *(N. splendida)* (the chest is red in the male, green in the female).

Polytelis—**Barraband's, rock pebblars** *(P. anthopeplus)*—The males of this genus are typically larger and brighter in color than females and young birds. Female Barraband's parakeets *(P. swainsonii)* lack the yellow feathers of the male. In rock pebblars, the ventral surface of the male's tail is black, whereas tail feathers of the female are margined and tipped in pink. The male Princess of Wales *(P. alexandrae)* is brighter in color and the bill is deeper red than the female. In many species, the male has an elongated spatula tip on the third primary.

Aprosmictus—**crimson-winged parakeet**—The male has a black mantle.

Alisterus—**king parrots**—Sexual dimorphism is present in plumage and beak color of some species. Some subspecies of green-winged king parrots *(A. chloropterus)* show dimorphism in the green patch on the wing that is absent in the female, but some subspecies are monomorphic. In Australian king parakeets *(A. scapularis)*, the male is red and the female's head is green.

Roratus—**eclectus parrots**—The male is brilliant emerald green with a yellow-orange beak. The female is red-maroon and purple with a black beak. The color difference is evident at the time of emergence of the first tail and contour feathers in chicks. The down of both sexes is black.

Tanygnathus—**great bills, blue napes, and Muller's parrots**—The beak of the male Muller's parrot *(T. mulleri)* is red, and the beak of the female is white. The beak of the male great-billed parrot *(T. megalorynchos)* is much larger than the female's.

Psittaculirostris—**fig parrots**—Most species are obviously dimorphic in plumage.

Psittrichas—**Pesquet's parrot**—Male has a red line behind the eye that is absent in the female.

Parrots of Afro-Asian Distribution

Psittacidae

Psittacinae

Monomorphic genera

Coracopis—**Vasa or black parrots**—Monomorphic in plumage; however, the tissues of the vent in males is hypertrophied, especially in breeding season.

Agapornis—**lovebirds**—Commonly available species are monomorphic. Some species show definitive dimorphism such as the Abyssinian lovebird *(A. taranta)* in which the male has a red patch on the forehead and lores that is absent in the female. The male Madagascar lovebird *(A. cana)* has a gray head, whereas the female has a green head.

Psittacus—**African gray parrots**—Very slight dimorphism is evident on close examination but should not be considered definitive. Females *(P. erithacus erithacus)* tend to be lighter gray than males and have red edging on the under tail coverts caudal to the vent. Tinmeh grays *(P. e. timneh)* are monomorphic.

Table continued on following page

TABLE 15–2 Sexual Dimorphic Characteristics of Some Psittacine Species
(Continued)

Parrots of Afro-Asian Distribution *(Continued)*
Psittacidae *(Continued)*
Dimorphic genera
    Psittacula—**ringnecks**—All male birds in the genus have a ring encircling the neck or a wide black moustache ring. In some species, this is lacking in the female and young, whereas in some it is less prominent. Adult male plumage may not be evident until 1½ to 2½ years of age. In some species, the beak color is different. The male derbyan parakeet *(P. derbyana)* and some subspecies of the moustache parakeet *(P. alexandri)* have a red beak, whereas the female's beak is black.
    Loriculus—**hanging parrots**—Adult birds are dimorphic in plumage and in some species in eye color. In most species, the forehead and/or crown of the male is blue or red and is green in the female.
    Poicephalus—**Senegal parrots and related species**—Some members of the genus show marked sexual dimorphism, whereas others are monomorphic. The male red-bellied parrot *(P. rufiventralis)* has a deep red-orange breast and abdomen, whereas the female's breast is greenish brown. The female Rüppell's parrot *(P. rueppellii)* is more brightly colored than the male, having a bright blue rump patch that is absent in the male. The Senegal parrot *(P. senegalus)* shows slight but unreliable dimorphism. The undertail coverts of the male are yellow or orange, whereas the female's are greenish yellow to greenish orange.
Parrots of South American Distribution
Psittacidae
  Psittacinae
    Monomorphic genera
      Ara—**macaws.**
      Anodorhynchus—**hyacinth macaw.**
      Aratinga—**conures.**
      Pyrrhura—**conures.**
      Nandayus—**Nanday conure.**
      Enidognathus—**slender-billed and Austral conures.**
      Cyanoliseus—**Patagonian conure.**
      Deroptyus—**hawkhead parrots.**
      Myiopsitta—**Quaker parakeets.**
      Rhynchopsitta—**thick-billed parrots.**
      Brotogeris—**bee-bee parakeets.**
      Pionus—**pionus parrots.**
      Pionites—**caiques.**
      Amazona—**Amazon parrots**—Most species are monomorphic. In the spectacled Amazon *(A. albifrons)*, the male has red marking on the cranial edge of the carpus and adjacent upper wing coverts on the dorsal side of the wing that are absent or reduced in the female. In the yellow-lored Amazon *(A. xantholora)*, the female is duller and lacks white on the head and red facial markings that are found in the male. The adult male yellow-faced Amazon *(A. xanthops)* has a patch of yellow-orange on the breast and abdomen that is reduced or absent in the female.
      Bolborhynchus—**mountain parakeets**—Only one species, the golden-fronted mountain parakeet *(B. aurifrons)* is dimorphic. The male has yellow markings on the lores, forehead, throat, and part of the cheek, whereas the female is predominantly green.
    Dimorphic genera
      Pionopsitta—**pileated parrot**—The male has a red head and the female has a green head. Dimorphism is evident in immature plumage. Other members of the genus are monomorphic and very rare in aviculture.
      Forpus—**parrotlets**—All species are dimorphic. In most species, the male will have coloration on the rump or wings, whereas the females are usually predominantly green.

Courtesy of Clubb SL. Nonsurgical means of sex determination in psittacine birds. In Bonagura JD, Kirk RW (eds): Kirk's Current Veterinary Therapy XII, Small Animal Practice. Philadelphia, WB Saunders, 1995, pp 1275–1278. Used by permission.

TABLE 15-3 Some Laboratories that Perform DNA or Chromosomal Gender Determinations

Avian Genetic Sexing Laboratory (chromosomal); 6551 Stage Oaks Drive, Suite 3, Barlette, TN 38134, (901) 388-9548

Research Associates Lab, Inc. (DNA); 100 Techne Center Drive, Suite 101, Milford, OH 45150, (513) 248-4700

Zoogen Inc. (DNA); 1756 Picasso Avenue, Davis CA 95616, (800) 995-BIRD, (916) 756-8089, fax (916) 756-5143

sides of the cloaca with the thumbs while holding the bird in a vertical position with the head down and the abdomen toward the examiner. In male ducks and geese, the phallus is covered with keratinized papillae. Two small labia-like structures are present in the female. The phallus can be palpated without eversion in the cloaca. No mass is palpable in female ducks and geese. Young gallinaceous birds are vent sexed in a similar way, except the birds are stimulated to defecate by gently pressing on the abdomen distal to the keel before the examination. Pigeons, doves, and passerine birds have prominent papillae of the ductus deferens. General anesthesia and a speculum are needed to visualize these structures.

NORMAL REPRODUCTION

Reproductive activity and secondary sex characteristics are under hormonal control. Gonadal and hypothalamic hormones act in a delicate balance, controlling sexual activity, spermatozoa production, and egg production. Avian reproductive hormones include follicle-stimulating hormone, luteinizing hormone, estrogen, progesterone, and testosterone.

Female Anatomy and Egg Production

Most female birds have a single ovary. It is located at the cranial pole of the left kidney. In immature birds, the ovary is flattened and triangular and may be white, yellow, or black (e.g., some cockatoos, macaws, and conures), with a faintly granular surface. The immature ovary may resemble a piece of fat. The active ovary has follicles in varying stages of development, appearing as a cluster of variably sized grapes. The normal postovulatory follicle lacks blood clots. During the nonbreeding season, the ovary and oviduct regress, and many small follicles will be present on the ovary.

The oviduct is very thin during reproductive inactivity, but it becomes long, wide, and tortuous during active egg laying. The parts of the oviduct include the infundibulum, magnum, isthmus, uterus, and vagina. The infundibulum engulfs the ovum and is the site of fertilization. The chalaziferous layer of albumen and paired chalazae are also produced in the infundibulum. Spermatozoa may be retained in glandular grooves. Just distal to the infundibulum is the magnum. Most of the albumen is deposited in the magnum. The isthmus is distal to the magnum and is the site where inner and outer shell membranes are added. The uterus is distal to the isthmus, and deposition of the shell and shell pigment occurs in the uterus. The vagina connects the uterus to the cloaca and contains spermatic fossulae, where sperm are stored.

Large amounts of calcium are expended with egg production for shell formation. During laying, intestinal absorption of calcium is markedly increased, and calcium may also be mobilized from bone. Approximately 10 days before egg formation, medullary spaces of the long bones may calcify. In psittacines, blood calcium levels can become extremely high, up to 30 mg/dl, during egg production. Psittacine birds should be fed a diet of 0.3% to 1% calcium, with a 1:1 to 2:1 calcium-to-phosphorus ratio. A slight increase in white blood cells (WBCs), packed cell volume (PCV), and total protein may also occur during laying.

Domestic chickens have a 24-hour lay interval. The lay interval for psittacines is generally 2 days. Most passerines lay at 24-hour intervals, but they can lay at 4- to 5-day intervals. Some species of birds are determinate layers (they lay a fixed number of eggs), such as budgies and crows. Many birds are indeterminate layers and will replace eggs that are broken or removed from the nestbox.

Psittacine reproductive activity is stimulated by the presence of a compatible mate, the presence of a nest box, the quality and quantity of food, and in some birds, an increasing photoperiod and the presence of other mating pairs. The size, shape, content, and location of the nest box in the aviary and the amount of darkness in the nest box affect reproductive activity.

The Egg

The structures of the egg are derived from the ovary or oviduct. Each structure serves a specific function. The yolk of the egg is the cytoplasm of the oocyte. Most of the contents of the yolk are synthesized in the liver and transported to the ovary in the blood. The yolk is yellow and separate from the albumen. The yolk contains maternal antibodies. The yolk provides nutrition for the developing embryo and passive immunity in the young chick. The germinal disc is a small, circular, white opaque spot on the surface of the yolk. This develops into the embryo in fertile eggs. Surrounding the yolk is the vitelline membrane, which protects the embryo from microorganisms and is derived from the ovary. Connecting the yolk to each end of the egg are the chalazae that stabilize the yolk in the center of the egg. The clear to whitish clear viscous fluid is albumen, which provides nutrition for the embryo and protects the embryo from microorganisms. Just under the shell are the inner and outer shell membranes, which protect the embryo from microorganisms and allow transpiration (passive diffusion of oxygen, carbon dioxide, and water) during embryo development. At the blunt end of the egg, the inner and outer shell membranes separate, forming the air cell that allows transpiration. The shell provides physical protection, protects the embryo from microorganisms, allows transpiration, regulates evaporation, and is a source of calcium carbonate for bone formation in the embryo. Pores are present in the shell. On the outside of the shell is the cuticle, which regulates evaporation and protects the embryo from microorganisms.

Male Anatomy

In male birds, the testes are located at the cranial pole of the kidneys, have a smooth surface, and vary in size, shape, and color. The testes of immature birds are small, bean shaped, and yellow to white. In some birds, they may be black or gray (e.g., some cockatoos, blue and gold macaws, golden conures, mynahs, and toucans). During the breeding season, the testes of mature birds may enlarge from 10% to 500%. The large testicles may be white, yellow, or gray, with a vascular surface. During the nonbreeding season, the testicles atrophy and appear similar to juvenile testicles.

Copulation occurs through eversion of the cloacal wall. Semen is deposited at the everted vaginal orifice of the oviduct. In birds that have a phallus, such as waterfowl and ratites, the phallus facilitates deposition of semen in the cloaca.

In many altricial birds, the male and female parent birds incubate and raise the young.

REPRODUCTIVE DISORDERS

Infertility

Infertility is the lack of egg production or laying repeatedly infertile eggs. Infertility can be the result of management problems or any disease process that affects the anatomy or physiology of the reproductive tract. Infertility is most commonly the result of management problems. Repeated production of infertile, but otherwise normal, eggs may be the result of same sex pairing, mate incompatibility, lack of or difficulty copulating, inexperience, male immaturity, loose perches, perches made of inappropriate materials (e.g., PVC or metal), malnutrition, obesity, aviary disturbances, inbreeding, genetic flaws, lameness or foot problems, heavy cloacal feathering, poor vision, reproductive tract infections, cloacal abnormalities, systemic disease, or male infertility. Production of some infertile eggs within a clutch can be normal under some circumstances. Infertile eggs are common at the beginning or end of the season and can be normal.

Hens may fail to lay eggs as a result of lack of appropriate stimuli, disturbances in the aviary, excessive or inappropriate drug therapies, mate incompatibility, pairing of same sex birds, immaturity, inbreeding, genetic flaws, malnutrition, obesity, stress, vision problems, reproductive tract infections, and other illnesses and toxicoses. Inappropriate nest box location, height, depth, width, entrance hole size, bedding, and box construction materials may result in a failure to produce eggs. Nest sites with aviary disturbances or excessive exposure to adverse weather may make some sites unacceptable to some birds, resulting in lack of egg production. Any disturbance in the aviary may result in lack of perceived security by the birds. Common disturbances include dogs, cats, rodents, temperature extremes, excessive or malicious human contact, automobile traffic, and housing of aggressive or antagonistic pairs within the aviary. Some species of birds (e.g., African gray parrots or budgies) are more productive when housed in flights located adjacent to one another, allowing visual and vocal contact with others of the same species. However, breeding may be inhibited under the same circumstances for some other species. Some species such as macaws do not nest and produce offspring every year in the wild.

Diagnosis of the etiology of infertility includes a review of management procedures, complete physical examinations, and diagnostic testing, which may include laparoscopy. Determine the sex of the birds with a reliable method of gender determination. Review management procedures, including housing, perches, nest box, nesting sites, pair bonding, mating behavior, nutrition, aviary disturbances, lack of visual barriers, lack of flock stimulants, extreme environmental temperatures, inbreeding, and excessive or inappropriate drug treatments. Make changes in management procedures while pursuing medical causes. Perform a complete physical examination, CBC, plasma biochemistries (including aspartate aminotransferase [AST], uric acid, total protein, calcium, etc.), and if the sex of the bird has not been determined by a reliable method, perform laparoscopy or DNA gender determination. During laparoscopy, determine the sex of the bird, visualize reproductive organs, visualize other celomic structures, and biopsy abnormalities. Endoscopy and testicular biopsy may reveal testicular abnormalities. Small round biopsy forceps are recommended (e.g., 5-Fr round) using a right and/or left lateral approach. A video camera is useful to observe the pair without interfering and inhibiting natural behavior and reproductive activity.

Make changes in management procedures for identified problems and treat medical problems. Confirm resolution of problems with follow-up observations.

Abnormal Eggs

Abnormal eggs may be the result of reproductive tract abnormalities, nutritional problems, or environmental effects. Abnormal eggs may produce normal chicks, but hatchability is decreased. Soft-shelled eggs may occur as a result of deficiencies in calcium, vitamin A, vitamin D, or trace minerals or because of uterine infection or pathology. Thin-shelled eggs may be the result of pathology of the oviduct or organochlorine pesticides in the environment or food. Rough-shelled eggs or overly thick-shelled eggs may be the result of uterine infection or pathology.

Production of multiple abnormal eggs warrants further investigation. Nutritional history and uterine culture are pursued. Collect samples for culture through the dilated cervix immediately after egg laying. If infection is suspected, antibiotics are infused into the uterus after sample collection. The choice of systemic antibiotics is based on culture sensitivity results.

Yolkless eggs may be the result of ectopic ovulation or ovarian or uterine pathology and may warrant endoscopy and visualization of the ovary and oviduct.

Egg Binding

Egg binding is most common in budgies, finches, canaries, cockatiels, and lovebirds. Common causes include malnutrition (calcium, vitamin A, protein, vitamin E, and selenium deficiencies), excessive egg production, malformed eggs, first-time egg laying, obesity, lack of exercise, stress, old age, and oviduct pathology or infection. Other causes include breeding birds out of season and persistent right oviduct. Clinical signs include depression, anorexia, wide stance, abdominal straining, and wagging of the tail, with or without leg paralysis. Canaries commonly have drooped wings.

The diagnosis and etiology of egg binding are based on history, physical examination, and radiology. Dietary insufficiencies must be sought from the history. Explore behaviors historically: previous egg laying, paper shredding, hiding under papers or in dark places, or nest building. On physical examination, an egg can often be palpated in the caudal abdomen. Eggs high in the oviduct and soft-shelled eggs may not be palpable, but the abdomen will be swollen and soft. Radiographs may reveal an egg (Fig. 13–21A and B) and polyostotic hyperostosis (medullary bone density). Eggs with a noncalcified shell may appear similar to peritonitis or an abdominal mass (Fig. 13–20A and B).

Stabilize depressed birds before initiating treatment for egg removal. Administer parenteral calcium, vitamin A, and vitamin D_3; administer dextrose via a feeding needle to anorectic birds; administer intravenous (IV), intraosseous (IO), or subcutaneous (SC) fluids if the bird is moderately depressed; lubricate prolapsed tissues and tissues surrounding the egg; and place the bird in a warm, moist environment (e.g., an incubator with moist towels, 85° to 95°F). Administer systemic antibiotics, possibly with rapidly acting steroids, if the bird is severely depressed. If the egg is not delivered within a few hours, prostaglandin E_2 (Prepidil) can be applied to the uterovaginal sphincter. Prostaglandins appear more effective than oxytocin. If this fails to result in egg delivery, the egg may be manipulated to aid in expulsion. Gentle, persistent pressure is applied to the egg to move it ventrally and caudally to the cloaca. Avoid pushing the egg against the kidneys. If the egg has not passed within a reasonable period of time (24 hours or more) or if the bird becomes depressed, perform ovocentesis. The bird is anesthetized and the egg is manipulated until the tip can be observed through the uterine opening into the cloaca and tapped through the cloaca. A large needle (18- to 22-gauge) is inserted into the egg, the contents of the egg are aspirated, and the egg is carefully collapsed with lateral digital pressure, avoiding pressure dorsally on the kidneys. Accessible eggshell fragments are removed with forceps. Remaining shell is usually expelled within several days. If the egg cannot be visualized with manipulation, the egg is held to the ventral body wall, and the contents of the egg are aspirated through the skin. The egg is gently imploded and the fragments are allowed to pass. The uterus is cultured and antibiotic therapy is begun changing as needed based on sensitivity results. Supportive care and calcium administration are continued until the shell is delivered. The uterus may be flushed with antibiotics for several days. Laparotomy is required if the uterus ruptures, if severe adhesions are present, if soft-shelled eggs are located anterior to the uterus, or if ectopic eggs are present.

Small birds (e.g., canaries and finches) are treated more aggressively because these birds often die within a few hours without aggressive therapy.

Egg-Related Peritonitis and Ectopic Eggs

Egg yolk peritonitis may result from septic or nonseptic yolk contamination of the body cavity. Yolk may be deposited into the body cavity as a result of ectopic ovulation or oviductal disease. Ectopic ovulation occurs when the infundibulum fails to engulf an ovum because of reverse peristalsis of the oviduct, trauma, or stress. Oviductal diseases that may result in ectopic ovulation include infectious salpingitis, rupture of the oviduct, cystic hyperplasia, and neoplasia.

Egg yolk peritonitis is most common in cockatiels, budgies, lovebirds, ducks, and macaws. Clinical signs include weight loss, depression, respiratory distress, anorexia, and ascites. Abdominal distention may or may not be present. Some birds abruptly stop laying, with fewer than the normal number of eggs. Waterfowl and gallinaceous birds frequently present with abdominal distention.

Diagnosis is based on physical examination and laboratory diagnostics. When peritonitis is suspected, abdominocentesis is performed (see Chapter 12). Aspirated fluid from septic yolk peritonitis appears yellow, green, or brown. Cytology of the fluid reveals inflammatory cells with a granular background. Yolk or fat globules may be noted. Intracellular bacteria or degenerate heterophils may be noted with septic peritonitis.

Treatment includes supportive care and antibiotic therapy, ideally based on culture and sensitivity results. Long-term antibiotic therapy may be necessary. Supportive care may include warmth, oxygen, fluid therapy, nutritional support, and corticosteroids. Corticosteroid therapy for 2 to 5 days appears to be beneficial in birds with egg-related peritonitis. Surgical intervention may be required with recurring ascites, when large amounts of yolk are present in the abdomen, or when adhesions develop. Stabilize birds with supportive care and antibiotics before surgery.

Chronic Egg Laying

Excessive or chronic egg laying is most common in budgies, cockatiels, and lovebirds. Excessive egg production can lead to calcium depletion, malnutrition, osteoporosis, and egg binding. Treatment includes behavioral modification and correction of nutritional deficits, if present. Medical therapy or surgery may be required to stop the egg laying.

Behavioral modification is effective for some birds. Do not remove eggs from the cage. Remove cagemates, nest boxes, nesting sites, and toys or other cage items the bird has a sexual affinity toward. Decrease exposure to light to 8 hours per day. Consider changing cages or location of the cage.

Medical therapy includes correction of the diet and vitamin and mineral supplementation as needed. Leuprolide, human chorionic gonadotropin, and medroxyprogesterone have been used to interrupt egg laying. Medroxyprogesterone administration has been associated with depression, polyuria, weight gain, liver damage, immunosuppression, and diabetes mellitus.

Salpingohysterectomy is used to permanently inhibit egg production in companion birds with no breeding intent.

Cloacal Prolapse

A cloacal prolapse may contain oviduct, ureter, phallus, intestines, or cloacal tissues or masses. Prolapses may be the result of straining, masses within the cloaca, egg binding, chronic irritation of the rectum, or sphincter problems. Common causes include egg binding, enteritis, and cloacitis. Phallus prolapse is commonly the result of trauma, infection, or extreme weather fluctuation.

Diagnosis is based on history and physical examination. Prolapse frequently follows straining, diarrhea, or egg laying. Palpate the abdomen for masses. Check for prolapse of the ureters or uterus. Check for cloacal tumors such as papillomas. Chronic cloacal prolapse in cockatoos may be associated with sexual behavior or may be idiopathic.

For treatment, the bird is anesthetized with isoflurane, and the caudal abdomen and cloacal regions are massaged to promote fecal evacuation. If fecal retention has occurred, administer parenteral fluids. Examine the cloaca. Diagnostic aids include a fecal wet amount, Gram's stain, culture, and radiographs. Suspected papillomatous lesions may be identified with the aid of a 5% acetic acid solution (e.g., apple cider vinegar). When applied to papillomatous tissues, the surface will blanch to white from the normal pink color.

Flush prolapsed mucosa with warm saline and cover it with a sterile lubricating jelly, then use a lubricated sterile swab to replace the tissues. Consider placing retention sutures, two simple transverse stay sutures perpendicular to the vent. A cloacapexy may be necessary in some birds to prevent recurrence of prolapse (see Chapter 14). Treat the underlying cause of the straining or prolapse.

If the oviduct is prolapsed, check for the presence of an egg. Consult the section on egg binding if an egg is present. If an egg is not present, flush the tissues with sterile saline and replace the tissues with a lubricated sterile swab. Oxytocin or prostaglandin may be applied to the oviduct to reduce swelling and control bleeding. A retention suture may be needed to prevent prolapse recurrence. If tissues appear desiccated or inflamed, replace the prolapsed tissue and administer antibiotics for 5 to 7 days, then re-evaluate the tissues. Amputate remaining necrotic areas, taking care to avoid the ureters.

For treatment of papillomas, see Chapter 9.

References and Additional Readings

Abbott UK, Brice AT, Cutler BA, et al. Embryonic development of the cockatiel (*Nymphicus hollandicus*). *J Assoc Avian Vet* 1991;5(4):207–209.

Abramson J, Speer BL, Thomsen JB. *The Large Macaw: Their Care, Breeding and Conservation.* Fort Bragg, CA, Raintree Publications, 1995.

Allen G. Hand raising endangered species birds in the home environment. *Proc Assoc Avian Vet* 1989;257–261.

Baumgartner R, Hatt JM, Dobeli M, et al. Endocrinologic and pathologic findings in birds with polyostotic hyperostosis. *J Avian Med Surg* 1995;9(4):251–254.

Clipsham R. Introduction to avicultural medicine. *Proc Assoc Avian Vet* 1989;223–238.

Clipsham R. Environmental preventive medicine: Food and water management for reinfection control. *Proc Assoc Avian Vet* 1990;87–105.

Clipsham R. Avicultural medical diagnostics and therapeutics. *Proc Parrot Mgmt Semin, Avian Res Fund* 1991;61–92.

Clipsham R. Preventive medical management of aviary diseases. *Proc Parrot Mgmt Semin, Avian Res Fund* 1991;23–56.

Clubb SL. Sex determination techniques. In Harrison GJ, Harrison LR (eds): *Clinical Avian Medicine and Surgery.* Philadelphia, WB Saunders, 1986, pp 613–619.

Clubb SL. Nonsurgical means of sex determination in psittacine birds. In Bonagura JD, Kirk RW (eds): *Kirk's Current Veterinary Therapy XII, Small Animal Practice.* Philadelphia, WB Saunders, 1995, pp 1275–1278.

Clubb SL. Aviculture medicine and flock health management. In Altman RB, Clubb SL, Dorrestein GM, Quesenberry K (eds): *Avian Medicine and Surgery*. Philadelphia, WB Saunders, 1997a, pp 101–116.

Clubb SL. Laws and regulations affecting aviculture and the pet bird industry. In Altman RB, Clubb SL, Dorrestein GM, Quesenberry K (eds): *Avian Medicine and Surgery*. Philadelphia, WB Saunders, 1997b, pp 45–53.

Clubb SL. Psittacine pediatric husbandry and medicine. In Altman RB, Clubb SL, Dorrestein GM, Quesenberry K (eds): *Avian Medicine and Surgery*. Philadelphia, WB Saunders, 1997c, pp 73–95.

Clubb SL, Clubb KJ, Schubot R. *Psittacine Aviculture*. Loxahatchee, FL, Avicultural Breeding and Research Center, 1992.

Dhillon AS, Jack O. Management of a psittacine aviary. *Proc Assoc Avian Vet* 1990;83–86.

Dhillon AS. Egg collection, sanitation and hatchery management. *Proc Assoc Avian Vet* 1991;144–145.

Dorrestein GM, van der Hage MH. Veterinary problems in mynah birds. *Proc Assoc Avian Vet* 1988;263–274.

Echols MS, Speer BL. A comprehensive plan for managing flock reproductive performance. *Sem Avian Exot Pet Med* 1996;5(4):205–213.

Ferris D. Breeding and rearing conures. *Proc Semin Parrot Breeding, Handrearing, and Viral Diseases Update, Avian Res Fund* 1993;35–38.

Flammer K. Aviculture management. In Harrison GJ, Harrison LR (eds): *Clinical Avian Medicine and Surgery*, Philadelphia, WB Saunders, 1986a, pp 601–612.

Flammer K. Sample weight gains of selected hand-raised psittacines. In Harrison GJ, Harrison LR (eds): *Clinical Avian Medicine and Surgery*. Philadelphia, WB Saunders, 1986b, pp 664–666.

Flammer K, Clubb SL. Neonatology. In Ritchie BW, Harrison GJ, Harrison LR (eds): *Avian Medicine: Principles and Application*. Lake Worth, FL, Wingers Publishing, 1994, pp 805–838.

Goodwin M, McGee ED. Herpes-like virus associated with a cloacal papilloma in an orange-fronted conure (*Aratinga canicularis*). *J Assoc Avian Vet* 1993;7(1):23–25.

Graham DL. Internal papillomatous disease: A pathologist's view, or cloacal papillomas—and then some! *Proc Assoc Avian Vet* 1991;141–143.

Hanson JT. Handraising large parrots: methodology and expected weight gains. *Zoo Biol* 1987;6:139–160.

Harlin RW. Pigeons. *Proc Assoc Avian Vet* 1995;361–374.

Halverson J. Nonsurgical methods of avian sex identification. In Altman RB, Clubb SL, Dorrestein GM, Quesenberry K (eds): *Avian Medicine and Surgery*. Philadelphia, WB Saunders, 1997, pp 117–121.

Harrison GJ. Reproductive medicine. In Harrison GJ, Harrison LR (eds): *Clinical Avian Medicine and Surgery*. Philadelphia, WB Saunders, 1986, pp 620–633.

Hicks KD. Ratite reproduction. *Proc Assoc Avian Vet* 1992;318–325.

Hillyer EV, Moroff S, Hoefer H, et al. Bile dict carcinoma in two out of ten amazon parrots with cloacal papillomas. *J Assoc Avian Vet* 1991;5(2):91–95.

Hines R, Kolattukuty PE, Sharley P. Pharmacological induction of molt and gonadal involution in birds. *Proc Assoc Avian Vet* 1993;127–134.

Hudelson KS. A review of the mechanisms of avian reproduction and their clinical applications. *Sem Avian Exot Pet Med* 1996;5(4):189–198.

Hudelson KS, Hudelson P. A brief review of the female avian reproductive cycle with special emphasis on the role of prostaglandins and clinical applications. *J Avian Med Surg* 1996;10(2):67–74.

Hudelson S, Hudelson P. Egg binding, hormonal control and therapeutic considerations. *Compendium on Continuing Education* 1993;15:427–432.

Ingram KA. Otoscopic technique for sexing birds. In Kirk R (ed): *Current Veterinary Therapy VII*. Philadelphia, WB Saunders, 1980.

Jennings J. Setting up the softbill aviary. *Proc Semin Parrot Breeding, Handrearing and Viral Diseases Update, Avian Res Fund* 1993;118–121.

Johnson AL. Reproduction in the female. In Sturkie PD (ed): *Avian Physiology*, ed 4. New York, Springer-Verlag, 1986, pp 403–431.

Johnson AL. Reproduction in the male. In Sturkie PD (ed): *Avian Physiology*, ed 4. New York, Springer-Verlag, 1986, pp 432–451.

Jordan R. *Parrot Incubation Procedures*. Pickering, Ontario, Silvio Mattacchione, 1990.

Joseph V, Ferrier W. A raptor management program. *J Assoc Avian Vet* 1990;4(1):16–18.

Joyner KL. Psittacine incubation and pediatrics. In Fowler ME (ed): *Zoo and Wild Animal Medicine Current Therapy 3*. Philadelphia, WB Saunders, 1993, pp 247–260.

Joyner KL. Theriogenology. In Ritchie BW, Harrison GJ, Harrison LR (eds): *Avian Medicine: Principles and Application*. Lake Worth, FL, Wingers Publishing, 1994, pp 748–804.

Kennedy FS, Sattler-Augustin S, Mahler JR. Oropharyngeal and cloacal papillomas in two macaws with a pancreatic and an intestinal adenocarcinoma with hepatic metastasis. *Proc Assoc Avian Vet* 1994;428–430.

King AS, McLelland J. *Birds: Their Structure and Function*. London, Balliere Tindall, 1984.

Lannom J. Breeding cockatoos. *Proc Parrot Mgmt Semin, Avian Res Fund* 1991;107–111.

Lightfoot TL. Clinical use and preliminary data on human chorionic gonadotropin administration in psittacines. *Proc Assoc Avian Vet* 1996;303–306.

Longo J. Breeding the toco toucan. *Proc Assoc Avian Vet* 1989;248–249.

Marshall R. Management of pigeon diseases. *Proc Assoc Avian Vet* 1990;122–135.

McCluggage D. Hysterectomy: A review of select cases. *Proc Assoc Avian Vet* 1992;201–206.

McDonald SE. Clinical experiences with cloacal papillomas. *Proc Assoc Avian Vet* 1988;27–30.

McDonald SE. Pre-purchase and post-purchase examination. *Proc Semin Parrot Breeding, Handrearing and Viral Diseases Update, Avian Res Fund* 1993;122–139.

Millam JR. Reproductive physiology. In Altman RB, Clubb SL, Dorrestein GM, Quesenberry K (eds): *Avian Medicine and Surgery*. Philadelphia, WB Saunders, 1997, pp 12–26.

Millam JR, Finney H. Leuprolide acetate can reversibly prevent egg laying in cockatiels. *Proc Assoc Avian Vet* 1993;46.

Morishita TY. Establishing a differential diagnosis for backyard poultry flocks. *Proc Assoc Avian Vet* 1990;136–146.

Morishita TY. Common reproductive problems in the backyard chicken. *Proc Assoc Avian Vet* 1995;465–467.

Muser KK. Neonates: Handrearing from day one. *Proc Semin Parrot Breeding, Handrearing and Viral Diseases Update, Avian Res Fund* 1993;53–65.

Muser KK. Psittacine nursery management. *Proc Semin Parrot Breeding, Handrearing and Viral Diseases Update, Avian Res Fund* 1993;40–52.

Nye RR. Dealing with the egg-bound bird. In Kirk RW (ed): *Current Veterinary Therapy IX, Small Animal Practice*. Philadelphia, WB Saunders, 1986, pp 746–747.

Olsen GH. Problems associated with incubation and hatching. *Proc Assoc Avian Vet* 1989;262–267.

Olsen GH, Clubb SL. Embryology, incubation, and hatching. In Altman RB, Clubb SL, Dorrestein GM, Quesenberry K (eds): *Avian Medicine and Surgery*. Philadelphia, WB Saunders, 1997, pp 54–71.

Olsen GH, Nicolich JM, Hoffman DJ. A review of some causes of death of avian embryos. *Proc Assoc Avian Vet* 1990;106–111.

Orosz SE. Avian reproductive medicine: A review. *Proc Assoc Avian Vet* 1990;365–368.

Ottinger MA, Bakst MR. Endocrinology of the avian reproductive system. *J Avian Med Surg* 1995;9(4):242–250.

Paster MB. Avian reproductive endocrinology. *Vet Clin North Am Small Anim Pract* 1991;1343–1360.

Phalen DN. Anatomy of the avian urogenital system. *Proc Found in Avian Med, Assoc Avian Vet* 1995;1–8.

Raines AM. How to evaluate a ratite facility to aid in diagnosing chick mortality. *Proc Assoc Avian Vet* 1994;97–102.

Ramey K, Moore N, Millam JR. Affiliative behavior in captive breeding amazon parrots. *Proc Assoc Avian Vet* 1994;434.

Ring L. Aviary design and management. *Proc Assoc Avian Vet* 1989;250–256.

Romagnano A. Avian obstetrics. *Sem Avian Exot Pet Med* 1996;5(4):180–188.

Rosskopf WJ, Woerpel RW. Avian obstetrical medicine. In Birchard SJ, Sherding RG (eds): *Saunders Manual of Small Animal Practice.* Philadelphia, WB Saunders, 1994, pp 1302–1311.

Rosskopf WJ, Woerpel RW. Cloacal conditions in pet birds with a cloacapexy update. *Proc Assoc Avian Vet* 1989;156–163.

Rosskopf WJ, Woerpel RW. Pet avian obstetrics. *Proc First Intl Conf Zool Avian Med* 1987;213–231.

Rosskopf WJ, Woerpel RW. Pet avian obstetrical medicine. *Proc Assoc Avian Vet* 1993;323–336.

Schmidt RE. Histology and pathology of the avian reproductive system. *Proc Found in Avian Medicine, Assoc Avian Vet* 1995;9–16.

Schubot RM, Clubb KJ, Clubb SL (eds): *Psittacine Aviculture, Perspectives, Techniques and Research.* Loxahatchee, FL, Avicultural Breeding and Research Center, 1992.

Speer BL. A clinical approach to psittacine infertility. *Proc Assoc Avian Vet* 1991;173–187.

Speer BL. Avicultural medical management. *Proc Parrot Management Semin, Avian Res Fund* 1991;125–152.

Speer BL. Avicultural medical management: An introduction to basic principles of flock medicine and the closed aviary concept. *Vet Clin North Am Small Anim Pract* 1991;1393–1404.

Speer BL. Clinical reproductive medicine. *Proc Found in Avian Med, Assoc Avian Vet* 1995;23–33.

Speer BL. The eclectus parrot: Medicine and avicultural aspects. *Proc Assoc Avian Vet* 1989;239–247.

Speer BL, Abramson J. Management and maintenance of a macaw breeding facility. *Proc Avic Conf, Assoc Avian Vet* 1992;2.1–2.17.

Stewart JS. Ratite incubation. *Proc Assoc Avian Vet* 1992;336–339.

Stonebreaker RF. Husbandry and medical management of the nursery. *Proc Assoc Avian Vet* 1991;161–166.

Taylor M. A morphologic approach to the endoscopic determination of sex in juvenile macaws. *J Assoc Avian Vet* 1989;3(4):199–201.

Taylor M. Endoscopic examination of ovarian morphology in juvenile psittacine birds: Preliminary findings. *Proc Assoc Avian Vet* 1988;33–34.

Thompson DR. Breeding amazons in captivity. *Proc Sem Parrot Breeding, Handrearing and Viral Diseases Update, Avian Res Fund* 1993;88–98.

VanDerHeyden N. Psittacine papillomas. *Proc Assoc Avian Vet* 1988;23–26.

Van Sant F. Resolution of a cloacal adhesion in a blue-fronted amazon. *Proc Assoc Avian Vet* 1992;162–164.

Voren H, Jordan R. *Parrots: Hand-Feeding and Nursery Management.* Pickering, Ontario, Silvio Mattacchione, 1992.

Wakenell PS. Obstetrics and reproduction of backyard poultry. *Sem Avian Exot Pet Med* 1996;5(4):199–204.

Wissman MA. Unusual c-section and hysterectomy in the isle of pines amazon. *Proc Assoc Avian Vet* 1991;265–266.

Wissman MA, Parsons B. Preparation for the breeding season. *Proc Assoc Avian Vet* 1992;387–389.

Worell A. Management and medicine of toucans. *Proc Assoc Avian Vet* 1988;253–262.

Chapter 16

Pediatrics

Chicks are altricial or precocial at hatching. At hatching, altricial birds have little or no down, have poor musculoskeletal development, and rely on parental feeding and warmth. Altricial birds include psittacines, passerines, toucans, pigeons, and doves. Raptors are semialtricial and require parental attention to survive. Precocial birds are covered with down at hatching and are able to stand, run, and occasionally fly soon after hatching. Precocial birds require minimal parental attention. Ducks, geese, gallinaceous birds, and ratites are precocial.

Chicks may be raised by their parents or by foster parents or be hand raised. Allowing the parents to rear their young saves labor and is often preferable for birds bred for breeding purposes or reintroduction into the wild. Parent birds may not provide optimal care or may traumatize offspring, especially with aviary disturbances. Nest boxes should have a small door that allows viewing of the chicks. Chicks should be monitored daily. Normal chicks have food in their crops and have yellowish-pink skin. Abnormalities to observe for include empty crops, listlessness, and feeling cool to the touch. These birds should be removed from the nest, examined and treated appropriately, and hand raised. Excellent parental nutrition is important for normal neonatal development.

Foster parenting means moving eggs or chicks from one nest to another. Foster parenting is used to increase productivity by allowing a desirable pair to lay more eggs, to raise young from neglectful or abusive parents, or when chicks are of different sizes in a nest. The foster nest should have chicks or eggs of similar size and age. However, fostering may spread disease.

Hand raising young birds is labor intensive, but birds that are hand raised often make better pets. Removing neonates and eggs for artificial incubation and hand raising increases production by allowing a pair of birds to lay additional clutches.

HAND RAISING

Many of the pediatric problems that occur in the nursery are husbandry related; the veterinarian can provide instruction in proper techniques to the aviculturist, as outlined below. Housing and nutrition profoundly affect the health of chicks. Neonates lack fully competent immune systems and are more susceptible to disease than are older birds. The basic concept of disease control through maintaining a closed aviary is discussed in Chapter 15. Nursery design, housing, bedding, disease control, chick identification, and record keeping are also discussed in Chapter 15. Records allow periodic evaluation of individual chicks, parents, and the aviary. A sample pediatric record is provided in Figure 16–1. A great deal of information is available about many aspects of hand raising birds (see references).

Nutrition

Nutritional requirements of psittacine chicks are not entirely known. Diets that work well for one aviary may not work well for another. Feeding techniques influence growth, including amount fed, frequency of feedings, and diet composition. Different species may have different nutritional requirements. In general, the protein content should be 18% to 22%; calcium content, 1%, and the calcium-to-phosphorus ratio, approximately 2:1. Birds older than 1 to 2 days should be fed a diet with 25% to 30% solids. Properly mixed commercial formulas should meet these requirements. Commercial diets appear to be superior to most homemade formulas. A more dilute formula is fed for the first day after hatching. Some commercial hand-feeding diets are listed in Table 16–1. Dilution of commercial diets with added foodstuffs will alter nutrient composition, and these changes may be detrimental.

Frequency of feeding depends on age, diet, and development of the birds. Table 16–2 lists recommendations for frequency of feedings of psittacine neonates. Birds younger than 1 week may benefit from around-the-clock feeding. Weak psittacines and soft-billed species may need to be fed around the clock. Older birds may be fed their last feeding between 10 p.m. and midnight and get their first feeding between 6 and 7 a.m.

The crop should be palpated before each feeding. It should be empty or almost empty between feedings, and it should be completely empty once daily.

Cleanliness and proper hygiene are important to the health of the hand-fed bird. Fresh formula should be mixed for each feeding—leftover formula should

---

TABLE 16–1 Some Commercial Hand-feeding Formulas

Exact Handfeeding Formula for all chicks and Exact Handfeeding Formula for macaws: Kaytee Products, Inc., PO Box 230, Chilton, WI 53014 (414) 849-2321; (800) 529-8331

Harrison's Juvenile Formulas: Harrison's Bird Diets, 7171 Mercy Rd., Ste 135, Omaha, NE 68106 (402) 397-9442; (800) 346-0269

Lakes Ultimate Avian Diet Hand-feeding Formula: Lakes Minnesota Macaws, Inc., 639 Stryker Ave., St. Paul, MN 55107 (800) 634-2473

Nutri-start Baby Bird Food: Lafeber Co., 24981 N. 1400 East Rd., Cornell, IL 61319 (815) 358-2301

Pretty Bird Hand-rearing Formula: Pretty Bird International, Inc., PO Box 177, 5810 Stacy Tr., Stacy, MN 55079 (800) 356-5020

Roudybush Hand-feeding Formula, Formula III, and Squab Formula: Roudybush, 3550 Watt Ave., Suite #8, Sacramento, CA 95821 (800) 326-1726

Topper Bird Ranch Baby Formula: Topper Bird Ranch, 1466 N. Carpenter Rd., Modesto, CA 95351 (209) 524-2828

Tropican Hand-feeding Formula: Rolf C. Hagen, Mansfield, MA 02048 (800) 724-2436

Zeigler Hand-feeding Formula for Medium and Large Hookbills: Zeigler Inc., PO Box 95, Gardners, PA 17324 (800) 841-6800

Identification _____ Species _____

Date of Hatch _____ Date of Hand Feeding Start _____

Formula _____

Age	Weight	Time	Volume fed	Comments

Figure 16–1. Pediatric record. (Courtesy of Speer BL. Avicultural medical management. *Proc Parrot Mgmt Semin* 1991; 125–152. Used by permission.)

TABLE 16–2 Suggested Feeding Frequencies in Psittacine Neonates

Birds 1 to 5 days old: feed 6 to 10 times daily
Birds with eyes closed: feed 4 to 6 times daily
Birds with eyes open: feed 3 to 4 times daily
Birds with feathers emerging: feed 2 to 3 times daily

---

not be refrigerated and later used. Opened containers of dry formula should be stored in sealed containers in the freezer.

The formula should be warmed to 101° to 104°F with hot water, hot plate, or coffeemaker. Heated formula is stirred with a clean finger to check for excessively hot areas of formula. A thermometer should be used to determine the temperature of the formula. Warming formula in microwave ovens often results in crop burns (see Chapter 4).

Catheter-tipped syringes work well for hand feeding. Syringes should be filled with warmed formula before feeding any birds. Syringes should not be dipped into the food for refilling once they have been used to feed a bird. The filled syringes may be placed in warm water to keep warm while feeding a group of birds. Separate syringes are used for each bird. The aviculturist or veterinarian should wash hands between birds or groups of birds. Syringes are separated, washed, disinfected, and allowed to dry between feedings. Quaternary ammonium compounds work well for disinfecting feeding syringes, which should be rinsed well to remove all residues of disinfectant.

The healthiest, most expensive, and most susceptible birds are fed first, before contact with any ill or possible carrier birds in the aviary. Healthy large psittacine chicks are also fed first, and conures, cockatiels, and budgies are fed last.

Touching the sides of the beak or under the chin will stimulate a feeding response. Neonates will bob their heads up and down. While the bird shows this feeding response, the head is gently supported and the food is administered (Fig. 16–2). Alternate sides of beak are used to feed the bird. If a feeding response is not displayed, there is an increased risk of tracheal aspiration during feeding.

Chicks should be weighed daily. The best time to weigh each bird is before the first feeding of the morning, when the crop is empty. Within 2 days after hatching, chicks should gain weight every day unless they are weaning or were overhydrated at hatching. The growth of the chick should be monitored and evaluated through comparison with established normal growth parameters from the aviary or other sources (Abramson, Speer, and Thomsen, 1995; Flammer, 1994; Hanson, 1987; Joyner, 1993; Schubot, Clubb, and Clubb, 1992). Lack of weight gain or weight loss indicates the need for a complete physical examination and diagnostic testing as needed to determine the etiology of the problem.

Several weeks before weaning, the bird should be offered a variety of foods, such as cooked vegetables, fruits, commercial formulated diet, spray millet, hulled seeds, soaked monkey chow, and peanut butter and jelly sandwiches. Vegetables and fruits should be so large that they cannot be ingested whole or chopped small enough to pass from the crop to the proventriculus. Large chunks of food or seeds with hulls may be consumed whole. Food should be easily accessible, in a bowl on the floor or at perch height. It is preferable to wean

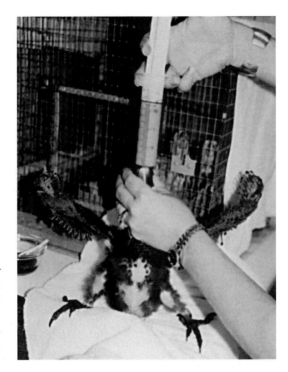

Figure 16–2. Touching the sides of the beak or under the chin will stimulate a feeding response. The head is gently supported, and the food is deposited in the caudal oropharynx and crop. (Photo courtesy of Jean Jordan, Adventures in Birds, Houston, TX. Used by permission.)

birds to a variety of commercially formulated diets with some vegetables and fruits. Acceptance of a varied diet may result in better acceptance of the foods offered when they leave the nursery. The same food should be continued by new owners.

Some birds wean themselves upon reaching the appropriate weight and development, but others require encouragement to wean. Birds of the appropriate weight, age, and development that are healthy are gradually weaned by decreasing food offered by syringe. The midday feeding is eliminated when the bird is at the appropriate age and development at the first sign of decreased interest. Then the morning feeding is eliminated, and the evening feeding is eliminated last. It is normal for weaning chicks to lose weight during weaning. The amount of weight loss varies depending on the weaning techniques and the species. Most chicks lose 10% to 15% of their body weight, with some chicks losing up to 20%.

Weaning is a stressful time for chicks. Fungal and bacterial infections are common. Clinical signs of problems include slowed crop emptying, depression, diarrhea, regurgitation, excessive weight loss, or a failure to wean. Many normal weaning chicks will regurgitate immediately after feeding if fed large amounts at this time when the crop is decreasing in size. If any abnormalities are noted, weaning is delayed and the problem is diagnosed and treated. In birds with severe weight loss, hand feeding can be resumed two or three times daily until adequate weight is gained. Severely ill birds may resist feeding or lack a feeding response; these ill birds are tube fed.

PHYSICAL EXAMINATION

The veterinarian should develop a systematic approach and use it every time a physical examination is performed. Evaluate the entire bird. A stamp, such as the one in Figure 1–5, may be useful to reinforce and record a complete physical examination.

Before physical examination, obtain a complete history. Review the chick's daily weights, daily volume of food fed, and daily crop emptying, and inquire about the egg, clutch, incubation, and hatching history. Inquire about the diet and method of hand feeding if the bird is hand fed. Observe hand feeding by the feeder, including mixing, heating, and feeding the formula if possible. Ask about the parents' diet, in parent-reared chicks. Obtain history of the aviary, including diseases occurring in the last few years, reproductive records on the parents, health status and diet of the parents, introduction of birds from other sources, and usage of antibiotics, antifungals, and anthelmintics.

Evaluate the environment. Note the size, shape, and material of the container used to house the chick. Examine the bedding material for abnormal feces, abnormal urates, regurgitated food, and blood. Learn about the temperature and humidity of the environment.

Observe the bird in its environment. Note the size and development, and compare it with chicks of the same clutch or same age and species if possible. Attitude and posture vary with the age, species, and development. Note abnormalities. Abnormal attitudes include hyperactivity, depression, dullness, and unusual vocalizations. Birds in excessively high environmental temperatures will pant and hold their wings away from their bodies. Chicks that are too cold will shiver and huddle and may have slow crop emptying. All chicks should be able to hold their heads up during feeding. Some unusual but normal behaviors include macaws reverting to behaviors seen in younger chicks during weaning, conures sleeping on their backs, young cockatoo chicks' reluctance to hold their head erect in the first few weeks of life except during feeding, and psittacine chicks frequently resting on their hocks and abdomen. Abnormalities to note include splay leg, scoliosis of the lower spine, opisthotonos, lateral deviation of the cervical spine, turned hocks, and bent toes.

Perform a complete physical examination with clean, dry, and warm hands in a warm room or under a heat lamp. If abnormalities are noted, consult appropriate sections of the text for additional information. When possible, examine the chick when the crop is empty to help prevent aspiration of crop contents. Examine the eyes for congenital abnormalities, discharge, swellings, scabs, and scars. Altricial birds hatch with eyes closed. In large psittacines, eyes generally open by 2 to 3 weeks of age and in smaller birds, by 1 week of age. Eyes still shut beyond the normal time may be the result of stunting, developmental anomaly, or sealing by exudate from an infection or dried food. A clear discharge may be seen when eyes open in normal birds. Congenital abnormalities include anophthalmia, microphthalmia, cataracts, retinal and ciliary body dysplasia, eyelid agenesis, cryptophthalmos, and ectropion. Discharges may be the result of corneal scratches, trauma, congenital abnormalities, accumulation of periorbital food, and infectious diseases (e.g., poxvirus, bacteria, *Mycoplasma, Chlamydia*).

Examine the nostrils, cere, and infraorbital sinus areas. The nares of some species of birds are closed at hatching but open within a few days. Observe for swelling, discharge, dried food, blood, and foreign bodies. Swelling around the eye or between the eyes and beak may be the result of sinusitis. Sinusitis or rhinitis may be the result of food in the nares or choana, choanal atresia, or infectious disease (e.g., bacterial, chlamydial, fungal, or viral).

The beak and oropharynx are difficult to examine in pediatric patients because the normal feeding response results in head motion. Observe for beak abnormalities and malformations (lateral deviations, shortened maxillas, prognathism, grooves or trauma to the rhamphotheca), exudates, plaques, accumulation of debris or food, discoloration, oropharyngeal ulcers, and ulceration of the lateral commissures of the beak. Check for a normal feeding response. Lack of a feeding response may be the result of weakness and disease.

Examine the ears. New World psittacines generally have closed ear canals at hatching that open at 10 to 30 days. The ears of precocial birds and Old World psittacines are usually open at hatching. Examine the ear with a strong light source, such as an endoscope. Abnormalities include presence of dried food or exudate on the skin or feathers near the opening, exudates in the ear canal, erythema, blood, and abnormally small ear openings. Stunting may result in delayed ear opening. Exudates may be the result of bacterial infection.

Examine the crop, esophagus, and trachea. Examine and palpate the crop for volume and character of contents, foreign bodies, clumps of food, abscesses, fibrous tissue from previous burns, air, and fluid. Observe for crop motility. Normal peristalsis is one to three contractions per minute in a crop partially filled with food. Crop stasis or delayed crop emptying is usually secondary to a generalized gastrointestinal dysfunction rather than to a primary crop disorder. Examine the skin surrounding the crop for discoloration, erythema, subcutaneous food, swellings, lumps, masses, scabs, and exudates.

Evaluate the head size in relation to body size and feathering. An abnormally large head in relation to body size, abnormal feathering, and large protruding eyes are often observed with undersized chicks or stunting.

Examine the abdomen, vent, and body. Examine the spine and carina (keel) for curvature. Evaluate subcutaneous muscle and fat mass over the back, toes, and wings. Pectoral muscle mass is a poor indicator of nutritional status before weaning. Palpate the abdomen. In normal chicks, the proventriculus and ventriculus are proportionally large and the abdomen protrudes slightly. Abnormalities include abdominal distention, palpable masses, open navels, and fecal or urate accumulation around the vent. Visualize abdominal contents through the translucent skin overlying the abdomen. Abnormalities include discoloration, hemorrhage, and ascitic fluid. The yolk sac should not be visible through the skin beyond 24 to 48 hours after hatching. The duodenal loop may be observed in some young chicks and should always contain ingesta.

Examine the legs and feet. Abnormalities include swellings, discolorations, cuts, abrasions, erythema, proliferative lesions, swollen joints, toe constrictions, neurologic deficits, fractures, and malformations (e.g., splay legs, perosis).

Examine the wings for symmetry, range of motion, and bony, soft tissue, and skin abnormalities. Abnormalities include swellings, bony abnormalities, enlarged joints, and ulcerations. Hydration status can be determined by observation of the basilic (wing) vein. Normal veins are turgid and refill immediately when depressed.

Examine the skin. Normal skin may be dry and flaky and is pink to pinkish-yellow, but varies among species. Overly dry or wrinkled skin may be the result of dehydration from illness, high environmental temperature, or low environmental humidity. A change in color to dark red may be the result of overheating, dehydration, or septicemia. Pale skin may be the result of anemia, hypothermia, shock, or illness. Other abnormalities include wounds, scabs, erythema, subcutaneous masses, hemorrhage, and soft tissue calcification.

Examine the feathers. Abnormalities in the pattern of feather development may be the result of stunted growth. Abnormalities include stress marks, retained feather sheaths, and bleeding, broken, missing, abnormally shaped, or damaged feathers. Antibiotic therapy may result in abnormal feather development. Multiple stress bars along feathers can indicate a repeated or ongoing problem and warrant a complete examination (see Chapter 8).

Auscult the heart and lungs. Abnormalities include murmurs, arrhythmias, dull heart sounds, overly loud heart sounds, abnormal heart and respiratory rates, and harsh, moist respiratory sounds.

DIAGNOSTICS

Pediatric diagnostics are similar to adult diagnostics with a few notable exceptions. Pediatric necropsy is discussed in Chapter 10.

Microbiology

Microbiology is a useful diagnostic tool in pediatric medicine. Chicks should be sterile at hatching, but they are rapidly colonized with bacteria from their environment. Bacterial and fungal cultures are useful to monitor the environment of the chick, including sanitation, management practices, and the presence of other diseases.

Cloacal, fecal, and crop Gram's stains and cultures are useful to determine the pattern of normal microflora for a nursery in normal chicks, to identify nursery management problems, to identify secondary bacterial or fungal infections, and to identify primary bacterial or fungal infections. Bacteria commonly cultured from healthy chicks include *Streptococcus, Staphylococcus, Lactobacillus, Corynebacterium, Escherichia coli, Enterobacter,* and *Klebsiella.* Bacteria cultured from the gastrointestinal tract may be the result of a primary infection or secondary infection or be nonpathogenic. If clinical signs of illness are present, antibiotic therapy is warranted when gram-negative bacteria are isolated (e.g., *E. coli, Klebsiella*). Evaluate the sanitation, management, and diet. Consult Chapter 12 for assistance in interpretive significance of isolated bacteria. Small numbers of yeast can also be found in the crop and cloacal samples of healthy chicks. Indications for gastrointestinal cultures include crop stasis, crop impaction, oral lesions, diarrhea, melena, hematochezia, and constipation.

Choana, trachea, conjunctiva, cornea, ear, and other sources are cultured when pathology is present. Rostral choanal cultures are useful to evaluate the microflora of the upper respiratory tract.

Gram's stains are quick and inexpensive, but some organisms may not be apparent. Gram's stains should be followed up with cultures. Yeast is present in some hand-feeding formulas and may be noted in crop, cloacal, and fecal Gram's stains, but will not show budding.

Hematology

Hematology in chicks is similar to adults with some notable exceptions. Contraindications for collection of blood samples include full crop, severe hypoproteinemia, anemia, severe depression, respiratory distress, extreme weakness, and when veins are inaccessible or are too small. Blood collection sites include the jugular, basilic (wing), and medial metatarsal veins. The jugular vein is the preferred site.

Chick hemograms differ from those of adults. Young chicks have lower PCVs (they can be in the low 20s, but are usually in the low 30s by 1 month of age). In general, young chicks have lower total protein (as low as 1 g/dl, but typically average 2 to 3 g/dl by 1 month of age). Red blood cell counts, hemoglobin concentrations, mean corpuscular hemoglobin, and mean corpuscular hemoglobin concentration are lower. Young chicks usually have higher WBC counts, and young chicks may have different leukocyte distributions (see Altman, Clubb, Dorrestein, and Quesenberry, 1997; Schubot, Clubb, and Clubb, 1992; Clubb, Schubot, and Joyner, 1990, 1991, 1991). Polychromatophils are abundant.

Plasma Biochemistries

Plasma biochemistry tests are useful diagnostic aids in pediatric patients, similar to adult birds. In general, 1% of the chick's body weight can be collected in blood (e.g., a 150-g chick can have up to 1.5 ml of blood taken in a single collection). Some differences exist in values between species and between different age groups of birds. In general, young chicks have lower total protein and lower albumin levels, may have higher alkaline phosphatase and creatine kinase (CK) levels, and may have lower uric acid levels and lower AST levels (see Altman, Clubb, Dorrestein, and Quesenberry, 1997; Clubb, Schubot, and Joyner, 1990, 1991a, 1991b; Schubot, Clubb, and Clubb, 1992). Phosphorus is often increased.

Radiography

Radiography is a useful diagnostic aid in pediatric patients. Isoflurane anesthesia is recommended. Use caution with manual restraint because of the lack of mineralization of the skeleton. If possible, the crop should be empty to help prevent aspiration. The proventriculus and ventriculus are large in proportion to the body, and intestinal loops may be filled with food. The liver and heart may also appear large in proportion to the rest of the body. Air sac spaces appear small because of the food-filled gastrointestinal tract. Growth plates disappear around weaning age in most birds. Aspiration pneumonia often has a caudodorsal lung distribution and caudal air sac involvement.

Endoscopy

Techniques and indications for endoscopy of pediatric patients are similar to adult birds. In pediatric patients, laparoscopy is complicated by the large size of the proventriculus and intestines. The chick should be fasted and the proventriculus gauged to be empty before surgery, if this procedure is deemed necessary in spite of the risks. Routine endoscopy is useful for crop, oropharyngeal, tracheal, ear, and cloacal examinations.

COMMON PROBLEMS

Ill neonates can quickly become dehydrated, hypoglycemic, hypothermic, and septicemic. Evidence of dehydration include dry, reddened, wrinkled skin; sunken facial features; and feeling sticky to the touch. Hypoglycemia results in depression. Supportive care is urgent when young chicks are ill. Supportive care is administered before collection of diagnostic samples in very ill birds. Place hypothermic patients in a warm, moist environment (e.g., an incubator set at 92° to 95°). Correct dehydration with IV or IO fluid therapy, similar to adults (see Chapter 1). Hypoglycemia is treated with 2.5% to 5% dextrose added to fluids. Primary and secondary bacterial infections are common in pediatric birds. When infection is suspected, begin antibiotic therapy with an antibiotic with minimal toxicity and good gram-negative activity (e.g., piperacillin or cefotaxime). Do not use aminoglycoside antibiotics in dehydrated patients. Waiting for culture results may be fatal.

Overgrowth of *Candida* is common in chicks receiving antibiotic therapy. Monitor chicks for *Candida* overgrowth with choanal, crop, or fecal Gram's stains. Consider prophylactic antifungal therapy in young birds being treated with antibiotics for prolonged periods of time (e.g., treatment of chlamydiosis).

Failure to Absorb the Yolk Sac

The yolk sac is a diverticulum of the intestine that supplies nourishment and maternal antibodies in the first few days of life. It is normally internalized into the abdomen before completion of hatching. Causes of failure to internalize the yolk sac include infection, improper incubation procedures, and idiopathic causes. When the yolk sac is not entirely internalized, the protruding yolk sac is prone to punctures and tears, which may result in hemorrhage or infection. The chick may absorb the yolk sac if left in the egg for several hours longer than normal. Support the neonate with oral lactated Ringer's solution administration with 2.5% dextrose added and ensure proper brooder temperature and humidity levels. If the sac is not absorbed within a few hours, gently clean the area with an iodine solution and lubricate the protruding sac and protect it with a nonstick wound dressing until the sac is fully absorbed. Large protrusions may be placed into the abdomen with a swab coated with a water-based sterile ointment. Then suture or seal the umbilicus with surgical glue. Very large external yolk sacs may require surgical removal.

The yolk is normally absorbed within 10 days after hatching. Clinical signs of failure to absorb the yolk material in the internalized sac include abdominal distention, dyspnea, exercise intolerance, depression, and anorexia. The abdomen has a doughy consistency, and the yolk sac may be visible through the abdominal skin and muscles.

Stunting

Chicks develop rapidly, and anything that interferes with metabolism can result in a decreased growth rate. Common causes of stunting include improper feeding, infection, and environmental or management problems. Improper feeding may be the result of inadequate caloric intake (inadequate volume, infrequent feedings, inadequate solids), unbalanced formula (calcium-to-phosphorus ratio imbalance, inadequate fat content, lack of essential amino acids), poor parental diet, or poor parenting. Common chronic infections resulting in stunting include gram-negative bacteria, yeast, polyomavirus, and PBFD. Environmental and management problems that often result in stunting include low or high environmental temperature or low humidity. Some other causes of stunting include ingestion of bedding, blood loss at hatching, assisted hatching, excessively wet or dry at hatching, and omphalitis.

Stunting appears to be most common in hyacinth macaws, palm cockatoos, and Queen of Bavaria conures, possibly as a result of different nutritional needs. These birds appear to perform better on a high-fat and high-fiber formulated diet, supplemented with nuts at weaning.

Diagnosis of the etiology of stunting includes exploring the diet and environmental conditions, performing a complete physical examination and choanal, crop, and cloacal Gram's stains. If obvious dietary deficiencies are present without abnormalities on the physical examination or Gram's stains, alter the diet and monitor the bird. Treat *Candida* infections noted on Gram's stains. If abnormalities are noted on the Gram's stains, submit samples for culture and sensitivity testing. Abnormalities noted on physical examination are pursued following guidelines listed in appropriate sections of this book.

If a diagnosis is not obvious, submit choanal, crop, and cloacal samples for bacterial and fungal cultures and submit samples for polyomavirus and PBFD probe testing.

Treatment for stunting entails treating the underlying cause. Ensure that excellent nutrition is provided.

Delayed Crop Emptying, Crop Stasis, Crop Foreign Bodies, or Crop Burns

See Esophagus and Crop Disorders, Chapter 4.

Splay Leg or Leg Deformities

See Limping, Lameness, or Leg Deformity, Chapter 7.

Constricted Toes

See Feet or Leg Lesions, Chapter 8.

Beak Deformities

See Beak Lesions, Chapter 8.

References and Additional Readings

Abramson J, Speer BL, Thomsen JB. *The Large Macaws: Their Care, Breeding and Conservation.* Fort Bragg, CA, Raintree Publications, 1995.

Altman RB. Avian neonatal and pediatric surgery. *Semin Avian Exot Pet Med* 1992;1(1):34–39.

Altman RB, Clubb SL, Dorrestein GM, Quesenberry K (eds): *Avian Medicine and Surgery.* Philadelphia, WB Saunders, 1997.

Blue-McLendon A. Pediatric disorders of ostriches. *Proc Assoc Avian Vet* 1993;269–271.

Bond MW. Avian pediatrics. *Proc Assoc Avian Vet* 1991;153–160.

Clipsham R. Pediatric management and medicine. *J Assoc Avian Vet* 1989;1(1):10–13.

Clipsham R. Avicultural medical diagnostics and therapeutics. *Proc Avian Pediatr Semin* 1991;61–92.

Clipsham R. Introduction to psittacine pediatrics. *Vet Clin North Am Small Anim Pract* 1991;21(6):1361–1392.

Clipsham R. Noninfectious diseases of pediatric psittacines. *Semin Avian Exot Pet Med* 1992;1(1):22–33.

Clipsham RC. Surgical correction of beaks. *Proc Assoc Avian Vet* 1990;325–333.

Clipsham RC. Correction of pediatric leg disorders. *Proc Assoc Avian Vet* 1991;200–204.

Clubb SL. Psittacine pediatric medicine. *ABVP Avian Specialty Core Review Course* 1993;159–165.

Clubb SL. Psittacine neonatology. In Kirk RW, Bonagura JD (eds): *Current Veterinary Therapy XI, Small Animal Practice.* Philadelphia, WB Saunders, 1992, pp 1142–1145.

Clubb SL, Clubb KJ. Psittacine pediatrics. *Proc Assoc Avian Vet* 1986;317–332.

Clubb SL, Clubb KJ. Psittacine pediatrics. *Proc Second European Symp Avian Med and Surg* 1989;283–299.

Clubb SL, Schubot RM, Joyner K, et al. Hematologic and serum biochemical reference intervals in juvenile eclectus parrots (*Eclectus roratus*). *J Assoc Avian Vet* 1990;4(4):218–225.

Clubb SL, Schubot RM, Joyner, K, et al. Hematologic and serum biochemical reference intervals in juvenile cockatoos. *J Assoc Avian Vet* 1991a;5(1):16–26.

Clubb SL, Schubot RM, Joyner K, et al. Hematologic and serum biochemical reference intervals in juvenile macaws (*Ara* sp.). *J Assoc Avian Vet* 1991b;5(3):154–162.

Dorrenstein GM. Avian pediatric pharmacology. *Semin Avian Exot Pet Med* 1993;2(3):110–115.

Flammer K. Pediatric medicine. In Harrison GJ, Harrison LR (eds): *Clinical Avian Medicine and Surgery.* Philadelphia, WB Saunders, 1986, pp 634–650.

Flammer K, Clubb SL. Neonatology. In Ritchie BW, Harrison GJ, Harrison LR (eds): *Avian Medicine: Principles and Application.* Lake Worth, FL, Wingers Publishing, 1994, pp 805–838.

Hagen M. Nutritional observations, hand-feeding formulas, and digestion in exotic birds. *Semin Avian Exot Pet Med* 1992;1(1):3–10.

Hanson JT. Hand-raising large parrots: Methodology and expected weight gains. *Zoo Biol* 1987;6:139–160.

Hicks KD. Ostrich pediatrics. *Semin Avian Exot Pet Med* 1993;2(3):136–141.

Joseph V. Raptor pediatrics. *Semin Avian Exot Pet Med* 1993;2(3):142–151.

Joyner KL. Avicultural pediatrics. *Proc Avian Pediatr Sem* 1988;83–92.

Joyner KL. Avicultural pediatrics. *Proc 10th Annual Mid-Atlantic States Avian Med Sem* 1989.

Joyner KL. Psittacine pediatric diagnostics. *Proc Assoc Avian Vet* 1990;60–74.

Joyner KL. Pediatric therapeutics. *Proc Assoc Avian Vet* 1991;188–199.

Joyner KL. Psittacine pediatric diagnostics. *Semin Avian Exot Pet Med* 1992;1(1):11–21.

Joyner KL. Psittacine incubation and pediatrics. In Fowler ME (ed): *Zoo and Wild Animal Medicine, Current Therapy 3.* Philadelphia, WB Saunders, 1993, pp 247–260.

Joyner KL, Swanson J, Hanson JT. Psittacine pediatric diagnostics. *Proc Assoc Avian Vet* 1990;60–82.

Lane RA, Rosskopf WJ, Allen KL. Avian pediatric hematology: Preliminary studies of the transition from the neonatal hemogram to the adult hemogram in selected psittacine species—African grey, amazons and macaws. *Proc Assoc Avian Vet* 1988;231–238.

Olsen GH, Duvall F. Commonly encountered hatching problems. *Proc Assoc Avian Vet* 1994;379–385.

Phillips AF, Clubb SL. Psittacine neonatal development. In Schubot RM, Clubb KJ, Clubb SL (eds): *Psittacine Aviculture, Perspectives, Techniques and Research.* Loxahatchee FL, Avicultural Breeding and Research Center, 1992.

Reavill DR. Psittacine pediatric emergency medicine. *Semin Avian Exot Pet Med* 1994;3(4):169–174.

Schubot R, Clubb SL, Clubb KJ. *Psittacine Aviculture.* Loxahatchee, FL, Avicultural Breeding and Research Center, 1992.

Shivaprasad HL. Neonatal mortality in ostriches: An overview of possible causes. *Proc Assoc Avian Vet* 1993;282–293.

Speer BL. Avicultural medical management: An introduction to basic principles of flock medicine and the closed aviary concept. *Vet Clin North Am Small Anim Pract* 1991;21(6):1393–1404.

Speer BL. Selected avian pediatric viral diseases. *Semin Avian Exot Pet Med* 1993;2(3):125–135.

Speer BL. Stunting in the large macaw. *Semin Avian Exot Pet Med* 1995;4(1):9–14.

Speer BL. Viral diseases of young birds. *Proc Avian Pediatr Semin Avian Res Fund* 1988;83–92.

Stonebreaker RF. Husbandry and medical management of the nursery. *Proc Assoc Avian Vet* 1991;161–166.

Takeshita K, Graham DL, Silverman S. Hypervitaminosis D in baby macaws. *Proc Assoc Avian Vet* 1986;341–346.

VanDerHeyden N. Avian pediatric physiology and medicine. *Proc ABVP Avian In-Depth Semin* 1994;61–69.

Voren H, Jordan R. *Parrots: Hand-Feeding and Nursery Management.* Pickering, Ontario, Silvio Mattacchione, 1992.

Wade JR. Ratite pediatric medicine and surgery. *Proc Assoc Avian Vet* 1992;340–353.

Worell AB. Nursery management. *Proc Semin Breeding, Rearing, and Marketing of Exotic Birds,* 1992.

Worell AB. Pediatric bacterial diseases. *Semin Avian Exot Pet Med* 1993;2(3):116–124.

Chapter 17

Formulary

Few pharmacologic studies have been performed on drugs commonly used in avian medicine. Most drug dosages in the literature are based on clinical experience or are extrapolated from use in other species. Suggested uses and dosages in this chapter are derived from the literature and personal experience. Every effort has been made to ensure that the information presented is accurate; however, the clinician assumes all responsibility for the use of all drugs. Consult references and product information provided by the manufacturer for additional precautions, toxicities, and possible drug interactions. Suggested drugs and dosages are for nonfood birds. Suggested doses may be suboptimal. Most drugs used in avian medicine are considered extra-label. Brand and manufacturers' names included are for reference purposes, not endorsement. Several drugs are available in generic form as well. Abbreviations are defined at the end of Table 17–1.

TABLE 17-1. Drugs Commonly Used in Avian Medicine

Drug	Route	Dosage	Comments
ANTIBIOTICS			
Amikacin (Amiglyde-V, Fort Dodge; Amikin, Bristol)	IM, IV	10–15 mg/kg q12h	Broad spectrum. Possible nephrotoxicity. Maintain adequate hydration. Synergistic with penicillins.
Amoxicillin (Amoxi-Inject, Amoxi-drops, SmithKline)	PO IM	150–175 mg/kg q8h 150 mg/kg q8h	Use limited to continuation of injectible amoxicillin therapy for cat bite wounds. Use limited to therapy for cat bite wounds.
Azithromycin (Zithromax, Pfizer)	PO	One drop of a 30 mg/ml suspension per g body wt q12h; 50–80 mg/kg q24h	Stable refrigerated for 3–4 wks. Do not use in birds with liver or kidney impairment. Administer on an empty stomach. May cause GI upset. For treatment of chlamydiosis, treat 3d, then off 4d for 6 wks. For treatment of mycoplasma, treat 3d, then off 4d for 21d. To make a 30 mg/ml suspension: mix 250 mg capsule with 8 ml lactulose.
Cefotaxime (Claforan, Hoechst)	IM, IV	75–100 mg/kg q4–8h	Broad spectrum, low toxicity, penetrates CSF. Active against many gram-negative and gram-positive organisms. Reconstituted stable for 10d refrigerated and 6mo frozen.
Cefoxitin (Mefoxin, Merck)	IM, IV	50–100 mg/kg q8–12h	Broad spectrum, low toxicity. Active against many gram-negative and gram-positive organisms. Reconstituted stable for 10d refrigerated, 6mo frozen.
Ceftazidime (Fortaz, Glaxo)	IM, IV	75–100 mg/kg q6–8h	Broad spectrum, penetrates CNS.
Ceftriaxone (Rocephin, Roche)	IM, IV	75–100 mg/kg q4–8h	Broad spectrum, low toxicity. Reconstituted stable for 10d refrigerated, 6mo frozen.
Ceftiofur (Naxcel, Upjohn)	IM	50–100 mg/kg q6h	Broad spectrum.
Cephalexin oral suspension (Keflex, Vista)	PO	Psittacines: 50–100 mg/kg q6–8h; cranes, emus: 35–50 mg/kg q6h; or 50–100 mg/kg q8h; quail, ducks: 35–50 mg/kg q2–3h	Spectrum includes many gram-positive, some gram-negative, and some anaerobes.
Cephalothin (Keflin, Lilly)	IM, IV	100 mg/kg q6h; quail, ducks: 100 mg/kg q2–3h	Not absorbed from GI tract.
Chloramphenicol (Parke-Davis; Fort Dodge)	PO	30–50 mg/kg q6–8h	Some gram-positive and gram-negative organisms sensitive, but many gram-negative avian isolates are resistant. Good tissue penetration. Avoid human skin contact.
	IM	80 mg/kg q8–12h; psittacines: 50 mg/kg q6–8h	Some gram-positive and gram-negative organisms sensitive, but many gram-negative avian isolates are resistant. Good tissue penetration. Avoid human skin contact.
Chlortetracycline (Aureomycin, American Cyanamid)	Feed	Psittacines: 1% in pelleted food as only source of food for 45d; small psittacines, finches: 0.5% in millet as only food source for 45d	For treatment of chlamydiosis. Monitor for *Candida* overgrowth with fecal Gram's stains.
	PO	1000–1500 mg/L of drinking water or 1500 mg/kg of soft food	Canaries for chlamydiosis. Treat for 30 days.

Table continued on following page

TABLE 17-1. Drugs Commonly Used in Avian Medicine (Continued)

Drug	Route	Dosage	Comments
Ciprofloxacin (Cipro, Miles)	PO, IM	15–20 mg/kg q12h	Broad spectrum. A 50 mg/ml suspension can be made by crushing a 500-mg tab and add to 10 ml water.
Doxycycline (Vibramycin, Pfizer)	PO	25–50 mg/kg q24h; African grays, cockatoos, macaws: 25 mg/kg q12–24h; cockatiels, Amazons: 40–50 mg/kg q12–24h	Drug of choice for treatment of chlamydiosis. Treat for 45d for treatment of chlamydiosis. Active against *Mycoplasma* and many gram-positive organisms. Most gram-negative bacteria are resistant. Regurgitation may occur with oral administration, especially in macaws. If vomiting occurs, split dose to q12h. If vomiting continues, decrease dose in 5 mg/kg intervals until vomiting stops. Monitor for *Candida* overgrowth with fecal Gram's stains. May interfere with calcium absorption with long-term administration.
Doxycycline (Vibravenos, Europe, Canada)	IM	Macaws: 75–100 mg/kg q5–7d for 45d; other psittacines: 25–50 mg/kg q5–7d for 45d	Causes muscle necrosis. Do not use vibramycin hyclate IM. Not available in the U.S. at this time.
Doxycycline (75 mg/ml from Mortar & Pestle)	IM	100 mg/kg q7d; cockatoos: 75 mg/kg q7d	Compounded by Mortar & Pestle and sold to veterinarians by prescription (injectable suspension).
Doxycycline (Vibramycin hyclate)	IV	25–50 mg/kg q24h for 3d	Used initially in acute severe chlamydiosis. Treatment is continued with oral doxycycline. Use within 6 hours of reconstitution, or freeze in small aliquots.
Enrofloxacin (Baytril, Haver/Diamond)	IM, PO	7.5–15 mg/kg q12h	Can use injectable orally. Excellent activity against most gram-negative, *Mycoplasma*, and some gram-positive bacteria. Resistance by *Pseudomonas* common. May eliminate clinical signs of chlamydiosis, but does not clear. Should not be used in birds with liver or kidney impairment.
Metronidazole (Flagyl, Searle)	PO	10–30 mg/kg q12h for 10d; canaries: 100 mg/L of drinking water or 100 mg/kg of soft food	For treatment of *Giardia, Hexamita*, and anaerobic bacterial infections. Contraindicated in finches.
Piperacillin (Pipracil, Lederle)	IM IM, IV	10 mg/kg q24h for 2d 100–200 mg/kg q6–8h	Excellent broad spectrum antibiotic. Effective against many gram-negative, gram-positive, anaerobic, and *Pseudomonas* spp. Parenteral administration only. Freeze in small vials and thaw as needed. Reconstituted stable for 24h at room T, 7d refrigerated, and 30d frozen. May be combined with amikacin (separate syringes) for synergistic effect.
Ticarcillin (Ticillin, SK Beecham; Ticar, SmithKline Beecham)	IM IM, IV	75–100 mg/kg q4–6h 150–200 mg/kg q6–8h	Amazon parrots. Broad spectrum. Effective against many gram-negative, gram-positive, anaerobic, and *Pseudomonas* spp. Parenteral administration only. Synergistic with amikacin.
Tobramycin (Nebicin, Lilly)	IM	2.5–5 mg/kg q12h	For resistant *Pseudomonas* spp.
Trimethoprim + sulfadiazine (Tribrissen, Cooper; Di-Trim, Syntex, 24% suspension)	IM	0.22 ml/kg q12–24h	Broad spectrum. Active against many gram-negative and gram-positive bacteria. Resistance by *Pseudomonas* common. Do not use in birds with liver or kidney impairment or in birds laying eggs.

Drug	Route	Dosage	Comments
Trimethoprim + sulfamethoxazole (Bactrim, Roche; Septra, Burrough Wellcome) (40 mg Trimethoprim + 200 mg sulfamethoxazole/5 ml)	PO	3 ml/kg q8–12h	Broad spectrum. Active against many gram-negative and gram-positive bacteria. Resistance by *Pseudomonas* common. Do not use in birds with liver or kidney impairment. GI upset and regurgitation common (especially in macaws) 1–3h after oral dose; combine with small amount of food or decrease dose.
Tylosin (Tylan, Elanco)	PO	250–400 mg/L of drinking water or 400 mg/kg of soft food	Used primarily for *Mycoplasma* infection. May be nebulized for respiratory infections; see Chapter 11.
	IM	10–40 mg/kg q6–8h; quail, pigeons, emus: 15–25 mg/kg q6–8h; cranes: 15 mg/kg q6–8h	
	Eye spray	Mix 1 ml injectable with 100 ml sterile water and apply q8–12h	Soluble powder can be mixed with sterile water 1:10 and used as an eye spray for *Mycoplasma* infection.

ANTIFUNGALS

Drug	Route	Dosage	Comments
Amphotericin B (Fungizone, Squibb)	IV	1.5 mg/kg q8–12h for 3–7d	Has been used in the treatment of aspergillosis. Nephrotoxic. Stable 1 wk after reconstitution refrigerated, 24h at room T. Can reconstitute and divide into small portions and freeze. Reconstitute with sterile water. Dilute 1:50 with 5% dextrose before IV administration or nebulization, making a concentration of 0.1 mg/ml.
	Intratracheal, air sac	1 mg/kg q8–12h	
	Nebulization	1 mg/ml saline for 15 min q12–24h for 5–7d, repeated every other wk	
Amphotericin B (3% cream)	Topical	q12h	Topical antifungal.
Chlorhexidine (Nolvasan, Fort Dodge)	PO	10–25 ml/gallon of drinking water	Used to prevent or treat mild GI candidiasis. Toxic to finches.
Clotrimazole (Lotrimin, Schering) 1% solution	Nebulization	30–45 min q24h for 3d, off 2d, repeat as needed	Has been used for treatment of aspergillosis when bird is stable and out of respiratory distress. May need for 1–4 mo. Use in combination with systemic antifungal. Suspend in polyethylene glycol (PEG 300). May be toxic to psittacines at this dose.
Fluconazole (Diflucan, Roerig)	PO	2–5 mg/kg q24h for 7–10d	Used for treatment of local or systemic candidiasis. May cause regurgitation. Has been used for treatment of aspergillosis at 2–5 mg/kg q24h or 20 mg/kg q48h, but may be toxic at higher doses. Generally less effective than itraconazole against aspergillosis except in cases involving privileged sites (brain, eye). Fungistatic, so long-term treatment is typically required for treatment of aspergillosis. For treatment of cryptococcosis in psittacines: 8 mg/kg 24h for 30d. Tablets can be crushed and added to nystatin to make a suspension.
Flucytosine (Ancobon, Roche)	PO	60 mg/kg q12h in birds >500 g; 150 mg/kg q12h in birds <500 g; psittacine neonates: 100–250 mg/kg q12h; raptors: 120 mg/kg q6h; prophylactic dose for raptors: 50 mg/kg q12h with amphotericin B	Has been used in the treatment of aspergillosis in raptors and psittacines, usually combined with amphotericin B or an azole. Has been used for prevention of aspergillosis in raptors and swans. Can be used to treat local or systemic candidiasis. May cause GI upset. Caution when used in birds with kidney or liver impairment.
Gentian violet	Topical	Paint lesions with 0.25%–0.5%	Topical antifungal for treatment of candidiasis.

Table continued on following page

TABLE 17–1. Drugs Commonly Used in Avian Medicine (Continued)

Drug	Route	Dosage	Comments
ANTIFUNGALS (Continued)			
Itraconazole (Sporanox, Janssen)	PO	5–10 mg/kg q12h for 4–5 wks; African grays: 5 mg/kg q24h	Dissolve capsule in 2 ml 0.1 N HCl (stable for 7d), then dilute in 18 ml orange juice or gavage with food to dose at appropriate dose. Drug of choice for the treatment of aspergillosis at this time. May be combined with amphotericin B. Do not use with CNS infections; fluconazole is recommended.
Ketoconazole (Nizoral, Janssen)	PO	20–30 mg/kg q12h for 14–30d	Used for treatment of candidiasis. Can be added to orange or pineapple juice, lactulose, or methylcellulose for administration.
Miconazole (Monistat, Janssen)	Topical IV Nebulization	20 mg/kg q8h Dilute in saline: 15–20 min q12h	Topical antifungal. For treatment of systemic mycoses, especially *Candida* and *Cryptococcus*. Has been used in conjunction with other antifungals for the treatment of aspergillosis in raptors.
Nystatin (Mycostatin)	PO	100,000–300,000 IU/kg q8–12h for 7–14d	Must come in contact with lesions to be effective. Not absorbed from the GI tract.
STA solution	Topical	As needed	Topical treatment for moist and fungal dermatitis.
ANTIPARASITICS			
Amprolium (Corid, Merck) (9.6% solution)	PO	2–4 ml/gallon of drinking water for 5d	Coccidiostat. Birds may not drink treated water. Clean environment to prevent reinfection. Mynah and toucan strains may be resistant.
Carbaril (Sevin, Southern Agricultural Insecticides)	Topical Nest box	Dust lightly 1–2 tsp, depending on size of box	Used for treatment of some ectoparasites. Used to control ants and mites, only when necessary. Remove after 24h.
Carnidazole (Spartrix, Wildlife)	PO	20–30 mg/kg	Used for treatment of trichomoniasis, hexamitiasis, and histomoniasis in pigeons and *Giardia* in cockatiels. May need to repeat in 10–14d.
Chloroquine (Aralen, Sandofi-Winthrop)	PO	Penguin: 10 mg/kg, then 5 mg/kg at 6, 18, 24h	Used for treatment of circulating forms of *Plasmodium*. Used in conjunction with primaquine phosphate. May cause vomiting, diarrhea, retinal damage, or seizures. Dissolve 500 mg tab in 5 ml sterile water.
Chlorsulon (Curatrem, MSD Ag Vet)	PO	20 mg/kg for 3tx, 2 wks apart	Used for treatment of flukes and tapeworms.
Clazuril (Appertex, Janssen)	PO	Pigeons, poultry: 5–10 mg/kg q24h for 3d, 2d off, then tx for 3d	Highly effective coccidiostat for poultry and pigeons.
Fenbendazole (Panacur, Hoeschst-Roussel)	PO	For ascarids: 20–50 mg/kg, repeat in 10d; for flukes and microfilaria: 20–50 mg/kg q24h for 3d; for capillaria: 20–50 mg/kg q24h for 5d. Anseriformes: 5–15 mg/kg q24h for 5d	For treatment for ascarids, some microfilaria, flukes, and *Capillaria*. Low margin of safety. Do not use during active feather development. Toxic when used in canaries, and possibly pigeons and some quail. Do not use in cockatiels.
Ivermectin (Ivomec, Merck)	IM, PO, topical	200 µg/kg, repeat in 10–14d	For treatment of nematodes, lice, mites. May be toxic to finches and waxbills.
Mebendazole (Telmintic, Telmin, Pitman-Moore)	PO	Psittacines: 25 mg/kg q12–24h for 5d; anseriformes: 5–15 mg/kg q24h for 2d	Used for treatment of nematodes (especially *Capillaria*), some cestodes, and trematodes. May be toxic in pigeons, raptors, pelicans, cormorants, and some finches and psittacines. Do not use during breeding season.

Drug	Dose	Route	Comments
Metronidazole (Flagyl, Searle)	10–30 mg/kg q12h for 10d; canaries: 100 mg/L of drinking water or 100 mg/kg of soft food	PO	For treatment of *Giardia, Hexamita, Trichomonas*, and anaerobic bacterial infections. Contraindicated in finches.
Oxfendazole (Syanthic, Benzelmin, Syntex)	10 mg/kg q24h for 2d	IM	Used to treat nematodes. Do not use in breeding season.
Piperazine (Vermizine, Agri-labs)	10–40 mg/kg	PO	For treatment of ascarids. May not be effective in psittacines or finches.
	Gallinaceous birds: 100–500 mg/kg, repeat in 10–14d; anseriformes: 45–200 mg/kg	PO	
Praziquantel (Droncit, Bayvet Haver)	10–20 mg/kg, repeat in 10–14d; toucans for flukes: 10 mg/kg q24h for 14d, then 6 mg/kg q24h for 14d	PO	For tapeworms and flukes.
	For flukes: 9 mg/kg q24h for 3d, then PO for 11d; for tapeworms: 9 mg/kg, repeat in 10d	IM	For tapeworms and flukes. Toxic to finches. Use with caution in young birds.
Primaquine (Winthrop) (26.3 mg tab = 15 mg active base)	0.03 mg/kg q24h for 3d	PO	For treatment of *Plasmodium* spp., usually with chloroquine in penguins. Dose based on mg of active base.
Pyrantel pamoate (Strongid T, Pfizer)	4.5 mg/kg, repeat in 10–14d	PO	For treatment of gastrointestinal nematodes.
Pyrethrins (0.150%)	Lightly mist	Topical	For treatment of external parasites resistant to carbaryl, primarily lice.
Pyrimethamine (Daraprim, Burroughs Wellcome)	0.5 mg/kg q12h for 14–28d	PO	For treatment of *Plasmodium*, toxoplasmosis, *Leucocytozoon* and *Sarcocystis*. Can mix 25 mg tab with 21 ml water and add 4 ml K-Y jelly to make a 1 mg/ml suspension. Can combine with sulfonamides (trimethoprim/sulfadiazine 30 mg/kg combined trimethoprim/sulfadiazine IM q12h) to enhance treatment of toxoplasmosis and *Sarcocystis*. Treat for at least 30 days when used for treatment of *Sarcocystis* and rebiopsy q4–8wks. Do not use for acute *Plasmodium* infection.
Quinacrine (Atabrine, Winthrop)	5–10 mg/kg q24h for 7d	PO	For treatment of *Giardia*, tapeworms, and *Plasmodium* in psittacines. Many *Plasmodium* spp. resistant. Give with food. Don't use with primaquine.
Ronidazole (Ridzol, Merck)	400 mg/kg of soft food or 400 mg/L of drinking water × 7d	PO	For treatment of *Cochlosoma* in passerines.
Sulfadimethoxine (Albon, SmithKline)	50 mg/kg q24h for 5d, off 3d, then tx for 5d	PO	Coccidiostat.
Thiabendazole (Equizole, MSD)	For ascarids: 250–500 mg/kg, repeat in 10–14d; for *Syngamus*: 100 mg/kg q24h for 7–10d	PO	For treatment of ascarids and *Syngamus*. May be toxic to ostriches, ducks, and cranes.
Trimethoprim + sulfamethoxazole, (Bactrim, Roche; Septra, Burroughs Wellcome) (40 mg trimethoprim + 200 mg sulfamethoxazole/5ml)	25 mg/kg q24h × 5d	PO	Used for treatment coccidia in mynahs and toucans.

Table continued on following page

TABLE 17–1. Drugs Commonly Used in Avian Medicine (Continued)

Drug	Route	Dosage	Comments
MISCELLANEOUS			
Acetic acid (apple cider vinegar)	PO	15 ml/qt of drinking water	For use in asymptomatic birds with gram-negative rods and/or yeast on oral or fecal Gram's stain.
Acetylsalicylic acid (aspirin, 5 gr)	PO	1 tab/250 ml of drinking water or 5 mg/kg q8h	Make fresh q2d. Anti-inflammatory, analgesic, anticoagulant, uricosuric. Contraindicated with tetracycline, insulin, or allopurinol therapy.
Activated charcoal, kaolin (Toxiban, Vet-A-Mix)	PO	2–8 g/kg as needed	Used to absorb some toxins from the GI tract. Can mix with hemicellulose to act as a bulk laxative to aid in passing ingested toxins.
Acyclovir (Zovirax, Burroughs Wellcome)	PO, IV, IM	80 mg/kg q8h; or mixed with food: up to 240 mg/kg of food	Antiviral. Commonly used to treat Pacheco's disease. Most effective when initiated before onset of clinical signs. IM injection causes severe muscle necrosis.
Adrenocorticotropic hormone, ACTH (Acthar, Amour; ACTH, Parke-Davis; H.P. Acthar, Amour)	IM	16–26 IU	Obtain baseline sample, administer ACTH, then sample at 1–2h. Stress of handling and venipuncture may invalidate results.
Allopurinol (Zyloprim, Burroughs Wellcome; Lopurin, Boots)	PO	Budgies: Crush 100 mg tab in 10 ml sterile water and give 1 ml/30 ml of drinking water, mixed fresh several times/day	Used in the treatment of gout. Maintain adequate hydration. In severe cases, decrease initial dose to 25% of recommended dose, and gradually increase over several days. Use with colchicine in severe cases of gout.
Aminopentamide (Centrine, Aveco)	IM, SC	0.05 mg/kg q12h, 5 doses max	Antiemetic, antidiarrheal, slows GI motility.
Aminophylline	IV, PO	10 mg/kg IV q3h	Used for lung edema. Can be given orally after initial response.
Amitriptyline (Elavil, Stuart; Endep, Roche)	PO	1–2 mg/kg q12–24h	Tricyclic antidepressant. Used for behavioral feather picking, but seldom effective.
Atropine	IM	0.2 mg/kg q3–4h; repeat as needed to control clinical signs	Anticholinergic for organophosphate or carbamate toxicosis. Does not cause pupil dilation. May increase viscosity of respiratory secretions and decrease gut motility. Not commonly used as a preanesthetic.
Buprenorphine (Buprenex, Reckitt & Colman)	IV, IO, IT	0.5 mg/kg	Used in cardiopulmonary resuscitation to restore cardiac function.
	IM	0.01–0.05 mg/kg	Used for postoperative analgesia.
Butorphanol tartrate (Torbugesic, Torbutrol, Fort Dodge; Stadol, Bristol)	IV, IM, PO	3–4 mg/kg as needed not to exceed q4h	Analgesic, antitussive. Used for abdominal and postoperative pain relief and with Amazon tracheitis.
Calcitonin (Calcimar, Rhone Poulenc Rorer; Macalcin, Sandoz)	IM	4 IU/kg q12h for 2 wks	Used for treatment of cholecalciferol rodent bait toxicosis (with steroids and activated charcoal if needed) and treatment of secondary hypercalcemia of neoplasia. Monitor calcium levels and diurese.
Calcium glubionate (Neo-Calglucon, Sandoz)	PO	150 mg/kg q12h; or 23 mg/30 ml of drinking water	For hypocalcemia.
Calcium gluconate (Vedco, Phoenix)	PO	1 ml/30 ml of drinking water	Used for calcium supplementation.
	IM	5–10 mg/kg q12h as needed	Used for calcium supplementation (eg, egg binding). Maintain hydration.
	IV	50–100 mg/kg slowly to effect	Used for hypocalcemic tetany. Dilute before administration. Maintain hydration.

Drug	Dosage	Route	Comments
Calcium lactate/glycerophosphate (Calphosan, Glenwood)	5–10 mg/kg 7d as needed	IM	For hypocalcemia.
Chlorhexidine solution, 2% (Nolvasan, Fort Dodge)	10–25 ml/gallon of drinking water	PO	Used to help control spread of viruses and treat milk flock candidiasis in psittacines. Not absorbed from the GI tract. Do not use in finches.
	1 ml mixed with 39 ml sterile water	Topical	Used for wound flush. Do not use in finches.
Cisapride (Propulsid, Janssen)	0.5–1.5 mg/kg q8h	PO	Used as a gastrointestinal stimulant for GI motility problems.
Clomipramine (Anafranil, Ciba Geneva)	0.5–1 mg/kg q12–24h	PO	Tricyclic antidepressant. Has been used to treat feather picking and self-mutilation in psittacines. Start with low initial dose and gradually increase over 4–5d. May cause regurgitation, drowsiness, or ataxia.
Colchicine (ColBenemid, Merck)	0.04 mg/kg q24h, gradually increase to q12h	PO, IV	Used for treatment of gout and hepatic fibrosis. Many metabolic side effects. Discontinue if vomiting or diarrhea occur. May potentiate gout formation.
Cyanocobalamin (Vitamin B₁₂)	250–500 μg/kg q7d	IM	May cause pink urates.
Deferoxamine mesylate (Desferal, Ciba-Geigy)	100 mg/kg q24h	SC, PO	Used for iron chelation in hemachromatosis. Monthly biopsies suggested to quantitate liver iron. May take 3 mo of treatment. May cause reddish urine. Do not use in birds with kidney disease.
Dexamethasone (Azium, Schering)	2–4 mg/kg q12–24h; raptors: 1 mg/kg	IM, IV	Anti-inflammatory. Higher dose for shock, head trauma, and gram-negative endotoxemia. High doses are immunosuppressive.
Dextrose	50–100 mg/kg, slowly to effect	IV	Used for treatment of hypoglycemia in birds with seizures.
Diazepam (Valium, Roche)	0.5–1 mg/kg q8–12h	IV, IM	Used for control of seizures.
	2.5–4 mg/kg as needed	PO	Used for feather picking and calming effect.
Digoxin (Cardoxin, Evsco; Lanoxin, Coopers)	0.02–0.05 mg/kg q24h	PO	Used for congestive heart failure in quaker (monk) parakeets, mynahs, and budgies. Monitor potassium, magnesium, and calcium levels and ECG. Toxic reactions include depression, ataxia, vomiting, and diarrhea. Lower dose with impaired kidney function.
Dimecasuccinic acid (DMSA, Aldrich Chemical)	25–35 mg/kg q12h 5d/wk for 3–5 wks	PO	Used for lead, gold, arsenic, and mercury toxicosis.
Dimercaprol (BAL, Beckton Dickinson)	2.5–5.0 mg/kg q4h for 2d, then q12h for 10d or until recovery	IM	Used for lead, gold, arsenic, and mercury toxicosis. Painful IM injection.
Dinoprost tromethamine (Lutalyse, Upjohn) (5 mg/ml injectable)	0.02–0.1 mg/kg once	IM, intracloacal	Prostaglandin F₂α. May be useful in cases of egg binding when the egg is in pelvic presentation and the uterovaginal sphincter is dilated. Use with caution; may result in uterine rupture, bronchoconstriction, increased blood pressure, and death. Prostaglandin E₂ may be better suited for use in egg binding in birds.
Doxapram (Dopram, Robins)	5–10 mg/kg once	IM, IV	Used as a respiratory stimulant.
Doxepin (Sinequan, Roerig; Adapin, Lotus)	0.5–1.0 mg/kg q12h	PO	Tricyclic antidepressant. May be beneficial in some cases of feather picking.
Edetate calcium disodium (Calcium Disodium Versenate, Riker)	35 mg/kg q12h for 5d, off 3–4d, then repeat	IM	Chelation therapy for heavy metal toxicosis (lead, zinc, etc). Use with caution in birds with liver or kidney impairment and discontinue if polyuria develops.
Epinephrine (Webster, Vedco, Butler) (1:1,000)	0.5–1.0 ml/kg	IT, IV, IC, IO	Used in cardiopulmonary resuscitation to restore cardiac function.
Ferric subsulfate	As needed	Topical	Used to control hemorrhage of nails or beak. Causes tissue necrosis.
Flunixin meglumine (Banamine, Schering)	1–10 mg/kg	IM, IV	Used as an anti-inflammatory, analgesic, and antipyretic (hyperthermia).
Furosemide (Lasix, Hoescht-Roussel)	0.15–2 mg/kg q12–24h	IM, IV	Used as a diuretic. Low margin of safety. Lories very sensitive.

Table continued on following page

TABLE 17–1. Drugs Commonly Used in Avian Medicine (Continued)

Drug	Route	Dosage	Comments
MISCELLANEOUS (Continued)			
Haloperidol (Haldol, McNeil-Barre-National)	IM PO	1–2 mg/kg q2–3wks 0.2 mg/kg q12h for birds <1 kg; 0.15 mg/kg q12–24h for birds >1 kg	Used for self-mutilation and feather picking. Discontinue if anorexia, ataxia, or vomiting occurs.
Human chorionic gonadotropin (Pregnyl, Organon)	IM	500–1000 IU/kg q3–6 wk as needed	Used to prevent egg laying and as a treatment for feather picking. Stable for 60d refrigerated after reconstitution. See Romagnano (1996) and Lightfoot (1996).
Insulin, NPH (NPH-ILENTIN-I, Lilly)	IM	0.5–3 units/kg	Used to treat diabetes mellitus. Monitor with glucose curve. May not work. Suggested initial doses for budgies: 0.002 U; and larger psittacines: 0.01–0.1 U.
Insulin, ultralente	IM	2 unit/bird (toco toucan)	Longer acting insulin used to treat diabetes mellitus.
Iodine (Lugol's solution)	PO	Mix 2 ml/20 ml of water to make stock solution; give 1 drop stock/250 ml of drinking water	Used to treat or prevent goiter. Mix dilute solution daily.
Iron dextran (Armedexan, Shering; Ferrextran 100, Fort Dodge; Pigdex 100, American Cyanamid; Imposil, Fisons)	IM	10 mg/kg, repeat in 7–10d if needed	For treatment of anemia and hemorrhage. Use cautiously in toucans, mynahs, and other birds prone to hemochromatosis.
Lactobacillus (Probiocin, Pioneer; Benebac, Pet Ag)	PO	1 pinch/day/bird or 1 tsp/quart hand feeding formula	Used for stimulation of normal flora regrowth.
Lactulose (Cephulac, Chronulac, Merrill Dow; Constilac, Cholac, Alra; Constulose, Enulose, Barre) (667 mg/ml susp)	PO	0.3–0.7 ml/kg q 8–12h	To retard absorption of toxins from the GI tract. May be used for carrier for oral medication. Commonly used with liver failure. Decrease dose if diarrhea occurs.
Levothyroxine (Thyroxine L, Butler)	PO	0.02 mg/kg q12–24h	Used for treatment of hypothyroidism. Thyroxine levels should be monitored.
Lugol's iodine	PO	Mix 2 ml/20 ml of water to make stock solution; give 1 drop stock/250 ml of drinking water	Used to treat or prevent goiter. Mix dilute solution daily.
Leuprolide (Lupron, Tap)	IM	0.375 mg/cockatiel	Used to reduce ovarian activity.
Mannitol (Webster)	IV	0.5 mg/kg slowly q24h	An osmotic diuretic used to treat brain edema, especially after head trauma.
Medroxyprogesterone acetate (Depo-Provera, Upjohn)	IM, SC	5–25 mg/kg, repeat in 4–6 wks if needed	Used to suppress ovulation and as an antipruritic. Seldom used. Side effects: obesity, diabetes mellitus, salpingitis, molt, polyuria/polydipsia, lethargy, thromboemboli, and liver impairment.
Methylprednisolone acetate (Depo-Medrol, Upjohn)	IM, PO	0.5–1 mg/kg	Used to control allergies and Amazon foot necrosis. Use orally once weekly, then taper off to once monthly, then stop.
Metoclopramide (Reglan, Robins)	IM, IV, PO	0.5 mg/kg q8–12h	Used for GI motility stimulant (delayed crop emptying, regurgitation, vomiting). Do not use with GI blockage or hemorrhage. May cause hyperactivity.
Mineral oil	Crop	5–10 ml/kg	Used to aid passage of grit and other GI foreign bodies. Gavage directly into the crop; oral administration may result in aspiration pneumonia. May be mixed with peanut butter 1:2 as bulk diet and cathartic.

Drug	Route	Dosage	Comments
Nalaxone (P/M Naloxone, Pitman-Moore, Mallinckrodt; Narcan, Dupont)	IV	2 mg q14–21h	Opiate and tranquilizer antagonist. Administer slowly.
Nortriptyline (Pamelor, Sandoz)	PO	2 mg/120 ml of drinking water	Tricyclic antidepressant. May be effective in treating some cases of feather picking. Dose should be decreased or discontinued if hyperactivity develops. Taper dose to discontinue.
Oxytocin	IM	0.5 IU/kg; may repeat in 60 min	Used with calcium gluconate for egg expulsion or alone to stop uterine bleeding. Do not use with ruptured uterus, if egg is adhered to the oviduct, or if passage of egg is mechanically inhibited (e.g., closed uterovaginal sphincter).
Pancreatic enzyme (Viokase, Prozyme, Pancrezyme)	In food	2400–4800 g/kg	Used for pancreatic insufficiency. Mix with food and let stand 30 min. Powder can be dosed at ⅛ tsp/kg.
D-Penicillamine (Cuprimine, Merck; Depen, Titratabs-Wallace)	PO	55 mg/kg q12h for 1–2 wk, off 1 wk, repeat as needed	Used for treatment of heavy metal (copper, lead, zinc, other) toxicosis. Administer on an empty crop and proventriculus. May be combined with EDTA calcium.
Polysulfated glycosaminoglycan (PSGAG) (Adequan, Luitpold)	IM, PO	5 mg/kg	Used for arthritis.
Potassium chloride	IV	0.1–0.3 mEq/kg	Used for potassium replacement. Monitor with electrocardiogram and electrolytes analysis.
Pralidoxime (2-PAM) (Protopam, Wyeth-Ayerst)	IM	10–100 mg/kg q24h	Used for organophosphate toxicosis. Use with atropine (at lower dose) and oxygen therapy. Up to 36h after exposure. Repeat as needed.
Prednisolone sodium succinate	IM, IV	Anti-inflammatory: 0.5–1 mg/kg once; for shock, trauma, endotoxemia, immunosuppression: 2–4 mg/kg	Higher doses are immunosuppressive. For CPR or head trauma use 10–20 mg/kg IV or IM q15min prn
Prostaglandin E₂ (Prepidil Gel, Upjohn Co, Sigma Chemical) (0.5 mg/2.5 ml gel)	Topical	1 ml/kg	Dilates uterovaginal sphincter. Allows expulsion of egg. Apply to the uterovaginal sphincter. Can be frozen in small aliquots.
Psyllium (Metamucil, Procter & Gamble)	PO	0.5 tsp/60 ml of baby food food gruel	For bulk diet
Selenium (Seltoc, Schering-Plough)	IM	0.06 mg Se/kg q3–14d	For neuromuscular disease in most species and cockatiels with tongue, jaw, and eyelid paralysis.
Silver sulfadiazine 1% (Silvadine, Marion Merrell Dow)	Topical	Apply q12–24h	For topical treatment of burns, ulcers, and wounds to help rehydrate wounds. Applied under a transparent dressing. Maintain hydration.
Sodium bicarbonate	IV	1–4 mEq/kg slowly over 15–30 min, not to exceed 4 mEq/kg	For metabolic acidosis. Best used when blood pH values are known.
Sodium iodide (20%)	IM	0.3 mg/kg	Used for treatment of goiter in budgies with respiratory distress. May continue with oral treatment.
Sodium sulfate (Glauber's salt) (GoLytely, Braintree)	PO	0.5–1 g/kg	Osmotic cathartic. May be used to evacuate the GI tract and to prevent absorption with heavy metal toxicosis. Do not use in birds with impaired GI function. Maintain hydration.
STA solution (Salicylic and tannic acid in ethylalcohol)	Topical	As needed	Topical treatment for moist and fungal dermatitis.
Sucralfate (Carafate, Marion)	PO	25 mg/kg q8h	Used for treatment of upper GI bleeding. Give 1h before food or other drugs.

Table continued on following page

TABLE 17–1. Drugs Commonly Used in Avian Medicine (Continued)

Drug	Route	Dosage	Comments
MISCELLANEOUS (Continued)			
Testosterone	IM	8 mg/kg q7d as needed.	Used as an anabolic steroid. Contraindicated in birds with liver or kidney disease.
	PO	Drinking water administration: 100 mg/30 ml of water, then use 5–10 drops/30 ml drinking water, mixed fresh daily for 5–10d	
Thiamine (Vitamin B₁)	PO	1–2 mg/kg q24h	Used in raptors, penguins, and cranes to treat deficiency.
	IM	1–3 mg/kg q7d	
Thyrotropin (TSH) (Dermathycin, Coopers; Thyrotropar, Armour)	IM	1–2 IU/kg	Used for thyroid stimulation testing. Difficult to obtain. Sample at time 0, then 4–6h after thyroid-stimulating hormone administration. Normal values are 2 times baseline.
Thyroxine (Synthroid)	PO	0.02 mg/kg q12–24h Drinking water administration: 0.1 mg/4–12 oz drinking water	Used for treatment of hypothyroidism. Monitor blood levels.
Vecuronium bromide (Norcuron, Organon) (4 mg/ml)	Topical	2 drops q15min for 3 tx, in eye	Used for pupillary dilation. Takes about 60 min. Pupils return to normal within 7h. Muscle relaxation may indicate toxicosis.
Vitamins A, D₃, E (100,000 IU vitamin A and 10,000 IU vitamin D₃/ml)	IM	0.1–0.2 ml/300 g q7d	Used for treatment of deficiency. Do not use in birds eating formulated diets. Compounded by Mortar & Pestle and sold via prescription.
Vitamin B complex	IM	1–3 mg thiamine/kg q7d	Used for treatment of deficiency.
	PO	1–2 g/kg of food; raptors, cranes, penguins: 1–2 mg/kg q24h	
Vitamin B₁₂	IM	200–500 g/kg q7d	Used for treatment of deficiency.
Vitamin E/selenium (Seltoc, Schering)	IM	0.06 mg Se/kg q3–14d	Used for treatment of deficiency.
Vitamin K₁ (Phytonadione)	IM	0.2–2.5 mg/kg q24h as needed; warfarin toxicosis 0.2–2.5 mg/kg q12h for 7d; other vit K inhibitors: for 21d	Used for coagulation impairment and for treatment of anticoagulant rodenticide toxicosis. Commonly administered before liver biopsy.
Yeast cell derivatives (Preparation H)	Topical	q24h	Used for stimulation of epithelialization of nonhealing wounds.

SOURCES OF COMPANION AVIAN VACCINATIONS

Pacheco's disease vaccine: Psittamune PDV, Biomune Co.
Salmonella typhimurium bacterin: Typhimune (for pigeons), Biomune Co.
Polyomavirus vaccine: Avian Polyomavirus Vaccine, Biomune Co.
Poxvirus vaccines: Biomune, Sterwin, Vineland, Sanofi, Maine Biological, Schering-Plough, Solvay.

IM = intramuscular; IV = intravenous; d = day; PO = by month; GI = gastrointestinal; qd = every day; qrh = every x hour; SC = subcutaneous; wks = weeks; PRN = as needed; mo = month; T = temperature; tsp = teaspoon; gr = grain; tx = treatments; IC = intracardiac; IT = intratracheal; X.Y% solution = XY mg/ml; IO = intraosseous; oz = ounces.

References and Additional Reading

Aguilar RF, Redig PT. Diagnosis and treatment of avian aspergillosis. In Bonagura JD, Kirk RW (eds): *Kirk's Current Veterinary Therapy XII, Small Animal Practice.* Philadelphia, WB Saunders, 1995, pp 1294–1299.

Barnes HJ. Parasites. In Harrison G, Harrison LR (eds): *Clinical Avian Medicine and Surgery.* Philadelphia, WB Saunders, 1986, pp 472–485.

Bauck L. Analgesics in avian medicine. *Proc Assoc Avian Vet* 1990;239–244.

Bauck L, Hoefer HL. Avian antimicrobial therapy. *Semin Avian Exot Pet Med* 1993;2(1):17–22.

Bicknese EJ. Review of avian sarcocystosis. *Proc Assoc Avian Vet* 1993;52–58.

Campbell TW. Mycotic diseases. In Harrison GJ, Harrison LR (eds): *Clinical Avian Medicine and Surgery.* Philadelphia, WB Saunders Co, 1986, pp 464–471.

Carpenter JW. Safety and efficacy of selected coccidiostats in cranes and implications for other avian species. *Proc Assoc Avian Vet* 1990;147–149.

Carpenter JW, Mashima TY, Rupiper DJ. *Exotic Animal Formulary.* Manhattan, KS, Greystone Publications, 1996.

Clark CH. Pharmacology of antibiotics. In Harrison GJ, Harrison LR (eds): *Clinical Avian Medicine and Surgery.* Philadelphia, WB Saunders Co, 1986, pp 319–326.

Clipsham R. Avian pathogenic flagellated enteric protozoa. *Semin Avian Exot Pet Med* 1995;4(3):112–125.

Clubb SL. Therapeutics. In Harrison GJ, Harrison LR (eds): *Clinical Avian Medicine and Surgery.* Philadelphia, WB Saunders, 1986, pp 327–355.

Clyde VL, Patton S. Diagnosis, treatment, and control of common parasites in companion and aviary birds. *Semin Avian Exot Pet Med* 1996;5(2):75–84.

Cornelissen H, Ducatelle R, Roels S. Successful treatment of a channel-billed toucan (*Ramphastos vitellinus*) with iron storage disease by chelation therapy: Sequential monitoring of the iron content of the liver during the treatment period by quantitative chemical and image analyses. *J Avian Med Surg* 1995;9(2):131–137.

Cross G. Antiviral therapy. *Semin Avian Exot Pet Med* 1995;4(2):96–102.

Degernes LA. Toxicities in waterfowl. *Semin Avian Exot Pet Med* 1995;4(1):15–22.

Dillon AS, Thacker HL, Winterfield RW. Toxoplasmosis in mynahs. *Avian Dis* 1982;26:455–449.

Doolen M. Adriamycin chemotherapy in a blue-front amazon with osteosarcoma. *Proc Assoc Avian Vet* 1994;89–91.

Dorrestein GM. Avian chlamydiosis therapy. *Semin Avian Exot Pet Med* 1993;2(1):23–29.

Dorrestein GM. Avian pediatric pharmacology. *Semin Avian Exot Pet Med* 1993;2(3):110–115.

Dorrestein GM. Chlamydiosis: A new approach in diagnosis and therapy. *Proc Assoc Avian Vet* 1989;29–37.

Dorrestein GM. Doxycycline formulations for avian use. *Proc Assoc Avian Vet* 1991;5–8.

Dorrestein GM. The pharmacokinetics of avian therapeutics. *Vet Clin North Am Small Animal Pract* 1991;21(6):1241–1264.

Dorrestein GM, van der Hage MH. Veterinary problems in mynah birds. *Proc Assoc Avian Vet* 1988;263–274.

Dorrestein GM, van Vurren C. Psittacosis control plan. *Proc Assoc Avian Vet* 1990;279–282.

Ehrenberg M, Rupiper D. Introduction to pigeon practice. *Proc Assoc Avian Vet* 1994;203–211.

Flammer K. An overview of antifungal therapy in birds. *Proc Assoc Avian Vet* 1993;1–4.

Flammer K. Antimicrobial therapy. In Ritchie BW, Harrison GJ, Harrison LR (eds): *Avian Medicine: Principles and Application.* Lake Worth, FL, Wingers, 1994, pp 434–456.

Flammer K. Avian antibacterial therapeutics. *Proc Assoc Avian Vet* 1988;109–118.

Flammer K. Clinical aspects of atoxoplasmosis in canaries. *Proc First Intl Conf Zoo and Avian Med* 1987;33–35.

Flammer K. Fluconazole in psittacine birds. *Proc Assoc Avian Vet* 1996;203–204.

Flammer K. New advances in avian therapeutics. *Proc Assoc Avian Vet* 1992;14–18.

Flammer K. Potential new methods for treating chlamydiosis in psittacine birds. *Proc Assoc Avian Vet* 1989;35–37.

Flammer K. Preliminary report on the use of doxycycline medicated feed in psittacine birds. *Proc Assoc Avian Vet* 1991;1–4.

Flammer K. A review of avian pharmacology. *ABVP Avian Specialty Core Review Course* 1993;111–123.

Flammer K. Treatment of chlamydiosis in psittacine birds in the United States. *J Am Vet Med Assoc* 1989;195:1537–1540.

Flammer K. Update on the clinical pharmacology of selected antimicrobial drugs in psittacine birds. *Proc Assoc Avian Vet* 1995;13–16.

Flammer K. An update on the diagnosis and treatment of avian chlamydiosis. In Kirk RW, Bonagura JD (eds): *Current Veterinary Therapy XI.* Philadelphia, WB Saunders, 1991, pp 1150–1153.

Flammer K. An update on psittacine antimicrobial pharmacokinetics. *Proc Assoc Avian Vet* 1990;218–220.

Flammer K. Use of amikacin in birds. *Proc First Intl Conf Zoo Avian Med* 1987;195–198.

Flammer K, Aucoin DP, Whitt DA, et al. Plasma concentrations of enrofloxacin in African grey parrots treated with medicated water. *Avian Dis* 1990;34:1017–1022.

Flammer K, Aucoin DP, Whitt DA. Intramuscular and oral disposition of enrofloxacin in African grey parrots following single and multiple doses. *Vet Pharm Ther* 1991;14:159–366.

France M, Gilson S. Chemotherapy treatment of lymphosarcoma in a moluccan cockatoo. *Proc Assoc Avian Vet* 1993;15–19.

Frazier DL, Jones MP, Orosz SE. Pharmacokinetic considerations of the renal system in birds: Part I. Anatomic and physiologic principles of allometric scaling. *J Avian Med Surg* 1995;9(2):92–103.

Frazier DL, Jones MP, Orosz SE. Pharmacokinetic considerations of the renal system in birds: Part II. Review of drugs excreted by renal pathways. *J Avian Med Surg* 1995;9(2):104–121.

Frazier DL, Jones MP, Schroeder ED, et al. Metabolic scaling of drug dosing regimens. *Proc Assoc Avian Vet* 1995;21–23.

Fudge A. Avian giardiasis: Syndromes, diagnosis and therapy. *Proc Assoc Avian Vet* 1985;155–164.

Fudge AM. Psittacine vaccines. *Proc Assoc Avian Vet* 1990;292–300.

Fudge AM. Psittacine vaccines. *Vet Clin North America, Small Animal Practice* 1991;21(6):1273–1279.

Fudge AM, McEntee L. Avian giardiasis: Syndromes, diagnosis, and therapy. *Proc Assoc Avian Vet* 1986;155–164.

Greiner EC, Ritchie BW. Parasites. In Ritchie BW, Harrison GJ, Harrison LR (eds): *Avian Medicine: Principles and Application.* Lake Worth, FL, Wingers, 1994, pp 1107–1029.

Greve JH. Parasitic diseases. In Fowler ME (ed): *Zoo and Wild Animal Medicine,* ed 2. Philadelphia, WB Saunders, 1986, pp 234–251.

Harlin RW. Pigeons. *Proc Assoc Avian Vet* 1995;361–373.

Harris JM. Avian client compliance. *Semin Avian Exot Pet Med* 1993;2(1):2–6.

Harrison GJ, Harrison LR (eds): *Clinical Avian Medicine and Surgery.* Philadelphia, WB Saunders, 1986.

Hines RS, Sharkey P, Friday RB. Itraconazole treatment of pulmonary, ocular and uropygial aspergillosis and candidiasis in birds: Data from five clinical cases and controls. *Proc Am Assoc Zoo Vet* 1990;322–327.

Hoefer HL. Antimicrobials in pet birds. In Bonagura JD, Kirk RW (eds): *Kirk's Current Veterinary Therapy XII—Small Animal Practice.* Philadelphia, WB Saunders, 1995, pp 1278–1283.

Hudelson KS. A review of the mechanisms of avian reproduction and their clinical applications. *Semin Avian Exot Pet Med* 1996;5(4):189–198.

Hudelson KS, Hudelson P. Egg binding, hormonal control, and therapeutic considerations. *Comp Cont Ed Vet Pract* 1993;15(3):427–432.

Hudelson KS, Hudelson P. A brief review of the female avian reproductive cycle with special emphasis on the role of prostaglandins and clinical applications. *J Avian Med Surg* 1996;10(2):67–74.

Huff DG. Avian fluid therapy and nutritional therapeutics. *Semin Avian Exot Pet Med* 1993;2(1):13–16.

Johnson-Delaney CA. Avian formulary. In Johnson-Delaney CA, Harrison LR (eds): *Exotic Companion Medicine Handbook for Veterinarians*. Lake Worth, FL, Wingers, 1996, pp 7–38.

Jones MP, Orosz SE, Frazier DL. Evaluation of the pharmacokinetic disposition of itraconazole in red-tailed hawks *(Buteo jamaicensis)*. *Proc Assoc Avian Vet* 1995;19–20.

Joseph V, Pappagianis D, Reavill DR. Clotrimazole nebulization for the treatment of respiratory aspergillosis. *Proc Assoc Avian Vet* 1994;301–306.

Joyner KL. Pediatric therapeutics. *Proc Assoc Avian Vet* 1991;188–199.

LaBonde J. The medical and surgical management of domestic waterfowl collections. *Proc Assoc Avian Vet* 1992;223–233.

LaBonde J. Toxicity in pet avian patients. *Semin Avian Exot Pet Med* 1995;4(1):23–31.

Lennox AM, Vanderheyden N. Haloperidol for use in treatment of psittacine self mutilation and feather plucking. *Proc Assoc Avian Vet* 1993;119–120.

Ley DH. Avian cryptposporidiosis. *Proc First Intl Conf Zoo Avian Med* 1987;299–303.

Lightfoot TL. Clinical use and preliminary data of chorionic gonadotropin administration in psittacines. *Proc Assoc Avian Vet* 1996;303–306.

Lumeij JT. Therapeutics for protozoal infections. *Proc Second European Symp Assoc Avian Vet* 1989;72–74.

Lumeij JT, Gorgevska K, Woestenborghs R. Plasma and tissue concentrations of itraconazole in racing pigeons *(Columba livia domestica)*. *J Avian Med Surg* 1995;9(1):32–35.

Lung NP, Romagnano A. Current approaches to feather picking. In Bonagura JD, Kirk RW (eds): *Kirk's Current Veterinary Therapy XII—Small Animal Practice*. Philadelphia, WB Saunders, 1995, pp 1303–1307.

MacWhirter P. Passeriformes. In Ritchie BW, Harrison GJ, Harrison LR, (eds): *Avian Medicine: Principles and Application*. Lake Worth, FL, Wingers, 1994, pp 1172–1199.

Marshall R. Avian anthelmintics and antiprotozoals. *Semin Avian Exot Pet Med* 1993;2(1):33–41.

McCluggage D. Parasitology in caged birds. *Proc Assoc Avian Vet* 1989;97–100.

Millam JR. Leuprolide acetate can reversibly prevent egg laying in cockatiels. *Proc Assoc Avian Vet* 1993;46.

Murphy J. Psittacine trichomoniasis. *Proc Assoc Avian Vet* 1992;21–24.

Norton TM, Greiner EC, Latimer KS, et al. Medical aspects of Bali mynahs *(Leucospar rothschildi)*. *Proc Am Assoc Zoo Vet* 1993;29–44.

Norton TM, Kollias GV, Gaskin JM, et al. Acyclovir (Zovirax) pharmacokinetics and the efficacy of acyclovir against Pacheco's disease in Quaker parakeets. *Proc Assoc Avian Vet* 1989;3–5.

Olsen GH. Common infectious and parasitic diseases of quail and pheasants. *Proc Assoc Avian Vet* 1993;146–150.

Orosz SE, Frazier DL. Antifungal agents: A review of their pharmacology and therapeutic indications. *J Avian Med Surg* 1995;9(1):8–18.

Orosz SE, Frazier DL, Schroeder EC, et al. Pharmacokinetic properties of itraconazole in blue-fronted Amazon parrots *(Amazona aestiva aestiva)*. *J Avian Med Surg* 1996;10(3):168–173.

Orosz SE, Schroeder EC, Cox SK, et al. The effects of formulation on the systemic availability of itraconazole in pigeons. *J Avian Med Surg* 1995;9(4):255–262.

Orosz SE, Schroeder EC, Frazier DL. Itraconazole: A new antifungal drug for birds. *Proc Assoc Avian Vet* 1994;13–16.

Page CD, Haddad K. Coccidial infections in birds. *Semin Avian Exot Pet Med* 1995;4(3):138–144.

Page CD, Schmidt RE, English JH, et al. Antemortem diagnosis and treatment of sarcocystosis in two species of psittacines. *J Zoo Wildl Med* 1992;23:77–85.

Panigrahy B, Senne DA. Diseases of mynahs. *J Am Vet Med Assoc* 1991;199:378–381.

Parenti E, Cerruti-Sola S, Turilli C, et al. Spontaneous toxoplasmosis in canaries *(Serinus canaria)* and other small passerine cage birds. *Avian Pathol* 1986;15:183–197.

Parrott R. Clinical treatment regimens with fluconazole. *Proc Assoc Avian Vets* 1991;15–16.

Parrott T. New clinical trials using acyclovir. *Proc Assoc Avian Vet* 1990;237–238.

Partington CJ, Gardiner CH, Fritz D, et al. Atoxoplasmosis in bali mynahs *(Leucospar rothschildi)*. *J Assoc Wildl Med* 1989;20:328–335.

Patton S. An overview of avian coccidia. *Proc Assoc Avian Vet* 1993;47–51.

Prus SE. Avian antifungal therapy. *Semin Avian Exot Pet Med* 1993;2(1):30–32.

Quesenberry KE. Avian antimicrobial therapeutics. In Jacobson E, Kolliass GV (eds): *Exotic Animals.* New York, Churchill Livingstone, 1988, pp 177–207.

Plumb DC. *Veterinary Drug Handbook,* ed 2. Ames, IA, Iowa State University Press, 1995.

Rae M. Endocrine disease in pet birds. *Semin Avian Exot Pet Med* 1995;4(1):32–38.

Rae M. Hemoprotozoa of caged and aviary birds. *Semin Avian Exot Pet Med* 1995;4(3):131–137.

Ramsay EC, Grindlinger H. Treatment of feather picking with clomipramine. *Proc Assoc Avian Vet* 1992;379–382.

Ramsay EC, Grindlinger H. Use of clomipramine in the treatment of obsessive behavior in psittacine birds. *J Assoc Avian Vet* 1994;8(1):9–15.

Redig PT. Avian aspergillosis. In Fowler ME (ed): *Zoo and Wild Animal Medicine, Current Therapy 3.* Philadelphia, WB Saunders, 1993, pp 178–181.

Redig PT, Duke GE: Comparative pharmacokinetics of antifungal drugs in domestic turkeys, red-tailed hawks, broad-winged hawks, and great horned owls. *Avian Dis* 1988;29:649–661.

Redig PT, Talbot B, Guarnera T. Avian malaria. *Proc Assoc Avian Vet* 1993;173–181.

Rich GA. Polyomavirus: What to do after the diagnosis. *Proc Assoc Avian Vet* 1996;299–301.

Ritchie BW. Avian therapeutics. *Proc Assoc Avian Vet* 1990;415–431.

Ritchie BW. Preventing viral infection. In *Avian Viruses, Function and Control.* Lake Worth, FL, Wingers, 1995, pp 105–126.

Ritchie BW, Harrison GJ. Formulary. In Ritchie BW, Harrison GJ, Harrison LR (eds): *Avian Medicine: Principles and Application.* Lake Worth, FL, Wingers, 1994, pp 457–478.

Ritchie BW, Harrison GJ, Harrison LR (eds): *Avian Medicine: Principles and Application.* Lake Worth, FL, Wingers, 1994.

Romagnano A. Avian obstetrics. *Semin Avian Exot Pet Med* 1996;5(4):180–188.

Rosenthal K, Stamoulis M. Diagnosis of congestive heart failure in an Indian Hill mynah bird *(Gracula religiosa). J Assoc Avian Vet* 1993;7(1):27–30.

Rosskopf WJ, Woerpel RW. Practical avian therapeutics. *Vet Clin North Am Small Animal Pract* 1991;21(6):1265–1272.

Rosskopf WJ, Woerpel RW, Albright M, et al. Pet avian emergency care. *Proc Assoc Avian Vet* 1991;341–356.

Rosskopf WJ, Woerpel RW, Asterino R. Successful treatment of avian tuberculosis in pet psittacines. *Proc Assoc Avian Vet* 1991;238–251.

Rupiper D, Briggs K, Ehrenberg M. Management of trichomoniasis, paramyxovirus-1, and salmonellosis in a pigeon loft. *Proc Assoc Avian Vet* 1994;241–247.

Schales C, Schales K. Galliformes. In Ritchie BW, Harrison GJ, Harrison LR (eds): *Avian Medicine: Principles and Application.* Lake Worth, FL, Wingers, 1994, pp 1218–1236.

Scholtens RG, New JC, Johnson S. The nature and treatment of giardiasis in parakeets. *J Am Vet Med Assoc* 1982;180:170–173.

Sedgewich CJ, Pokras M, Kaufman G. Metabolic scaling: Using estimated energy costs to extrapolate drug dosages between species and different individuals of diverse body sizes. *Proc Am Assoc Zoo Vet* 1990;249–254.

Sellers LM, Sundberg JA. A study of compounded doxycycline for IM use in cockatiels. *Proc Assoc Avian Vet* 1992;384–386.

Sikarskie JG. The use of ivermectin in birds, reptiles, and small mammals. In Kirk RW (ed): *Current Veterinary Therapy IX—Small Animal Practice.* Philadelphia, WB Saunders, 1986, pp 743–745.

Smith SA. Diagnosis and treatment of helminths in birds of prey. In Redig PT, Cooper JE, Remple JD, et al (eds): *Raptor Biomedicine.* Minneapolis, University of Minnesota Press, 1993, pp 21–27.

Smith SA. Parasites of birds of prey: Their diagnosis and treatment. *Semin Avian Exot Pet Med* 1996;5(2):97–105.

Stadler CK, Carpenter JW. Parasites of backyard game birds. *Semin Avian Exot Pet Med* 1996;5(2):85–96.

Trees AJ. Parasitic conditions in poultry 1: Protozoal diseases. In Boden E (ed): *Poultry Practice.* Philadelphia, Bailliere Tindall, 1993, pp 59–71.

Trees AJ. Parasitic diseases. In Jordan FTW (ed): *Poultry Diseases,* ed 3. Philadelphia, Bailliere Tindall, 1990, pp 226–253.

Trees AJ, Beesley W. Parasitic conditions in poultry 2: Helminths and arthropods. In Boden E (ed): *Poultry Practice.* Philadelphia, Bailliere Tindall, 1993, pp 73–85.

Tully TN. Formulary. In Altman RB, Clubb SL, Dorrestein GM, et al (eds): *Avian Medicine and Surgery.* Philadelphia, WB Saunders, 1996, pp 671–688.

Turner R. Trexan (naltrexone hydrochloride) use in feather picking in avian species. *Proc Assoc Avian Vet* 1993;116–118.

VanDerHeyden N. Aspergillosis in psittacine chicks. *Proc Assoc Avian Vet* 1993;207–212.

VanDerHeyden N. Avian tuberculosis: Diagnosis and attempted treatment. *Proc Assoc Avian Vet* 1986;203–214.

VanDerHeyden N. Identification, pathogenicity and treatment of avian hematozoa. *Proc Assoc Avian Vet* 1985;163–174.

VanDerHeyden N. Update on avian mycobacteriosis. *Proc Assoc Avian Vet* 1994;53–61.

VanDerHeyden N. New strategies in the treatment of avian mycobacteriosis. *Semin Avian Exot Pet Med* 1997;6(1):25–33.

Ward FP. Parasites and their treatment in birds of prey. In Fowler ME (ed): *Zoo and Wild Animal Medicine,* ed 2. Philadelphia, WB Saunders, 1986, pp 425–430.

Westerhof I, Pellicaan CHP. Effects of different application routes of glucocorticoids on the pituitary-adrenocortical axis in pigeons (*Columba livia domestica). J Avian Med Surg* 1995;9(3):175–181.

Wheler C. Avian anesthetics, analgesics, and tranquilizers. *Semin Avian Exot Pet Med* 1993;2(1):7–12.

Wheler CL, Machin KL, Lew LJ. Use of antibiotic-impregnated polymethylmethacrylate beads in the treatment of chronic osteomyelitis and cellulitis in a juvenile bald eagle (*Haliaeetus leucocephalus). Proc Assoc Avian Vet* 1996;187–194.

Worell A. Management and medicine of toucans. *Proc Assoc Avian Vet* 1988;253–262.

Worell AB. Therapy of noninfectious avian disorders. *Semin Avian Exot Pet Med* 1993;2(1)42–47.

Wright J. Reports of untoward reactions of birds to pharmaceuticals. *J Assoc Avian Vet* 1989;3(4):190.

Zwart P. Pigeons and doves. In Fowler M (ed): *Zoo and Wild Animal Medicine,* ed 2. Philadelphia, WB Saunders, 1986, pp 440–445.

Appendix 1

Sources of Equipment and Pharmaceuticals

EQUIPMENT

Anesthesia Monitors

Dynax
Medical Engineering & Development Corp.
Silogic Design Ltd.

Band Removal Equipment

Donna G Corp.
L&M Animal Farms

Beak Repair Materials

Ellman International Inc.

Cast Material and Orthopedic Supplies

Fitz Enterprises
Hexcel Medical Products
IMEX Veterinary Inc.
Jorgensen Laboratories Inc.
Kirschner Medical Corp.
Seaberg Co.
3M Animal Care Products

Collars

E-Jay International
Veterinary Specialty Products Inc.

Critical Care Units and Incubators

Animal Care Products
Avian Engineering Inc.
AvTech Systems
D&M Bird Farm
Dean's Animal Supply Inc.
Joe Freed's Avian "Pet"iatric Supply
Lyon Electric Company Inc.
Snyder Manufacturing Co.
Thermocare Inc.

Radiosurgical Equipment

Cameron-Miller
Ellman International Inc.
Summit Hill Labs

Endoscopes

Karl Storz Veterinary Endoscopy

Endotracheal Tubes, Ayres T-Pieces, and Bain's Systems

Bivona Inc.
Matrix Medical Inc.
Summit Hill Labs
Veterinary Specialty Products Inc.

Feeding Needles and Tubes

Corners Limited
E-Jay International
IAW Research Institute
Joe Freed's Avian "Pet"iatric Supply
Lafeber Co.
Popper & Sons Inc.
Professional Specialties Inc.

Gram Scales

D&M Bird Farm
Henry Schein Inc
Joe Feed's Avian "Pet"iatric Supply
Lafeber Co.
Lyon Electric Co., Inc.
Northgate Veterinary Supply
Ohaus Corp.
Veterinary Specialty Products Inc.

Grinding Tools

General hardware stores
Joe Freed's Avian "Pet"iatric Supply
Lyon Electric Company Inc.
Veterinary Specialty Products Inc.

Heating Pads and Platforms

ASI Sales
Gorman-Rupp Industries Division
Safe and Warm Inc.
Valentine Equipment Co.
Veterinary Specialty Products Inc.

Hematology, Cytology, and Gram's Stain Kits

AJP Scientific
American Scientific Products
Baxter Diagnostics Inc.
Difco Laboratories
Fisher Scientific
Harleco
Mid-Atlantic Biomedical
Miles Laboratories Inc.
Scott Laboratories
Veterinary Specialty Products Inc.

Magnifying Loupes

Aseptico
Carl Zeiss Inc.
General Scientific Corp.
Lafeber Co.
MDS Medical Diagnostic Services Inc.

Microchips and Equipment

American Veterinary Identification Devices (AVID)

Microsurgical Microscopes and Equipment

General Scientific Corp.
Prescott's Inc.
Solvay Animal Health Inc.

Mouth Speculums

Joe Freed's Avian "Pet"iatric Supplies
Lafeber Co.
Veterinary Specialty Products Inc.

Nebulizers

D&M Bird Farm
DeVilbiss
Dynax
Joe Freed's Avian "Pet"iatric Supply
Thermocare Inc.

Nets

Aviary West
Beckman Net Co.

Restraint Devices

Henry Schein Inc.
Silverdust
Veterinary Specialty Products Inc.

Surgical Drapes (Clear)

Johnson & Johnson
3M Animal Care Products
Veterinary Specialty Products Inc.

Surgical Instruments

Arista Surgical Supply Co.
Sontec Instruments

Tissue Glue

Ellman International Inc.
3M Animal Care Products
Tri-Point Medical
Veterinary Specialty Products Inc.

EQUIPMENT COMPANY ADDRESSES, NUMBERS

AJP Scientific
(800) 922–0223

American Scientific Products
(800) 922–5227

American Veterinary Identification
  Devices (AVID)
3179 Hamner Ave., Ste. 5
Norco, CA 91760
(909) 371–7505

Animal Care Products
(800) 327–7306

Arista Surgical Supply
67 Lexington Ave.
New York, NY 11010
(800) 223–1984

Aseptico
Kirkland, WA 98083
(800) 426–5913

ASI Sales
12712 Carmenita Rd.
Santa Fe Springs, CA 90670

Avian Engineering Inc.
Arlington, TX 76096
(800) 687–1863

Aviary West
Hacienda Heights, CA 91745
(818) 330–8700

AvTech Systems
San Diego, CA 92126
(619) 695–9640
Fax (619) 695–9720

Baxter Diagnostics Inc.
Scientific Division
1430 Waukegan Rd
McGaw Park, IL 60085–6787
(708) 689–8410
(800) 633–7369

Beckman Net Co.
3729 Ross St.
Madison, WI 53797

Bivona Inc.
Gary, IN 46406
(302) 645–2226

Cameron-Miller
Chicago, IL 60609
(312) 523–6360

Carl Zeiss Inc.
Thornwood NY
(800) 442–4020

Corners Ltd.
Kalamazoo, MI 49007
(800) 456–6780

D&M Bird Farm
538 Mountain View Rd.
El Cajon, CA 92021
(619) 588–7897
Fax (619) 588–0689

Dean's Animal Supply Inc.
Orlando, FL 32869
(407) 256–8387

Dentsply International Inc.
York, PA

Dynax
A Division of AMC, Inc.
4109 Spring Grove Ave.
PO Box 14703
Cincinnati, OH 45250–0703
(513) 681–3900
Fax (513) 921–5220

E-Jay International
Glendora, CA 91740

Ellman International Inc.
Hewlett, NY 11557
(516) 569–1492
Fax (516) 569–0054

Fisher Scientific
Houston, TX 77099
(800) 766–7000

General Scientific Corp.
Ann Arbor, MI 48103
(313) 996–9200
Fax (313) 662–0520

Henry Schein Inc.
Port Washington, NY 11050
(800) 443–2756

Hexcel Medical Products
6700 Sierra Ln.
Dublin, CA 94566
(510) 847–9500

IAW Research Institute
PO Box 6385
Burbank, CA 91510

IMEX Veterinary Inc.
Longview, TX 75604
(800) 828–4639

Joe Freed's Avian "Pet"iatric Supply
1018 W 63rd South
Witchita, KS 67217
(316) 524–1154
Fax (316) 524–1778

Johnson & Johnson Medical
PO Box 90130
Arlington, TX 76004–3130
(800) 433–5170
(817) 465–3141

Jorgensen Laboratories Inc.
1450 North Van Buren Ave.
Loveland, CO 80538

Karl Storz Veterinary Endoscopy
175 Cremona Dr.
Goleta, CA 93117
(800) 955–7832
Fax (805) 685–2588
michelem@ksvea.com

Kirschner Medical Corp.
Timonium, MD 21093
(800) 638–7622

L&M Animal Farms
Pleasant Plain, OH 45162
(800) 332–5623
(513) 877–2131

Lafeber Co.
24981 N 1400 East Rd.
Cornell, IL 61319
(815) 358–2301
Fax (815) 358–2352

Lyon Electric Company Inc.
2765 Main St.
Chula Vista, California 91911
(619) 585–9900
Fax (619) 420–1426
lyonelect@aol.com

Matrix Medical Inc.
Orchard Park, NY 14127
(716) 662–6650

MDS Medical Diagnostic Services
Inc.
PO Box 1441
Brandon, FL 33509
(813) 653–1180

Medical Engineering &
Development Corp.
Jackson, MI 49201
(517) 783–5851

Miles Laboratories Inc.
Elkhart, IN 46515

Northgate Veterinary Supply
San Rafael, CA 94903
(800) 338–4641

Ohaus Corp.
Florham Park, NJ 07932
(201) 377–9000

Popper & Sons Inc.
Biomedical Instrument Division
New Hyde Park, NY 11040
(516) 248–0300
Fax (516) 747–1188

Prescott's Inc.
Monument, CO 80132
(719) 481–3353
(800) 438–3937

Professional Specialties Inc.
Linstrom, MN 55045
(612) 583–2914

Safe & Warm Inc.
Seattle, WA 98117
(800) 421–3237
Fax (206) 789–9527

Scott Laboratories
(800) 821–7254

Seaberg Company Inc.
South Beach, OR 97366
(541) 967–4726
(800) 818–4726

Silverdust Bird Positioner
PO Box 159
El Granada, CA 94122

Snyder Manufacturing Co.
Denver, CO 80222
(303) 756–1932
(800) 422–1932

Solvay Animal Health Inc.
Mendota Heights, MN 55120
(612) 681–9556
(800) 247–1139

Sontec Instruments
7248 S. Tucson Way
Englewood, CO 80112
(303) 790–9411
(800) 821–7496
Fax (303) 792–2606

Summit Hill Labs
Navesink, NJ 07752
(201) 291–3600

Thermocare Inc.
PO Drawer YY
Incline Village, NV 89450

3M Animal Care Products
St Paul, MN 55144–1000
(612) 733–1110
(800) 848–0829
Fax (612) 737–5360

Tri-Point Medical
Raleigh, NC 27604
(919) 876–7800

Valentine Equipment Co.
Chicago, IL 60609

Veterinary Specialty Products Inc.
PO Box 812005
Boca Raton, FL 33481
(561) 362–7340
(800) 362–8138
Fax (561) 362–9982

SOURCES OF CLIENT EDUCATION MATERIALS

Association of Avian Veterinarians
PO Box 210732
Bedford, TX 76095–0732
(817) 428–7900
Fax (817) 485–4800

Harrison's Bird Diets
7171 Mercy Rd, Ste. 135
Omaha, NE 68106
(800) 346–0269
Fax (402) 397–9454

Lafeber Co.
24981 N 1400 East Rd.
Cornell, IL 61319
(815) 358–2301

Wingers Publishing Inc.
PO Box 6863
Lake Worth, FL 33466–6863
(800) 946–4782
Fax (407) 641–0234

PHARMACEUTICAL COMPANIES

Alra Laboratories, Inc.
3850 Clearview Ct.
Gurnee, IL 60031
(708) 244–9440
(800) 248–ALRA
Fax (708) 244–9464

American Cyanamid Co.
One Cyanamid Plaza
Wayne, NJ 07470
(609) 799–0400
(800) 422–0222
Fax (609) 799–2159

Armour Pharmaceutical Co.
500 Arcola Rd
PO Box 1200
Collegeville, PA 19426–0107
(800) 727–6737

Barre-National Inc. and NMC
7205 Windsor Blvd.
Baltimore, MD 21244

Biomune Inc.
Lenexa, KS
(913) 894–0230
Fax (913) 894–0236

Bristol-Myers Squibb Co.
PO Box 4500
Princeton, NJ 08543–4500
(609) 897–2000
(800) 332–2056

Cibageneva Pharmaceuticals
Ciba-Geigy Corp.
556 Morris Ave.
Summit, NJ 07901
(800) 525–8747
(303) 466–2400
Fax (303) 469–6467

Coopers Animal Health Inc.
A Pitman-Moore Co.
421 E. Hawley St.
Mundelein, IL 60060
(708) 949–3300
(800) 525–9480
Fax (708) 949–2311

DuPont Pharma
DuPont Merck Plaza
Centre Road
Wilmington, DE 19805
(302) 992–5000
(302) 992–4240

Elanco
Eli Lilly Co.
Lilly Corporate Center
Indianapolis, IN 46285
(317) 276–3000
(800) 782–8977
Fax (317) 276–4471

Fisons Animal Health
1221 Nicollet Mall #230
Minneapolis, MN 55403
(800) 654–3839

Fort Dodge Laboratories, Inc.
800 Fifth St. NW
Fort Dodge, IA 50501
(515) 955–4600

Goechst-Roussel Agri-Vet Co.
Rt. 202–206
PO Box 2500 BedI
Somerville, NJ 08876–1258
(908) 247–4838
Fax (908) 231–4452

Humco Labs
Texarkana, TX
(800) 866–3967

Janssen Pharmaceutic Inc.
1125 Trenton-Harbourton Rd.
PO Box 200
Titusville, NJ 08560–0200
(800) JANSSEN
(609) 730–2000
Fax (609) 730–3044

Lilly and Co.
Eli Lilly and Co.
Lilly Corporate Center
Indianapolis, IN 46285
(317) 276–2000
(800) 782–8977
Fax (317) 276–4471

Lotus Biochemical Corp.
PO Box 3586
Radford, VA 24143
(800) 455–5525
Fax (800) 962–2200

Luitpold Pharmaceuticals, Inc
Animal Health Division
One Luitpold Dr.
Shirley, NY 11967
(516) 942–4000
(800) 458–0163
Fax (516) 924–1731

Maine Biological Labs Inc.
PO Box 255
Waterville, ME 04903
(207) 873–3989

Mallinckrodt Veterinary Inc.
421 E Hawley St.
Mundelein, IL 60060
(708) 949–3300
(800) 525–9480
Fax (708) 949–2311

Marion Merrell Dow Inc.
9300 Ward Pky.
PO Box 8480
Kansas City, MO 64114–0480
(800) 552–3656

McNeil Consumer Products Co.
Division of McNeil PPC Inc.
Camp Hill Rd.
Fort Washington, PA 19034
(215) 233–7000

Merck Agvet Division
PO Box 2000
Rahway, NJ 07065–0912
(908) 855–3800
Fax (908) 855–9366

Merck & Co., Inc.
PO Box 4
West Point, PA 19486–0004
(800) 637–2579

Miles Inc.
Agricultural Division
12707 West 63rd St.
PO Box 390
Shawnee, KS 66201
(913) 631–4800
(800) 255–6517
Fax (913) 632–2803

Mortar and Pestle
3701 Beaver Ave.
Des Moines, IA 50310
(800) 279–7054

Organon Inc.
375 Mount Pleasant Ave.
West Orange, NJ 07052
(201) 325–4500
(800) 631–1253
Fax (201) 325–4699

Parke-Davis
Division of Warner-Lambert Co.
201 Tabor Rd.
Morris Plains, NJ 07950
(800) 223–0432
Fax (201) 540–2284

Pfizer Inc.
US Animal Health Operations
235 E 42nd St.
New York, NY 10017
(212) 573–2323
Fax (212) 573–1601

Pharmacia
7001 Post Rd.
Dublin, OH 43017
(614) 764–8100

Pittman Moore Inc.
421 E. Hawley St.
Mundelein, IL 60060
(708) 949–3300
(800) 525–9480
Fax (708) 949–2311

Rhone Merieux Inc.
115 Transtech Dr.
Athens, GA 30601
(706) 548–9292
(800) 934–4447

Rhone-Poulenc Rorer
   Pharmaceuticals Inc.
500 Arcola Rd.
Collegeville, PA 19426–0107
(610) 454–8000

Riker Labs Inc.
3M Pharmaceuticals
3M Center 275–3W–01
PO Box 33275
St Paul, MN 55133–3275
(800) 328–0255

AH Robins Company Inc.
1407 Cummings Dr.
Richmond, VA 23220
(610) 688–4400

Roche Laboratories
340 Kingsland St.
Nutley, NJ 07110
(800) 526–0625

JB Roerig Division
Pfizer Inc.
235 East 42nd St.
New York, NY 10017–5755
(800) 438–1985

Sandoz Pharmaceuticals
(210) 503–7500
Fax (201) 503–8265

Sanofi Winthrop Pharmaceuticals
90 Park Ave.
New York, NY 10016
(212) 551–4000
(800) 446–6267

Sanofi Animal Health
7101 College Blvd.
Overland Park, KS 66210
(913) 451–3434

Schering Corp.
of Schering-Plough Corp.
Galloping Hill Rd.
Kenilworth, NJ 07033
(908) 298–4000
(800) 222–7579
Fax (908) 820–6400

Schering-Plough Animal Health
PO Box 529
Galloping Hill Rd.
Kenilworth, NJ 07033
(908) 298–4000
(800) 648–2118
Fax (908) 709–2807

SmithKline Beecham Animal Health
Whiteland Business Park
812 Springdale Dr.
Exton, PA 19341–2803
(800) 366–5288
Fax (215) 363–3286

Sterwin Laboratories Inc.
Rt. 113, PO Box 537
Millsboro, DE 19966–0537
(800) 633–0462

Syntex Animal Health Inc.
Division of Syntex Agribusiness Inc.
4800 Westown Pkwy, Ste. 200
West Des Moines, IA 50265
(515) 224–2400
(800) 247–2210
Fax (515) 224–2482

Tri-point Medical
Raleigh, NC
(919) 876–7800

The Upjohn Company
Animal Health Division
7000 Portage Rd.
Kalamazoo, MI 49001
(616) 365–6736

Vet-A-Mix Animal Health
604 W Thomas Ave.
Shenandoah, IA 51601
(712) 246–4000
(800) 813–0004
Fax (712) 256–5245

Vineland Laboratories
2285 E Landis Ave.
Vineland, NJ 08360
(800) 225–0270

Whitehall Labs
New York, NY
(800) 322–3129

Wildlife Pharmaceuticals Inc.
1401 Duff Dr. Ste. 600
Fort Collins, CO 80524
(970) 484–6267

Appendix 2

Typical Weights of Common Adult Pet Birds

Order	Group	Species	Weight
Psittaciformes	Cockatoos	Citron	283–514 g°
		Goffin's	221–386 g
		Greater Sulphur-Crested	608–1200 g
		Lesser-Sulphur-Crested	251–412 g
		Major Mitchell's	300–452 g
		Moluccan	640–1025 g
		Palm (Goliath)	990–1057 g
		Rose-Breasted	281–390 g
		Umbrella	458–756 g
	Macaws	Blue and Gold	892–1294 g
		Buffon's	1080–1534 g
		Green-Winged	1058–1529 g
		Hyacinth	1185–1529 g
		Military	774–1065 g
		Scarlet	1058–1464 g
		Yellow-Collared	223–308 g
	Parrots	African Grey	300–380 g
		Blue-Fronted Amazon	275–510 g
		Blue-Headed Pionus	238–278 g
		Double Yellow-Headed Amazon	545 g
		Eclectus	383–524 g
		Hispaniolan Amazon	268 g
		Mealy Amazon	600–685 g
		Orange-Winged Amazon	440–470 g
		Senegal	125–150 g
		Yellow-Fronted Amazon	260–460 g
	Smaller Species	Budgerigar	30–60 g
		Blue-Crowned Conure	84–96 g
		Jandaya Conure	118–128 g
		Pennant's Parakeet	180–200 g
		Red-Crowned Parakeet	60–75 g
		Love Birds (various species)	50–70 g
Anseriformes		Domestic Duck	2–3 kg
		Domestic Goose	4–5 kg
		Canada Goose	3.5–4.5 kg
Apodiformes		Hummingbirds	2.5–5 g
Columbiformes		Collared Dove	150–220 g
		Diamond Dove	40 g
		Domestic Pigeon	260–350 g
Falconiformes		Harris Hawk	574–1000 g
		Kestrel	145–282 g
		Peregrine Falcon	560–1500 g
		Red-Tailed Hawk	698–1350 g
		Sparrow Hawk	150–300 g
Galliformes		Domestic Fowl	1.75–4 kg
		Domestic Turkey	4–15 kg
		Japanese Quail	18–42 g
Gruiformes		Crowned Crane	3.5–4 kg
Passeriformes		Canary	12–29 g
		English Robin	20–30 g
		Glossy Starling	74–82 g
		Goldfinch and Green Finch	15–20 g
		Greater Indian Hill Mynah	180–240 g
		House Sparrow	25–30 g
		Java Sparrow	24–30 g
		Zebra Finch	10–16 g

°Weights are the lowest female weight to the highest male weight.

From Altman RB, Clubb SL, Dorrestein GM, Quesenberry K (eds): *Avian Medicine and Surgery*. Philadelphia, WB Saunders Co, 1996, p 1027.

Appendix 3

Plants Reported to Cause Toxic Reactions in Pet Birds, Waterfowl, and Game Fowl

Avocado (*Persea americana*)	Maternity plant (*Klanchoe* spp)
Bishops weed (*Ammi majus*)	Milkweed (*Asclepias* spp)
Black locust (*Robina pseudoacacia*)	Nightshade (*Solanum* spp)
Blue-green algae (*Microcystis aeruginosa*)	Oak (*Quercus* spp)
Burdock (*Arctium minus*)	Oleander (*Nerium oleander*)
Camel bush (*Trichodesma incanum*)	Parsley (*Petroselinum sativum*)
Castor bean (*Ricinus communis*)	Philodendron (*Philodendron scandens*)
Clematis (*Montana rubens*)	Poinsettia (*Euphorbia pulcheriama*)
Coffee bean (*Sesbania drumundii*)	Pokeweed (*Phytolacca americana*)
Diffenbachia (*Diffenbachia* spp)	Precatory bean (*Abrus precatoius*)
Elephant's ear (*Colocasia* or *Alocasia* spp)	Rhododendron (*Rhododendron simsii*)
Ergot (*Claviceps purpurea*)	Tobacco (*Nicotiana* spp)
Lily of the valley (*Convallaria majalis*)	Virginia creeper (*Parthenocissus quinquefolio*)
Locoweed (*Astragalus emoryanus*)	Yew (*Taxus media*)

From Labonde J. Avian toxicology. *Vet Clin North Am Small Anim Pract* 1991;21(6):1339.

Appendix 4

Some Plants Considered Safe for Use in Aviaries

House Plants*	Outdoor Plants†
African violet *(Saintpaulia* sp)	American bittersweet
Aloe plant *(Aloe vera)*	Autumn olive
Areca palm *(Chrysalidocarpus lutescens)*	Bamboo
Australian laurel *(Pittosporum tobira)*	Barberry
Bamboo palm *(Chamaedorea erumpens)*	Bayberry
Begonias *(Begonia* sp)	Beech (American, European)
Bird's nest fern *(Asplenium nidus)*	Bladdernut
Boston fern *(Nephrolepis exaltata)*	Blueberry
Bottle brush fern *(Asparagus densiflorus)*	Comfrey
Canary Island palm *(Phoenix canariensis)*	Coralberry
Christmas cactus *(Schlumbergera bridgesii)*	Cotoneaster firethorn
Coffee tree *(Coffea arabica)*	Crabapple
Corn plant *(Dracaena deremensis)*	Dogwood
Creeping fig *(Ficus pumila)*	Elderberry (common, European, red)
Danish ivy *(Cissus rhombifolia)*	Fir (balsam, Douglas, subalpine, white)
Devil's ivy *(Epipremnum aureum)*	Grape vine
Dragon tree *(Dracaena marginata)*	Huckleberry
European fan palm *(Chamaerops humilis)*	Marigold
Fiddle leaf fig *(Ficus lyrata)*	Nasturtium
Fig tree *(Ficus benjamina)*	Pine (ponderosa, spruce, Virginia, white)
Flame nettle *(Coleus* sp)	Pyracantha
Hawaiian schefflera *(Schefflera arboricola)*	Raspberry
Indian laurel *(Ficus retusa)*	Rose
Jade plant *(Crassula argentea)*	Snowberry
Kangaroo vine *(Cissus antarctica)*	Spruce (black, Norway, red, white)
Lace fern *(Asparagus plumosus)*	Viburnum
Lady palm *(Raphis excelsa)*	Wax plant
Maidenhair fern *(Adiantum* sp)	White poplar
Ming fern *(Asparagus retrofractus)*	Willow
Mother fern *(Asplenium bulbiferum)*	
Mother-in-law's tongue *(Sansevieria trifasciata)*	
Norfolk pine *(Araucaria heterophylla)*	
Paradise palm/Kentia palm *(Howea foresterana)*	
Parlor palm *(Chamaedorea elegans)*	
Pepperomia *(Pepperomia* sp)	
Prayer plant *(Maranta leuconeura)*	
Purple passion *(Gynura aurantiaca)*	
Rubber tree *(Ficus elastica)*	
Spider plant *(Chlorophytum comosum)*	
Umbrella tree/Schefflera *(Brassaia actinophylla)*	
Wandering Jew *(Tradescantia* sp)	

*From Johnson CA. Better safe than sorry. *Bird Talk Magazine,* October, 1987.
†From *Birds USA,* 1996/97, p. 147.

Appendix 5

The Skeletal Anatomy of Birds

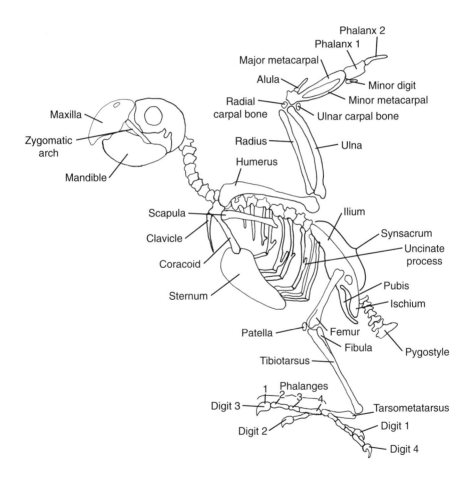

Appendix 6

The Visceral Anatomy of Birds

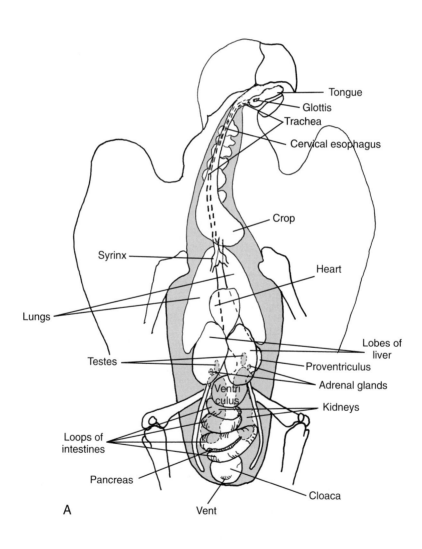

Tongue
Glottis
Trachea
Cervical esophagus
Crop
Syrinx
Heart
Lungs
Lobes of liver
Testes
Proventriculus
Adrenal glands
Ventriculus
Kidneys
Loops of intestines
Pancreas
Cloaca
A
Vent

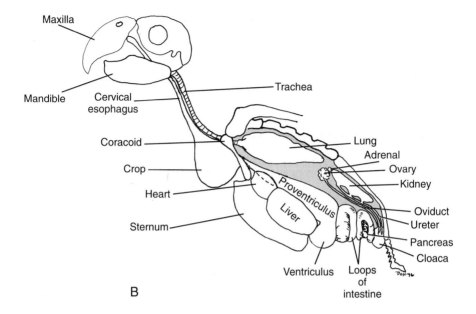

B

Appendix 7

The Major Blood Vessels and Nerves of the Wings and Legs of Birds

The ventral aspect of the wings and the medial aspect of the legs are illustrated. The dotted lines represent a passage behind the bones.

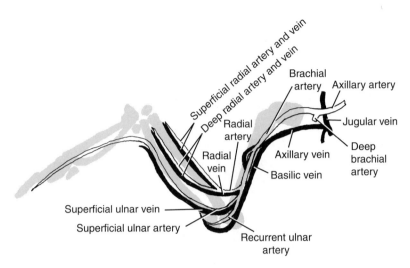

THE MAJOR BLOOD VESSELS OF THE MEDIAL (VENTRAL) RIGHT WING

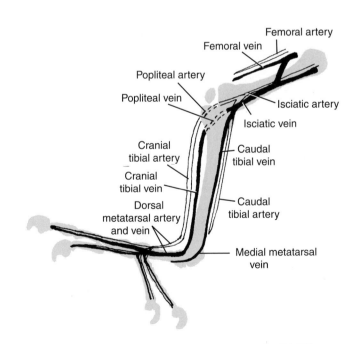

THE MAJOR VESSELS OF THE MEDIAL RIGHT LEG

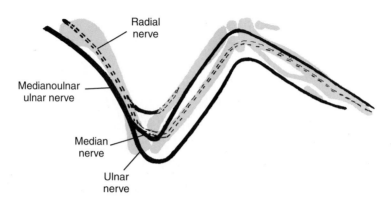

THE MAJOR NERVES OF THE MEDIAL (VENTRAL) LEFT WING

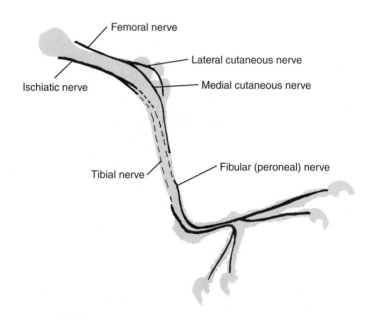

THE MAJOR NERVES OF THE MEDIAL LEFT LEG

Index

Note: Page numbers in *italics* refer to illustrations; page numbers followed by t refer to tables